The Menopause:
Clinical, Endocrinological
and Pathophysiological
Aspects

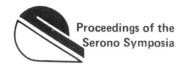

Proceedings of the Serono Symposia

Recent Titles

*At the time of going to press these titles were in preparation.

The Menopause: Clinical, Endocrinological and Pathophysiological Aspects

Proceedings of the
Serono Symposia, Volume 39

Edited by

P. Fioretti

Istituto di Clinica Ostetrica e Ginecologica
Università di Pisa
Spedall Rlunltl S. Chiara
Via Roma
Pisa, Italy

L. Martini

Istituto di Endocrinologia
Università degli Studi di Milano
Via A. del Sarto
Milan, Italy

G.B. Melis

Istituto di Clinica Ostetrica e Ginecologica
Università di Pisa
Spedali Riuniti S. Chiara
Via Roma
Pisa, Italy

S.S.C. Yen

Department of Reproductive Medicine
Research Center, School of Medicine
University of California, San Diego,
La Jolla, California, USA

1982

ACADEMIC PRESS
A Subsidiary of Harcourt Brace Jovanovich, Publishers
London New York
Paris San Diego San Francisco São Paulo
Sydney Tokyo Toronto

ACADEMIC PRESS INC. (LONDON) LTD.
24–28 OVAL ROAD
LONDON NW1

U.S. Edition published by
ACADEMIC PRESS INC.
111 FIFTH AVENUE
NEW YORK, NEW YORK 10003

British Library Cataloguing in Publication Data

The Menopause: clinical, endocrinological and
    pathophysiological aspects.–(Proceedings of the
    Serono symposia, ISSN 0308–5503; v. 39)
    1. Menopause–Congresses
    I. Fioretti, P.   II. Series
    612'.665   RG186

ISBN 0-12-256080-9
LCCCN 81–69584

Typeset in 10/11pt IBM (Press Roman) by
RDL., 26 Mulgrave Road, Sutton, Surrey
Printed by T. J. Press (Padstow) Ltd., Padstow, Cornwall

PREFACE

Nowadays the human life-span is longer than ever before, so that more than one third of living women are of climacteric or postclimacteric age; what's more, women's importance in the socio-economic and cultural fields is also greater. Consequently, troubles related to the menopause are the object of ever-increasing interest. Therefore the Congress at Viareggio, a pretty town by the sea near Pisa (Italy), was organized to review present knowledge about medical and non-medical problems at the climacterium.

Investigators, psychologists, sociologists, sexologists and andrologists from all over the world have studied the physiological, pathological, clinical and psychological aspects which characterize the pre- and postmenopausal period in the life of women and aging males.

Anatomy, metabolism, endocrinology and, in general, the physiological homeostasis of the female organism at this stage were all examined. Subsequently pathological alterations were discussed in relation to their frequency during the climacterium. Therefore many of the presentations discussed cardiovascular diseases, alterations of calcium metabolism, low urinary tract diseases and breast and endometrial pathology. Psychological problems were also examined with regard to social and sexological behaviour; moreover, their role in the common complaints of postmenopausal women was the object of discussion. The usefulness of current therapy and the risk/benefit ratio was subsequently evaluated. In particular, it was found that non-steroidal agents seemed to represent an interesting therapeutic approach.

Apart from the many reports, we are grateful to all those who contributed to the success of the Congress, mainly the members of the Scientific Committee, who supplied us with the best advice with particular regard to the Symposium programme. We gratefully acknowledge our Sponsors' contributions and the Serono Symposia and Biodata for their help in the organization. We also wish to express our appreciation to the members of the Local Organizing Committee (A. M. Paoletti, V. Mais, M. Gambacciani, F. Menchini-Fabris, M. Mariani, F. Strigini, F. Fruzzetti and G. Guarnieri) who were helpful during both the Congress and its preparation.

It is our hope that this volume, which contains papers from all the different speakers, will be useful to investigators of the climacterium and to women who will be helped to face this period of their lives more positively.

December 1981   THE EDITORS

CONTENTS

Section III

Morphology of the Ageing Ovary

Section IV

Breast Disease in Premenopausal and Postmenopausal Age

Section V

Genital Diseases, Hormones and the Menopause

Section VI

Clinical Pathology of the Postmenopause

Section VII

The Aged Couple: Sexual Behaviour and Social Problems

Section VIII

Therapeutic Approaches to Climacteric Disturbances: Benefits and Risks

CONTRIBUTORS

F. AGRIMONTI Clinica Medica B, Università di Torino, Turin, Italy

V. AIMONE Ente Ospedaliero S. Anna, Via Genova 3, 10126 Turin, Italy

M. F. AKSU Departments of Obstetrics and Gynaecology, Cerrahpasa Faculty of Medicine, University of Istanbul, Istanbul, Turkey

V. ALOISIO Cattedra di Patologia Medica 2, Università di Pisa, Pisa, Italy

J. ANDOR Women's Hospital, School of Medicine, University of Basle, Basle, Switzerland

A. ANGELI Clinica Medica Generale e Terapia Medica B, Università degli Studi, Torino, Via Genova 3, 10126 Turin, Italy

M. ATLAS Division of Obstetrics and Gynaecology, The Sheba Medical Centre Tel-Hashemer, Sackler School of Medicine, Tel-Aviv University, Tel-Aviv, Israel

C. BABUNA Departments of Obstetrics and Gynaecology, Istanbul Faculty of Medicine, University of Istanbul, Istanbul, Turkey

M. A. BACIGALUPO Istituto di Fisiologia ed Anatomia, Istituto di Zootecnica, Università di Milano, Milan, Italy

G. BAGGIANI Geriatric Department, Santa Chiara Hospital of Pisa, Pisa, Italy

G. C. BALBONI Institute of Human Anatomy, University of Florence, Florence, Italy

E. BARTOCCIONI Laboratrio di Endocrinologia Molecolare, Istituto di Clinica Ostetrica e Ginecologica, Università Cattolica del Sacro Guore, Largo Gemelli 8, 00168 Rome, Italy

L. BASCHIERI Cattedra di Patologia Medica 2, University of Pisa, Pisa, Italy

C. BASILE FASOLO Post-graduate School of Andrology, 1st Medical Clinic, Pisa University, Pisa, Italy

F. BATTAGLIA Department of Obstetrics and Gynaecology, Catholic University, Largo Gemelli 8, 00168 Rome, Italy

P. BELFORTE Ospedale Ostetrico Ginecologico Sant'Anna, Turin, Italy

G. P. BERNINI Postgraduate School of Endocrinology, Pisa, Italy

L. BERTA Patologia Speciale Medica B, Università di Torino, Strada San Vito 34, 10133 Turin, Italy

S. BETTOCCHI 1′ Clinica Ostetrica e Ginecologica, Università di Bari, Bari, Italy

B. BIANCHI Post-graduate School of Andrology, 1st Medical Clinic, Pisa University, Pisa, Italy

A. BOMPIANI Istituto di Clinica Ostetrica e Ginecologica, Università Cattolica del S. Cuore, Rome, Italy

P. A. BOSSOLO Clinica Medica I "A Ferrata", Università di Pavia, Pavia, Italy

F. BOTTIGLIONI Institute of Obstetrics and Gynaecology, University of Bologna, 40138 Bologna, Italy

P. BRUNETTI Medical Pathology, Perugia University, School of Medicine, 06100 Perugia, Italy

I. BRUNORI DE LUCA Clinica Ostetrica e Ginecologica, Università di Pisa, Pisa, Italy

F. CAMINIT Department of Obstetrics and Gynaecology, School of Medicine, University of Cagliari, Cagliari, Italy

C. CAMPAGNOLI Ospedale Ostetrico Ginecologico Sant'Anna, Turin, Italy

S. CAMPBELL Department of Obstetrics and Gynaecology, King's College Hospital Medical School, Denmark Hill, London SE5 8RX, UK

S. CAMPO Catholic University, Department of Obstetrics and Gynaecology, Largo A. Gemelli 8, Rome, Italy

N. CAPPELLI Clinica Ostetrica e Ginecologica, Università di Pisa, Pisa, Italy

A. CARUSO Catholic University, Department of Obstetrics and Gynaecology, Largo A. Gemelli 8, Rome, Italy

L. CASARELLA Department of Obstetrics and Gynecology, Catholic University, Largo Gemelli 8, 00168 Rome, Italy

M. M. CASELLATO Laboratorio di Fisiologia ed Anatomia, Istituto di Zootecnica, Università di Milano, Milan, Italy

P. CASTROGIOVANNI Cattedra di Psicologia dell'Università di Pisa, Pisa, Italy

M. CASULINI Clinica Medica Generale e Terapia Medica B, Università degli Studi, Torino, Via Genova 3, 10126 Turin, Italy

P. CAVALLO-PERIN Cattedra di Semeirotica Medica, Department of Internal Medicine, University of Turin, Turin, Italy

I. CORRADI Istituto di Clinico Psichiatrica dell'Università di Pisa, Pisa, Italy

F. CROZE Institute of Medicine, Radioimmunoassay Laboratory, University of Liège, Liège, Belgium

P. CUGINI I' Patologia Medica, University of Rome, Rome, Italy

S. DANERO Clinica Ostetrica e Ginecologica, University of Siena, Siena, Italy

N. D'ANTONA Clinica Ostetrica e Ginecologica, University of Siena, Siena, Italy

R. DARGENIO Catholic University Department of Obstetrics and Gynaecology, Largo A. Gemelli 8, Rome, Italy

D. De ALOYSIO Institute of Obstetrics and Gynaecology, University of Bologna, 40138 Bologna, Italy

R. De CATERINA CNR Clinical Physiology Institute, University of Pisa, Pisa, Italy

J. N. DE FOSSE Centre d'Exploration Fonctionelle et d'Etude de le Réproduction (CEFER), Marseille, France

S. DEL BELLO Clinica Medica Generale e Terapia Medica B, Università degli Studi, Torino, Via Genova 3, 10126 Turin, Italy

V. DE LEO Clinica Ostetrica e Ginecologica, Università degli Studi di Siena, Siena, Italy

M. DE MURTAS Department of Obstetrics and Gynaecology, School of Medicine, University of Cagliari, Cagliari, Italy

A. M. DOLFIN Ospedale Ostetrico Ginecologico Sant'Anna, Turin, Italy

G. H. DONKER Department of Obstetrics and Gynaecology, University Hospital Utrecht, Utrecht, The Netherlands

J. DUVIVIER Department of Clinical Biochemistry, University of Liège, Liège, Belgium

R. EREZ Department of Psychiatry and Endocrinology, Cerrahpasa Faculty of Medicine, University of Istanbul, Istanbul, Turkey

F. FACCHINETTI Istituto di Clinica Ostetrica e Ginecologica, Via G. B. Mascagni, Siena, Italy

V. FACCHINI Istituto di Clinica Ostetrica e Ginecologica, Università degli Studi, Via Roma 35, 56100 Pisa, Italy

G. FACHINI Istituto di Patologia Generale dell'Università di Milano, Milan, Italy

P. FALASCHI Istituto di Clinica Medica Generale V, Università di Roma, Rome, Italy

A. M. FAZZARI Clinica Medica Generale e Terapia Medica B, Università degli Studi, Torino, Via Genova 3, 10126 Turin, Italy

L. FEDELI Centre of Nuclear Medicine, Perugia University, School of Medicine, 06100 Perugia, Italy

J. P. FELBER Division de Biochimie Clinique, Département de Médicine, CHUV, 1011 Lausanne, Switzerland

E. FERRARI Clinica Medica I "A. Ferrata", Università di Pavia, Pavia, Italy

L. FERRUZZI Ospedale Ostetrico Ginecologico Sant'Anna, Turin, Italy

P. FILIPPONI Institute of Clinical Medicine, Perugia University School of Medicine, 06100 Perugia, Italy

P. FIORETTI Istituto di Clinica Ostetrica e Ginecologica, Università degli Studi, Via Roma 35, 56100 Pisa, Italy

P. FIORILLO Department of Obstetrics and Gynaecology, Catholic University, Largo Gemelli 8, 00168 Rome, Italy

E. J. FOLKERD Department of Chemical Pathology, St. Mary's Hospital Medical School, London, W2 1PG, UK

G. FRAIESE Istituto di Clinica Medica Generale V, Università di Roma, Rome, Italy

R. FRAIRIA Clinica Medica Generale e Terapia Medica B, Università degli Studi, Torino, Via Genova 3, 10126 Turin, Italy

S. FRANCESCHI Istituto di Ricerche Farmacologiche "Mario Negri", Via Eritrea 62, 20157 Milan, Italy

F. FRANCHI Postgraduate School of Endocrinology, Pisa, Italy

P. FRANCHIMONT Institute of Medicine, Radioimmunoassay Laboratory, University of Liège, Liège, Belgium

H. FRANKE Medizinische Poliklinik, University of Würzburg, Würzburg, West Germany

F. FRUZZETTI Istituto di Clinica Ostetrica e Ginecologica, Università degli Studi, Via Roma 35, 56100 Pisa, Italy

G. GAIDANO Patologia Speciale Medica B, Università di Torino, Strada San Vito 34, 10133 Turin, Italy

M. GAMBACCIANI Istituto di Clinica Ostetrica e Ginecologica, Università degli Studi, Via Roma 35, 56100 Pisa, Italy

M. GANGEMI Obstetrical and Gynaecological Department, University of Padua, Padua, Italy

N. GARCEA Catholic University, Department of Obstetrics and Gynaecology, Largo A. Gemelli 8, Rome, Italy

T. GARGIULO Primario Divisione Ostetrica e Ginecologica, Ospedale dei Poveri Infermi, CEVA (CN), Italy

G. GASPERETTI CNR Clinical Physiology Institute, University of Pisa, Pisa, Italy

M. GASPERI Division de Biochimie Clinique, Départment de Medicine, CHUV, 1011 Lausanne, Switzerland

S. GELLER Centre d'Exploration Fonctionelle et d'Etude de la Réproduction (CEFER), Marseille, France

A. R. GENAZZANI Cattedra di Patologia Ostetrica e Ginecologica, Università degli Studi di Siena, Siena, Italy

G. L. GESSA Istituto di Farmacologia Medica, Università di Cagliari, Cagliari, Italy

J. GINSBURG Academic Department of Medicine, Royal Free Hospital Medical School, Pond Street, London NW3, UK

I. GRANIER Fondation de Recherche en Hormonologie, Paris, France

G. GUARNIERI Istituto di Clinica Ostetrica e Ginecologica, Università degli Studi, Via Roma 35, 56100 Pisa, Italy

E. S. E. HAFEZ Department of Gynaecology and Obstetrics, C. S. Mott Center for Human Growth and Development, Wayne State University School of Medicine, Detroit, Michigan, USA

F. HALBERG Chronobiology Laboratories, University of Minnesota, Minneapolis, USA

M. T. HAZEE-HAGELSTEIN Institute of Medicine, Radioimmunoassay Laboratory, University of Liège, Liège, Belgium

K. HENDERSON Institute of Medicine, Radioimmunoassay Laboratory, University of Liège, Liège, Belgium

C. J. HILLYARD Endocrine Unit, Royal Postgraduate Medical School, Hammersmith Hospital, Ducane Road, London W12 OHS, UK

H. H. HUANG Research Laboratories, Mercy Hospital and Medical Center, Stevenson Expressway at King Drive, Chicago, Illinois 60616, USA

J. HUSTIN Departments of Gynaecology and Obstetrics, University of Liège, Liège, Belgium

S. IACOBELLI Laboratorio di Endocrinologia Molecolare, Istituto di Clinica Ostetrica e Ginecologica, Università Cattolica del Sacro Cuore, Largo Gemelli 8, 00168 Rome, Italy

F. IANNOTTA Divisione "B" di Medicina Generale, Ospedale Regionale di Varese Biometria, Farmitalia Carlo Erba, Milan, Italy

P. INAUDI Cattedra di Patologia Ostetrica e Ginecologica, Università degli Studi die Siena, Siena, Italy

S. INNOCENTI Department of Obstetrics and Gynaecology, University of Pisa, Pisa, Italy

H. S. JACOBS St. Mary's Hospital Medical School, London W2, UK

V. H. T. JAMES Department of Chemical Pathology, St. Mary's Hospital Medical School, London W2 1PG, UK

U. JÄNNE Department of Obstetrics and Gynaecology, Biochemistry and Clinical Chemistry, University of Oulu, Oulu, Finland

S. L. JEFFCOATE Chelsea Hospital for Women, London SW3, UK

E. A. JOHNS Department of Chemical Pathology, St. Mary's Hospital Medical School, London W2 1PG, UK

D. L. JONES Department of Chemical Pathology, St. Mary's Hospital Medical School, London W2 1PG, UK

A. KAUPPILA Departments of Obstetrics and Gynaecology, Biochemistry and Clinical Chemistry, University of Oulu, Oulu, Finland

P. M. KICOVIC Reproductive Medicine Programme, Medical Unit, Organon, Oss, The Netherlands

R. J. B. KING Hormone Biochemistry Department, Imperial Cancer Research Fund Laboratories, P.O. Box 123, Lincoln's Inn Fields, London WC2A 3PX, UK

S. KIVINEN Department of Obstetrics and Gynaecology, University of Oulu, Oulu, Finland

E. KOKKO Department of Biochemistry and Clinical Chemistry, University of Oulu, Oulu, Finland

R. LAMBOTTE Department of Gynaecology and Obstetrics, University of Liège, Liège, Belgium

T. LANTTO Department of Obstetrics and Gynaecology, University of Oulu, Oulu, Finland

R. LA ROSA Clinica Ostetrica e Ginecologica, Università degli Studi di Siena, Siena, Italy

C. LA VECCHIA Istituto di Ricerche Farmacologica "Mario Negri" Via Eritrea 62, 20157 Milan, Italy

C. LEMASSON Centre d'Exploration Fonctionelle et d'Etude de la Réproduction (CEFER), Marseille, France

H. M. LEMON Division of Oncology, Department of Internal Medicine, University of Nebraska, Omaha, USA

M. LENCI Catholic University, Department of Obstetrics and Gynaecology, Largo A. Gemelli 8, Rome, Italy

G. LENTI Cattedra di Clinica Medica A, Department of Internal Medicine, University of Turin, Turin, Italy

L. LENTINI Institute of Clinical Medicine, Perugia University School of Medicine, Perugia, Italy

S. L. LIGHTMAN St.Mary's Hospital Medical School, London W2, UK

T. LIPPI Cattedra di Patologia Medica 2, University of Pisa, Pisa, Italy

P. LONGO Laboratorio di Endocrinologia Molecolare, Istituto di Clinica Ostetrica e Ginecologica, Università Cattolica del Sacro Cuore, Largo Gemelli 8, 00168 Rome, Italy

G. LUGARO, M. M. CASELLATO, E. MANERA and M. A. BAGIGALUPO Laboratorio di Fisiologia ed Anatomia, Istituto di Zootecnica, Università di Milano, Milan, Italy

M. LUISI Postgraduate School of Endocrinology, Pisa, Italy

G. MAGRINI Clinical Biochemistry Division, Medical Department, CHUV, Lausanne, Switzerland

A. K. MAGUIRE St. Mary's Hospital Medical School, London W2, UK

V. MAIS Istituto di Clinica Ostetrica e Ginecologica, Università degli Studi, Via Roma 35, 56100 Pisa, Italy

B. M. MANDELLI Clinica Medica I "A. Ferrata" Università di Pavia, Pavia, Italy

E. MANERA Laboratorio di Fisiologia ed Anatomia, Istituto di Zootecnica, Università di Milano, Milan, Italy

D. MANGO Department of Obstetrics and Gynaecology, Catholic University, Largo Gemelli 8, 00168 Rome, Italy

D. MARCHESONI Obstetric and Gynaecological Department, University of Padua, Padua, Italy

P. MARCHETTI Laboratorio di Endocrinologia Molecolare, Istituto di Clinica Ostetrica e Ginecologica, Università Cattolica del Sacro Cuore, Largo Gemelli 8, 00168 Rome, Italy

S. MARIOTTI Cattedra di Patologia Medica 2, University of Pisa, Pisa, Italy

L. MARTINI Department of Endocrinology University of Milan, Via Andrea del Sarto 21, 20129 Milan, Italy

E. MARTINO Cattedra di Patologia Medica 2, University of Pisa, Pisa, Italy

A. MASERI CNR Clinical Physiology Institute, University of Pisa, Pisa, Italy

C. MAZZI Department of Endocrinology, St. Antony Hospital, Gallarate, Italy

P. G. McDONOUGH Department of Obstetrics and Gynaecology, Medical College of Georgia, Augusta, Georgia 30912, USA

G. McGARRICK Chelsea Hospital for Women, London SW3, UK

H. MEDEN-VRTOVEC Department of Gynaecology and Obstetrics, University of Ljubljana, Slajmerjeva 3, Ljubljana, Yugoslavia

J. MEITES Department of Physiology, Neuroendocrine Research Laboratory, Michigan State University, East Lansing, Michigan 48824, USA

G. B. MELIS Istituto di Clinica Ostetrica e Ginecologica, Università degli Studi, Via Roma 35, 56100 Pisa, Italy

G. F. MENCHINI FABRIS Post-graduate School of Andrology, 1st Medical Clinical, Pisa University, Pisa, Italy

G. MOGGI Clinica Ostetrica e Ginecologica dell'Università di Pisa, Pisa, Italy

F. MONZANI Cattedra di Patologia Medica 2, University of Pisa, Pisa, Italy

G. MORRA Cattedra di Clinica Medica A, Department of Internal Medicine, University of Turin, Turin, Italy

E. MOTZ Cattedra di Patologia Medica 2, University of Pisa, Pisa, Italy

B. MOZZANEGA Obstetrical and Gynaecological Department, University of Padua, Padua, Italy

S. MURRU Clinica Ostetrica e Ginecologica del'Università di Pisa, Pisa, Italy

K. NAHOUL Fondation de Recherche en Hormonologie, Paris, France

G. B. NARDELLI Obstetric and Gynaecological Department, University of Padua, Padua, Italy

A. NASI Department of Obstetrics and Gynaecology, School of Medicine, University of Cagliari, Cagliari, Italy

V. NATOLI Laboratrio di Endocrinologia Molecolare, Istituto di Clinica Ostetrica e Ginecologica, Università Cattolica de Sacro Cuore, Largo Gemelli 8, 00168 Rome, Italy

C. NAVELLO Patologia Speciale Medica B, Università di Torino, Strada San Vito 34, 10133 Turin, Italy

I. NICOLETTI Institute of Clinical Medicine, Perugia University School of Medicine, 06100 Perugia, Italy

C. T. NOEL Department of Chemical Pathology, St. Mary's Hospital Medical School, London W1 1PG, UK

G. PAGANO Cattedra di Semeiotica Medica, Department of Internal Medicine, University of Turin, Turin, Italy

A. M. PAOLETTI Istituto di Clinica Ostetrica e Ginecologica, Università degli Studi, Via Roma 35, 56100 Pisa, Italy

D. PARRINI Clinica Ostetrica e Ginecologica, University of Siena, Siena, Italy

W. PASINI Unit of Psychosomatic Gynaecology and Sexology Medical School, University of Genève, Geneva, Switzerland

J. R. PASQUALINI Fondation de Recherche en Hormonologie, Paris, France

F. PETRAGLIA Cattedra di Patologia Ostetrica e Ginecologica, University of Siena, Siena, Italy

G. PINOTTI Divisione "B" di Medicina Generale, Ospedale Regionale di Varese Biometra Farmitalia Carlo Erba, Milan, Italy

E. PISI 1st Institute of Special Medical Pathology and Clinical Methodology, University of Bologna, Bologna, Italy

E. PISU Cattedra di Semeiotica Medica, Department of Internal Medicine, University of Turin, Turin, Italy

F. PIVA Department of Endocrinology, University of Milano, Via Andrea del Sarto 21, 20129 Milano, Italy

C. POLLINI Divisione "B" di Medicina Generale, Ospedale Regionale di Varese Biometria Farmitalia Carlo Erba, Milan, Italy

P. POMPEI Istituto di Clinica Medica Generale V, Università di Roma, Rome Italy

J. POORMAN Department of Obstetrics and Gynaecology, University Hospital Utrecht, Utrecht, The Netherlands

D. POPOVIC Department of Gynaecology and Obstetrics, Clinical Centre Dedinje, Belgrade, Yugoslavia

L. PRELATO Ospedale Ostetrico Ginecologico Sant'Anna, Turin, Italy

E. PUCCI Post-graduate School of Endocrinology, Pisa, Italy

J. PUSCH Medizinische Poliklinik, University of Würzburg, Würzburg, West Germany

M. J. REED Department of Chemical Pathology, St. Mary's Hospital Medical School, London W2 1PG, UK

Ch. RENARD Institute of Medicine, Radioimmunoassay Laboratory, University of Liège, Liège, Belgium

L. RIBONI Laboratorio di Chimica degli Ormoni, CNR Via Mario Bianco 9, 20131 Milan, Italy

M. G. RICCI-DANERO Clinica Ostetrica e Ginecologica, Università degli Studi di Siena, Siena, Italy

L. P. RIVA Department of Endocrinology, St. Antony Hospital, Gallarate, Italy

C. ROBYN Human Reproduction Research Unit, Université Libre de Bruxelles, Hôpital Saint-Pierre, 322 Rue Haute, 1000 Brussels, Belgium

A. ROCCO Istituto di Clinica Medica Generale V, Università di Roma, Rome, Italy

E. ROVERO Patologia Speciale Medica B, Università di Torino, Strada San Vito 34, 10133 Turin, Italy

A. RUJU 2 Divisione Radiologica OORR, Pisa, Italy

F. SANTEUSANIO Institute of Clinical Medicine Perugia University School of Medicine, 06100 Perugia, Italy

P. A. SANTORI Institute of Clinical Medicine, Perugia University School of Medicine, 06100 Perugia, Italy

G. SCAMBIA Laboratorio di Endocrinologia Molecolare, Istituto di Clinica Ostetrica e Ginecologica, Università Cattolica del Sacro Cuore, Largo Gemelli 8, 00168 Rome, Italy

D. SCAVO I Patologia Medica University of Rome, Rome, Italy

H. P. G. SCHNEIDER Department of Obstetrics and Gynaecology, The University of Münster, Münster, West Germany

P. SCHNEIDER 1st Women's Hospital, School of Medicine, University of Vienna, Vienna, Austria

R. SCHOLLER Fondation de Rercherche en Hormonologie, Paris, France

A. SCHRAMM Medizinische Poliklinik, University of Würzburg, Würzburg, West Germany

P. SCIRPA Department of Obstetrics and Gynaecology, Catholic University, Largo Gemelli 8, 00168 Rome, Italy

M. SELCI Clinica Chirurgica dell'Università, Pisa, Italy

F. P. SELVAGGI 1 Clinica Ostetrica e Ginecologica e Insegnamento di nefrologia di interesse chirurgico, Università di Bari, Bari, Italy

K. SEMM Department of Gynaecology and Obstetrics, University of Kiel and Michaelis Midwifery School, Kiel, West Germany

M. SERIO Endocrinology Unit, University of Florence, Florence, Italy

D. M. SERR Division of Obstetrics and Gynaecology, The Sheba Medical Centre TeP-Hashomer, Sackler School of Medicine, Tel-Aviv University, Tel-Aviv, Israel

G. B. SERRA Istituto di Clinica Ostetrica e Ginecologica, Università Cattolica del S. Cuore, Rome, Italy

G. SICA Istituto di Istologia ed Embriologia Generale, Università Cattolica S. Cuore, Via della Pineta Sacchelti 644, Rome, Italy

P. SICCARDI Catholic University, Department of Obstetrics and Gynaecology, Largo A. Gemelli 8, Rome, Italy

N. C. SIDDLE Department of Obstetrics and Gynaecology, King's College Hospital Medical School, University of London, Denmark Hill, London SE5 8RX, UK

D. SILVESTRI Laboratorio di Endocrinologia del CNR dell'Università di Pisa, Pisa, Italy

I. SIMEONE Centre de Gériatrie, Départment de Medicine et de Psychiatrie, Université de Genève, Geneva, Switzerland

I. SIMONETTI CNR Clinical Physiology Institute, University of Pisa, Pisa, Italy

J. W. SIMPKINS Physiology Department, JHMHC, J125, University of Florida, Gainesville, Florida 32601, USA

R. SORBO Cattedra di Clinica Medica A, Department of Internal Medicine, University of Turin, Turin, Italy

R. W. STEGER Department of Obstetrics and Gynaecology, University of Texas Health Science Center, San Antonio, Texas 78284, USA

J. C. STEVENSON Endocrine Unit, Royal Postgraduate Medical School, Hammersmith Hospital, Ducane Road, London W12 0HS, UK

F. STRIGINI Clinica Ostetrica e Ginecologica, Pisa, Italy

J. R. SWINHOE Academic Department of Medicine, Royal Free Hospital Medical School, Pond Street, London NW3, UK

G. TETI Clinica Ostetrica e Ginecologica dell'Università di Pisa, Pisa, Italy

J. H. H. THIJSSEN Department of Obstetrics and Gynaecology, University Hospital Utrecht, Utrecht, The Netherlands

P. T. THO Reproductive Endocrin Division, Department of Obstetrics and Gynaecology, Medical College of Georgia, Augusta, Georgia 30912, USA

L. TODROS Patologia Speciale Medica B, Università di Torino, Strada San Vito 34, 10133 Turin, Italy

G. TOGNONI Istituto di Ricerche Farmacologiche "Mario Negri" Via Eritrea 62 20157 Milan, Italy

P. TOUSIJN Ospedale Ostetrico Ginecologico Sant'Anna, Turin, Italy

P. T. TOWNSEND Department of Obstetrics and Gynaecology, King's College Hospital Medical School, University of London, Denmark Hill, London SE5 8RX, UK

R. TREVOUX Rue de l'Assomption 31, Paris XVIᵉ, France

K. TSCHERNE Women's Hospital, School of Medicine, University of Graz, Graz, Austria

A. TUDISCO Istituto di Ricerche Farmacologiche "Mario Negri" Via Eritrea 62, 20157 Milan, Italy

R. TUIMALA Departments of Obstretrics and Gynaecology, Biochemistry and Clinical Chemistry, University of Oulu, Oulu, Finland

G. V. UPTON Wyeth International Limited, P.O. Box 8616, Philadelphia, Pennsylvania 19101, USA

C. VALENZANO Patologia Speciale Medica B, Università di Torino, Strada San Vito 34, 10133 Turin, Italy

W. H. M. VAN DER VELDEN Department of Gynaecology and Obstetrics, St. Joseph Hospital, Eindhoven, The Netherlands

G. VAUDAGNA Cattedra di Patologia Medica 2, University of Pisa, Pisa, Italy

A. VERMEULEN Department of Endocrinology and Metabolic Diseases, Academic Hospital, University of Chent, Ghent, Belgium

R. VIHKO Departments of Obstetrics and Gynaecology, Biochemistry and Clinical Chemistry, University of Oulu, Oulu, Finland

A. S. VILLECCO 1st Institute of Special Medical Pathology and Clinical Methodology, University of Bologna, Bologna, Italy

E. VÖGELIN Women's Hospital, Schook of Medicine, University of Basle, Basle, Switzerland

B. VRTOVEC Department of Gynaecology and Obstetrics, University of Ljubljana, Slajmerjeva 3 Ljubljana, Yugoslavia

M. I. WHITEHEAD Department of Obstetrics and Gynaecology, King's College Hospital, Medical School, University of London, Denmark Hill, London SE5 8RX, UK

M. A. H. M. WIEGERINCK Department of Obstetrics and Gynaecology, University Hospital Utrecht, Utrecht, The Netherlands

O. M. YOUNG Department of Obstetrics and Gynaecology, King's College Hospital Medical School, University of London, Denmark Hill, London SE5 8RX, UK

M. ZANISI Department of Endocrinology, University of Milan, Via Andrea del Sarto 21, 20129 Milan, Italy

R. ZECCA Clinica Ostetrica e Ginecologica dell'Università di Pisa, Pisa, Italy

SECTION I

NEUROENDOCRINOLOGY OF THE MENOPAUSE

CENTRAL NERVOUS SYSTEM NEUROTRANSMITTERS DURING THE DECLINE OF REPRODUCTIVE ACTIVITY

J. Meites*, H. H. Huang, J. W. Simpkins and R. W. Steger

Department of Physiology, Neuroendocrine Research Laboratory, Michigan State University, East Lansing, Michigan, USA

INTRODUCTION

A number of neurotransmitters in the hypothalamus have been demonstrated to exert important influences on secretion of pituitary hormones, including the gonadotropins (Meites *et al.*, 1977, Müller *et al.*, 1977). Most is known about the actions of dopamine (DA), norepinephrine (NE) and serotonin (5-HT), all three of which are highly concentrated in the hypothalamus. Acetylcholine, histamine, gamma aminobutyric acid (GABA), brain opiates (endorphins and encephalins), melatonin, neurotensin, substance P, bombesin, etc., were also reported to influence secretion of pituitary hormones, but their physiological role in regulating secretion of these hormones remains to be established. It is generally believed that the hypothalamic neurotransmitters influence pituitary hormone secretion by regulating the release of the hypothalamic peptidergic releasing or release-inhibiting hormones (GnRH or LHRH, TRH, somatostatin, etc.) into the portal vessels where they are carried to, and act directly on, the pituitary. In general, NE has been shown to stimulate release of gonadotropins, whereas 5-HT has

*Aided by US Public Health Service grants AG00416 from the National Institute on Aging, AM04784 from the National Institute for Arthritis, Metabolism and Digestive Diseases, and CA10771 from the National Cancer Institute.

Serono Symposium No. 39, "The Menopause: Clinical, Endocrinological and Pathophysiological Aspects", edited by P. Fioretti, L. Martini, G. B. Melis and S. S. C. Yen, 1982. Academic Press, London and New York.

been found to inhibit release under most conditions. Contradictory results have
been reported for DA, the precursor of NE, on release of gonadotropins.

The female rat comes into puberty at 35–45 days of age, and exhibits regular
4–5 day estrous cycles for the first 8–12 months of life. The decline in reproductive functions has been described by us previously (Meites *et al.*, 1978).
First there is an irregularity of estrous cycles which are lengthened by 1–4 days.
This is usually seen at 10–15 months of age in our rats. By 10–18 months of
age, most rats enter a "constant estrous" state, and exhibit ovaries with well-
developed follicles, some cystic, but no ovulations and no corpora lutea. Rats
at this stage show a loss of ability to release LH and FSH cyclically and an
increase in prolactin secretion. From the "constant estrous" condition, some
of the rats enter into a "pseudopregnant-like" state, characterised by the presence
of numerous corpora lutea that actively secrete progesterone stimulated by the
high serum levels of prolactin. Prolactin is luteotropic in the rat. We have no evidence that the corpora lutea originate from follicles that have actually ruptured,
and have observed entrapped ova in the corpora lutea of luteinised follicles.
The oldest rats, 2–3 years of age, show an "anestrous" syndrome, with inactive
appearing ovaries containing only small or under developed follicles, and little evidence of estrogen secretion as indicated by the appearance of an atrophic reproductive tract. The pituitaries of these "anestrous" rats are frequently tumorous,
and secrete large amounts of prolactin and almost no gonadotropins. Many
old female rats develop mammary tumours, believed to be associated with the
high secretion of prolactin. It has been demonstrated that when the ovaries of
old non-cycling female rats were transplanted to young ovariectomised rats,
they became functional and the rats exhibited estrous cycles (Peng and Huang,
1972). The principal cause, therefore, for the loss of estrous cycles in aging
female rats lies in the failure of the hypothalamo-pituitary system to produce
a cyclic surge of gonadotropins every 4–5 days as in young rats.

We postulated quite early on that the hypothalamic neurotransmitters and the
releasing or release-inhibiting hormones probably played a key role in determining
the decline or reproductive functions in the aging rat. We reported (Clemens
et al., 1969) that direct electrical stimulation of the preoptic area of the hypothalamus or injection of epinephrine or progesterone could induce ovulation
and reinitiate estrous cycles in old non-cycling female rats. Subsequently we
observed that administration of L-DOPA, iproniazid (a monoamine oxidase
inhibitor that prevents metabolism of catecholamines and 5–HT), ACTH, ether
stress, some prostaglandins, and other agents could induce resumption of estrous
cycles in old "constant estrus" and "pseudopregnant-like" female rats (Meites
et al., 1978). GnRH was found to be present in the hypothalamus, but apparently
the neural signals necessary to induce cyclic release of GnRH and of LH and FSH
by the pituitary every 4 or 5 days were not forthcoming. A number of studies
indicated that the hypothalamus of old rats did not respond normally to stimuli
that usually release gonadotropins. Thus castration of old female rats resulted
in a significantly smaller elevation of serum LH than in young castrated rats.
Stress, which elicits an acute release of LH in young rats, was much less effective
in producing release of LH in old rats. Young ovariectomised, estrogen-primed
rats responded to subsequent estrogen or progesterone administration with a
marked surge of serum LH and FSH, whereas similarly treated old female rats
showed only a small elevation of these hormones.

In view of the above observations, it was of interest to compare the concentration and metabolism of DA and NE in the hypothalamus of old and young rats, and to determine whether these showed any relationship to the decline in reproductive functions with aging.

COMPARISON OF HYPOTHALAMIC CONCENTRATIONS AND METABOLISM OF NE AND DA IN OLD AND YOUNG FEMALE RATS

Multiparous female Long-Evans rats (Blue Spruce Farms, Altamount, NY) were housed in steel cages in an air-conditioned and temperature-controlled $(24 \pm 2\,^\circ C)$ room. Light was provided from 0600 to 2000 h daily. The rats were maintained on a complete diet of Wayne Lab Blox (Allied Mills, Chicago, Illinos) and tap water *ad libitum.* When rats reached 18-20 months of age, daily vaginal smears were taken and recorded, and animals exhibiting constant vaginal cornification for 20 days or longer were considered to be in "constant estrus", and used for experimentation. Four month old rats of the same strain, showing regular 4-day estrous cycles were used for comparison.

For measurements of steady state concentrations of norepinephrine (NE) and dopamine (DA), intact and ovariectomised old and young rats were killed, and their brains were removed rapidly and placed on dry ice. For measurements of NE and DA metabolism (turnover), the rats were first injected i.p. with 250 mg alpha-methyl-paratyrosine (α-MpT/kg body weight) or its 0.9% NaCl vehicle, and 45 min later, the rats were killed and the brains were rapidly removed and placed on dry ice. The anterior hypothalamus was dissected form each rat by making cuts rostral to the optic chiasma, at the hypothalamic sulci, and caudal to the tuber cinereum. The posterior hypothalamus was dissected by making cuts rostral to the tuber cinereum, caudal to the mammillary bodies, and at the hypothalamic sulci. The hypothalamic cubes were 2-3 mm deep.

Hypothalamic NE and DA were assayed by the radioenzymatic method of Coyle and Henry (1973), using catecholamine-0-methyltransferase isolated from rat liver by a modification of the method of Nikodijevic *et al.* (1970). The assay was sensitive to 320 pg of DA and 500 pg of NE, and linear to at least 4 ng for both catecholamines. Results are expressed as ng of DA and NE per gram wet weight. Analysis of variance and Newman-Keul's multiple range tests were used to analyze the results. The results were considered to be significant if $P < 0.05$.

Figure 1 shows that the steady state concentration of anterior hypothalamic NE was significantly lower in old CE rats than in young rats on proestrous or estrous day (1210 ± 62 vs 1543 ± 123 and 1509 ± 98 ng/g wet weight, respectively). Forty-five minutes after α-MpT injection, NE decreased by $28 \pm 3\%$ in old rats, by $41 \pm 0.3\%$ in young proestrous rats, and by $42 \pm 4\%$ in young estrous rats. Ten days after ovariectomy, steady state concentrations of anterior hypothalamic NE were not altered in old or young rats (1227 ± 143 vs 1619 ± 59 ng/g wet weight, respectively). However, 45 min after α-MpT injection, NE decreased by $53 \pm 3\%$ in young rats, but only by $34 \pm 3\%$ in old rats. This indicates that NE metabolism after ovariectomy was increased significantly in the anterior hypothalamus of young rats, but only slightly in old rats.

The steady state concentration of anterior hypothalamic DA and percentage of DA depletion after α-MpT treatment were the same in both old and young

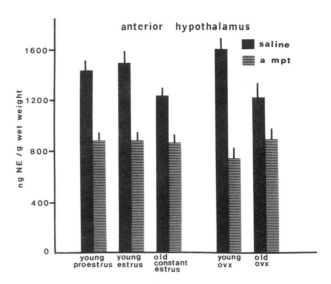

Fig. 1. NE steady state concentration in the anterior hypothalamus before and after α-MpT treatment of intact and ovariectomised old and young rats. Vertical lines = SEM; N = 6. (Huang, Simpkins and Meites, unpublished).

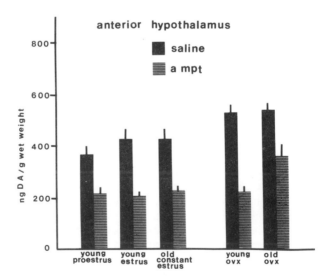

Fig. 2. DA steady state concentration in the anterior hypothalamus before and after α-MpT treatment of intact and ovariectomised old and young rats. Vertical lines = SEM; N = 6. (Huang, Simpkins and Meites, unpublished).

rats (Fig. 2). Ten days after ovariectomy, the steady state concentration of anterior hypothalamic DA rose similarly in both old and young rats. However, the percentage DA depletion after α-MpT treatment was significant only in young rats ($69 \pm 4\%$ vs $46 \pm 6\%$ and $51 \pm 3\%$, respectively), and not in old rats

(48 ± 1% vs 48 ± 6%). This indicates that DA metabolism in the anterior hypothalamus of ovariectomised young rats was greater than in the anterior hypothalamus of ovariectomised old rats. The steady state concentration of posterior hypothalamic NE and DA, and percentage NE and DA depletion after α-MpT treatment did not differ between old and young rats, and were not altered by ovariectomy (Figs 3 and 4).

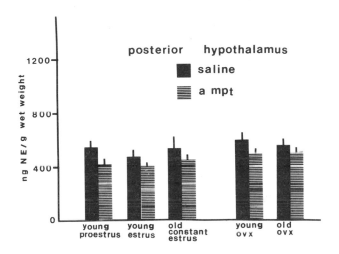

Fig. 3. NE steady state concentration in the posterior hypothalamus before and after α-MpT treatment of intact and ovariectomised old and young rats. Vertical lines = SEM; N = 6. (Huang, Simpkins and Meites, unpublished).

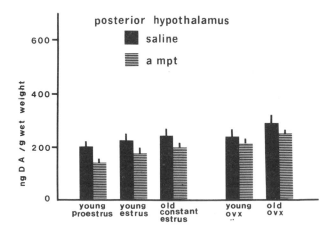

Fig. 4. DA steady state concentration in the posterior hypothalamus before and after α-MpT treatment of intact and ovariectomised old and young rats. Vertical lines = SEM; N = 6. (Huang, Simpkins and Meites, unpublished).

These results show that in intact old constant estrous female rats which fail
to ovulate, there is a reduction in steady state concentration and metabolism
of NE in the anterior but not in the posterior hypothalamus, as compared with
that in young cycling rats on days of proestrus or estrus. This is believed to
largely account for the failure of these old rats to exhibit a cyclic release of
LHRH from the hypothalamus and of LH and FSH from the pituitary (Huang
et al., 1978). It has been shown that there is a rise in NE metabolism in the
anterior hypothalamus just prior to the surge of LH and FSH on the afternoon
of proestrus which induces ovulation in the young cycling female rat (Kalra
and McCann, 1973). Administration of 6-hydroxy-DA to inhibit the rise of
NE on the afternoon of proestrus prevents the surge of LH and FSH and inhibits
ovulation (Simpkins *et al.,* 1979).

The present observations show that after ovariectomy there was a significant
rise in the metabolism of NE in the young, but not in the old rats. The rise in
NE metabolism in the young ovariectomised rats is in agreement with many
previous reports (Anton–Tay and Wurtman, 1971), and is believed to account
in part for the increase in gonadotropin secretion seen after ovariectomy. The
failure of the old rats to show a similar increase in anterior hypothalamic NE
metabolism after ovariectomy is believed to largely account for the significantly
reduced increase in serum LH and FSH seen in old rats.

An increase in hypothalamic DA metabolism is not essential for the proestrous surge of gonadotropins and is not seen during the estrous cycle. In the
present study the steady state concentration of DA in the anterior hypothalamus
of old intact or ovariectomized rats did not differ from that found in young
rats, although the metabolism of DA was greater in the young than in the old
ovariectomised rats. This latter may reflect a greater rate of conversion of DA
to NE in the young ovariectomised rats.

Serum LH and FSH in these old rats failed to show a cyclic surge as in young
rats, and the rise in serum LH and FSH after ovariectomy was significantly lower
than in young rats after ovariectomy. This is in agreement with previous results
reported by our laboratory (Meites *et al.,* 1978), and illustrates the lower capacity
of old female rats to release gonadotropins. Induction of ovulation and estrous
cycles in old constant estrous rats by direct stimulation of the preoptic area of
hypothalamus or by adminstration of L-DOPA or iproniazid (Clemens *et al.,*
1969) indicates that the normal stimulus to cyclic release of GnRH from the
hypothalamus is missing in these rats. Other work suggests that the uptake of
estrogen by the preoptic area of the hypothalamus may be reduced in old female
rats (Peng and Peng, 1973), and this also may be true for progesterone. The
reduced ability of estradiol or progesterone to induce release of LH and FSH
in old ovariectomised, estrogen-primed female rats may be related both to the
decrease in hypothalamic uptake of these steroids as well as to reduced NE
activity.

COMPARISON OF HYPOTHALAMIC CONCENTRATIONS AND
METABOLISM OF NE, DA AND SEROTONIN (5–HT) IN OLD
AND YOUNG MALE RATS

The aging male rat shows many parallels in its neuroendocrine reproductive
patterns to those of the aging female rat. Thus, in old male rats, radioimmunoassays

of serum LH, FSH and testosterone show a significant decline, whereas serum
prolactin shows a significant rise, when compared with related serum values
in young male rats (Meites *et al.*, 1978). As in female rats, the decline in ability
to secrete gonadotropins and increase in release of prolactin has been shown
to be related to changes in concentration and metabolism of hypothalamic neurotransmitters.

Figure 5 shows that concentrations of DA and NE in the medial basal hypothalamus are reduced in 21 month old as compared with 3–4 month old male
Wistar rats. The metabolism of DA is also greater in young than in old rats.
Similar differences in concentration of DA and NE were found in the remainder
of the hypothalamus between old and young rats, and the metabolism of NE
was greater in the young than in the old rats (Fig. 6). Figure 7 shows that hypothalamic concentrations of 5-HT were similar in old and young rats, but metabolism of this neurotransmitter was greater in the old rats.

The lower hypothalamic NE and higher 5-HT concentrations and/or metabolism in the old as compared to the young male rats is believed to largely account
for the reduction in secretion of LH, FSH and testosterone by the old rats.
Whereas NE stimulates gonadotropin release, 5-HT has been reported to inhibit
gonadotropin release under most conditions (Meites *et al.*, 1977). DA is believed
to be the principal hypothalamic inhibitor of prolactin release (Meites *et al.*,
1977; Müller *et al.*, 1977), and the reduction in DA concentration and metabolism in the medial basal hypothalamus in the old rats probably mainly accounts
for the rise in serum prolactin values. Serotonin is a potent stimulator of prolactin release in rats (Meites *et al.*, 1977), and is also probably responsible in
part for the increase in prolactin secretion. Thus the secretory patterns of LH,
FSH, prolactin and the changes in hypothalamic NE and DA concentration
and/or metabolism in old male and female rats appear to be essentially similar.

In general the reproductive decline in male rats is more gradual than in aging

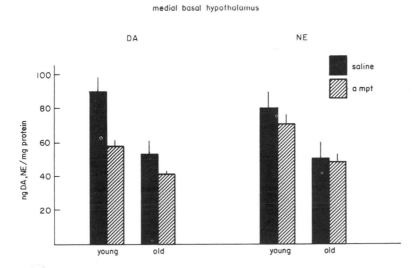

Fig. 5. DA and NE steady state concentrations in medial basal hypothalamus before and
after α-MpT treatment of young and old male rats. Vertical lines = 1 SEM. Each bar = the
mean of 6–8 determinations (after Simpkins *et al.*, 1979).

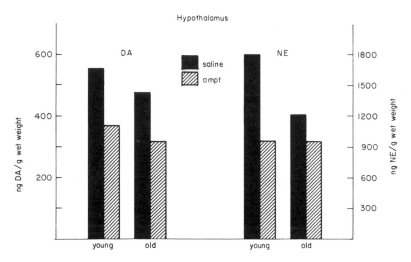

Fig. 6. DA and NE steady state concentrations in remainder of hypothalamus before and after α-MpT treatment of young and old male rats. See Fig. 5 for further explanation (after Simpkins *et al.*, 1979).

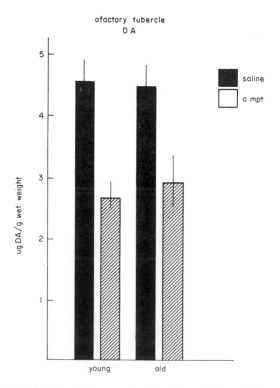

Fig. 7. Serotonin (5-HT) steady state concentration in hypothalamus before and 30 min after administration of 75 mg pargyline HCl/kg body weight. Vertical lines represent 1 SEM. Each bar represents mean of 7–10 determinations (after Simpkins *et al.*, 1979).

female rats, and testosterone and sperm production may continue to the end of life, provided the animals remain in good health. There is some evidence that in addition to the changes in hypothalamic function, the pituitary of aging male rats may secrete less gonadotropins in response to stimulation by GnRH, and less testosterone in response to injections of gonadotropins (Meites *et al.*, 1978).

The causes for the decline in hypothalamic DA and NE activity in aging male and female rats, and the increase in hypothalamic 5-HT activity in old male rats are not yet clear. There is some evidence for selective loss of neurons in old female fats in the medial preoptic area, in the anterior hypothalamic area, and in the arcuate nucleus, regions concerned with secretion of gonadotropins and prolactin (Hsu and Peng, 1978). There also is some evidence for an increase in hypothalamic monoamine oxidase and catecholamine-O-methyl-transferase activities, the two major enzymes responsible for metabolising catecholamines and 5-HT (Robinson *et al.*, 1972; Lytle and Altar, 1979). Changes also may occur in the activity of tyrosine hydroxylase, the rate limiting enzyme for conversion of tyrosine to catecholamine, and in tryptophan hydroxylase, the rate limiting enzyme for conversion of tryptophan to 5-HT (Lytle and Altar, 1979). In addition, there may be a loss of receptors for catecholamines and other neurotransmitters in the hypothalamus of aging animals (Makman *et al.*, 1979). There may be other causes for aging changes in the activity of hypothalamic neurotransmitters as well.

NEUROENDOCRINE RELATIONSHIPS IN THE REPRODUCTIVE DECLINE IN WOMEN

A number of important differences are exhibited by women in the pre- and postmenopausal states when compared with aging female rats. In women approaching the menopause, the menstrual cycles tend to become irregular, but these are usually shortened rather than lengthened (Talbert, 1977; Schiff and Wilson, 1978). Ovulations become fewer and there is a tendency to form cystic follicles, as in the rat. However, the ovaries of women approaching the menopause show a reduced response to gonadotropins and a decrease in secretion of ovarian hormones, resulting in increased secretion by the pituitary of FSH and LH (Rebar and Yen, 1979). In postmenopausal women, the follicles gradually disappear, and the ovaries become fibrotic and secrete but little steroid hormones, resulting in a further increase in secretion of FSH and LH. Therefore the primary cause for cessation of menstrual cycles in aging women appears to be in the ovaries rather than in the hypothalamic-pituitary system. However, the high secretion of gonadotropins in these women does not necessarily imply that the hypothalamic-pituitary system functions normally. The ability of this system to respond to stimulus that normally evokes release of gonadotropins or other pituitary hormones has not been adequately compared between young and older women. Dillman (1971) has hypothesised that the hypothalamic threshold to stimuli that influence many physiological processes is reduced in elderly human subjects.

The relationship of hypothalamic neurotransmitters to secretion of pituitary hormones is not as well defined in human beings as in animal species. Intravenous infusion of DA into normal women was reported to depress LH and prolactin concentrations in the blood (Leblanc *et al.,* 1975), but there is little evidence as yet that catecholamines have a definite role in the release of gonadotropins in human subjects. There is evidence that the preoptic area of the hypothalamus, which is important for regulation of gonadotropin release in the rat, is not essential for cyclic release of gonadotropins in primates; cyclic control of gonadotropins in primates appears to lie in the pituitary and medial basal hypothalamus (Knobil and Plant, 1978). As in the rat, there is evidence for a decrease in catecholamines in selective areas of the brains of human subjects, including the hypothalamus, and also for an increase in monoamine oxidase and catecholamine-O-methyltransferase (Robinson *et al.,* 1972, Lytle and Altar, 1979). Administration of L-DOPA, the precursor of the catecholamines, was reported to initiate menstrual bleeding in some postmenopausal women (Kruse-Larson and Garde, 1971), but there were no observations as to whether this altered estrogen secretion or induced ovulation. It is obvious that further work is necessary to clarify the relationship of hypothalamic neurotransmitters to release of gonadotropins in human subjects, and to their possible role in reproductive senescence.

REFERENCES

Anton–Tay, F. and Wurtman, R. J. (1971). *In* "Frontiers in Neuroendocrinology" (L. Martini and W. F. Ganong, Eds), 45–66. Oxford University Press, London and New York.

Clemens, J. A., Amenomori, Y., Jenkins, T. and Meites, J. (1969). *Proceedings of the Society of Experimental Biology and Medicine* **132**, 561.

Coyle, J. T. and Henry, D. (1973). *Journal of Neurochemistry* **21**, 61.

Dillman, V. M. (1971). *Lancet* **1**, 1211.

Hsu, H. K. and Peng, M. T. (1978). *Gerontology* **24**, 434.

Huang, H. H., Steger, R. W., Bruni, J. F. and Meites, J. (1978). *Journal of Endocrinology* **103**, 1955.

Kalra, S. P. and McCann, S. M. (1973). *Endocrinology* **93**, 356.

Knobil, E. and Plant, T. M. (1978). *In* "Frontiers in Neuroendocrinology" (W. F. Ganong and L. Martini, Eds), 249–264. Raven Press, New York.

Kruse–Larson, C. and Garde, K. (1971). *Lancet* **1**, 707.

Leblanc, H. Lachelin, G.C.L., Abu–Fadil, S. and Yen, S.S.C. (1975). *Journal of Clinical Endocrinology and Metabolism* **43**, 668.

Lytle, L. D. and Altar, A. (1979). *Federations Proceedings* **38**, 2017.

Makman, M. H., Ahn, H. S., Thal, L. J., Sharpless, N. S., Dvorkin, B., Horowitz, S. G. and Rosenfeld, M. (1979). *Federation Proceedings* **38**, 1922.

Meites, J., Simpkins, J., Bruni, J. and Advis, J. (1977). *IRCS Journal of Medical Sciences* **5**, 1.

Meites, J., Huang, H. H. and Simpkins, J. W. (1978). *In* "The Aging Reproductive System" (E. L. Schneider, Ed.), 213–236. Raven Press, New York.

Müller, E. E., Nistico, G. and Scapagnini, U. (1977). "Neurotransmitters and Pituitary Function." Academic Press, New York.

Nikodijevic, B., Senoh, S., Daly, J. W. and Creveling, C. R. (1970). *Journal of Pharmacology Experimental Therapy* **174**, 83.

Peng, M. T. and Huang, H. H. (1972). *Fertility and Sterility* **23**, 535.

Peng, M. T. and Peng, Y. M. (1973). *Fertility and Sterility* **24**, 534.

Rebar, R. W. and Yen, S.S.C. (1979). *In* "Endocrine Rhythms" (D. T. Krieger, Ed.), 259–298. Raven Press, New York.

Robinson, P. S., Nies, A., Davis, J. N., Bunney, W. E., Davis, J. M., Colburn, R. W., Bourne, H. R., Shaw, D. M. and Coppen, A. J. (1972). *Lancet* **1**, 290.

Schiff, J. and Wilson, E. (1978). *In* "The Aging Reproductive System" (E. L. Schneider, Ed.), 9–28. Raven Press, New York.

Simpkins, J. W., Huang, H. H., Advis, J. P. and Meites, J. (1979). *Biology of Reproduction* **20**, 625.

Talbert, G. B. (1977). *In* "The Aging Reproductive System" (E. L. Schneider, Ed.), 318–356. Raven Press, New York.

STUDIES ON THE DIFFERENTIAL CONTROL OF LH
AND FSH RELEASE

F. Piva, M. Zanisi and L. Martini

*Department of Endocrinology, University of Milan, Via Andrea del Sarto,
Milan, Italy*

INTRODUCTION

It has long been known that, in women, the patterns of secretion of LH and of
FSH are substantially different (Wide *et al.*, 1973). Figure 1 shows the pattern of
LH secretion before and after the menopause in normal women. It is apparent that,
during the fertile period, LH shows a typical elevation at mid-cycle. It is also clear
that, after the menopause, LH is released in elevated quantities, with no further
signs of cyclicity. Figure 1 also shows that, usually, the mid-cycle LH peak reaches
levels which are much higher than those found after the menopause. Figure 2
shows the pattern of FSH secretion. As for LH, during the fertile period there is
a rise of FSH at mid-cycle; however, the FSH peak is minor when compared to
the LH peak. After the menopause, serum FSH levels are significantly increased,
and reach concentrations which are much higher than those found at mid-cycle.
This paper will concentrate on some experimental work performed in the author's
laboratory and aimed at explaining some of the neuro-endocrine mechanisms which
may entertain the different patterns of secretion of the two gonadotropins.

EFFECTS OF CASTRATION ON GONADOTROPIN RELEASE

In 1973, Zanisi *et al.* reported that castration, performed in adult female rats,
exerts substantially different effects on LH and FSH secretion. As may be seen in

Serono Symposium No. 39, "The Menopause: Clinical, Endocrinological and Pathophysiological Aspects", edited by P. Fioretti, L. Martini, G. B. Melis and S. S. C. Yen, 1982. Academic
Press, London and New York.

F. Piva et al.

Fig. 3, it is clear that FSH levels increase immediately after ovariectomy; significantly higher levels of this gonadotrophin are found in the serum as early as one day following gonadectomy; this phase of rapid increase is then followed by a subsequent less dramatic elevation, which lasts up to the end of the experimental period. On the contrary, the hypersecretion of LH induced by ovariectomy develops more slowly; serum LH levels begin to be significantly different from pre-castration values only 7 days after ovariectomy. Similar results have been reported by Ramirez and Sawyer (1974), Cooper *et al.* (1974) and Brown-Grant and Greig (1975). Additional differences in the mode of secretion of the two gonadotropins have been found following sex steroid treatment. Zanisi and Martini (1975) have shown that the administration of oestrogens to adult ovariectomized female rats brings about a total suppression of LH secretion at different intervals after castration, but exerts only minor effects on FSH release. An interpretation of these results is probably provided by the recent demonstration that the fluid of the ovarian follicles (De Jong and Sharpe, 1976; Marder *et al.*, 1977; Schwartz and Channing, 1977; Chappel *et al.*, 1980) and the ovarian vein plasma (De Paolo *et al.*, 1979; Shander *et al.*, 1980) contain a hypothetical substance, called inhibin or folliculostatin, which specifically blocks the secretion of FSH with little or no activity on LH. If one accepts this view, it might be postulated that FSH is under a dual feedback control (sex steroids and folliculostatin) while LH is only controlled by sex steroids. Whether cessation of the production of folliculostatin may also explain the hypersecretion of FSH found in postmenopausal women remains to be ascertained.

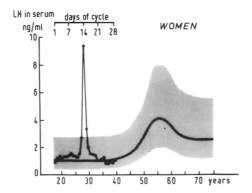

Fig. 1.   Serum LH levels in women of different ages (Wide *et al.*, 1973).

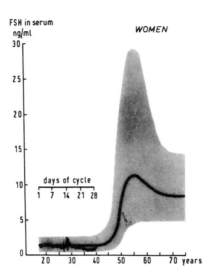

Fig. 2. Serum FSH levels in women of different ages (Wide *et al.*, 1973).

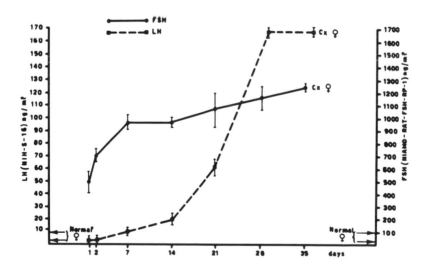

Fig. 3. Effect of castration (Cx) on serum levels of FSH and LH (measured by radioimmuno-assay) of adult ♀ rats killed at different times after gonadectomy.

EFFECTS OF NEUROTRANSMITTERS ON GONADOTROPIN RELEASE

Additional information regarding the mechanisms underlining the differential control of the secretion of the two gonadotropins has been derived from neuroendocrinological studies recently performed by Borrell *et al.* (1979) and by Piva *et al.* (1980). These authors have tried to interrupt neuronal inputs to the amygdala using a pharmacological approach. It is known that the amygdala is largely innervated by neuronal pathways which originate in the mid-brain. A series of putative or classical neurotransmitters has been identified in the neuronal terminals reaching the amygdala (e.g., acetylcholine, dopamine, norepinephrine, epinephrine, serotonin, GABA, histamine, substance P, enkephalins, LHRH, etc.). The bilateral implantation into the basomedial nucleus of the amygdala of a drug like phenoxybenzamine which inhibits α-adrenergic receptors is followed by a significant increase of serum LH levels and by an even more significant increase in serum FSH (Fig. 4). The implantation in the same area of the β-blocker propranolol is followed only by an increase of LH secretion without any concomitant alteration of FSH (Fig. 5). The implantation of atropine, a typical antimuscarinic drug, is also followed by a significant elevation of the release of LH with no simultaneous alterations in FSH secretion (Fig. 6). These results underline the existence of a complex neuronal circuit involved in the control of gonadotropin secretion; this circuit comprises mid-brain, amygdalar and hypothalamic components (Fig. 7). The data also suggest that the amygdala must be considered an important station for the differential control of the secretion of the two gonadotropins.

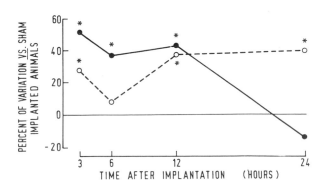

Fig. 4. Effects of implants of *Phenoxybenzamine* into the basomedial portion of the amygdala on serum LH and FSH levels of adult castrated ♀ rats. •—• LH; ○---○ FSH; * significant vs sham implanted animals.

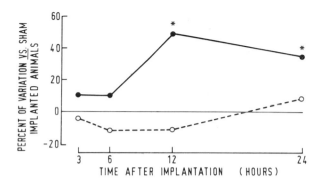

Fig. 5. Effects of implants of *Propanolol* into the basomedial portion of the amygdala on serum LH and FSH levels of adult castrated ♀ rats. ●—● LH; ○- - -○ FSH; * significant vs sham implanted animals.

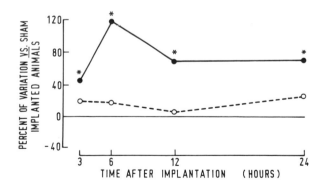

Fig. 6. Effect of implants of *Atropine* into the basomedial portion of the amygdala on serum LH and FSH levels of adult castrated ♀ rats. ●—● LH; ○---○ FSH; * significant vs sham implanted animals.

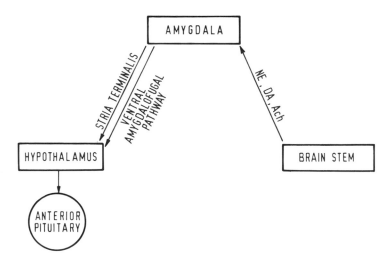

Fig. 7. Interrelationships of different nervous structures in the control of anterior pituitary function.

PROGESTERONE METABOLITES AND GONADOTROPIN RELEASE

It has been reported by this and other laboratories that in the brain and in the anterior pituitary of female rats progesterone is converted into 5α-pregan-3, 20-dione (dihydroprogesterone, DHP), into 5α-pregan-3α-ol-20-one (3α-ol) and 5α-pregnan-3β-ol-20-one (3β-ol) through the action of a 5α-reductase 3-hydroxy-steroid dehydrogenase system (Karavolas and Nuti, 1976; Stupnicka *et al.*, 1977). The same structures are also able to convert progesterone into 20α-hydroxy-progesterone (Robinson and Karavolas, 1973). This compound may subsequently be reduced to the corresponding 5α-reduced metabolites (Nowak and Karavolas, 1974. Fig. 8). The work of Stupnicka *et al.* (1977) has indicated that the 5α-reductase activity of the anterior pituitary gland shows oestrous linked variations; moreover, in the anterior pituitary, this enzymatic activity is highly increased following castration and brought back to normal by the administration of sex steroids. These variations of the activity of the 5α-reductase in conditions in which the feedback signals to the pituitary are diminished or increased have led us to postulate that the conversion of progesterone into its corresponding 5α-reduced metabolites might play some important function in the modulation of the feedback effects of progesterone. Different types of experiments have been performed in order to verify this hypothesis. In one experiment, castrated female rats were implanted in the median eminence with small amounts of oestrogens prior to the systemic administration of progesterone or of the corresponding 5α-reduced metabolites. Serum level of LH and FSH were measured subsequently with specific radioimmunoassay. It is apparent from Fig. 9 that, in animals so prepared, progesterone and DHP are able to significantly increase the release of LH without modifying the release of FSH. On the contrary, 3α-ol and 3β-ol, which are ineffective in releasing LH, do increase the secretion of FSH (Martini *et al.*, 1979). In another experiment, castrated female rats were treated systemically with oestradiol for 5 days and subsequently injected with progesterone, 20α-hydroxy-progesterone (20α P), or 5α-pregnan-3α, 20α-diol (3α-20α-DHP). It is obvious from Fig. 10 that all three steroids increased LH secretion; progesterone, under the conditions of the present experiment, was also able to enhance FSH release. On the contrary, 20α-hydroxy-progesterone was ineffective on the secretion of FSH, while the 5α-reduced metabolites of 20α-hydroxyprogesterone were even inhibitory on the secretion of this gonadotropin (Zanisi and Martini, 1979). These studies underline profound divergences in the secretory responses of the anterior pituitary when submitted to the effects of different progestagens. The data moreover underline that sex steroids may play an important role in the control of the secretion of the two gonadotropins.

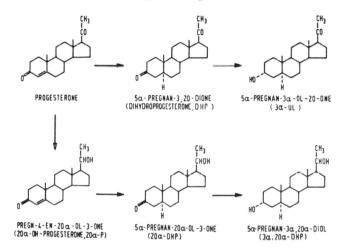

Fig. 8.

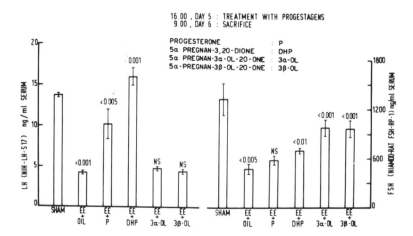

Fig. 9. Effect of treatment with 100 μg/rat of progesterone and of its metabolites on serum levels of LH and FSH of castrated ♀ rats implanted in the median eminence with ethinyl oestradiol (EE) 5 days earlier.

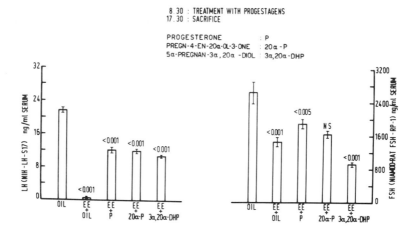

Fig. 10. Effect of treatment with 100 μg/rat of progesterone and of its metabolites on serum levels of LH and FSH of castrated ♀ rats treated for 5 days with 0.4 μg of ethinyl oestradiol (EE).

CONCLUSIONS

The present data indicate that the neuronal regulation and the feedback control of the two gonadotropins are substantially different for LH and FSH. The data indicate that the amygdala may be one of the centers where the differential control of the secretion of the two gonadotropins is modulated. Additional work is needed to fully understand the role of sex steroids and of folliculostatin.

REFERENCES

Borrell, J., Piva, F. and Martini, L. (1979). *Acta Endocrinologica* **90**, 385.
Brown-Grant, K. and Greig, F. (1975). *Journal of Endocrinology* **65**, 389.
Chappel, S. C., Holt, J. A. and Spies, H. G. (1980). *Proceedings of the Society for Experimental Biology and Medicine* **163**, 310.
Cooper, K. J., Fawcett, C. P. and McCann, S. M. (1974). *Endocrinology* **95**, 1293.
De Jong, F. H. and Sharpe, R. M. (1976). *Nature* **263**, 71.
De Paolo, L. V., Shander, D., Wise, P. M., Barraclough, C. A. and Channing, C. P. (1979). *Endocrinology* **105**, 647.
Karavolas, H. J. and Nuti, K. M. (1976). *In* "Subcellular Mechanisms in Reproductive Neuroendocrinology" (F. Naftolin, K. J. Ryan and I. J. Davies, Eds) 305–326. Elsevier, Amsterdam.
Marder, M. L., Channing, C. P. and Schwartz, N. B. (1977). *Endocrinology* **101**, 1639.
Martini, L., Celotti, F., Juneja, H., Motta, M. and Zanisi, M. (1979). *In* "Central Regulation of the Endocrine System" (K. Fuxe, T. Hokfelt and R. Luft, Eds) 273–295. Plenum Publishing Corporation, New York.

Nowak, F. V. and Karavolas, H. J. (1974). *Endocrinology* **94**, 994.

Piva, F., Borrell, J., Limonta, P., Gavazzi, G. and Martini, L. (1980). *Acta Endocrinologica* **93**, 1.

Ramirez, V. D. and Sawyer, C. H. (1974). *Endocrinology* **94**, 987.

Robinson, J. A. and Karavolas, H. J. (1973). *Endocrinology* **93**, 430.

Schwartz, N. B. and Channing, C. P. (1977). *Proceedings of the National Academy of Sciences, USA* **74**, 5724.

Shander, D., Anderson, L. D. and Barraclough, C. A. (1980). *Endocrinology* **106**, 1047.

Stupnicka, E., Massa, R., Zanisi, M. and Martini, L. (1977). *In* "Clinical Reproductive Neuroendocrinology" (P. O. Hubinont, M. L'Hermite and C. Robyn, Eds) 88–95. Karger, Basel.

Wide, L., Nillius, S. J., Germzell, C. and Roos, P. (1973). *Acta Endocrinologica* Supplementum **174**, 1.

Zanisi, M. and Martini, L. (1975). *Acta Endocrinologica* **78**, 683.

Zanisi, M. and Martini, L. (1979). *Proceedings of the Society for Experimental Biology and Medicine* **161**, 66.

Zanisi, M., Motta, M. and Martini, L. (1973). *In* "Hypothalamic Hypophysiotropic Hormones" (C. Gual and E. Rosemberg, Eds) 24–32. Excerpta Medica, Amsterdam.

INTERRELATIONSHIP BETWEEN PROLACTIN SECRETION AND OVARIAN ACTIVITY

C. Robyn

Human Reproduction Research Unit, Université Libre de Bruxelles,
Hôpital Saint-Pierre, Rue Haute, Bruxelles, Belgium

INTRODUCTION

The relationship between prolactin and the ovary is complex. Prolactin secretion is sensitive to ovarian steroids while follicular growth, maturation and ovarian steroidogenesis are influenced by prolactin.

SEX STEROIDS IN THE CONTROL OF PROLACTIN SECRETION

Prolactin secretion is under the permanent inhibitory influence of the hypothalamus; dopamine released from the nerve endings in the median eminence of the hypothalamus is a major prolactin inhibiting factor (PIF) of physiological significance (Mc Leod and Lamberts, 1978). It acts via specific dopamine receptors which are equivalent to post-synaptic receptors (Caron *et al.*, 1978). In teleost fish, dopaminergic fibres descending from the median eminence make synaptic contact with cells of the anterior lobe of the pituitary gland (Ingleton *et al.*, 1977). With evolution, these direct contacts disappeared and dopamine was transferred by the portal circulation from the median eminence to the adenohypophysis.

It has been shown recently that, *in vitro*, the lactotrophs, isolated from all hypothalamic influences, can generate calcium dependent action potentials (Dufy

Serono Symposium No. 39, "The Menopause: Clinical, Endocrinological and Pathophysiological Aspects", edited by P. Fioretti, L. Martini, G. B. Melis and S. S. C. Yen, 1982. Academic Press, London and New York.

et al., 1979a). Such spontaneous activities are inhibited by dopamine agonists and stimulated by TRH, by dopamine antagonists, and also by oestrogens (Dufy *et al.*, 1979b). Ion exchange through cell membranes appears to play an important role in the control of prolactin secretion. Dopamine antagonists (neuroleptics, butyrophenones, reserpine, etc.) and dopamine agonists (ergot alcaloid derivatives, L-DOPA, etc.) act directly at the pituitary level to suppress or to reinforce the inhibitory influence on prolactin secretion via the dopaminergic pathway (Mc Leod and Robyn, 1977; Mc Leod and Lamberts, 1978).

Thyrotropin releasing hormone (TRH), the hypothalamic hormone releasing thyrotropin, also releases prolactin (both *in vivo* and *in vitro*); TRH acts via specific receptors on TSH and prolactin cells (Schally *et al.*, 1973). It has clearly been shown that TRH is internalized in the cytoplasm of pituitary cells (Tixier-Vidal *et al.*, 1978). The effect of TRH on prolactin secretion is under dopaminergic control. Treatment with dopamine agonists suppresses the release of prolactin as induced by TRH (Frantz *et al.*, 1973). Serotonin and enkephalins or endorphins stimulate prolactin secretion. Most of the data support the concept that the effects of these substances are not direct effects but mediated by the dopaminergic pathway.

Inside the hypothalamus, there is a close relationship between dopaminergic fibres and fibres of the luteinizing hormone releasing hormone (LHRH) neurons (Fuxe *et al.*, 1978). However, it has been established that dopamine and LHRH are released by different neurons (Kizer *et al.*, 1975). Prolactin stimulates the turnover of dopamine in the hypothalamic tuberoinfundibular neurons (Fuxe *et al.*, 1978). This effect predominates in all hyperprolactinaemic states, including lactation. The increase of circulating prolactin associated with nursing does not appear to be entirely due to a decrease of dopamine in the portal blood: on the contrary, quite soon after the onset of suckling, the dopamine concentration in the portal blood increases. This is probably the result of an increased dopamine turnover, a consequence of the hyperprolactinaemia associated with nursing.

Oestrogens exert major effects on prolactin secretion (Jacobi *et al.*, 1977), in that they stimulate the release and the synthesis of prolactin. Oestradiol antagonizes the action of dopamine on the lactotrophs (Labrie *et al.*, 1978). It has been recently shown that oestrogens interact with anterior pituitary dopamine receptors (Schaeffer and Hsueh, 1979). Oestradiol, when directly applied to prolactin cells, provokes action potentials firing; dopamine does not suppress this oestrogen-induced electrical activity (Dufy *et al.*, 1979b). Furthermore, oestrogens stimulate the mitoses of cells in the adenohypophysis; the most sensitive cells appear to be the lactotrophs (Jacobi *et al.*, 1977). During gestation in women and in the chimpanzee, serum levels of prolactin increase progressively; this increase is parallel to that of circulating oestrogens (Robyn *et al.*, 1977). In species where there is no significant increase in circulating oestrogens during pregnancy (the rat, the sheep, the Rhesus monkey, etc.), there is also no significant change in circulating prolactin levels (Rigg *et al.*, 1977). Even transient increases in serum oestradiol levels, as seen during the preovulatory phase of the menstrual cycle in women (Vekemans *et al.*, 1977) or in the Mangabey monkey (Aidara *et al.*, 1978), are followed by a significant increase of serum prolactin.

In animals, chronic treatment with oestrogens induces the development of pituitary tumours secreting prolactin; this is yet further evidence for the mitogenic effects of oestrogens on the lactotrophs (El Etreby and Fath El Bab, 1977). It has been shown that, when bromocriptine is administered together with oestrogens, this dopamine agonist prevents the development and growth of these pituitary tumors. This is indirect evidence for the anti-tumoral effect of bromocriptine.

In women, there are significant changes in serum prolactin levels with age (Vekemans and Robyn, 1975). A significant increase takes place at the time of the menarche and a significant fall occurs at the menopause. Such changes are closely related to similar changes in circulating oestrogens. In men, serum levels of prolactin fluctuate around the same average value throughout lifetime. Prolactin secretion is relatively more sensitive to oestrogens in postmenopausal than in premenopausal women. The effects of a low oral dose of two synthetic oestrogens on serum prolactin levels, ethinyloestradiol and moxestrol (Roussel Laboratoires, Paris), have been tested in postmenopausal women. A double blind cross-over design has been used; three women received ethinyloestradiol first and three received moxestrol first. Serum LH, FSH and prolactin were measured in blood samples collected before, during and after treatment and also during the interval between the steroid administration. Similarly, the eosinophilic and the caryopycnotic indexes were evaluated in samples of vaginal smears. There was no significant effect during the first period of treatment but there was an effect on the endocrine parameters during the second one. Thus, the data were combined in order to compare the endocrine effects of 25 μg ethinyloestradiol with those of 5 μg moxestrol. Both treatments resulted in a significant decrease of serum LH and FSH and in a significant increase of serum prolactin and the oestrogenic indexes of the vaginal smears. It can be concluded that 5 μg/day moxestrol administered orally exerts significant oestrogenic effects; these are only slightly less important than those obtained with 25 μg ethinyloestradiol. The most striking endocrine effect is that obtained with 25 μg ethinyloestradiol on serum prolactin levels; after 1 week of treatment, serum levels of prolactin were increased to pre-menopausal levels. After interruption of ethinyloestradiol administration, serum prolactin levels fell progressively; after 1 week they were again within the pretreatment values.

The sensitivity of prolactin secretion to oestrogens varies according to the type of oestrogens administered. Conjugated oestrogens seem to be much less effective than unconjugated oestrogens. A daily oral dose of 1.2 mg oestrone sulphate and 0.8 mg oestradiol sulphate, administered during 4 weeks, has no significant effect on serum prolactin levels (Robyn *et al.*, 1978). Similarly, a daily oral dose of 6 mg oestriol administered during 4 weeks is also ineffective on serum prolactin levels (L'Hermite *et al.*, 1979). The daily oral dose of ethinyloestradiol inducing a significant increase of serum prolactin levels is larger in pre-menopausal than in postmenopausal women (Robyn *et al.*, 1978); during 21 days of treatment with 50 μg in pre-menopausal women, serum prolactin levels remained within the values obtained during a control cycle investigated in the same women. In premenopausal women, a significant increase of serum prolactin was reported with daily oral doses of 100 μg or more (Reymond and Lemarchand–Beraud, 1976).

It has been reported recently that progesterone exerts an inhibitory influence on prolactin secretion, at least when prolactin secretion is stimulated by oestrogens (Libertum *et al.*, 1979). Cramer *et al.* (1979) have shown that the administration of large doses of progesterone to rats results in an increase of the dopamine content of the portal blood. During the menstrual cycle in the Mangabey monkey, serum prolactin levels increase within 48 h after the oestradiol peak (Aidara *et al.*, 1978). Thereafter, they decline during the luteal phase, when progesterone levels are high. But at the end of the cycle they rise again, when the progesterone peak is over (Aidara *et al.*, 1978). Progestogens such as chlormadinone, norgestrel and norethisterone acetate were reported to have no significant effect on prolactin secretion in women (Robyn *et al.*, 1978).

It has been shown very recently that decidual cells of the human endometrium containing immunoreactive prolactin (Mena and Grosvenor, 1980); prolactin is present in these cells when decidualization is the consequence of an intra- or extrauterine pregnancy or that of a prolonged treatment with a progestogen such as lynoestrenol (Orgametril®, Organon®). Furthermore, decidualized endometrium produces prolactin during *in vitro* incubation (Golander *et al.*, 1978; Riddick *et al.*, 1978). Further studies are required to elucidate the mechanism of the induction of prolactin synthesis in the endometrium and to understand its possible role during implantation and in the transfer of prolactin into the amniotic fluid during pregnancy.

THE EFFECTS OF PROLACTIN ON THE OVARY

Prolactin interferes with follicular maturation and ovulation. Hyperprolactinaemia is associated with disorders of the menstrual cycle: amenorrhoea, anovulatory cycles, cycles with short luteal phase. Such disorders occur whatever the cause of the hyperprolactinaemia may be: lactation, a pituitary adenoma secreting prolactin, treatment with a dopamine antagonist, etc. (Robyn *et al.*, 1980).

Ovarian follicles of similar size contain less granulosa cells when collected from hyperprolactinaemic women than from normoprolactinaemic women (Mc Natty, personal communication). However, such an alteration in follicular growth is not due to a direct effect of prolactin on the ovary. Major effects of prolactin excess seem to be exerted at the hypothalamic level. Prolactin increases dopamine turnover in the tubero-infundibular neurons and the concentration of dopamine in portal blood (Gudelsky and Porter, 1980). This is a short feedback mechanism by which prolactin inhibits its own secretion (Advis *et al.*, 1977; Fuxe *et al.*, 1978). For various reasons, in hyperprolactinaemic states, prolactin's self-control over its own secretion does not function, although the increased dopamine turnover can be shown. In pathological hyperprolactinaemia associated with amenorrhoea, the pulsatile release of LH, and thus likely that of LH–RH, is suppressed or even completely abolished (Bohnet and Schneider, 1977). Similar alterations of the pulsatile release of LH have also been reported in lactational hyperprolactinaemia (Wright *et al.*, 1980). In the case of the pituitary stalk section in the Rhesus monkey, hyperprolactinaemia and amenorrhoea prevail (Knobil, 1980). The pulsatile release of LH is abolished. When LH–RH is injected i.v. at regular intervals, follicular growth recurs normally; ovulation takes place again with normal corpus luteum activity (Knobil, 1980). Similarly, in the case of amenorrhoea due to hyperprolactinaemia, i.v. injections of LH–RH at 90 min intervals for several days restore follicular growth and ovulation (Leyendecker *et al.*, 1979). Dopamine stimulates the degradation of LH–RH by rat synaptosomes (Marcano De Cotte *et al.*, 1980). The mechanism seems to be physiological and calcium dependent, it requires the structural integrity of the nerve endings and fluctuates with the reproductive state of the animal. Thus, it appears from all these data that the major effect of pro-lactin excess is the suppression of the pulsatile release of LH-RH, probably a con-sequence of the increased dopamine turnover in the median eminence. When the alteration of the pulsatile release is only partial, some follicular growth may persist, luteinization may still occur but the cycles may be impaired: short luteal phase and poor progesterone secretion (Robyn *et al.*, 1976).

This is apparent in types of hyperprolactinaemia: pathological (L'Hermite *et al.*, 1978), lactational (Delvoye *et al.*, 1980) and pharmacological (Robyn *et al.*, 1976, 1977; L'Hermite *et al.*, 1978). Prolactin may also exert direct effects at the ovarian level as was initially suggested. This concept was based on the observation that in hyperprolactinaemic women, the ovaries were much more sensitive to gon-adotropins after initiation of bromocriptine therapy than before treatment (Besser and Thorner, 1975). However, it should be remembered that bromocriptine therapy quite rapidly results in normalizing serum prolactin levels and restoration of follicular growth is immediate. Thus, the ovaries become obviously more sensitive to gonad-otropins. However, it is well established that in cases of anovulation, ovarian sen-sitivity to gonadotropins is no different in hyperprolactinaemic than in normopro-lactinaemic women (Kemmann *et al.*, 1977). Aono *et al.* (1978) reported no inhibition by sulpiride hyperprolactinaemia of the ovarian response to exogenous gonadotropins. The only demonstration of a direct effect of prolactin on the ovary has been reported by McNatty *et al.* (1974, 1977). When granulosa cells from human Graafian follicles are incubated with physiological concentration of prolactin, they produce optimal amounts of progesterone. When they are incubated with increasing concentrations of prolactin, above this limit, they produce decrea-sing amounts of progesterone. These data cannot be extrapolated to the produc-tion of oestrogens by the growing follicles under the influence of prolactin excess. However, such abusive interpretation of McNatty's data has often been used to support the concept that prolactin exerts direct effects on the growing follicles. Using immunohistochemical techniques, Nolin (1978) has indicated the presence of prolactin in luteal cells and in dietyate oöcytes of primordial and maturing ovarian follicles in the rat. Hamada *et al.* (1980) recently showed that high levels of prolactin inhibit ovulation by using the *in vitro* perfused rabbit ovary pre-paration.

REFERENCES

Advis, J. P., Hall, T. R., Hodson, C. A., Mueller, G. P. and Meites, J. (1977). *Proceedings of the Society of Experimental Biology and Medicine* **155**, 567.

Aidara, D., Tahiri, Z. and Robyn, C. (1978). *In* "60th Annual Meeting of the Endocrine Society, Endocrinology Suppl. to Vol. 102, p.350." Abstract No. 550.

Aono, T., Yasuda, M., Shioji, K., Kondo, K. and Kurachi, K. (1978). *Acta Endo-crinologica.* **89**, 142.

Besser, G. M. and Thorner, M. O. (1975). *Pathologie Biologie* **23**, 779.

Bohnet, H. G. and Schneider, H. P. G. (1977). *In* "Prolactin and human repro-duction" (P. G. Crosignani and C. Robyn, Eds), 153–159. Academic Press, London and New York.

Caron, M. G., Beaulieu, M., Raymond, V., Gagne, B., Drouin, J., Lefkowitz, R. J. and Labrie, F. (1978). *Journal of Biology and Chemistry* **253**, 2244.

Cramer, O. M., Parket, C. R. and Porter, J. C. (1979). *Endocrinology* **105**, 929.

Delvoye, P., Delogne-Desnoeck, J. and Robyn, C. (1980). *Clinical Endocrinology* (in press).

Dufy, B., Vincent, J. D., Fleury, H., Du Pasquier, P., Gourdji, D. and Tixier-Vidal, A. (1979a). *Science* **204**, 509.

Dufy, B., Vincent, J. D., Fleury, H., Du Pasquier, P. and Gourdji, D. (1979b). *Nature* **282**, 855.

El Etreby, M. F. and Fath El Bab, M. R. (1977). *Histochemistry* **53**, 1.

Frantz, A. G., Habif, D. V., Hyman, G. A., Shu, H. K., Sassin, J. F., Zimmerman, E. A., Noel, G. L. and Kleinberg, D. L. (1973). *In* "International Symposium on human prolactin" (J. P. Pasteels and C. Robyn, Eds), 120–135. Excerpta Medica, Amsterdam.

Fuxe, K., Andersson, K., Hökfelt, T., Agnati, L. E., Ögren, S. O., Eneroth, P., Gustafsson, J. A. and Skett, P. (1978). *In* "Progress in prolactin physiology and pathology" (C. Robyn and M. Harter, Eds) 95–109. Elsevier/North Holland, Biomedical Press, Amsterdam.

Golander, A., Hurlet, T., Barrett, J., Hizi, A. and Handwerger, S. (1978). *Science* **202**, 311.

Gudelsky, G. A. and Porter, J. C. (1980). *Endocrinology* **106**, 526.

Hamada, Y., Schlaff, S., Kobayashi, Y., Santulli, R., Wright, K. H. and Wallach, E. E. (1980). *Mature* **285**, 161.

Ingleton, P. M., Batten, T. F. C. and Ball, J. N. (1977). *Journal of Endocrinology* **73**, 9P.

Jacobi, J., Lloyd, H. M. and Meares, J. D. (1977). *Journal of Endocrinology* **72**, 35.

Kemmann, E., Gemzell, C. A., Beinert, W. C., Beling, C. B. and Jones, J. R. (1977) *American Journal of Obstetrics and Genecology* **129**, 145.

Kizer, J. S., Arimura, A., Schally, A. V. and Brownstein, M. J. (1975). *Endocrinology* **96**, 523.

Knobil, E. (1980). *Recent Progress Hormone Research* (in press).

Labrie, F., Beaulieu, M., Caron, M. G. and Raymond, V. (1978). *In* "Progress in prolactin physiology and pathology" (C. Robyn and M. Harter, Eds) 121–136. Elsevier/North Holland, Biomedical Press, Amsterdam.

Leyendecker, G., Struve, T. and Plotz, E. J. (1979). *In* "61th Annual Meeting of the Endocrine Society" Abstract No. 926.

L'Hermite, M., Caufriez, A., Badawi, M., Sugar, J., Schwers, J., Robyn, C., Cordova, T., Ayalon, D., Legros, J. J. and Stevenaert, A. (1978). *In* "Progress in prolactin physiology and pathology" (C. Robyn and M. Harter, Eds) 398–414. Elsevier/North Holland, Biomedical Press, Amsterdam.

L'Hermite, M., Badawi, M., Michaux-Duchene, A. and Robyn, C. (1979). *Clinical Endocrinology* **11**, 173.

Libertum, C., Kaplan, S. E. and De Nicola, A. F. (1979). *Neuroendocrinology* **28**, 64.

Marcano De Cotte, D., De Menezes, C. E. L., Bennett, G. W. and Edwardson, J. A. (1980). *Nature* **283**, 487.

Mc Leod, R. M. and Robyn, C. (1977). *Journal of Endocrinology* **72**, 273.

Mc Leod, R. M. and Lamberts, S. W. J. (1978). *Endocrinology* **103**, 200.

Mc Leod, R. M. and Lamberts, S. W. J. (1978). *In* "Progress in prolactin physiology and pathology" (C. Robyn and M. Harter, Eds) 111–119. Elsevier/North Holland, Biomedical Press, Amsterdam.

Mc Natty, K. P., Sawers, R. S. and Mc Neilly, A. S. (1974). *Nature* **250**, 653.

Mc Natty, K. P., Mc Neilly, A. S. and Sawers, R. S. (1977). *In* "Prolactin and human reproduction" (P. G. Crosignani and C. Robyn, Eds), 109–118. Academic Press, London and New York.

Mena, F. and Grosvenor, C. E. (1980). *In* "Sixth International Congress of Endocrinology". Abstract No. S34.

Nolin, J. (1978). *Endocrinology* **102**, 402.

Reymond, M. and Lemarchand-Beraud, T. (1976). *Clinical Endocrinology* **5**, 429.

Riddick, D. H., Luciano, A. A., Kusmik, W. E. and Maslar, I. A. (1978). *Life Science* **23**, 1913.

Rigg, L. A., Lein, A. and Yen, S. S. C. (1977). *American Journal of Obstetrics and Gynecology* **129**, 454.

Robyn, C., Vekemans, M., Caufriez, A. and L'Hermite, M. (1976). *IRCS, Medical Science* **4**, 14.

Robyn, C., Delvoye, P., Van Exter, C., Vekemans, M., Caufriez, A., Denayer, P., Delogne-Desnoeck, J. and L'Hermite, M. (1977). *In* "Prolactin and human reproduction" (P. G. Crosignani and C. Robyn, Eds), 71–96. Academic Press, London and New York.

Robyn, C., Vekemans, M., Delvoye, P. and L'Hermite, M. (1978). *In* "International Symposium on Hormonal Contraception" (A. A. Haspels and C. R. Kay, Eds), 98–125. Excerpta Medica, Amsterdam and Oxford.

Robyn, C., Delvoye, P., Meuris, S., Vekemans, M., Caufriez, A. and L'Hermite, M. (1980). *In* "International Congress of Endocrinology, Melbourne" (in press).

Schaeffer, J. M. and Hsueh, J. W. (1979). *Journal of Biology and Chemistry* **254**, 5606.

Schally, A. V., Arimura, A. and Kastin, A. J. (1973). *Science* **179**, 341.

Tixier-Vidal, A., Brunet, N. and Gourdji, D. (1978). *In* "Progress in prolactin physiology and pathology" (C. Robyn and M. Harter, Eds) 29–43. Elsevier/North Holland, Biomedical Press, Amsterdam.

Vekemans, M. and Robyn, C. (1975). *British Medical Journal* **4**, 738.

Vekemans, M., Delvoye, P., L'Hermite, M. and Robyn, C. (1977). *Journal of Clinical Endocrinology and Metabolisim* **44**, 989.

Wright, P. J., Geytenbeek, P. E., Clarke, I. J. and Findlay, J. K. (1980). *In* "Sixth International Congress of Endocrinology". Abstract No. 884.

β-LIPOTROPIN (βLPH) and β-ENDORPHIN (βEP) IN FERTILE AND POSTMENOPAUSAL WOMEN

A. R. Genazzani[1], F. Facchinetti[1], S. Danero[2], D. Parrini[2], F. Petraglia[1] and N. D'Antona[2]

[1] *Cattedra di Patologia Ostetrica e Ginecologica, University of Siena, Italy.*
[2] *Clinica Ostetrica e Ginecologica, University of Siena, Italy*

INTRODUCTION

It has been clearly established for some years that some pituitary hormones present different plasma concentrations during the various periods of life in the human female. In particular, LH and FSH plasma levels, which are very low during prepuberty (Janner *et al.*, 1972), increase during pubertal development and reach adult values at the end of sexual maturation (Genazzani *et al.*, 1978). Furthermore, the cyclic changes in gonadotropin plasma levels which characterize the menstrual cycle (Apter *et al.*, 1978) also start during the same period. FSH and LH levels increase at the end of the fertile period, and reach the highest concentrations after the menopause (Wide *et al.*, 1973).

Plasma prolactin (PRL) levels increase slightly during pubertal development to reach adult levels during the reproductive period (Aubert *et al.*, 1977). After the menopause they show a decline, and this pattern has been shown to be closely related to the concomitant fall in plasma oestrogens (Robyn *et al.*, 1977). ACTH plasma concentrations have been found to be constant from early infancy until old age, as are plasma cortisol (F) levels (Jensen and Blichert-Toft, 1971). The recent discovery in anterior pituitary cells of a 31 000 dalton (31K) common precursor molecule for ACTH and β-lipotropin (βLPH) (Mains *et al.*, 1977), and

Serono Symposium No. 39, "The Menopause: Clinical, Endocrinological and Pathophysiological Aspects", edited by P. Fioretti, L. Martini, G. B. Melis and S. S. C. Yen, 1982. Academic Press, London and New York.

the observations suggesting the ACTH and βLPH or its derivative β-endorphin (βEP; βLPH 61–91) are secreted concomitantly (Guillemin *et al.*, 1977; Nakao *et al.*, 1978; Krieger *et al.*, 1979), seem to indicate that plasma ACTH and resting basal opioid levels may present a similar pattern throughout life. The present paper describes the behaviour pattern of plasma βLPH and βEP levels in healthy females from 17 to 87 years of age, in comparison with those of ACTH and other pituitary (LH, FSH), ovarian (oestradiol-E$_2$) and adrenal (cortisol-F, dehydroepiandrosterone sulphate – DHAS) hormones measured in the same samples.

MATERIALS AND METHODS

Subjects

One hundred healthy women between 17 and 87 years of age, 41 of them with regular menstruation (17–45 year age group; at day 4–8 of the menstrual cycle) and 59 postmenopausal subjects (46–87 year age group) were examined. After overnight fasting, a blood sample was collected from each subject at 9 a.m. in a cold syringe with 5000 KIU Trasylol (Bayer, Basel, CH) and heparin. The samples were rapidly centrifuged and the plasma stored at $-70°$C until time of assays. No sample was defrosted more than once.

Assays

ACTH, LH, FSH and F plasma levels were measured by radioimmunoassay (RIA) using commercially available kits (ACTH and F: CIS, Saluggia, Vercelli; LH and FSH: Biodata, Rome, Italy). DHAS was measured directly in diluted plasma by RIA using an antiserum purchased from Dr G. Abraham (Rolling Hills, Ca, USA). E$_2$ RIA was performed after plasma extraction with ethyl–ether (1 : 10); the rabbit antiserum was supplied by CIS, tritiated molecules from NEN (Boston, Mass, USA) and standard hormones from Vister (Milan, Italy: E$_2$) or Merck (Darmstadt, Germany: DHAS).

The steroid RIAs were characterized by overnight incubation at $4°$C and dextran-coated charcoal separation (Facchinetti and Genazzani, 1978). βLPH and βEP were extracted from 2.5 ml of plasma with 150 mg glass powder (Corning Glass, New York, USA: 100 mesh) on a rotary mixer for 1 h (Facchinetti and Genazzani, 1979). After washing with water (twice) and 1 N HCl (once) the powder was resuspended and extracted twice with 1 ml acetone-1 N HCl (9:1). The extract was dried under nitrogen, dissolved in 0.5 ml acetic acid 0.1 M, 0.01% BSA and applied to a Sephadex G-75 column (1.5 x 45 cm) eluted with the same solution. Two different peaks containing respectively βLPH and βEP were collected in accordance with the partition coefficient of cold βLPH and βEP added to a charcoal-treated plasma. The fractions were freeze-dried, redissolved in 0.4 ml of 0.04 M phosphate buffer pH 7.4, and subjected to RIA (Facchinetti and Genazzani, 1979).

The materials employed and the RIA characteristics are reported elsewhere (Facchinetti and Genazzani, 1979). In summary, an 18 h incubation at $4°$C with the antiserum (donated by Dr C. Pert, NIH, Bethesda, Ma, USA, and employed for both βLPH and βEP RIA at the respective dilutions of 1 : 3400 and 1 : 6800) was followed by the addition of I^{125}-labelled peptides (6000 cpm/tube); the reaction was interrupted after 48 h with a goat anti-rabbit gamma globulin serum (1 : 10). Sensitivity of the RIA was 11 pg for βLPH and 4 pg for βEP.

RESULTS

Gonadotropins and Oestradiol

LH and FSH plasma levels (mU/ml) showed constant values up to 40 years of age (Fig. 1), followed by progressive increases from the 46–50 year old age group onwards (LH: 42.1 ± 10.8; FSH: 46.7 ± 12.0), reaching the highest concentrations at 56–70 years (LH: 70.2 ± 13.6; FSH: 98.0 ± 25.6). LH and FSH plasma levels remained more or less stable up to the 71–80 year old age group (LH: 70.0 ± 26.0; FSH: 100.0 ± 34.1) and then declined in subjects over 80 years of age (LH: 20.4 ± 10.5; FSH: 44.8 ± 20.2).

E_2 plasma levels (pg/ml) showed the highest concentrations in the 17–30 year old age group (135.1 ± 13.0). During the fertile period, the concentrations of this hormone declined slightly and at 46–50 years (93.4 ± 11) they were significantly lower than at 17–30 years ($P < 0.05$). E_2 plasma concentrations continued to decrease with age, reaching the lowest levels after 60 years (61–65 year old age group: 48.0 ± 6.7; $P < 0.01$ in comparison with the 46–50 year old age group). No further changes occurred in late menopause and in elderly subjects.

ACTH and Cortisol (F)

ACTH plasma levels (pg/ml) failed to show any significant differences from 17 to 70 years (Fig. 2); the different groups of pre- and postmenopausal subjects showed average ACTH values (± SE) varying from 75.1 ± 12.0 at 17–30 years, to 112.6 ± 21.4 at 61–65 years. ACTH concentrations were only found to be significantly lower (35.1 ± 7.0) in the over 81 year olds compared to the levels found in the 61–65 and 17–30 year old age groups. F concentrations did not present any statistically significant changes throughout life; they varied randomly between a maximum of 142.5 ± 18.1 ng/ml at 41–45 years, and a minimum of 89.5 ± 16.6 ng/ml at 56–60 years.

βLPH and βEP

Plasma levels of the two opioids were characterized by significant changes between the various age groups (Fig. 3). βLPH (pg/ml) increased significantly from the 17–30 year old age group (114.9 ± 10.6) to the 41–45 year old age group (143.7 ± 10.6; $P < 0.02$), and subsequently decreased significantly in the 46–50 year old age group (110.8 ± 11.4; $P < 0.05$) and remained more or less stable until old age. Significantly higher concentrations were found in subjects over 80 years of age (168.7 ± 28.5).

βEP plasma levels (pg/ml) showed a similar pattern to that of βLPH, but with more significant differences between the various groups. They increased from the

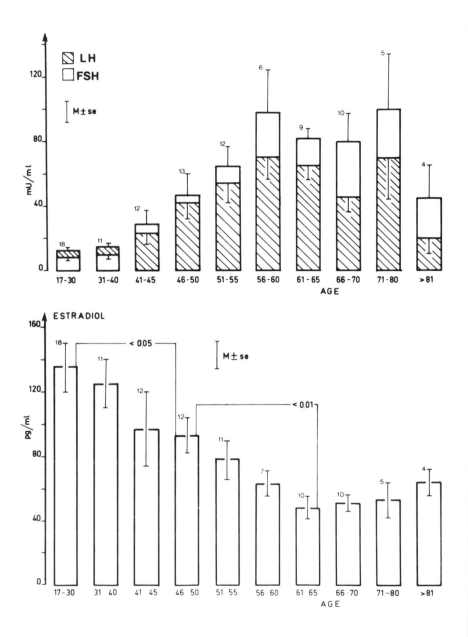

Fig. 1. Plasma concentrations (M ± SE) of LH (closed bars) and FSH (open bars; upper part), and Oestradiol (lower part) in the different age groups. The statistical analysis is reported.

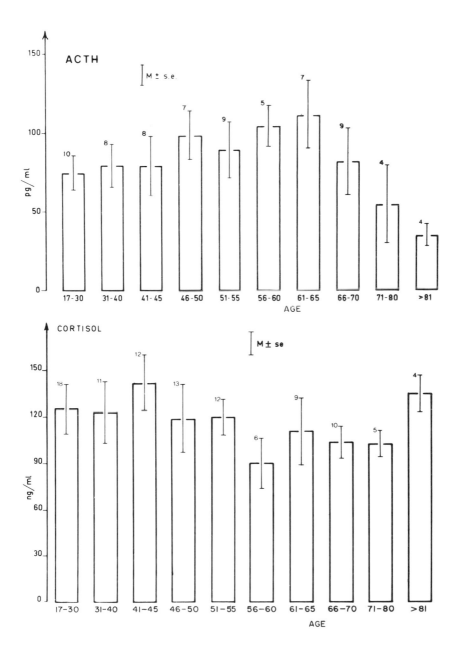

Fig. 2. Plasma concentrations (M ± SD) of ACTH and Cortisol in the different age groups. The statistical analysis is reported.

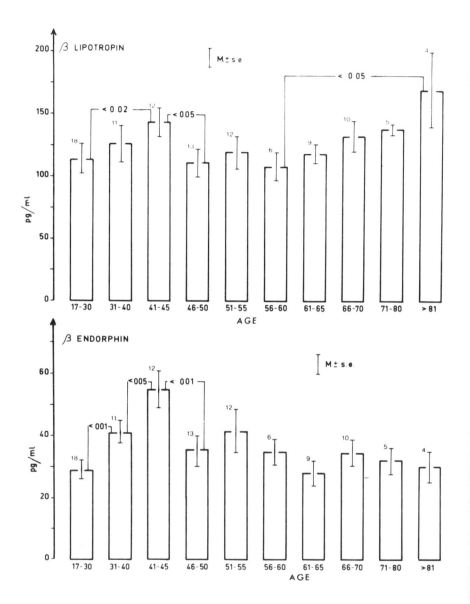

Fig. 3. Plasma concentrations (M ± SE) of β-lipotropin and β-endorphin in the different age groups. The statistical analysis is reported.

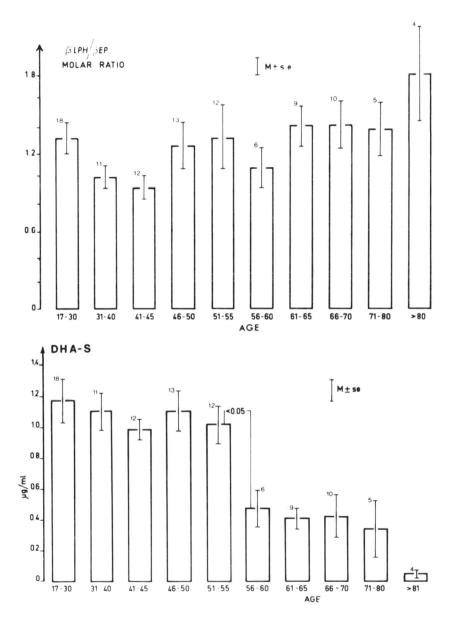

Fig. 4. βLPH/βEP molar ratio and DHA-S plasma levels in the different age groups. The statistical analysis is reported.

17-30 year old age group (24.2 ± 3.1) to the 31-40 year old age group (41.2 ± 3.0; $P < 0.01$), reaching the highest levels in the 41-45 year old age group (54.7 ± ± 0.6; $P < 0.05$). The βEP concentrations in the 46-50 year old age group were found to be significantly lower (35.3 ± 5.5; $P < 0.001$) and remained at more or less constant levels until old age.

βLPH/βEP molar ratio and DHA-S

The βLPH/βEP ratio of molar concentrations (MR) ranged as mean values from 0.93 ± 0.09 (41-45 years) to 2.43 ± 0.61 (81-87 years), but no significant differences were found between the different groups (Fig. 4). DHA-S plasma levels (μg/ml) were stable in the fertile and early menopausal period (1.18 ± 0.12 at 17-30 years; 1.01 ± 0.12 at 51-55 years). They then decreased from the 56-60 year old age group (0.47 ± 0.12) to the elderly, where the lowest values were found in the over 80 year olds (0.048 ± 0.018 μg/ml; $P < 0.01$ in comparison with the 56-60 year old age group).

DISCUSSION

The behaviour patterns of plasma gonadotropins and E_2 confirm those previously reported by other authors (Longcope, 1971; Wide et al., 1973). Similarly, in accordance with the observation of Jensen and Blichert-Toft (1971), ACTH plasma levels remain stable until old age, and this pattern is also confirmed by the analogous trend of F concentrations.

The finding of a significant decrease in plasma DHA-S after 55 years of age, confirms previous observations (Milewich et al., 1978) and indicates that after the menopause, as in the period prior to and during puberty (Genazzani et al., 1978), there is a dissociation between plasma glucocorticoids and Δ_5 adrenal androgen levels. The observation that plasma ACTH does not evidence similar changes during pubertal developments has led several authors (Parker and Odell, 1977; Grumbach et al., 1978) and ourselves (Genazzani et al., 1978) to hypothesize the existence of other factor(s) responsible for the development of adrenal androgen-secreting cells. However, ACTH remains the hormone responsible for the secretory activity of these cells (Genazzani et al., 1979). Thus, the decrease in DHA-S in climacteric females could possibly be explained by a concomitant reduction in the so-called adrenal androgen stimulating hormone (AASH) (Parker and Odell, 1977; Grumbach et al., 1978; Genazzani et al., 1979). The striking finding of this study is the progressive and significant increase of βLPH and βEP plasma levels throughout fertile life, followed by a sudden drop after menopause to levels which are similar to those observed in 17-30 year old subjects. These data therefore clearly demonstrate the existence of a dissociation between basal ACTH and opioid plasma levels.

Previous reports showing a concomitant, dynamic secretion of both opioids and ACTH in response to stressing stimuli or pharmacological treatments (Guillemin et al., 1977; Nakao et al., 1978; Krieger et al., 1979) are not contradictory to our observations, since our data indicate that resting levels of the three peptides do not present parallel changes throughout life.

The reduction in βEP levels after 45 years of age is more pronounced than that of βLPH, and this observation is supported by evidence of the existence of a highly significant negative correlation between plasma βEP concentrations and age, while βLPH does not present any correlation of this type (Fig. 5). A significant negative correlation was observed in the same patients, however, between DHA-S and age (Fig. 5). The homogeneous pattern of βEP and DHA-S plasma levels is also confirmed by the positive correlation (< 0.001) between the two hormones in subjects over 40 years of age (Fig. 6).

It remains to be clarified whether the decrease in plasma opioid levels after the menopause, and in particular the reduction in βEP, are due to changes in their MCRs (Foley *et al.*, 1979) or in the enzymes responsible for the breakdown of proopiocortin (Graf *et al.*, 1977). Moreover, one may also take into account the hypothesis of the disappearance of the contribution from sources other than the anterior pituitary, in maintaining the circulating opioid pool (Bruni *et al.*, 1979).

In conclusion, the present study indicating a decrease in circulating opioid levels in the menopausal period, may offer a biochemical basis to explain the change in mood and in responsiveness to nociceptive stimuli typical of climateric females.

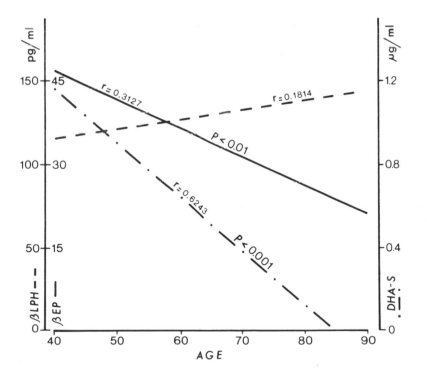

Fig. 5. Regression line (calculated by the least squares' method) between β-lipotropin (- - -), β-endorphin (—) and dehydroepiandrosterone sulphate (-·-·-) with age. Correlation coefficients are reported.

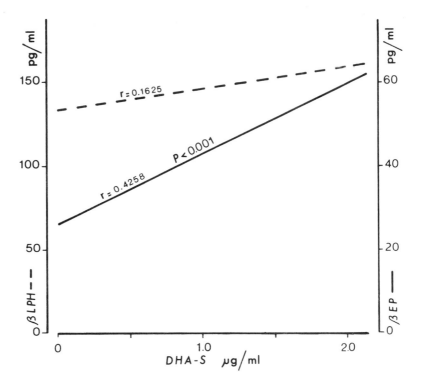

Fig. 6.   Regression line between plasma concentrations of βLPH and βEP with those of DHA-S in subjects over 40 years of age. Correlation coefficients are reported.

ACKNOWLEDGEMENT

This work was partially supported by the CNR project "Biology of Repro-duction".

REFERENCES

Apter, D., Wiinikka, L. and Wihko, R. (1978). *Journal of Clinical Endocrinology and Metabolism* **47**, 944–954.
Aubert, M. L., Sizonenko, P. C., Kaplan, S. L. and Grumbach, M. M. (1977). *In* "Prolactin and Human Reproduction" (P. G. Crosignani and C. Robyn, Eds) pp. 5–19. Serono Symposia, Academic Press, London.
Bruni, J. F., Watkins, W. B. and Yen, S. S. C. (1979). *Journal of Endocrinology and Metabolism* **49**, 649–650.
Facchinetti, F. and Genazzani, A. R. (1978). *Journal Nuclear Medicine and Allied Science* **22**, 61–66.
Facchinetti, F. and Genazzani, A. R. (1979). *In* "Radioimmunoassay of Drugs and Hormones in Cardiovascular Medicine" (A. Albertini, M. Da Prada and B. A. Peskar, Eds), pp. 347–353. Elsevier/North-Holland, Biomedical Press, Amsterdam.
Foley, K. M., Kourides, I. A., Inturrisi, C. E., Kaiko, R. G., Zaroulis, C. G., Posner,

J. B., Houde, R. W. and Li, C. H. (1979). *Proceedings of the National Academy of Sciences of the USA* **78**, 5377–5381

Genazzani, A. R., Pintor, C., Facchinetti, F., Carboni, G., Pelosi, U. and Corda, R. (1978). *Clinical Endocrinology* **8**, 15–25.

Genazzani, A. R., Pintor, C., Facchinetti, F., Inaudi, P., Maci, D. and Corda, R. (1979). *Journal of Steroid Biochemistry* **11**, 571–577.

Graf, L., Kenessey, A., Berzetei, I. and Ronai, A. Z. (1977). *Biochemical and Biophysical Research Communications* **78**, 111–114.

Grumbach, M. M., Richards, G. E., Conte, F. A. and Kaplan, S. (1978). *In* "The Endocrine Function of the Human Adrenal Gland" (V. H. T. James, M. Serio, G. Giusti and L. Martini, Eds), pp. 583–611. Academic Press, London.

Guillemin, R., Vargo, T., Rossier, J., Minick, S., Ling, N., Rivier, C., Vale, W. and Bloom, F. (1977). *Science* **197**, 1367–1369.

Janner, M. R., Kelch, R. P., Kaplan, S. L. and Grumbach, M. M. (1972). *Journal of Clinical Endocrinology and Metabolism* **34**, 521–530.

Jensen, H. K. and Blichert-Toft, M. (1971). *Acta Endocrinologica* **66**, 25.

Krieger, D. T., Liotta, A., Suda, T., Goodgold, A. N. and Condon, E. (1979) *Journal of Clinical Endocrinology and Metabolism* **48**, 566–571.

Longcope, C. (1971). *American Journal of Obstetrics and Gynecology* **111**, 778–782.

Mains, R. E., Eipper, B. A. and Ling, N. (1977). *Proceeding of the National Academy of Science of USA* **74**, 3014–3018.

Milewich, L., Gomez-Sanchez, C., Madden, J. D., Bradfield, D. J., Parker, P. M., Smith, S. L., Carr, B. R., Edman, C. D. and MacDonald, P. C. (1978). *Journal of Steroids Biochemistry* **9**, 1159–1164.

Nakao, K., Nakai, Y., Oki, S., Horii, K. and Imura, H. (1978). *Journal of Clinical Investigation* **62**, 1395–1398.

Parker, L. and Odell, W. D. (1977). *Clinical Research* **25**, 299–303.

Robyn, C., Delvoie, P., Van Exter, C., Vekemans, M., Laufriez, A., Denayer, P., Delogne-Desndeck, S., and L'Hermite, M. (1977). *In* "Prolactin and Human Reproduction" (P. G. Crosignani and C. Robyn, Eds), pp. 71–96. Serono Symposia, Academic Press, London.

Wide, L., Nillius, S. J., Gemzell, C. and Roos, P. (1973). *Acta Endocrinologica* **174**, suppl. 1.

OPPOSITE EFFECT OF METHYLDOPA AND BROMOCRIPTINE ON PROGESTERONE INDUCED LH AND PRL RELEASE IN POSTMENOPAUSAL WOMEN

I. Nicoletti[1], P. Filipponi[1], L. Fedeli[3], L. Lentini[1], P. A. Santori[1], F. Santeusanio[1] and P. Brunetti[2]

Institutes of Clinical Medicine[1] and Medical Pathology[2], Centre of Nuclear Medicine[3], Perugia University School of Medicine, Perugia, Italy

INTRODUCTION

The concept that catecholamines are involved in the release of pituitary gonadotropins was proposed more than 30 years ago (Sawyer *et al.*, 1947) but the stimulatory or inhibitory role of catecholaminergic mechanisms in the control of LH secretion has yet to be established in either man or the laboratory animal. In normal cycling and hypogonadal women dopamine administration induces a significance reduction of LH and PRL plasma levels (Leblanc *et al.*, 1976; Lachelin *et al.*, 1977; Judd *et al.*, 1978). In animal models, while norepinephrine seems to have a stimulatory effect (Sawyer, 1975), dopamine may have stimulatory (Schneider and McCann, 1970; Kamberi *et al.*, 1970; Rotszejn *et al.*, 1977) or inhibitory (Fuxe *et al.*, 1976; Drouva and Gallo, 1977) effects on gonadotropin release.

It is known that progesterone administration elicits an LH surge in oestrogen primed postmenopausal or ovariectomized women (Odell and Swerdloff, 1968; Nillius and Wide, 1971). The concurrent increase of PRL levels (Rakoff and Yen,

Serono Symposium No. 39, "The Menopause: Clinical, Endocrinological and Pathophysiological Aspects", edited by P. Fioretti, L. Martini, G. B. Melis and S. S. C. Yen, 1982. Academic Press, London and New York.

1978) and experimental evidence of hypothalamic tyrosine-hydroxilase inhibition, in oestrogen primed castrated rats, by progesterone (Beattie and Soyka, 1973), suggested that a fall in hypothalamic dopamine may account for the progesterone induced LH release (Rakoff and Yen, 1978).

Catecholamine depleting drugs, however, block the stimulatory effect of progesterone on gonadotropin release in oestrogen primed castrated rats (Kalra *et al.*, 1972; Kalra and McCann, 1973). These contradictory data have prompted us to investigate the effect of catecholamine depleting (methyldopa) or dopamine agonist (bromocriptine) drugs on LH and PRL response to progesterone in oestrogen primed postmenopausal women.

Table I. Basal hormonal data (mean ± SE) in the three groups of examined women.

	LH mIU/ml	FSH mIU/ml	PRL ng/ml	E_2 pg/ml
Group 1	71.4 ± 6.1	121.9 ± 14.0	6.9 ± 0.8	18.3 ± 3.6
Group 2	78.1 ± 3.2	118.5 ± 17.7	5.0 ± 0.7	21.4 ± 4.3
Group 3	84.1 ± 14.0	108.4 ± 21.9	5.5 ± 0.8	17.9 ± 4.1

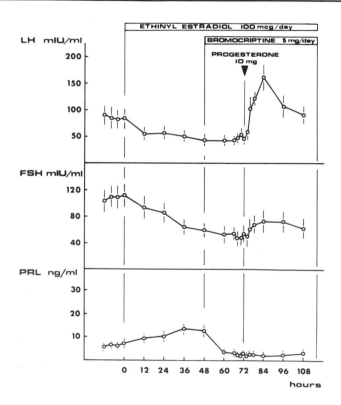

Fig. 1. Concurrent LH and PRL release in response to progesterone in oestrogen primed postmenopausal women (mean ± SE, N = 4).

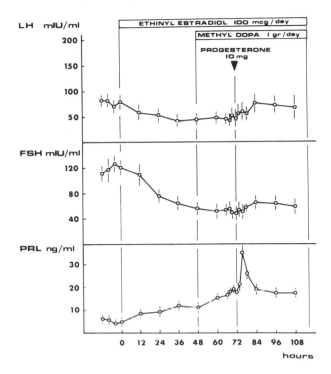

Fig. 2. Effect of methyldopa administration (250 mg/6 h) on progesterone induced LH and PRL release in oestrogen primed postmenopausal women (mean ± SE, N = 4).

MATERIALS AND METHODS

Twelve postmenopausal women (aged 51–68) volunteered for this study. All subjects had not received steroids or any medication for at least one month prior to the initiation of the study, the women, matched for age and body weight, were divided into three groups. All the women received 10 mg of progesterone i.m. after 72 h of oestrogen priming (accomplished by oral administration of ethinyloestradiol in a daily dose of 100 mcg). No other drug was administered to Group 1 women (controls); in Group 2, methyldopa (250 mg/6 h) was administered, starting 24 h before progesterone administration. Group 3 women received bromocriptine (2.5 mg/12 h) starting 24 h before progesterone administration.

In all subjects serum samples were obtained, by i.v. catheter, at 15 min intervals 1 h prior to commencing ethinyloestradiol, at 12 h intervals during oestrogen priming, at 15 min intervals 1 h prior to progesterone administration and 2, 4, 6, 12, 24 and 36 h thereafter. Serum LH (Midgley, 1966), FSH (Midgley, 1967), PRL (Sinha *et al.*, 1973), E_2 (Hotchkiss *et al.*, 1971) and P (Abraham *et al.*, 1972) were determined by radioimmunoassay. Circulating E_2 levels were not measured during the test, since the antibody of our assay does not cross-react with ethinyloestradiol. Statistical analysis was performed by the two-tailed *t*-test.

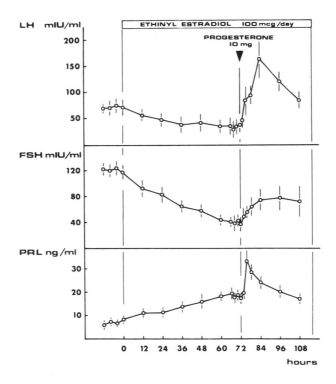

Fig. 3. Effect of bromocriptine (2.5 mg/12 h) on progesterone induced LH and PRL release in oestrogen primed postmenopausal women (mean ± SE, N = 4).

RESULTS

Serum concentrations (mean ± SE) of LH, FSH, PRL and E_2 in the basal state were similar in the three groups (Table I). After 72 h of oestrogen administration, serum levels of LH and FSH were markedly reduced in all three groups ($P < 0.01$); a significant increase of PRL was also observed at 48th hour of oestrogen treatment ($P < 0.01$). The maximal increase in serum progesterone, after administration of 10 mg i.m. ranged in physiological levels and was also similar in the three groups (Group 1: 0.34 ± 0.02 to 3.6 ± 0.9; Group 2: 0.26 ± 0.04 to 3.9 ± 0.5; Group 3: 0.28 ± 0.06 to 3.4 ± 0.3).

Progesterone administration evoked a marked release of LH and PRL in Group 1 women (Fig. 1). In methyldopa treated patients, PRL release was similar to controls but LH output was significantly ($P < 0.01$) reduced (Fig. 2). In Group 3 (bromocriptine treated women), progesterone induced LH surge was unaffected by dopamine agonist, while PRL levels were markedly suppressed ($P < 0.01$; Fig. 3). FSH levels slightly increased after progesterone administration; the smaller increase was observed in methyldopa treated subjects but the difference between groups was not significant.

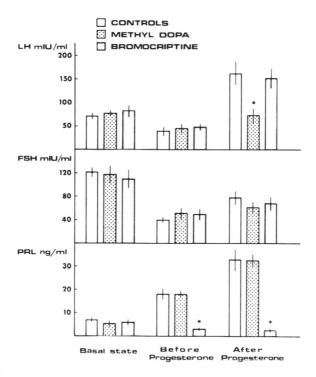

Fig. 4. Comparison of methyldopa and bromocriptine effect on LH, FSH and PRL levels in response to progesterone in oestrogen primed postmenopausal women. The "after progesterone" data refer to the maximal increase of the examined parameters, * P < 0.01.

DISCUSSION

The results of our study indicate that catecholamine depleting and dopamine agonist drugs have a dissociate effect on PRL and LH release in response to progesterone in oestrogen primed postmenopausal women (Fig. 4).

The positive feedback of progesterone on LH and PRL was attributed to a reduction of hypothalamic dopamine (Rakoff and Yen, 1978). Dopamine (Leblanc *et al.*, 1976; Judd *et al.*, 1978, Judd *et al.*, 1979) and dopamine agonists (Lachelin *et al.*, 1977; Travaglini *et al.*, 1979) have been shown to reduce the release of both PRL and LH in humans; the site of the inhibitory effect of dopamine seems to be at hypothalamic GnRH secreting neurons (Lofstrom *et al.*, 1977; Miyachi *et al.*, 1973) for LH release and at pituitary level (McLeod *et al.*, 1969) for PRL.

In our subjects however, bromocriptine administration induced a marked and sustained decrease of PRL levels while LH release in response to progesterone was unaffected. Therefore, since a pharmacological activation of dopamine receptors is not followed by reduction or abolition of progesterone induced LH release, it is unlikely that a fall of dopaminergic hypothalamic activity is responsible for the positive feedback of progesterone on pituitary gonadotropins.

Methyldopa administration was followed by a significant reduction of LH release in response to progesterone in our subjects; it is known that this drug reduces the CNS levels of catecholamines (Sjoerdsma *et al.*, 1963) and inhibits catecholaminergic neurotransmission (Kopin, 1968). If catecholaminergic control of gonadotropin release is mainly inhibitory, through hypothalamic dopamine, (Fuxe *et al.*, 1976; Quigley *et al.*, 1979) the administration of catecholamine depleting drugs should be followed by an evident release of LH and FSH; the absence of LH or FSH increase during methyldopa administration and the significant reduction of LH release in response to progesterone, as observed in our study, seem to indicate that catecholaminergic neurons are involved in progesterone positive feedback in oestrogen primed postmenopausal women.

Although contradictory data still exist, there is evidence that noradrenergic neurons stimulate GnRH release in the rat (Rubinstein and Sawyer 1970; Sawyer, 1975; McCann and Moss, 1975). Adrenergic blockers and catecholamine synthesis inhibiting drugs clearly lower LH in castrated animals (Ojeda and McCann, 1973). Furthermore, α-blocking drugs or selective destruction of catecholaminergic neurons by 6-OH-dopamine, have a blocking effect on progesterone induced gonadotropin release in ovariectomized rats (McCann, 1974).

Our observations suggest that, despite the inhibitory effect of pharmacological doses, endogenous dopamine is not a tonic inhibitor of LH release. The positive feedback of progesterone on gonadotropin release seems, therefore, to be mediated through an activation of catecholaminergic neurons, rather than through a reduction of hypothalamic dopamine in oestrogen primed postmenopausal women.

ACKNOWLEDGEMENTS

The authors express their gratitude to Mr Fausto Taragnoloni and to Mr Alvaro Cini for their excellent technical assistance. This study was supported by Italian CNR grant No. 78.02009.04.

REFERENCES

Abraham, G. E., Swerdloff, R., Tulchinsy, D. and Odell, W. D. (1972). *Journal of Clinical Endocrinology and Metabolism* 35, 458.
Beattie, C. W. and Soyka, L. F. (1973). *Endocrinology* 93, 1453.
Drouva, S. V. and Gallo, R. (1977). *Endocrinology* 100, 792.
Fuxe, K., Hokfelt, T., Agnati, L., Lofstrom, A., Everitt, B. J., Johansson, O., Jonsson, G., Wuttke, W. and Goldstein, M. (1976). *In* "Neuroendocrine regulation of fertility" (Anand-Kumar, Ed.) 124–140. Karger, Basel.
Hotchkiss, J., Atkinson, L. E. and Knobil, E. (1971). *Endocrinology* 89, 177.
Judd, S. J., Rakoff, J. S. and Yen, S. S. C. (1978). *Journal of Clinical Endocrinology and Metabolism* 47, 494.
Judd, S. J., Rigg, L. A. and Yen, S. S. C. (1979). *Journal of Clinical Endocrinology and Metabolism* 49, 182.

Kalra, P. S. and McCann, S. M. (1973). *Progress in Brain Research* **39**, 185.
Kalra, P. S., Kalra, S. P., Krulich, L., Fawcett, C. P. and McCann, S. M. (1972). *Endocrinology* **90**, 1168.
Kamberi, I. A., Mical, R. S. and Porter, J. C. (1970). *Endocrinology* **88**, 1003.
Kopin, I. J. (1968). *Annual Review of Pharmacology* **8**, 377.
Lachelin, G. C. L., Leblanc, H. and Yen, S. S. C. (1977). *Journal of Clinical Endocrinology and Metabolism* **44**, 728.
Leblanc, H., Lachelin, G. C. L., Abu Fadil, S. and Yen S. S. C. (1976). *Journal of Clinical Endocrinology and Metabolism* **43**, 668.
Lofstrom, A., Eneroth, P., Gustafsson, J. A. and Skett, P. (1977). *Endocrinology* **101**, 1559.
McCann, S. M. (1974) *In* "Handbook of Physiology" Section 7, "Endocrinology" Vol. 4. "The pituitary gland", Part 2 (E. Knobil and W. H. Sawyer, Eds) 489–517. American Physiology Society, Washington.
McCann, S. M. and Moss, R. L. (1975). *Life Science* **16**, 833.
McLeod, R. M., Abad, A. and Eidson, L. L. (1969). *Endocrinology* **84**, 1475.
Midgley, A. R. Jr (1966). *Endocrinology* **79**, 10.
Midgley, A. R. Jr (1967). *Journal of Clinical Endocrinology and Metabolism* **27**, 295.
Miyachi, Y., Mecklenburg, R. S. and Lipsett, M. B. (1973). *Endocrinology* **93**, 492.
Nillius, S. J. and Wide, L. (1971). *Acta Endocrinologica (Kbh).* **67**, 362.
Odell, W. D. and Swerdloff, S. R. (1968). *Proceeding of National Academic of Science* **61**, 529.
Ojeda, S. E. and McCann, S. M. (1973). *Neuroendocrinology* **12**, 295.
Quigley, M. E., Judd, S. J., Gilliand, G. B. and Yen, S. S. C. (1979). *Journal of Clinical Endocrinology and Metabolism* **48**, 718.
Rakoff, J. S. and Yen, S. S. C. (1978). *Journal of Clinical Endocrinology and Metabolism* **47**, 918.
Rotsztejn, W. H., Charli, J. L., Pattou, E. and Kordon, C. (1977). *Endocrinology* **101**, 1475.
Rubinstein, L. and Sawyer, C. M. (1970). *Endocrinology* **86**, 998.
Sawyer, C. H. (1975). *Neuroendocrinology* **17**, 97.
Sawyer, C. H., Markee, J. E. and Hollinshead, W. H. (1947). *Endocrinology* **41**, 395.
Schneider, H. P. G. and McCann, S. H. (1970). *Endocrinology* **87**, 249.
Sinha, Y. N., Selby, F. W., Lewis, U. J. and Wanderlaan, W. P. (1973). *Journal of Clinical Endocrinology and Metabolism* **36**, 509.
Sjoerdsma, A., Vendsalu, A. and Engelman, K. (1963). *Circulation* **28**, 492.
Travaglini, P., Ballabio, M., Elli, R., Scaperrotta, R. C., Moriondo, P. and Faglia, G. (1981). *Journal Endocrinological Investigation* **4** (Suppl. 1), 441.

PROLACTIN, GROWTH HORMONE AND THYROTROPIN RESPONSES TO THE THYOROTROPIN-RELEASING HORMONE AND LEVODOPA IN POSTMENOPAUSE

L. P. Riva and C. Mazzi

Department of Endocrinology, St. Antony Hospital, Gallarate, Italy

INTRODUCTION

Prolactin (PRL), growth hormone (GH) and thyrotropin (TSH) secretion in postmenopause does not seem to have been definitively explained. Available data, mostly obtained from heterogeneous groups, which often include very old subjects and which are not always subdivided into appropriate age groups, are often contradictory, either as to hormone basal levels or as to their responses to dynamic tests. PRL secretion does not appear to be particularly influenced by age and its response to TRH may be normal. Contrasting results have been reported with regard to GH response to tests. For TSH, a steadiness of basal levels in different ages is present, while its response to TRH was found to be either similar to that of young subjects or reduced. For these reasons, it still seemed useful to examine PRL, GH and TSH secretion in postmenopause.

METHODS

This study was carried out on 10 non-obese women who had been in post-menopause for at least 4 years, aged 49–60 (mean 55). A comparison was made with results obtained in 17 non-obese menstruating women in the early folli-

Serono Symposium No. 39, "The Menopause: Clinical, Endocrinological and Pathophysiological Aspects", edited by P. Fioretti, L. Martini, G. B. Melis and S. S. C. Yen, 1982. Academic Press, London and New York.

cular phase, aged 18–40 (mean 32). None of the subjects had ever been hospitalized for severe illness or endocrine disorders; and none had received psychoactive drugs. All had documented normal response to oral glucose tolerance test (OGTT) and normal secretion of the thyroid gland and pituitary hormones, and besides the gonadotropins found in postmenopausal women at levels typical of this age. Serum PRL, GH and TSH levels were evaluated under basal conditions together with dynamic tests which allowed us to judge pituitary function.

PRL and TSH levels were measured 20, 40, 60 and 90 min after i.v. administration of TRH (200 μg). PRL and GH levels were measured 15, 30, 45, 90 and 120 min after oral administration of L-DOPA (500 mg). Hormone values were determined by a radioimmunological method, using materials supplied by Biodata (Milano). The F test for significance was used for the comparison of mean values.

RESULTS

The results in Fig. 1 show PRL secretion after TRH and L-DOPA administration; in Fig. 2, GH secretion after the L-DOPA test is shown and in Fig. 3, TSH levels after TRH administration are shown. A summary of the results is shown in Table I.

In the two age groups, differences between PRL, GH and TSH basal levels are not evident. The measured levels of these hormones during tests are very much alike; only the percentage GH increase after L-DOPA is greater, but not significantly, both in eumenorrhoic women (+ 530%) and in postmenopausal women (+ 325%).

DISCUSSION

No difference exists in the PRL basal levels between eumenorrhoic and postmenopausal women, according to Friesen *et al.* (1973), De Rivera *et al.*(1976), Yamaji *et al.* (1976) and Jaffe (1978). It is right to point out that others (Robyn *et al.*, 1977; Del Pozo *et al.*, 1977) have shown, in contrast, a progressive decline in PRL levels with age; and this secretion is reported to be parallel to the fall in ovarian steroidogenesis. However, the PRL pituitary reserve in older women is normal at least till 60 years of age. The data are similar to those obtained by Jacobs *et al.* (1973), Franchimont *et al.* (1976) and Yamaji *et al.* (1976), with a wide individual variability of the PRL response in the older group. Also oestrogen administration to postmenopausal women has been shown to enhance PRL levels. The PRL percentage increases with the two stimuli, TRH and oestrogens, within a similar range. In this investigation the maximum increase after TRH is + 577%; while it is + 514% and + 496% in two women (aged respectively 54 and 53) during oestrogen treatment (Yen *et al.*, 1974), but + 86% in five women aged 52–78 (Robyn and Vekemans, 1976). The present study, besides a stimulation test, considers the inhibition test by means of L-DOPA. PRL response shown by postmenopausal women is very similar to that obtained in eumenorrhoic women, confirming that PRL concentrations are not affected by age. It may be suggested that pituitary PRL biosynthesis is preserved in the postmenopause.

GH basal levels are also in the same order of magnitude, irrespective of age.

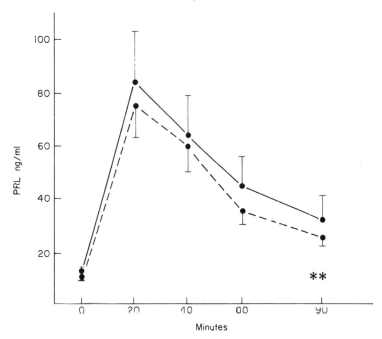

Response to TRH

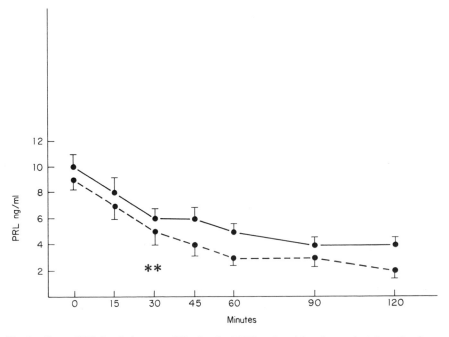

Response to Levodopa

Fig. 1. Serum PRL levels (mean ± SE) after i.v. TRH and oral levodopa administration in eumenorrhoic and in postmenopausal subjects. - - - eumenorrhoea; ——— postmenopause ** *P* < 0.01.

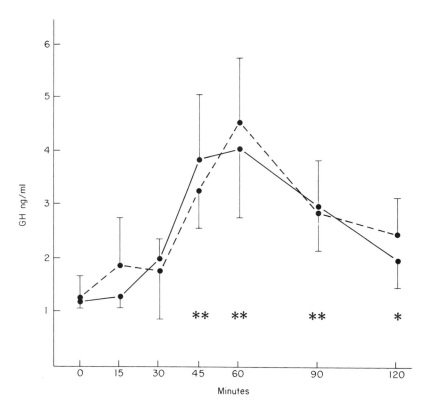

Fig. 2. Serum GH levels (mean ± SE) after levodopa administration in eumenorrhoic and in postmenopausal subjects. - - - eumenorrhoea; ———— postmenopause. * P < 0.05; ** P < 0.01.

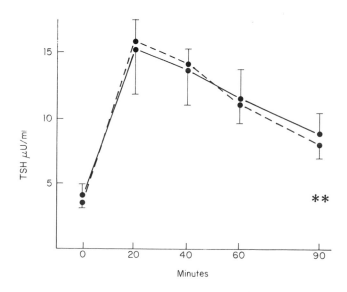

Fig. 3. Serum TSH levels (mean ± SE) after TRH administration in eumenorrhoic and in postmenopausal subjects. - - - eumenorrhoea; ———— postmenopause. ** P < 0.01.

Table I. Effects of TRH (200 µg i.v.) and levodopa (500 mg orally) on serum TSH (µU/ml), GH (ng/ml) and PRL (ng/ml) levels (means ± SE), in women with eumenorrhoea (17 subjects) and in postmenopause (10 subjects).

TRH i.v.

	TRH response						PRL response					
	Eumenorrhoea			Postmenopause			Eumenorrhoea			Postmenopause		
	Baseline	Peak	%	Baseline	Peak	%	Baseline	Peak	%	Baseline	Peak	%
	3.7 ± 0.3	15.8 ± 1.5[a]	+327	3.8 ± 1.1	15.6 ± 3.4[a]	+310	11.3 ± 1.3	76.8 ± 10.7[a]	+579	12.4 ± 1.8	84.0 ± 19.1[a]	+600

Oral levodopa

	GH response						PRL response					
	Eumenorrhoea			Postmenopause			Eumenorrhoea			Postmenopause		
	Baseline	Peak	%	Baseline	Peak	%	Baseline	Peak	%	Baseline	Peak	%
	1.0 ± 0.1	6.3 ± 1.0[a]	+530	1.2 ± 0.1	5.1 ± 1.1[a]	+325	9.0 ± 0.7	2.0 ± 0.4[a]	−78	10.0 ± 0.9	3.0 ± 0.5[a]	−66

[a] $P < 0.01$ versus baseline levels.

These results agree with the research of Danowski *et al.* (1969), Taylor *et al.* (1969) and Muggeo *et al.* (1974). On the other hand they are in contrast to the data of others who found that the GH level either significantly increased (Franchimont, 1971; Legros *et al.*, 1973; Blichert-Toft, 1975) or significantly decreased in older non-obese women rather than in younger ones (Finkelstein *et al.*, 1972; Vidalon *et al.*, 1973). The presence or absence of a GH sleep-peak was not consistently related to the occurrence of slow-wave sleep (Carlson *et al.*, 1972; Blichert-Toft, 1975). With regard to GH response to stimuli in postmeno-pausal subjects, different data have been reported. Significant progressive decrease of GH levels either as peak or as response areas were observed after insulin toler-ance tests (Muggeo *et al.*, 1974). Statistically significant differences were reported in the GH mean peak levels during OGTT between young women (20-30 years of age) and non-obese subjects during the sixth decade of life (Danowski *et al.*, 1969) or during the fifth and sixth decades of life (Vidalon *et al.*, 1973). Never-theless, the GH sensivity to dopaminergic stimulus seems to be normally pre-served, at least till 60 years of age.

The behaviour of TSH levels during postmenopause is similar to that shown by Freychet *et al.* (1968) and Snyder and Utiger (1972), who found unmodified basal or TSH stimulated levels of TSH is spite of changes in age. It is noteworthy that the mean Δ TSH response to TRH reported by Snyder and Utiger (1972) in aged females (40-59 years) is $16.0 \pm 2.5 \, \mu U/ml$, which closely parallels that found here, which is $11.8 \pm 2.3 \, \mu U/ml$. Since these authors used $400 \, \mu g$ of TRH as a stimulus, once again this would confirm that a dose of $200 \, \mu g$ is practically maxi-mal stimulation. Evidently the normality of TSH secretion in very old subjects also reduces the incidence of thyroid diseases in old age, as pointed out by former research (Pellegrini and Piotti, 1954; Baschieri *et al.*, 1961; Lloyd and Goldberg, 1961).

REFERENCES

Baschieri, L., De Luca, F. and Negri, M. (1961). *Giornale di Gerontologia* **9**, 111.
Blichert-Toft, M. (1975). *Acta endocrinologica* **78**, Suppl. 195, 60.
Carlson, H. E., Gillin, J., Gorden, P. and Snyder, F. (1972). *Journal of Clinical Endocrinology and Metabolism* **34**, 1102.
Danowski, T. S., Tsai, C. T., Morgan, C. R., Sieracki, J. C., Alley, R. A., Robbins, T. J., Sabeh, G. and Sunder, J. H. (1969). *Metabolism* **18**, 811.
Del Pozo, E., Hiba, J., Lancranjan, I. and Kunzig, H. J. (1977). *In* "Prolactin and Human Reproduction", Serono Symposium No. 11 (P. G. Crosignani and C. Robyn, Eds), 61-69. Academic Press, London and New York.
De Rivera, J. L., Lal, S., Ettigi, P., Hontela, S., Muller, H. F. and Friesen, H. G. (1976). *Clinical Endocrinology* **5**, 273.
Finkelstein, J. W., Roffwarg, H. P., Boyar, R. M., Kream, J. and Hellman, L. (1972). *Journal of Clinical Endocrinology and Metabolism* **35**, 665.
Franchimont, P. (1971). *In* "Sécrétion normale et pathologique de la somato-trophine et des gonadotrophines humaines", p. 64. Masson et Cie. Paris.
Franchimont, P., Dourcy, C., Legros, J. J., Reuter, A., Vrindts-Gevaert, Y., Van Cauwenberge, J. R., Remacle, P., Gaspard, U. and Colin, C. (1976). *Annales d'endocrinologie* **37**, 127.

Freychet, P., Rosselin, G. and Grenier, N. (1968). *In* "Actualités Endocrinologiques" (J. Decourt and G. Dreyfus, Eds), 217–227. L'Expansion Scientifique Francaise, Paris.

Friesen, H. G., Fournier, P. and Desjardins, P. (1973). *In* "Clinical Obstetrics and Gynecology" (H. J. Osofsky and G. Schaefer, Eds) Vol. 16, 25–45. Harper and Row, Hagerstown.

Jacobs, L. S., Snyder, P. J., Utiger, R. D. and Daughaday, W. H. (1973). *Journal of Clinical Endocrinology and Metabolism* **36**, 1069.

Jaffe, R. B. (1978). *In* "Reproductive Endocrinology" (S.S.C. Yen and R. B. Jaffe, Eds) 261–220. W. B. Saunders Company, Philadelphia.

Legros, J. J., Meurisse, J. and Franchimont, P. (1973). *In* "Les endocrines et le troisième âge" (H. P. Klotz, Ed.) 5–15. L'Expansion Scientifique Francaise, Paris.

Lloyd, W. H. and Goldberg, I.J.L. (1961). *British Medical Journal* **2**, 1257.

Muggeo, M., Crepaldi, G., Fedele, D., Tiengo, A., Dusi, U. and Garotti, C. (1974). *Giornale di Gerontologia* **22**, 1075.

Pellegrini, G. and Piotti, L. E. (1954). *Bollettino della Società medico-chirurgica di Pisa* **22**, 177.

Robyn, C. and Vekemans, M. (1976). *Acta endocrinologica* **83**, 9.

Robyn, C., Delvoye, P., Van Exter, C., Vekemans, M., Caufriez, A., de Nayer, P., Delogne-Desnoeck, J. and L'Hermite, M. (1977). *In* "Prolactin and Human Reproduction", Serono Symposium, No. 11 (P. G. Crosignani and C. Robyn, Eds), 71–96. Academic Press, London and New York.

Snyder, P. J. and Utiger, R. D. (1972). *Journal of Clinical Endocrinology and Metabolism* **34**, 1096.

Taylor, A. L., Finster, J. L. and Mintz, D. H. (1969). *Journal of Clinical Investigation* **48**, 2349.

Vidalon, C., Khuruna, R. C., Chae, S., Gegick, C. G., Stephan, T., Nolan, S. and Danowski, T. S. (1973). *Journal of the American Geriatrics Society* **21**, 253.

Yamaji, T. Shimamoto, K., Ishibashi, M., Kosaka, K. and Orimo, H. (1976). *Acta endocrinologica* **83**, 711.

Yen, S.S.C., Ehara, Y. and Siler, T. M. (1974). *Journal of Clinical Investigation* **53**, 652.

SECTION II
ENDOCRINE ASPECTS OF THE MENOPAUSE

THE PHYSIOLOGY OF THE PERIMENOPAUSAL YEARS:
THE IMPORTANCE OF PROGESTERONE AND PROLACTIN

G. V. Upton

Wyeth International Limited, Philadelphia, Pennsylvania, USA

INTRODUCTION

The "over-40" time of life can be a troublesome period for women and many symptoms can appear that are little understood and consequently frightening, particularly if the woman still has a "normal menses". The menopause does not constitute a disease process and cessation of menstruation is not a life-threatening situation. However, numerous related and sometimes aberrant physiological changes can occur during the transitional years into and beyond the menopause that can mimic organic disorders. It is important to stress that the menopause is a point in time. The period preceding and just after the menopause is called the perimenopause during which time the waning and cessation of ovarian function occurs. Since the rate of ovarian decline can vary markedly many years may be involved. A better understanding of the physiology of women in the perimenopause is essential for the proper management of symptoms and signs with hormonal replacement therapy. The subtle interplay of hormones during this transitional period is masked by an almost imperceptible estrogen and progesterone decline accompanied by many apparently innocuous symptoms, all of which are influenced by age and the changing sensitivity of target tissues. The symptoms experienced during the perimenopause can be quite indefinite. Fatigue, insomnia, depression and nervousness are common complaints and may be interpreted as responses to the vicissitudes of life. Few women attach any significance to the

Serono Symposium No. 39, "The Menopause: Clinical, Endocrinological and Pathophysiological Aspects", edited by P. Fioretti, L. Martini, G. B. Melis and S. S. C. Yen, 1982. Academic Press, London and New York.

lengthening or shortening of cycles. Estrogen fluctuations and anovulation proceed unnoticed until marked estrogen deprivation is manifest with quite objective signs such as vasomotor instability, depression, bone loss, and genital tissue atrophy that can progress to the extreme point of urinary incontinence. Surely these latter changes are most undesired and compelling reasons for using prophylactic therapy. Selected studies on the physiology of the perimenopause and the importance of progesterone and prolactin in these years are presented in this review.

THE ESTROGEN YEARS

The reproductive life of women can be arbitrarily divided into the following five stages that represent a gradual rise and fall in estrogen (Upton, 1980):

(1)   The *premenarche* or *prepuberty*, the developmental years of the child.
(2)   The *menarche*, the first bleeding and the onset of menstruation, a single point in time.
(3)   The *menstrual* or ovulatory, encompassing three phases:
   (a)   The *postmenarche*, the initial years of menstruation, noted for great variability in menstrual intervals.
   (b)   The *menstrual*, marked by cyclic regularity (approximate age 20 to 40 years).
   (c)   The *perimenopause*, encompassing the time preceding and just after the menopause (sometimes called the premenopause). A transitional phase characterised by unusually long or short cycles that are often interspersed. Symptoms of estrogen deficiency frequently first appear at this time (usually after age 40).
(4)   The *menopause*, a single point in time representing the last "bleed". Frequently, however, "menopause" is used loosely to signify a range of time.
(5)   The *postmenopause*, encompassing all time after the permanent cessation of the menses.

Some years ago, Treloar *et al.* (1967) showed that each woman's cycle variability in her perimenopausal years is the mirror image of that found in her post-menarchal years. Figure 1 summarises these data on 2700 women and 25 285 woman years of menstrual experience. As shown in Fig. 1, increased variation in menstrual intervals occurs immediately following menarche and just before the menopause. Transitions into and out of the comparative regularity of "middle life" occur over a period of many years during both the postmenarchal and perimenopausal experience; however, the perimenopausal transition is accomplished more gradually than the postmenarchal changes and represents passage from the most regular cyclic period of life to the most variable.

THE ENDOCRINE PROFILE OF THE PERIMENOPAUSE

Cyclic variations during the perimenopause may be due to irregular maturation of residual follicles or to anovulatory uterine bleeding following estrogen withdrawal without evidence of corpus luteum function (Sherman *et al.*, 1976). The continuous decline in estrogen and absence of ovarian progesterone results in the

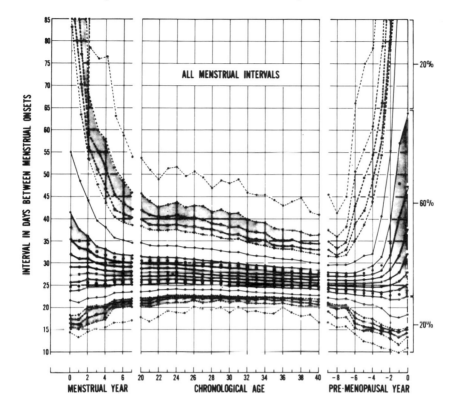

Fig. 1. Contours for the frequency distribution of all menstrual intervals in three zones of experience. Percentages shown on the right and shaded areas represent the largest similar variation groups. (Adapted from Treloar *et al.* (1967) with permission of the authors and reprinted with permission of the *International Journal of Gynaecology and Obstetrics* 17:6, 531, 1980).

typical deficiency symptoms such as hot flushes, headaches, insomnia, depression and nervousness that are so disconcerting and puzzling to the woman who is still menstruating.

A recent study serves to illustrate the gradual change in hormone levels in the aging woman. Reyes *et al.* (1977) did a cross-sectional study of 58 ovulating women in different age groups and of 18 postmenopausal women. Women 20–29 years of age (N = 15) had a 25–32 day cycle range; women 40–44 years of age (N = 15) had a cycle range of 23–34 days, while those 45–50 years of age (N = 12) had a range of 24–34 days. Not a great difference! Yet seven of these 27 women experienced hot flushes and night sweats. Figure 2 compares the hormonal profiles of these two groups of perimenopausal women with a group of young women 20–29 years of age. Table I presents the mean hormonal levels of postmenopausal women for comparison.

The only remarkably distinct hormonal change is the erratic and elevated level of follicle stimulating hormone (FSH) in the 45–50 group. In the 40–44 group,

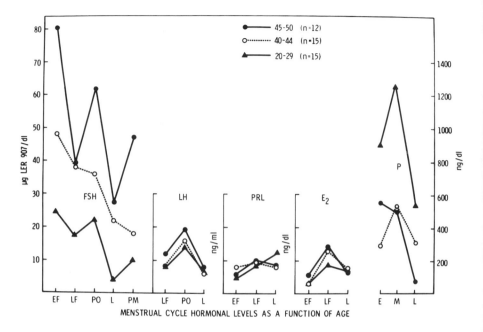

Fig. 2. Follicle-stimulating hormone (FSH), luteinising hormone (LH), prolactin (PRL) and estradiol (E₂) in perimenopausal women at the early follicular (EF), follicular (F), late follicular (LF), periovulatory (PO), luteal (L) and premenstrual (PM) phases of the cycle. Progesterone (P) levels at the early (E), middle (M) and late (L) luteal phases in the same group. FSH and LH and prolactin were measured by radioimmunoassay with human pituitary gonadotropin (LER 907) as a standard. [Adapted from Reyes *et al.* (1977) with permission of the authors and reprinted with permission of the *International Journal of Gynaecology and Obstetrics* **17**:6, 531, 1980].

Table I.

Mean hormone levels in the postmenopausal woman (N = 18)

FSH	=	$336 \pm 21 \ \mu g/dl$
LH	=	$34 \pm 0.9 \ \mu g/dl$
PRL	=	$5.1 \pm 0.2 \ ng/ml$
E_2	=	$1.0–2.8 \ ng/dl^{a}$
P	=	$2–34 \ ng/dl$

[a] Only 6/18 women had detectable levels. (Adapted from Reyes *et al.* (1977) with permission of the authors and reprinted with permission of the *International Journal of Gynaecology and Obstetrics* **17**:6, 531, 1980).

there was a loss of the normal periovulatory FSH peak and the plasma FSH levels declined steadily throughout the menstrual cycle, with no erratic, fluctuating levels as in the older group.

The luteinizing hormone (LH) levels peaked at the periovulatory period in all premenopausal subjects. The LH levels of the 45-50 group were significantly higher in the follicular phase than those seen in the 20-29 year-old women, mirroring the estrogen trend. Postmenopausal LH levels (Table I) were approximately two to three times as high as those LH levels seen in the 45-50 group.

Estrogen levels rose gradually during the late follicular phase in both the 40-44 and 45-50 groups. Luteal progesterone showed a decrease with age. The prolactin (PRL) levels in both older groups were similar to those in younger women and were directly proportional to the circulating estrogen concentrations. In postmenopausal women there was a marked and persistent hypoestrogenism, resulting in a marked decline in PRL levels (Table I). To provide a broader view, Fig. 3 shows FSH levels after the menopause showing the gradual FSH decline with time (Chakravarti *et al.*, 1976). Figure 4 shows the PRL levels throughout life. The plasma PRL levels peak at about age 30 and then decrease with age (Robyn and Vekemans, 1976; del Pozo *et al.*, 1977). These studies illustrate that the very gradual hormonal changes, coupled with the many apparently innocuous symptoms, can mask the dynamics of the physiology during the transition into the post-menopause.

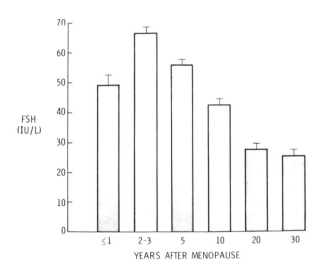

Fig. 3. Follicle-stimulating hormone (FSH) levels in 60 women at various times after menopause who never received any replacement therapy. (Adapted from Chakravarti *et al.* (1976) with permission of the authors). N = 6; age range = 49-91 years.

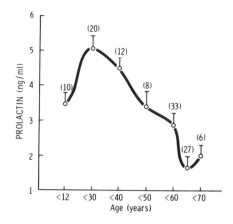

Fig. 4. Plasma prolactin levels at various ages throughout life in women not receiving replacement therapy. (Adapted from del Pozo *et al.* (1977) with permission of the authors and Robyn and Vekemans (1976) with permission of the authors).

THE MISSING INGREDIENT

The thinking has been that without a uterus all a woman needs is estrogen replacement, but this viewpoint disregards the influence of age on steroid metabolism, on tissue and organ sensitivity and the secretory function of the ovary. Such considerations make the dosage, the potency and the type of estrogen administered an important factor and also raise the question as to whether the role of progesterone is confined to the uterus.

Ovariectomy leads to an increased release of pituitary FSH and LH, and accelerates hypothalamic norepinephrine (NE) synthesis and turnover, suggesting that gonadal steroids may influence catecholamine (CA) synthesis in the brain (Anton-Tay *et al.*, 1970; Bapna *et al.*, 1971). Beattie *et al.* (1972) extended these observations by administering estrogen and progesterone, alone and in combination, to ovariectomised rats. They found that progesterone had an inhibitory, and estrogen, a stimulatory effect on hypothalamic tyrosine hydroxylase (the enzyme that converts tyrosine to DOPA). Thus the increase in brain CA synthesis after ovariectomy may be due to an increase in the activity of the rate-limiting step, tyrosine hydroxylase, and to the absence of ovarian progesterone.

Reports by Hsueh *et al.* (1975) have shown that progesterone reduces the number of estrogen cytoplasmic receptors by interfering with their replenishment. The reduction results in a lessened sensitivity of uterine tissue to estrogen. These studies underline two important points:

(1)   That progesterone can affect the turnover of biogenic amines and, consequently, sympathetic outflow. Progesterone does have effects other than on the uterus and specifically can affect hypothalamic centers.

(2)   That progesterone modulates the effects of estrogen by reducing the number of estrogen receptors. The widespread effects of estrogen throughout the

body are well known, and progesterone can effectively modulate these effects at the cellular level.

Additionally, progesterone through its anti-estrogenic activity, can modify the consequences of hyperestrogenism. Its effects on the autonomic system, CNS, cerebral coritcal function and its behaviour have been demonstrated clinically (Carter Little *et al.*, 1974; Herrman and Beach, 1978). Its influence on vasomotor function (Bullock *et al.*, 1975) is not surprising in the light of these studies. Progesterone's positive effect in preventing any decrease in bone mineral content (Lindsay *et al.*, 1978) and therefore, increasing bone formation, makes it inclusion in replacement therapy an important consideration.

THE HOT FLUSH

Vasomotor instability is a common symptom in the perimenopause. The subjectivity of the vasomotor flush has obscured its etiology, particularly when it occurs in a menstruating woman who has no obvious estrogen deficiency.

Since estrogen (Speroff *et al.*, 1978), progestin (Bullock *et al.*, 1975) and clonidine (Clayden *et al.*, 1974) have each been successful in relieving vasomotor symptoms to varying degrees (Fig. 5), the common denominator shared by these factors must reside somewhere between the endocrine and central nervous systems.

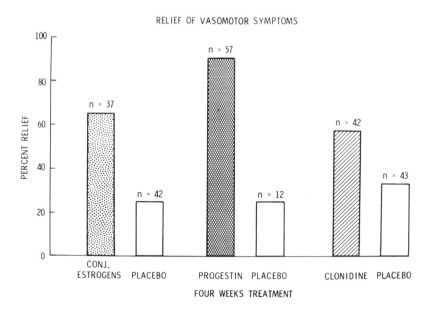

Fig. 5. The percent relief of vasomotor symptoms in women on placebo compared to those taking conjugated estrogen, progestin and clonidine over 4 weeks of treatment. The majority of women were postmenopause (either surgical or spontaneous). Progestin alone relieved vasomotor symptoms in 89% of the women compared to conjugated estrogen in 65% and clonidine in 58%. (Reprinted with the permission of the *International Journal of Gynaecology and Obstetrics* 17:6, 531, 1980).

G. Upton

It is known that modification of the synthesis, release, or metabolism of brain CAs interferes with the secretion of hormones from the anterior pituitary (Munson, 1963; Everett, 1964; Scharrer, 1976).

Available evidence suggests that the hypothalamic hormones that control the synthesis and release of the pituitary hormones must also be involved in the turnover of NE. It also has been shown that pituitary hormones can directly affect NE turnover and metabolism in the rat heart (Landsberg and Axelrod, 1968). Hartman's experiments showing that central noradrenergic neurons innervate cerebral and hypothalamic blood vessels further strengthened the interdependent relationship between the biogenic amines, the hypophysiotropic hormones and the cardiovascular system (Hartman, 1973).

Two recent studies offer firm clinical evidence that autonomic response can be correlated with the occasion of the actual flush. Molnar (1975) measured temperature changes with thermocouples and recorded continuous electrocardiograms during menopausal hot flushes in one 59 year old woman. The heart rate increased immediately at the onset of the episode (Fig. 6). Body temperature was normal or depressed, while sweat prints indicated profuse sweating on the forehead and nose. Internal temperatures were low in spite of warm digits and rising cheek temperatures, indicating a disorder of the thermoregulatory function.

Sturdee *et al.* (1978a) studied similar effects in eight menopausal and six premenopausal women during hot flushes. The study supplied strong evidence for an increase in sympathetic drive at the onset of the flush. An acute rise in skin temperature, peripheral vasodilatation, a transient increase in heart rate, fluctuations in the electrocardiographic (ECG) baseline, and a decrease in skin resistance accompanied the hot flush in the menopausal women. In contrast, the induced

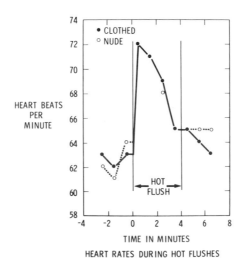

HEART RATES DURING HOT FLUSHES

Fig. 6. The increase in heart rate during eight hot flushes in one woman, age 59 years. Heart rate accelerated 13% at the onset of the flush and showed immediately thereafter. (Reproduced from Molnar (1975) with permission of the author and reprinted with permission of *International Journal of Gynaecology and Obstetrics* 17:6, 531, 1980).

warming (artificial as it may have been) of the premenopausal women was not accompanied by changes in heart rate or ECG baseline.

These clinical studies suggest that the "hot flush" is partly a thermo-vascular phenomenon with vasodilatation responsible for some of the signs and symptoms. Yen (1977) speculated that since prostaglandins can be released by sympathetic stimulation, they may be responsible for the vasodilatation. Looking still further, estrogen deficiency may induce changes in prostaglandins and catecholamines, producing a regional vasodilatation including that of the brain. It is speculated that CA function diminishes with age. Thus, reduced sensitivity and higher set point of the hypothalamic axis may lessen the effect of the interaction between CA and prostaglandins on vascular tone. Recently, Casper *et al.* (1979) and Meldrum *et al.* (1980) have shown that flush episodes are associated with pulsatile release of LH. Since LH release is controlled by hypothalamic secretion of luteinizing hormone releasing hormone, the link between neuro-endocrines, biogenic amines and flush episodes is strengthened. It becomes clearly evident that whatever the etiology of vasomotor flush may be, disorder of thermo-vascular and neuro-endocrine function play an intimate role, and both are modified by the aging process.

THE ASSOCIATION OF STEROIDS AND CANCER

Steroid hormones in themselves are not primary carcinogens. However, they may act as co-factors in stimulating some latent primary carcinogenic factor. Berenblum (1978) postulated that hormones operate as modifying factors and can influence carcinogenesis by (1) preparative action on target tissue, (2) permissive influence on the carcinogenic process and (3) conditional influence on a hormone-dependent tumor. Therefore, stimulation of the tissue is important but the timing of the hormonal event and the endocrine status at that time are all contributory and essential factors.

Recognition that adenomatous hyperplasia is a precursor of cancer associated with endogenous or exogenous estrogens in women at risk, underlined the importance of the relationship between risk factors, estrogens and cancer (Gusberg, 1980). Estrogen has long been associated with endometrial and breast cancer but a causal relationship has not been established. Much of the evidence stems from epidemiologic studies, some of it is clinical and some is experimental or based on pure theoretical grounds; none of it is conclusive. The consensus is that exposure to unopposed endogenous or exogenous estrogen for prolonged periods renders the subject susceptible to or at least at greater risk to carcinogenic factors, when they do exist.

During the perimenopause a woman's chances of long periods of unopposed estrogen stimulation increase. As Treloar *et al.* (1967) pointed out, the menstrual intervals of women in the perimenopause become intermittently lengthened. The luteal phases become shorter, the incidence of anovulation increases, and women may be exposed to persistent unopposed estrogen secretion for prolonged periods of time (Sherman and Korenman, 1974). Progesterone is notably absent. If unopposed estrogen is prescribed for menopausal symptoms to these women in this transitional phase, there is a very good chance that they will receive too much estrogen.

Table II. Sequential estrogen/progestogen therapy.

Investigator	Publication year	No. of pts.	Days on P[c]	Duration of study (years)	Results
Aylward et al.	1978	19	10	< 1	No endometrial hyperplasia
Budoff and Sommers	1979	74	7–10	< 5	2–3% with hyperplasia
Campbell et al.	1978	58	7–10	< 2	1–2% with cystic glandular hyperplasia
Gambrell	1978	126[a]	7–10	5	120 became normal
Gambrell	1979	148	7–10	2	4% with breast cancer
Hammond et al.	1979	72	7–10	5	No adverse effects
Nachtigal et al.	1979	84	7	10	No increased risk of breast cancer or endometrial Ca
Stryker	1977	276	7–10	< 15	1% incidence hyperplasia
Studd et al.	1979	58[b]	10	< 5	2% incidence cystic hyperplasia
Sturdee et al.	1978	102	7–10	< 1	No abnormal findings
Thom et al.	1979	200	7–13	> 4	2% hyperplasia
Whitehead and Campbell	1977	15[a]	7–10	2	All normal
Whitehead	1978	76	7–10	4	1–2% incidence hyperplasia
Whitehead et al.	1979	75	5–7	> 4	2–3% incidence hyperplasia
	Total	1383			

[a]Pre-existing endometrial pathology; [b]Pre-existing endometrial pathology in some patients; [c] = Progestogen.

THE AEGIS OF PROGESTERONE

A protective role for progesterone (or progestogen) against endometrial cancer and breast cancer has been postulated by several investigators who have based their opinion on their clinical observations (Sherman and Korenman, 1974; Stryker, 1977; Whitehead and Campbell, 1977; Gambrell, 1978, 1979; Whitehead, 1978; Aylward *et al.*, 1978; Campbell *et al.*, 1978; Sturdee *et al.*, 1978; Budoff and Sommers, 1979; Hammond *et al.*, 1979; Nachtigall *et al.*, 1979; Studd *et al.*, 1979; Thom *et al.*, 1979; Whitehead *et al.*, 1979; Patterson *et al.*, 1980).

Table II shows a listing of results from recently published studies by investigators who utilized sequential estrogen/progestogen therapy each month in peri- and postmenopausal women. The incidences of cancer of the breast or endometrium are listed. Although not shown in Table II, each observation was matched with untreated controls or with patients treated with unopposed estrogen. In every study, treatment with sequential estrogen/progestogen therapy did not increase the risk, and most often, greatly reduced the incidence of carcinoma when compared with controls and unopposed estrogen treated groups. Figure 7 depicts results from some of the studies from Table II. In each instance, controls (untreated or high dose estrogen treated) are compared to their respective estrogen and progesterone treated group. Where one may argue the statistics of a given trial, it is Important to appreciate the obvious trend that has developed. Certainly 1383 patients are a substantive number upon which to base a reasonable hypothesis.

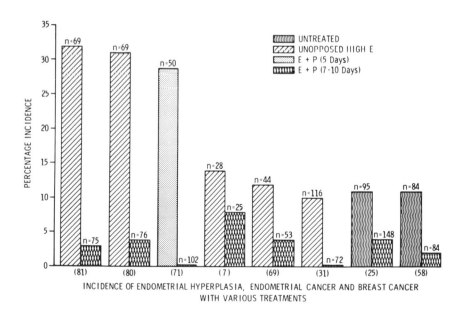

Fig. 7. Treatment of peri- and postmenopausal women in various trials are compared with the corresponding percentage incidence of endometrial hyperplasia and cancer that occurred in each group. (E = Estrogen, P = progestin).

It has previously been demonstrated (Hsueh *et al.*, 1975) that progesterone reduces the number of estrogen receptors and this property provides the basis for its protective action against hyperestrogenism.

Rather substantive reports emphasise the protective role of progesterone (Gambrell, 1974, 1977, 1978, 1978). Gambrell (1974, 1977) points out that the co-administration of progesterone (progestogen) may interrupt a series of progressive hyperplastic changes resulting from unopposed estrogen by producing more complete endometrial shedding (Fig. 8). This hypothesis presents convincing reason for using combination estogens plus progestogen therapy. It is

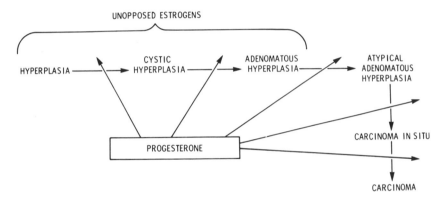

PREVENTION OF ADENOCARCINOMA OF ENDOMETRIUM

Fig. 8. The hypothetical protective effect of progesterone that interrupts a series of progressive hyperplastic changes resulting from unopposed estrogen by producing more complete endometrial shedding. (Reproduced from Gambrell (1974) with permission of the author and reprinted with permission of the *International Journal of Gynaecology and Obstetrics* **17**:6, 531, 1980).

also remarkable that some investigators (Gambrell, 1978; Whitehead and Campbell, 1977; Studd *et al.*, 1979) have clinically observed a reversal of endometrial pathology when combination therapy has been instituted reinforcing the concept that progestogen is protective. It is agreed that diagnosis of adenomatous hyperplasia calls for therapy with progestogen. However, several more severe grades are managed better with hysterectomy. One does not recommend steroid treatment for a virulent tumor. But combination therapy in many instances appears to play a protective role as shown by the recent study of Weiss and Sayvetz (1980). They found that combination oral contraceptives were protective. When menopausal patients went on to use unopposed estrogens for 2-3 years, the protection was lost.

THE PROLACTIN CONNECTION

It is known that circulating estrogen levels are directly proportional to prolactin levels (Nagasawa, 1979; Reyes *et al.*, 1977). Therefore, high levels of unopposed endogenous estrogen will also result in high prolactin levels. High PRL levels are known to be associated with secondary amenorrhea and galactorrhea (Friesen, 1976; Frantz, 1978). PRL may directly influence steroid secretion in the ovary modulating LH receptors (Furth, 1973).

The importance of PRL is magnified by the implication of elevated levels as a risk factor in breast cancer. In both animals and humans, PRL does promote the development and growth of mammary tumors (Furth, 1973; Meites, 1973; Welsh and Nagasawa, 1977). The incidence of breast cancer increases in women treated for long periods with drugs such as reserpine that stimulate prolactin release (Ettigi *et al.*, 1973; Armstrong *et al.*, 1974; Heinonen *et al.*, 1974). Furthermore, prolactin has been shown to stimulate human breast tumor growth in tissue culture (Burke and Goffney, 1978; Shafie and Brooks, 1977). Specific prolactin receptor sites have been demonstrated in normal breast tissue (Frantz, 1978) and in cancerous breast tissue (Kirschner, 1977; Partrige and Hachnel, 1979).

Prolonged elevation of PRL levels has also been shown to increase dehydro-epiandrosterone sulphate production by the adrenals (Vermeulen and Ando, 1976) providing an additional source for increased endogenous estrogen. Not all exogenous estrogens will induce high prolactin levels. The elevation of PRL depends on the dose of estrogen, duration of therapy, potency of estrogen, and the age and weight of the subject (Upton, 1980). Grattarola (1964) found that women with recent breast cancer had a higher incidence of anovulatory cycles and a higher incidence of primary and secondary sterility compared to normal women. These women were obviously being exposed to unopposed estrogen and consequently high PRL. The absence of progesterone implies that a possible protective agent was missing. Attempts to establish that higher levels of prolactin exist in breast cancer patients have been consistently unrewarding perhaps because the patients had already been treated surgically and/or chemotherapeutically (Cole *et al.*, 1977; Jones *et al.*, 1977). The studies of Kwa *et al.* (1974, 1976) and of Henderson *et al.* (1975) demonstrate that PRL levels were higher in members of breast-cancer families compared with controls. Thus, the propensity to higher levels seems to be present and perhaps is a genetic predisposition.

AGE AND OBESITY

Other factors can modulate estrogen levels. Most prominent, particularly in the aging woman, is age itself and obesity (MacDonald *et al.*, 1978; Upton, 1980). As the women ages, ovarian function declines and finally ceases. However, extra-ovarian sources provide amounts of estrogen such that many older women continue to have significant levels beyond the menopause (Judd *et al.*, 1974a; Upton, 1980). Adipose tissue has the ability to convert the precursor Δ^4-androstenedione, to estrone sulphate and estrone (Grodin *et al.*, 1973a, 1973b). The efficiency of this conversion increases with age (Hemsell *et al.*, 1974; Korenman *et al.*, 1978; MacDonald *et al.*, 1978) and is correlated with body weight (MacDonald *et al.*, 1978).

In some postmenopausal patients, ovarian androgen contribution may be significant (Judd *et al.*, 1974b). Testosterone can be aromatised in fat tissue to 17-β estradiol and to a lesser degree, to estrone (Judd *et al.*, 1974a). Although the fractional conversion of testosterone to estradiol increases, the production rate is low and thus estradiol by this pathway, is insignificant (Longcope, 1974). It is known that fat women (MacDonald *et al.*, 1978) convert a much larger fraction of androstenedione to estrone than non-fat women. Thus, excess adipose tissue can increase the amount of available estrogen. This source of estrogen assumes greater importance when ovarian function ceases.

DIET

Countries that have a high incidence of breast cancer are usually those with higher standards of living whose diets include greater dietary fat and caloric intake (Hankin and Rawlings, 1978) [it is known that a high fat diet in rodents will promote the development of mammary tumors (Kent, 1979)]. Curiously, the incidence of breast cancer in these affluent populations also increases with age (Hankin and Rawlings, 1978; Lipsett, 1979). In contrast, low risk countries show the exact opposite trends. For example, breast cancer in American women is six times that of Japanese women. Americans consume 300% more fat than do Japanese (Kent, 1979). It is also known that prolactin release in high-risk women may be abnormal (Hill *et al.*, 1976). Hill and Wynder (1976) demonstrated that changing women from a Western diet to a vegetarian one was accompanied by a reduction in the nocturnal release of PRL, a decrease in prolactin levels and a shortening of the menstrual cycle.

When Japanese women migrated to the United States, their rate of breast cancer increased significantly with succeeding generations (Haenszel and Kurihara, 1968; Kent, 1979; Lipsett, 1979). In addition, the ratio of urinary estriol to estradiol and estrone is lower in the high risk groups than lower risk groups. Moreover, plasma androstenedione and testosterone levels in postmenopausal Japanese are much lower than in Caucasian women (Kent, 1979). All of these factors are interrelated. The consequences of aging, in addition to liver enzyme changes and reduced organ sensitivity, are the well-known reduction in estrogen and absence of progesterone. The high fat diet leads to obesity and then to increased levels of unopposed estrogen (Hankin and Rawlings, 1978) and consequently high PRL (Kent, 1979; Nagasawa, 1979; Upton, 1980). Thus, a vicious cycle is formed (Fig. 9). The woman is at risk from her excess unopposed estrogen

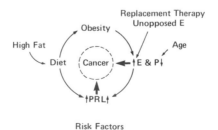

Risk Factors

Fig. 9. The schematic diagram depicts the risk factors that have been hypothesized as contributory in the etiology of cancer.

provided by her adipose tissue and her high fat diet feeds this internal fire. Should she seek therapy for perimenopausal symptoms from her physician, she may likely receive estrogen replacement which adds more fuel to her already primed cancer predisposition.

CONCLUSIONS

The physiology of women in the perimenopause is marked by great variability and usually by very gradual hormonal changes.

Progesterone (progestogen) does have effects other than on the uterus that have been little appreciated. Specifically, it has pronounced effects on hypothalamic centers subserving endocrine, cardiovascular and thermoregulatory function. Progestogen provides a protective effect against endometrial and breast cancer through its anti-estrogenic actions at a cellular level. It can further aid in protecting against bone loss.

Prolactin remains an insidious intruder and must be a consideration when administering replacement therapy. The choice of a weak, low-dose estrogen that will not increase PRL, combined with cyclic progestogen (7–10 days), is the preferred regimen.

Age, obesity and diet are all contributory risk factors for the potential development of cancer and should also be weighed carefully when treating the aging woman.

REFERENCES

Anton-Tay, F., Anton, F. S. M. and Wurtman, R. J. (1970). *Neuroendocrinology* **6**, 265.

Armstrong, B., Stevens, N. and Doll, S. R. (1974). *Lancet* **2**, 672.

Aylward, M., Parker, A., Maddock, J., Protheroe, A. and Ward, A. (1978). *Postgraduate Medical Journal* **54** (Suppl. 2), 74.

Bapna, J., Neff, N. H. and Costa, E. (1971). *Endocrinology* **89**, 1345.

Beattie, C. W., Rodgers, C. H. and Soyka, L. F. (1972). *Endocrinology* **91**, 276.

Berenblum, I. (1978). *Journal of the National Cancer Institute* **60**, 723.

Budoff, P. and Sommers, C. (1979). *The Journal of Reproductive Medicine* **22** (5), 241.

Bullock, J. L., Massey, F. M. and Gambrell, R. D., Jr (1975). *Obstetrics and Gynecology* **46**, 165.

Burke, R. E. and Gaffney, E. V. (1978). *Life Sciences* **23**, 901.

Campbell, S., McQueen, J., Minardi, J. and Whitehead, M. I. (1978). *Postgraduate Medical Journal* **54** (Suppl. 2), 59.

Carter Little, B., Matta, R. J. and Zahn, T. P. (1974). *Journal of Nervous and Mental Disease* **159**, 256.

Casper, R. F., Yen, S. S. C. and Wilkes, M. M. (1979). *Science* **205**, 823.

Chakravarti, S., Collins, W. P., Forecast, J. D., Newton, J. R., Oram, D. H. and Studd, J. W. W. (1976). *British Medical Journal* **2**, 784.

Clayden, J. R., Bell, J. W. and Pollard, P. (1974). *British Medical Journal* **1**, 409.

Cole, E. N., England, P. C., Sellwood, R. A. and Griffiths, K. (1977). *European Journal of Cancer* **13**, 677.

del Pozo, E., Hiba, J., Lancranjan, I. and Kunzig, H. J. (1977). *In* "Prolactin and Human Reproduction" (P. G. Crosignani and C. Robyn, Ed.), p. 61. Academic Press, London and New York.

Ettigi, P., Lal, S. and Friesen, H. (1973). *Lancet* 2, 266.

Everett, J. W. (1964). *Physiology Review* 44, 373.

Frantz, A. G. (1978). *The New England Journal of Medicine* 298, 210.

Friesen, H. G. (1976). *Research in Reproduction* 8, 3.

Furth, J. (1973). *In* "Human Prolactine" (J. L. Pasteels and C. Robyn, Eds), p. 233. International Congress Series, Excerpta Medica (No. 308). Amsterdam.

Gambrell, R. D., Jr (1974). *In* "The Menopausal Syndrome" (R. B. Greenblatt, V. B. Mahesh and P. G. McDonough, Eds), p. 147. Medcom Press, New York.

Gambrell, R. D., Jr (1977). *The Journal of Reproductive Medicine* 18(6), 301.

Gambrell, R. D., Jr (1978). *Obstetrics and Gynecology News*, Jan. 15.

Gambrell, R. D. Jr (1979). *Acta Obstetrica Gynecologica Scandinavica* Suppl. 88, 73.

Grattarola, R. (1964). *Cancer* 17, 1119.

Grodin, J. M., Siiteri, P. K. and MacDonald, P. C. (1973a). *In* "The Menopause and Aging" (K. J. Ryan and D. C. Gibson, Ed.), p. 15, DHEW Publication No. 73 (NIH).

Grodin, J. M., Siiteri, P. K. and MacDonald, P. C. (1973b). *Journal of Clinical Endocrinology and Metabolism* 36, 207.

Gusberg, S. B. (1980). *The New England Journal of Medicine* 302(13), 729.

Haenszel, W. and Kurihara, M. (1968). *Journal of the National Cancer Institute* 40, 43.

Hammond, B., Jelovsek, R., Lee, L., Creasman, T. and Parker, T. (1979). *American Journal of Obstetrics and Gynecology* 133, 603.

Hankin, J. H. and Rawlings, V. (1978). *American Journal of Clinical Nutrition* 31, 2005.

Hartman, B. K. (1973). *In* "Frontiers in Cathecholamine Research" (E. Usdin and S. H. Snyder, Eds), p. 91. Pergamon Press, New York

Heinonen, O. P., Shapiro, S., Tuominen, L. and Turunen, M. (1974). *Lancet* 2, 675.

Hemsell, D. L., Grodin, J. M., Brenner, P. F., Siiteri, P. K. and MacDonald, P. C. (1974). *Journal of Clinical Endocrinology and Metabolism* 38, 476.

Henderson, B. E., Gerkins, V., Rosario, I., Casagrande, J. and Pike, M. C. (1975). *New England Journal of Medicine* 293, 790.

Herrman, W. M. and Beach, R. C. (1978). *Postgraduate Medical Journal* 54 (Suppl. 2), 82.

Hill, P. and Wynder, E. (1976). *Lancet* 2, 806.

Hill, P., Wynder, E. L., Kumar, H., Helman, P. Rona, G. and Kuno, K. (1976). *Cancer Research* 36, 4102.

Hsueh, A. J. W., Peck, E. J. Jr and Clark, J. H. (1975). *Nature* 254, 337.

Jones, M. K., Ramway, I. D., Booth, M. and Collins, W. P. (1977). *Clinical Oncology* 3, 177.

Judd, H. L., Judd, G. E. and Lucas, W. E. (1974a). *Journal of Clinical Endocrinology and Metabolism* 39, 1020.

Judd, H. L., Lucas, W. E. and Yen, S. S. C. (1974b). *American Journal of Obstetrics and Gynecology* 118, 793.

Kent, S. (1979). *Geriatrics* 34, 83.

Kirschner, A. (1977). *Cancer* 39, 2716.

Korenman, S. G., Sherman, B. M. and Korenman, J. C. (1978). *Clinics in Endocrinology and Metabolism* 7, 625.

Kwa, J. G., Engelsman, E., DeJong-Bakker, M. and Cleton, F. J. (1974). *Lancet* **1**, 433.

Kwa, J. G., Cleton, F., DeJong-Bakker, M., Bulbrook, R. D., Hayward, J. L. and Wang, D. Y. (1976). *International Journal of Cancer* **17**, 441.

Landsberg, L., and Axelrod, J. (1968). *Circulation Research* **22**, 559.

Lindsay, R., Hart, D. M., Purdie, D., Ferguson, M. M., Clark, A. S. and Kraszewski, A. (1978). *Clinical Science and Molecular Medicine* **54**, 193.

Lipsett, M. B. (1979). *Cancer* **43**, 1967.

Longcope, C. (1974). *In* "The Menopausal Syndrome" (R. B. Greenblatt, V. B. Mahesh and P. G. McDonough, Eds), p. 6. Medcom Press, New York.

MacDonald, P. C., Edman, C. D., Hemsell, D. L., Porter, J. C. and Siiteri, P. K. (1978). *American Journal of Obstetrics and Gynecology* **130**, 448.

Meites, J. (1973). *In* "Human Prolactin" (J. L. Pasteels and C. Robyn, Eds), p. 105, International Congress Series, Excerpta Medica (no. 308), Amsterdam.

Meldrum, D. R., Tataryn, I. V., Frumar, M., Erlik, Y., Lu, H. and Judd, L. (1980). *Journal of Clinical Endocrinology and Metabolism* **50**(4), 685.

Molnar, G. W. (1975). *Journal of Applied Physiology* **38**, 499.

Munson, P. (1963). *In* "Advances in Neuroendocrinology" (A. V. Nalbandov, Ed.), p. 427. University of Illinois Press, Urbana, Illinois.

Nachtigall, E., Nachtigall, R. H., Nachtigall, D. and Beckman, E. (1979). *Journal of The American College of Obstetricians and Gynecologists* **54**(1), 74.

Nagasawa, H. (1979). *European Journal of Cancer* **15**, 267.

Partridge, R. K. and Hachnel, R. (1979). *Cancer* **43**, 643.

Patterson, M. E. L., Wade-Evans, T., Sturdee, D. W., Thom, H. and Studd, J. W. W. (1980). *British Medical Journal* **5**, 822.

Reyes, F. I., Winter, J. S. and Faiman, C. (1977). *American Journal of Obstetrics and Gynecology* **129**, 557.

Robyn, C. and Vekemans, M. (1976). *Acta Endocrinologica* **83**, 9.

Scharrer, B. (1976). *American Zoology* **7**, 161.

Shafie, S. and Brooks, S. C. (1977). *Cancer Research* **37**, 792.

Sherman, M. and Korenman, G. (1974). *Cancer* **33**, 1306.

Sherman, B. M., West, J. H. and Korenman, S. G. (1976). *The Journal of Clinical Endocrinology and Metabolism* **42**, 629.

Speroff, L., Glass, R. H. and Kase, N. G. (1978). *In* "Clinical Gynecologic Endocrinology and Infertility" Second Edition (L. Speroff, R. H. Glass and N. G. Kase, Eds), p. 65. Williams and Wilkins, Baltimore, Maryland.

Stryker, J. C. (1977). *Clinical Obstetrics and Gynecology* **20**(1), 155.

Studd, J. W. W., Thom, M. H., Paterson, M. E. L. and Wade-Evans, T. (1979). *In* "First International Congress on Hormones and Cancer" Oct. 3–6, 1979 (S. Iacobelli, R. J. B. King, H. R. Lindner and M. E. Lippman, Eds). Raven Press, New York, (in press).

Sturdee, D. W., Wade-Evans, T., Paterson, M. E. L., Thom, M. and Studd, J. W. W. (1978a). *British Medical Journal* **1**, 1575.

Sturdee, D. W., Wilson, K. A., Pipili, E. and Crocker, A. D. (1978b). *British Medical Journal* **2**, 79.

Thom, H., White, P. J., Williams, R. M., Sturde, D. W., Paterson, M. E. L., Wade-Evans, T. and Studd, J. W. W. (1979). *The Lancet* **455**.

Treloar, A. R., Boynton, R. E., Behn, B. G. and Brown, B. W. (1967). *International Journal of Fertility* **12** (Part 2), 77.

Upton, G. V. (1980). *International Journal of Gynecology and Obstetrics* **17**(6), 531.

Vermeulen, A. and Ando, S. (1976). *Clinical Endocrinology* **8**, 295.

Weiss, N. S. and Sayvetz, T. A. (1980). *New England Journal of Medicine* **302**, 551.

Welsh, C. W. and Nagasawa, H. (1977). *Cancer Research* **37**, 951.

Whitehead, M. I. (1978). *Maturitas* **1**, 87.

Whitehead, M. I. and Campbell, S. (1977). *Acta Obstetrica Gynecologica Standinavica* Suppl 65, 91.

Whitehead, M. I., McQueen, J., King, R. J. B. and Campbell, S. (1979). *Journal of the Royal Society of Medicine* **72**, 322.

Yen, S. S. C. (1977). *The Journal of Reproductive Medicine* **18**, 287.

SHORT TERM EFFECT OF GONADECTOMY ON
PITUITARY SECRETION IN FEMALES

P. Fioretti, G. Guarnieri, V. Mais, A. M. Paoletti, M. Gambacciani,
F. Fruzzetti, V. Facchini, T. Gargiulo[1], F. Facchinetti[2], G. B. Melis.

*Clinica Ostetrica e Ginecologia Università di Pisa; Divisione di Ostetrica,
Ospedale di Cerva (CN)[1]; Clinica Ostetrica e Ginecologica,
Università di Siena, Italy[2].*

INTRODUCTION

Ovarian failure is followed by long-term modifications of endocrine balance in animals and in humans, since ovarian secretion exerts well-known effects on the function of many districts (Fuxe *et al.*, 1969; Löfström *et al.*, 1977; Judd *et al.*, 1979). It has been demonstrated that the hypothalamic-pituitary-thyroid axis undergoes activation of its function during hyperoestrogenic states such as pregnancy and steroid therapy (Man *et al.*, 1969). On the contrary, inhibitory effects on thyroid hormone metabolism may be observed during menopause or in subjects with ovarian failure (Rubenstein *et al.*, 1973). As for adrenal function, cortisol secretion shows significant increase through pregnancy as well as during steroid supplementation, since in these conditions the levels and the production rate of transcortine, the specific cortisol binding protein, are high (Westphal, 1971). Adrenal steroids also show different patterns of production and/or metabolism during reproductive life in females (Vermeulen, 1976). In addition, many reproductive disorders are associated with alterations of adrenal androgen secretion (Yen, 1978). Growth hormone (GH) and prolactin (PRL) plasma levels also

Serono Symposium No. 39, "The Menopause: Clinical, Endocrinological and Pathophysiological Aspects", edited by P. Fioretti, L. Martini, G. B. Melis and S. S. C. Yen, 1982. Academic Press, London and New York.

show significant variations either in physiological or in pathological conditions depending on the levels of circulating steroids (Jacobs *et al.,* 1977; Löfström *et al.,* 1977; Schaeffer and Hsuech, 1979). In fact estradiol levels directly influence central nervous system (CNS) concentrations of dopamine (DA), which is the most important neurotransmitter regulating GH and PRL release (Fluckiger *et al.,* 1976; McLeod and Lamberts, 1978). Since the above modifications regard long-term effects of steroids on the endocrine system, the acute effects of premenopausal ovariectomy (OVR) on hypothalamic–pituitary secretion were evaluated in this paper. Pharmacological treatment by means of oestrogens was performed with the purpose of underlining some mechanism regulating the post-castration release of pituitary hormones.

MATERIALS AND METHODS

Twenty-three normally menstruating women, 31–42 years of age, were admitted to this study. They had not received endocrine active drugs for at least 3 months until they were hospitalized for surgical treatment. Total hysterectomy was performed with bilateral OVR as a part of treatment for uterine fibroids, endometriosis and pelvic inflammatory diseases. All patients did not present post-operation major complications. Pentazocine and amplicilline were the only medications used after surgery. Endocrine studies were performed in 19 subjects by serial determination of circulating pituitary hormones and/or steroids either in basal conditions or after acute stimulation tests with LHRH (Relisorm, Serono, Italy) and metoclopramide (Plasil, Lepetit, Italy), according to the following experimental protocol: OVR was performed during the early follicular phase in five subjects, whereas subjects of the other two groups (each one of seven subjects) were operated respectively during periovulatory period and middle luteal phase. Morning blood samples were withdrawn either 2 and 3 days before OVR or every day from the 7th to the 14th day after surgery. In the first group of five subjects operated during the early follicular phase, combined acute tests with LHRH ($10~\mu g$ i.v.) and metoclopramide (5 mg i.v.) were performed the day before OVR and 7, 14 and 21 days after operation. Blood samples were collected through a poliethylene catheter inserted in an antecubital vein and kept open by the slow infusion of saline solution, either before ($-60, -40, -20, 0$ min) or after (15, 30, 45, 60, 90 min) acute injection with the drugs. Four other subjects were castrated during the early follicular phase of their menstrual cycle. Blood samples were withdrawn either 2 and 3 days before OVR or between the 7th and the 14th day after OVR. LHRH test was performed as in control subjects. In addition, pharmacological treatment with oral ethynil oestradiol ($100~\mu g$ daily) was performed during the second week after OVR. All heparinized blood samples were centrifuged immediately after collection and separated plasma was deep frozen until assayed. Circulating levels of GN (gonadotropins i.e. LH, FSH), prolactin (PRL), oestradiol (E_2), progesterone (P), oestrone (E_1), dehydroepiandrosterone (DHEA) and its sulphate (DHEA-S), androstenedione (A), testosterone (T) and dihydrotestosterone (DHT) were measured by specific radioimmunoassay (RIA) methods. While proteic hormones were directly assayed in the plasma using previously described RIA methods (Melis *et al.,* 1977; Fioretti *et al.,* 1978), E_2 and P were measured after plasma extraction with diethylether (Fioretti *et al.*, 1974). Other steroid hormones were assayed after plasma purification by means of celite chromathography (Facchinetti and Genazzani, 1978).

RESULTS

All results are reported as mean ± standard error (M ± SE). Before OVR, plasma GN and PRL levels were within the limit of normal range for premenopausal women (Fig. 1). In all subjects, OVR was followed by a prompt and significant increase in plasma GN. From basal pre-OVR values of 6.5 ± 2 mU/ml, plasma LH levels started increasing significantly ($P < 0.05$) on the 10th day after operation with values of 11.2 ± 2.5 mU/ml; a further rise was observed until the 21st day with values of 28.9 ± 6.5 mU/ml ($P < 0.01$): these last values were about five-fold greater than pre-operation values.

Plasma FSH levels increased more promptly than those of LH. From preoperation values of 7.6 ± 0.6 mU/ml, they rose to 33.8 ± 2.2 mU/ml on the 6th day after

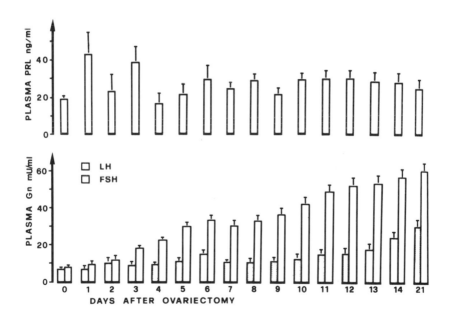

Fig. 1. Diagrams indicate daily mean values of prolactin (PRL, upper graph), LH (on the left of lower graph) and FSH (on the right of lower graph) in 23 female subjects before OVR (day 0) and from the 1st to the 21st day after OVR. Gonadotropins (GN) show progressively increasing levels during post-operation period. On the 21st day FSH values were about nine-fold higher and LH values were about five-fold higher than the pre-operation ones. PRL levels show irregular variations and particularly high levels were measured just after surgery. The results are expressed as mean ± standard error (M ± SE).

OVR ($P < 0.01$) and showed a *plateau* on the 7th and 8th day; thereafter, they started to increase until the 21st day after OVR with values of 69.1 ± 5.3 mU/ml ($P < 0.001$) which were about nine-fold higher than preoperation values.

Plasma PRL levels showed irregular variations during the same period. Starting from basal pre-operation values of 19.1 ± 2.0 ng/ml, higher levels were measured just after surgery with values of 42.9 ± 14.5 ng/ml and 38.6 ± 10 ng/ml respectively on the 1st and the 3rd day. Thereafter decreased levels were observed, but they

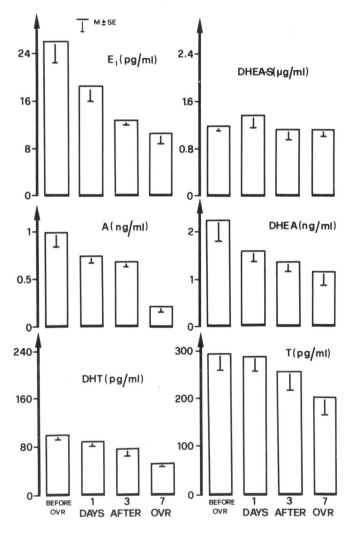

Fig. 2. Diagrams represent post-operation patterns of several circulating steroids before OVR and 1, 3 and 7 days after operation. OVR was performed during follicular phase. Significant decreased levels ($P < 0.02$) were shown by oestrone (E_1), androstenedione (A), dehydrotestosterone (DHT) and dehydroepiandrosterone (DHEA) levels. Minor variations were shown by DHEA-sulphate and testosterone. The values are expressed as M ± SE.

were significantly higher ($P < 0.05$) on the 21st day in comparison to preoperation values (Fig. 1).

The patterns of FSH and PRL varied according to the different phase of the menstrual cycle in which OVR was performed. During the 2nd week after operation a greater increase of FSH was observed when OVR was performed during the follicular phase rather than during the luteal phase. On the contarary PRL circulating levels showed a higher increase when operation was performed during the luteal phase of the cycle.

As for other hormonal parameters, GH plasma levels as well as TSH and thyroid hormones measured in the subjects operated during follicular phase, failed to show any significant difference after OVR in comparison to pre-operation values. On the contrary, plasma steroid levels showed consistent modifications in the

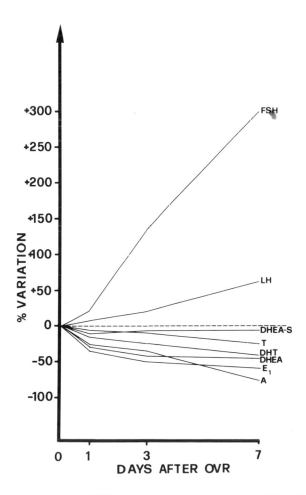

Fig. 3. Diagram compares post OVR gonadotropin increase to steroid (mainly adrenal) decrease. A significant correlation between LH increase and A decrease may be observed.

same subjects. E_2 levels showed a sharp decrease just after operation: starting
from values of 79 ± 5 pg/ml, they fell to values of 17 ± 3 pg/ml within 24 h of the
operation. Minor modifications were shown by P levels, which varied from pre-
operation values of 650 ± 89 pg/ml to post-operation values of 430 ± 54 pg/ml.
Blood concentrations of E_1, A, DHT, DHEA and T showed a significant decrease
during the first week after operation, whereas DHEA-S was unaltered (Fig. 2).
When the percentage variation of GN and steroid hormones during post-operation
period over pre-operation values was considered a significant correlation between
LH increase and A decrease was observed (Fig. 3), while FSH release was correlated to E_2 disappearance.

As for pituitary stimulation tests, LHRH injection was followed by a significant
release of both LH and FSH, as observed during the low estrogenic phase of menstrual cycle (Figs. 4 and 5). A progressive amplification of LHRH-induced GH
release was seen through the post-operation period. The peak values of LH were
respectively 18 ± 5.3 mU/ml (before OVR), 28.5 ± 8.5 mU/ml (7 days after OVR),
65 ± 7.2 mU/ml (14 days after OVR) and 68.1 ± 10.8 mU/ml (21 days after
OVR; Fig. 4). The peak values of FSH were 12 ± 3.5 mU/ml (before OVR),
54.2 ± 7.9 mU/ml (7 days after OVR), 112 ± 9.5 mU/ml (14 days after OVR) and
135 ± 23.5 mU/ml (21 days after OVR; Fig. 5).

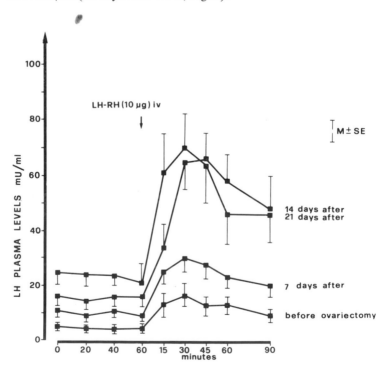

Fig. 4. LH response to LHRH stimulation test performed before, 7, 14 and 21 days after
OVR. Arrow indicates LHRH (10 μg i.v. bolus) injection. A progressive increased response to
stimulus was observed. The values are expressed as M ± SE.

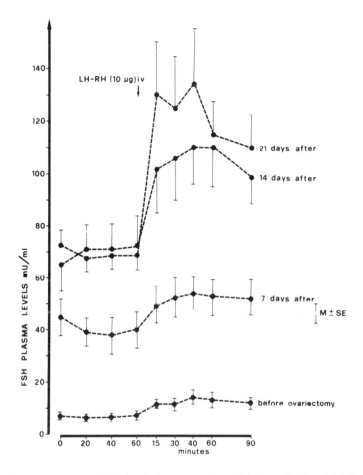

Fig. 5. FSH response to LHRH stimulation test performed before, 7, 14 and 21 days after OVR. Arrow indicates LHRH (10 μg i.v. bolus) injection. Peak values were progressively increased through post-operation. The values are expressed as M ± SE.

The percentage GN increase after LHRH stimulation was calculated considering the increased basal levels after OVR. LH percentage increase was higher ($P < 0.05$) on the 21st day after OVR rather than on the 7th and 14th days, however, the normal postmenopausal response to LHRH stimulation (as tested in 10 subjects) was even higher. On the contrary, FSH percentage increase after LHRH, was higher ($P < 0.05$) on the 21st day after OVR in comparison either with other tests performed in the same subjects or with the values obtained in postmenopausal subjects.

Before OVR, PRL response to metoclopramide was comparable to the one obtained in normally mestruating women during the follicular phase of the cycle, with a peak at 30 min from stimulation (values of 198 ± 22.8 ng/ml). After 7 days from OVR the response was slightly reduced with peak values of 170.2 ± 15.3 ng/ml. PRL concentrations of 203.2 ± 18.5 ng/ml and 205 ± 30.5 ng/ml were observed after 30 min from stimulations performed respectively on the 14th and 21st post-operation day. The statistical analysis showed that only peak values of PRL after metoclopramide injection on the 7th and 21st day after OVR were significantly different ($P < 0.05$).

The group of patients treated with ethyniloestradiol (EE_2) at the dose of 100 μg daily from the 7th to the 14th post-castration day showed GN levels similar to the untreated group until the start of treatment (the 7th day after OVR; Fig. 6). Thereafter a progressive decrease of both GN was observed and LH values of 7.3 ± 3.9 mU/ml were measured on the 14th day after OVR (like pre-operation levels) whereas FSH concentrations of 14.5 ± 2.4 mU/ml were measured on the same day, these last values being even higher than the pre-operation ones (Fig. 6). In the same subjects, plasma PRL levels were higher than either pre-operation values or post-castration control values. The pituitary response to LHRH stimulation performed on the 14th day (after 7 days of EE_2 treatment) was different from the one observed on the same day in untreated subjects and it was comparable to pre-operation tests. However, LH peak values in treated subjects after 45 min from stimulation were higher (38 ± 11.7 mU/ml) than the corresponding pre-operation values (18 ± 5.3 mU/ml)

DISCUSSION

Acute gonadectomy seems to be accompanied by a series of modifications of GN, PRL and steroids. As for GN, OVR induced a prompt and large increase of both LH and FSH in animals and in humans during the first two weeks after operation (Ostergard et al., 1970; Yen and Tsai, 1972; Zanisi and Martini, 1975b; Hunter et al., 1977; Martini, 1978). Although the most accepted opinion on the regulation of gonadotropin secretion sustains that a single central factor, e.g. LHRH, affects both LH and FSH (Carmel et al., 1975; Fink et al., 1975), other peripheral factors differentially influence GN release. Inhibin seems to exert a more inhibitory action on FSH secretion rather than on LH, whereas steroids affect GN release according either to different pathophysiological conditions or to their amount (Motta et al., 1968; Odell and Swerdloff, 1968; Yen and Tsai, 1972; Zanisi and Martini, 1975a). These observations suggest that FSH and LH post-OVR patterns may depend on the combined effects played by peripheral factors. A more rapid and large release of FSH was observed just after OVR, since combined actions of steroids and inhibin rapidly stop with activation of negative feedback. The partial independence of LH from inhibin, as supported by experimental studies, might explain its slow increase (Martini, 1978; Piva et al., 1978). OVR during follicular phase was seen to be followed by a prompt and much greater GN rise in comparison to the one observed when OVR was performed during luteal phase (Yen and Tsai, 1972). The amount of circulating E_2 and P during luteal phase could blunt post-castration rise of GN with an inhibitory mechanism greater than during follicular phase (Yen and Tsai, 1972; Martini, 1978; Piva et al., 1978). In our experiments, only FSH post-castration rise showed a clear-cut relationship with the phase of cycle in which OVR was performed, whereas LH rise was similar in all groups of subjects. Since the LH assay and the age of our subjects were different from those of other authors' experiments (Franchimont et al., 1973; Yen

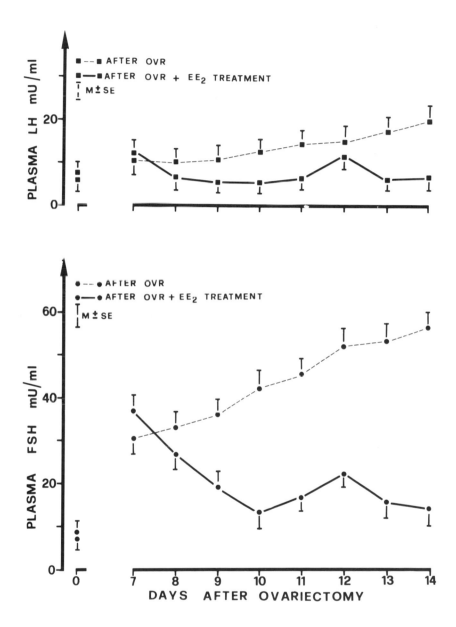

Fig. 6. Gonadotropin post-castration patterns in five subjects operated without additional treatment (dotted line) and during oral therapy (four subjects) with EE_2 (100 μg daily from the 7th to the 14th day). The treatment was able to counteract gonadotropin post-castration rise (see results). The values are expressed as M ± SE.

and Tsai, 1972), discrepancies might be due to these methodological differences. However, inhibin has been isolated from human follicular fluid (Chari, 1977; Hopkinson *et al.*, 1977). It seems to be produced during follicular maturation in greater amount than during luteal phase (Welschener *et al.*, 1977), and its circulating levels might be higher during the first half of the cycle (Chari, 1977). So, larger FSH release when OVR was performed during follicular phase might also depend on the different effect of inhibin feed-back, whereas the largest steroid secretion during luteal phase could minimize the role of inhibin (Zanisi and Martini, 1975c; Piva *et al.*, 1978). As is well known, circulating steroids show significant modifications after OVR because of either the acute lack of ovarian secretion or the surgery-induced stress. Although the levels of oestrogens, particularly E_2, represent the main factor affecting GN secretion (McLeod and Lamberts, 1978), some experimental (Neill and Smith, 1974; Zanisi and Martini, 1975c) and clinical data (Yen and Tsai, 1972) suggest that also adrenal androgens may physiologically participate in the feed-back control of GN release (Baird and Guevara, 1969). Our experiments show that a clear relationship correlates LH post-castration increase to the decrease of A, and suggest that this steroid may possibly represent another factor modulating post-castration GN rise (Baird *et al.*, 1969; Zanisi and Martini, 1975b). Secretion patterns of GN express both release and synthesis of gonadotropins induced by OVR (Yen and Tsai, 1972; Chen *et al.*, 1977). Moreover, the pituitary sensitivity, defined as the response to acute pulse of LHRH (10 μg), represents the releasing capacity of pituitary (Yen *et al.*, 1972a, b). It has been shown that pituitary sensitivity progressively increases during post-castration period, (Siler and Yen, 1973; Fink *et al.*, 1975). After OVR, FSH release seems to be progressively stimulated until the 21st day; at this time, the percentage change in response to exogenous LHRH seems to be even greater than in postmenopausal women. On the contrary, LH release is less evident and its percentage change after LHRH pulse is lower than the corresponding change observed in postmenopausal women. These data confirm that the endogenous LHRH differentially affects storage/release ratio of LH and FSH. This view also seems to be sustained by experiments performed by means of EE_2 treatment. This drug was able to suppress LH and FSH basal levels but, after LHRH pulse, LH release was greater than pre-operation response to the same test. In rats, castration is followed by plasma GN release (Piva *et al.*, 1978) and by reduction of LHRH content in median eminence (Gross, 1980). The sequential increased secretory activity of LHRH neurons into median eminence was limited by oestradiol benzoate administration (Gross, 1980). If these results could be extrapolated to humans, the inhibitory effects of EE_2 could be mediated through the inhibition of endogenous LHRH. However, oestrogens are also able to stimulate pituitary LH synthesis (Wang *et al.*, 1976). Thus, basal or stimulated GN release depend on the combined central and peripheral effects of ovarian factors (Motta *et al.*, 1968; Chen *et al.*, 1977).

As for other pituitary hormones, OVR does not seem to affect either GH or TSH and thyroid hormone secretion. In spite of their well-known relationships, sex hormones affect thyroid function indirectly by acting on liver metabolism with progressive activation of thyroxin binding globulin synthesis (Glinoer *et al.*, 1977). Actually, the controversial reports on the effects of pregnancy on TSH circulating levels are probably due to individual variation in addition to methodological problems (for review see Baschieri *et al.*, in this volume). Basal or stimulated levels of thyroid hormones and TSH show a progressive decrease through the postmenopausal period but it is unclear whether this decrease is due to the lack of oestrogens or to age (Rubenstein *et al.*, 1973; Hayward *et al.*, 1978; Bigazzi *et al.*, 1980). All these findings suggest that acute OVR probably cannot modify the thyroid axis since the above mechansim has to still be activated. In contrast some authors (Galvanini *et al.*, 1975; Chen and Walfish, 1978; Roti *et al.*, 1978) have seen modifications of thyroid function after OVR. However, the discrepancy may be due either to a different length of observation or to stress and pharmacological factors.

As for PRL and GH secretion, the data presented here seems to suggest either indirect or no effects of OVR on the release ot both hormones. In contrast to its regulatory mechanism (Fuxe *et al.*, 1969), GH plasma levels show no significant alterations relative to levels of circulating steroids; as expected, GH post-OVR levels are stable. PRL levels undergo significant modifications through reproductive life showing increased levels in the hyperoestrogenic states (Robyn *et al.*, 1977). Oestrogens are able either to act directly on the pituitary gland or to interfere with hypothalamic mechanisms regulating PRL secretion (Fuxe *et al.*, 1969). OVR would be expected to be followed by a reduction of PRL levels, since the oestrogens were decreased. In contrast, higher levels were seen during post-operation and particulary during the first week after surgery. Indeed, the PRL response to metoclopramide stimulation appeared to be unaltered in comparison to pre-OVR values. All these results lead us to suggest that different factors (environmental factors, anxiety, drugs, steroids) may influence the post-OVR pattern of PRL.

ACKNOWLEDGEMENTS

This work was partially supported by CNR (Rome, Italy) through the project "Biology of Reproduction" and Grant Nos 79.01891.04 and 80.00445.04.

REFERENCES

Baird, B. T. and Guevara, A. (1969). *Journal of Clinical Endocrinology and Metabolism* 29, 149.
Baird, B. T., Uno, A. and Melby, S. C. (1969). *Journal of Endocrinology* 45, 135.
Bigazzi, M., Sardano, G., Martino, E., Vaudagna, G., Ronga, G., Pinchera, A. and Baschieri, L. (1980). *Journal of Endocrinological Investigation* 3, 367.
Carmel, P. C., Araki, S. and Ferin, M. (1975). *In* "Program of 57th Meeting Endocrine Society", p. 104.
Chen, H. J. and Walfish, P. G. (1978). *Journal of Endocrinology* 78, 225.
Chen, H. T., Generau, J. and Meites, J. (1977). *Proceedings of the Society of Experimental Biology and Medicine* 156, 127.
Chari, S. (1977). *Endokrinologie* 70, 98.
Facchinetti, F. and Genazzani, A. R. (1978). *Journal of Nuclear Medicine and Allied Sciences* 22, 419.
Fink, G., Aiyer, M. S., Jameson, M. G. and Chiappa, S. A. (1975). *In* "Hypothalamic Hormones" (M. Motta, P. G. Crosignani and L. Martini, Eds.), p. 139. Academic Press, London, New York and San Francisco.

Fioretti, P., Genazzani, A. R., Facchinetti, F., Nasi, A., Melis, G. B. and Paoletti, A. M. (1974). *In* "Atti del LVI Congresso Nazionale della Società Italiana di Ostetricia e Ginacologia", p. 637.

Fioretti, P., Melis, G. B., Paoletti, A. M., Parodo, G., Caminiti, F., Corsini, G. U., and Martini, L. (1978). *Journal of Clinical Endocrinology and Metabolism* **47**, 1336.

Flückiger, E., Markö, M., Doepfener, W. and Nierdercer, W. (1976). *Postgraduate Medicine* **52**, Suppl. 1, 57.

Franchimont, P., Becher, H., Ernould, C., Thys, M., Demoulin, J., Borugnignon, L., Ugros, R., and Valke, A. (1973). *Annales d'Endocrinologie* **34**, 477.

Fuxe, K., Hokfelt, T. and Nilsson, O. (1969). *Neuroendocrinology* **5**, 107.

Galvanini, G., Ferrari, M., Adami, S., Cominacini, L., Aguggiaro, S., Pollini, G. P., Menestrina, F. and Lo Cascio, V. (1975). *Minerva Medica* **70**, 2251.

Glinoer, D., Gershengorn, M. C., Dubois, A. and Robbins, J. (1977). *Endocrinology* **100**, 807.

Gross, D. S. (1980). *Endocrinology* **106**, 1442.

Hayward, J. L., Greenwood, F. C., Glober, G., Stermmerma, G., Bulbrook, R. D., Wang, D. Y. and Kumaokas, S. (1978). *European Journal of Cancer* **14**, 1221.

Hopkinson, C. R. N., Damne, E., Stur, G., Fritz, E., Kaiser, S. and Hirshansen, C. (1977). *Journal of Reproduction Fertility* **50**, 93.

Hunter, D. J., Julier, D., Frankin, M. and Green, E. (1977). *Obstetrics and Gynaecology* **49**, 180.

Jacobs, J., Lloyd, M. M. and Meares, J. D. (1977). *Journal of Endocrinology* **72**, 35.

Judd, H. L., Judd, G. E., Lucas, W. E. and Yen, S. S. C. (1974). *Journal of Clinical Endocrinology and Metabolism* **39**, 1020.

Judd, S. J., Rigg, L. A. and Yen, S. S. C. (1979). *Journal of Clinical Endocrinology and Metabolism* **49**, 182.

Löfström, A., Eneroth, P., Gustafsson, J. A. and Skett, P. (1977). *Endocrinology* **101**, 1559.

Man, E. B., Reid, W. A., Hellegers, A. E. and Jones, W. S. (1969). *American Journal of Obstetrics and Gynecology* **103**, 328.

Martini, L. (1978). *In* "Proceedings of the 8th Congress of Gynecology and Obstetrics" (C. MacGregor, Ed.) p. 345. Excerpta Medica, Amsterdam.

McLeod, R. M. and Lamberts, S. W. J. (1978). *Endocrinology* **103**, 200.

Melis, G. B., Mameli, M., Cardia, S., Genazzani, A. R., Milia, A., Nasi, A., Paoletti, A. M., Puddu, R. and Fioretti, P. (1977). *Acta Europea Fertilitatis* **8**, 283.

Motta, M., Fraschini, F., Giuliani, G. and Martini, L. (1968). *Endocrinology* **83**, 1101.

Neill, J. D., and Smith, M. S. (1974). *In* "Current Topics in Experimental Endocrinology" (V. H. T. James and L. Martini, Eds). Vol. 2, p. 73. Academic Press, London, New York and San Francisco.

Odell, W. D. and Swerdloff, R. S. (1968). *Proceedings of the National Academy of Sciences USA* **61**, 529.

Ostergard, D., Parlow, A. and Townsend, D. (1970). *Journal of Clinical Endocrinology* **31**, 43.

Piva, P., Motta, M., and Martini, L. (1978). *In* "Metabolic Basis of Endocrinology" (L. J. DeGroot, Ed). p. 67. Grune and Stratton, New York.

Robyn, C., Delvoye, P., Van Exter, C., Vekernans, M., Canfrier, A., de Najer P., Delogne-Desnoeck, J., and L'Hermite, M. (1977). *In* "Prolactin and Human Reproduction" (P. G. Crosignani and C. Robyn, Eds) p. 71. Academic Press, London, New York and San Francisco.

Roti, E., Christianson, D., Harris, A. R., Braverman, L. E. and Vagenakis, A. G. (1978). *Endocrinology* **103**, 1662.

Rubenstein, H. A., Butler, V. P. Jr and Weiner, S. C. (1973). *Journal of Clinical Endocrinology and Metabolism* **37**, 247.

Schaeffer, J. M., and Hsuech, J. M. (1979). *Journal of Biology Chemistry* **254**, 5606.

Siler, T. M., and Yen, S. S. C. (1973). *Journal of Clinical Endocrinology and Metabolism* **37**, 491.

Vermeulen, A. (1976). *Journal of Clinical Endocrinology and Metabolism* **42**, 247.

Wang, F., Losley, B. L., Lein, A. and Yen, S. S. C. (1976). *Journal of Clinical Endocrinology and Metabolism* **42**, 718.

Welschener, R., Hermans, W. P., Dullaart, J. and de Jong, F. M. (1977). *Journal of Reproduction and Fertility* **50**, 129.

Westphal, U. (1971). *In* "Steroid Protein Interaction" (U. Westphal, Ed.), p. 216. Springer-Verlag, Berlin.

Yen, S. S. C. (1978). *In* "Reproductive Endocrinology: Physiology, Pathophysiology and Clinical management" (Yen, S. S. C., and Yaffe, R. B., Eds.) p. 324, Saunders Company, Philadelphia, London, Toronto.

Yen, S. S. C. and Tsai, C. C. (1972). *Journal of Clinical Endocrinology and Metabolism* **34**, 298.

Yen, S. S. C., Vanderberg, G., Rebar, R. and Ehara, Y. (1972a). *Journal of Clinical Endocrinology and Metabolism* **35**, 931.

Yen, S. S. C., Tsai, C. C., Naftolin, F., Vanderberg, G. and Ajabar, L. (1972b). *Journal of Clinical Endocrinology and Metabolism* **34**, 671.

Zanisi, M. and Martini, L. (1975a). *Journal of Steroid Biochemistry* **6**, 1021.

Zanisi, M. and Martini, L. (1975b). *Acta Endocrinologica* **78**, 683.

Zanisi, M. and Martini, L. (1975c). *Acta Endocrinologica* **78**, 689.

INHIBIN PRODUCTION BY THE OVARY

P. Franchimont, K. Henderson, F. Croze, M. T. Hazee-Hagelstein and Ch. Renard

Institute of Medicine, Radioimmunoassay Laboratory, University of Liège, Belgium

INTRODUCTION

Inhibin may be defined as a peptidic factor of gonadal origin that specifically or selectively lowers the rate of secretion of FSH. This substance has been detected and partially purified from ovarian extracts (Hopkinson *et al.*, 1975, 1977; Chappel *et al.*, 1979), porcine (Marder *et al.*, 1977; Welschen *et al.*, 1977; Lorenzen *et al.*, 1978) and human (Chari *et al.*, 1979) follicular fluid as well as the culture medium of granulosa cells (Erickson and Hsueh, 1978).

In this paper, we intend to describe the assay of inhibin, to quantify the concentration of inhibin in follicular fluids and to approach the mechanism of inhibin secretion by granulosa and luteal cells.

ASSAY OF INHIBIN

The assay of inhibin already described by Lee *et al.* (1979) is based on the inhibition of LHRH-induced FSH secretion by dispersed pituitary cells (Franchimont *et al.*, 1979a). Anterior pituitary cells from adult male Wistar rats are dispersed using the trypsin method of Hopkins and Farquhar (1973). The dispersed cells are suspended in 3 ml Dulbecco Modified Eagle's Medium (DMEM) (Dulbecco and Freeman, 1959), supplemented with 5% horse serum, 2.5% foetal calf serum, 1% glutamine and 1% non-essential amino acids and then distributed in culture

Serono Symposium No. 39, "The Menopause: Clinical, Endocrinological and Pathophysiological Aspects", edited by P. Fioretti, L. Martini, G. B. Melis and S. S. C. Yen, 1982. Academic Press, London and New York.

dishes. Each culture dish (Falcon Plastics) contains 1×10^6 cells and is incubated at 37 °C in a water-saturated atmosphere of 95% air and 5% CO_2 for 3 days. After this period, samples of standard and unknowns are added to five culture dishes for each concentration. The total volume of incubation was 1.6 ml. The incubation was continued for a further 3 days. After this period, the media were removed, and the culture plates were washed and then incubated for a further 6 h in DMEN with the samples at the same concentrations and with luteinizing hormone-releasing hormone (LHRH) at a final concentration of 10^{-8} M. Each concentration of the samples is tested in 5-plicate in basal conditions and under the stimulatory effect of LHRH.

The reference preparation is derived from ovine testicular lymph (OTL) given an arbitrary potency 1 U/mg. The inhibin standard is added to dispersed rat anterior pituitary cell culture over a dose range of 250 to 2.000 μg ml^{-1}.

Active preparations extracted from rete testis fluid have been extensively

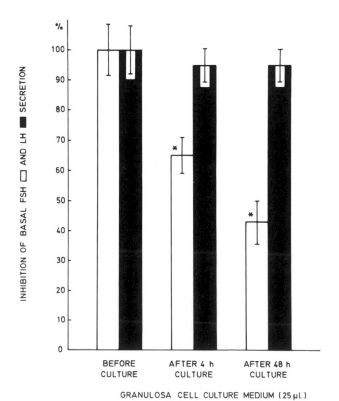

Fig. 1. Effect of 25 μl granulosa cell culture medium on basal FSH and LH secretion by 10^6 dispersed anterior pituitary cells after 3 days of incubation. Unprimed culture medium is used as control and basal FSH and LH secretion in its presence represents 100%. Media of 4 h and 48 h cultures of granulosa cells significantly decrease basal FSH secretion without affecting LH secretion. Each bar represents the mean ± 1 standard deviation. *$P < 0.001$.

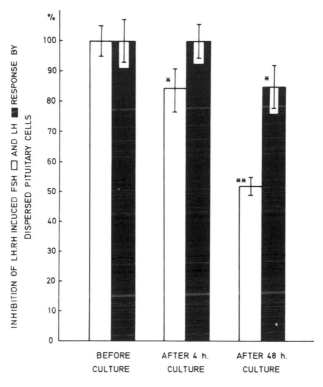

Fig. 2. Effect of 25 μl granulosa cell culture medium on LHRH-induced FSH and LH release by 10[6] dispersed anterior pituitary cells. Unprimed culture medium is used as control and LHRH-induced FSH and LH release in its presence represents 100%. Medium of 4 h culture of granulosa cells significantly decreases FSH release without affecting LH. Medium of 48 h culture significantly depresses both FSH and LH release but the effect is much more marked for FSH than for LH. Each bar represents the mean ± 1 standard deviation. *$P < 0.01$; **$P < 0.001$.

described previously (Franchimont *et al.*, 1978). Follicular fluids and culture medium are always pretreated with charcoal–dextran for the purpose of removing the sex steroids. Charcoal treatment involved the addition of activated charcoal (NORIT A 1%) pretreated with dextran (0.1%). The samples are mixed at 4° for 16 h followed by centrifugation at 3.000 g. The supernatants are filter-sterilized by passing through a 0.45 μm cellulose millipore filter before use.

The concentrations of follicular fluid in the pituitary cell culture medium range from 1% to 5% (v/v) whereas the concentrations of granulosa and luteal cells culture medium are between 3% and 60% (v/μ). Control values are obtained using the same concentration of granulosa or luteal cell culture medium before any contact with the cells. Each amount of standard or unknowns and each volume of biological fluid are assayed five times at several concentrations. Specificity of the method is ascertained in two ways (Franchimont *et al.*, 1979b). First, inhibin activity is defined by absence of effect on LH secretion in basal conditions after 3 days of incubation with inhibin preparations (Fig. 1). Furthermore, a preferential inhibitory effect on FSH secretion must be observed after stimulation of pituitary cells by LRRH (Fig. 2). Second, the secretion of pituitary hormones such as prolactin and TSH should not be affected by inhibin.

The precision and parallelism (Borth, 1976) for inhibin assay were evaluated. The FSH concentrations are expressed as percentage of control (no added inhibin). Fig. 3 represents the mean curve from 15 individual curves of inhibition of LHRH-induced FSH release by increasing amounts of OTL standard (OTLS$_6$)*. The mean slope (b) is equal to 27.7 (19.4 – 34.2) and the significance of regression (Finney's g) is always higher than 0.01. RTF$_1$A, a preparation of inhibin extracted from rete testis fluid with a M.W. higher than 10 000 (Franchimont *et al.*, 1978) and follicular fluid induce a dose dependent inhibition of LHRH-induced FSH

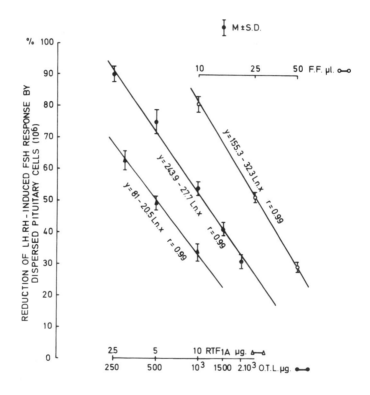

Fig. 3. Reduction of LHRH-induced FSH release by increasing amounts of several preparations of inhibin. Ordinate : reduction of FSH secretion expressed as percentage of the control value (100%) ± 1 SD. Abscisa : bovine follicular fluid (FF) fraction 1[A] of rete testis fluid (RTF$_1$ A) and the standard : OTL.

*Kindly provided by Professor B. Hudson, Howard Florey Institute of Experimental Physiology and Medicine, University of Melbourne, Australia.

secretion. Variations in their slopes (G_2) are not significant and, therefore, curves are considered as parallel. Index of precision (λ) is ranged between 0.06 to 0.19. Inhibin preparations also decrease basal FSH concentrations in a dose dependent manner. But the inhibition curves are less steep (b = 19.3) and less precise (λ between 0.41 - 0.15). For these reasons, LHRH-induced FSH release was chosen as the end point of inhibin assay.

INHIBIN IN OVARIAN VEIN AND FOLLICULAR FLUID

In female monkeys (Channing *et al.*, 1980) and rats (De Paolo *et al.*, 1979) inhibin activity is found in ovarian vein. In rats, the FSH-inhibiting activity in ovarian venous plasma varies inversely with peripheral plasma FSH concentrations. In monkeys, removal of large follicles from ovaries is followed by a decrease in FSH inhibiting activity of ovarian venous plasma and consequently there is a significant rise in serum FSH. Furthermore, in several animal species, inhibin activity has been found by *in vivo* assays in the follicular fluid pretreated with charcoal to remove sex steroids (De Jong and Sharpe, 1976; Marder *et al.*, 1977; Welschen *et al.*, 1977; Lorenzen *et al.*, 1978).

Data from the literature are contradictory concerning the levels of ovarian inhibin during follicular development. According to Lorenzen *et al.* (1978), the concentration of inhibin diminishes with the growth of the follicle in the pig. In contrast, Welschen *et al.* (1977) found inhibin in small bovine follicles (5-10 mm in diameter) and maximum concentrations were reached in medium and large (11-20 mm in diameter) follicles. By assaying inhibin *in vitro*, we have found that the concentration of inhibin is higher in small follicles from which a small volume of fluid is collected. In contrast, when the volume of follicular fluid increases, the concentration of inhibin decreases (Fig. 4).

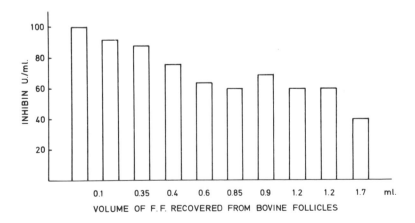

Fig. 4. Concentration of inhibin expressed in U/ml in follicular fluid according to the volume collected from individual antral follicles.

P. Franchimont et al.

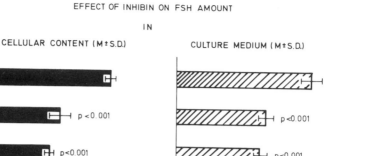

EFFECT OF INHIBIN ON FSH AMOUNT

IN

CELLULAR CONTENT (M±S.D.)   CULTURE MEDIUM (M±S.D.)

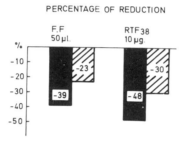

PERCENTAGE OF REDUCTION

Fig. 5. Effect of 50 μl of steroid-free bovine follicular fluid (FF) and 10 μg of ram rete testis fluid (RTF_{38}) on amounts of FSH cell content and in culture medium after 3 days of incubation. Bar C : control values observed in the absence of inhibin preparations. The upper part of the graph indicates absolute FSH amounts ± SD and the lower part represents the reduction of FSH amounts in cellular content (black columns) and culture medium (hatched columns) expressed as percentage, the control values representing 0%. Under these experimental conditions, no effect was observed on LH intracellular and culture medium contents.

In vitro, various preparations of inhibin (extract of RTF, follicular fluid from mare, etc.) lead to a concomitant reduction in the quantity of FSH in the culture medium and within the cells after 72 h of incubation in the absence of LHRH. This action is more marked on the cell content than on the quantities of FSH released into the culture medium (Fig. 5). Under our chosen experimental conditions, no effect was observed on the quantities of LH present in either the culture medium or the cells. These actions on the quantities of FSH in the two compartments show that inhibin preparations tested have an effect on FSH synthesis under basal conditions. In fact, if the actions were limited to an inhibition of FSH release, the level of FSH would be reduced in the culture medium whereas the quantities of FSH in the cells would remain the same or be even greater than in the control cells (Franchimont *et al.*, 1978).

MECHANISMS OF INHIBIN SECRETION

To investigate the mechanism of inhibin secretion, monolayer granulosa and luteal cell culture were carried out. Indeed, Erickson and Hsueh (1978) had showed that the granulosa cells in culture secrete a substance that acts directly on pituitary cell culture and preferentially suppresses FSH secretion. The methods were extensively described by one of us (Henderson and Moon, 1979). Granulosa cells are obtained from bovine large antral follicles (7-15 mm). The harvested cells are pooled, washed three times with Minimum Essential Medium with Earle's Salts (EMEM) and supplemented with Hepes buffer (20 mM), glutamine (2 mM), antibiotics and non-essential amino acids. Each dish contained 10^{-6} cells which are cultured at $36\,^{\circ}$C in a humidified incubator on 15 mm diameter round plastic coverslips in 1 ml culture medium consisting of 10% (v/μ) foetal bovine serum and 90% EMEM without Hepes but supplemented with glutamine, antibiotics and non-essential amino acids.

Luteal cells are obtained from bovine corpora lutea. Small fragments of corpora lutea are incubated for 20 min at $37\,^{\circ}$C with stirring in Hanks' Balanced Salt Solution supplemented with glutamine (2 mM), Hepes (20 mM) and antibiotics and contain 0.2% collagenase (Ig/c II, Sigma). The medium is decanted and the released cells are collected by low speed centrifugation and stored at $4\,^{\circ}$C. The remaining fragile tissue fragments are incubated again in the same medium containing 0.2% collagenase. All the released cells are pooled together, filtered through sterile gauze and washed four times to remove any trace of collagenase. Culture of 10^6 cells are set up exactly as described for the granulosa cells.

Pregnant mare serum gonadotropin (PMSG) has predominantly FSH like activity and induces ovarian follicular development in intact as well as hypophysectomized immature rats. In order to induce a follicular development 10 IU PMSG were injected subcutaneously to 21 day old female rats. Animals were killed 3 days later. Pseudopregnant corpora lutea were induced by sequential injection of 50 IU PMSG and 25 IU HCG s.c. at days 10 and 7 respectively before sacrifice. Rat dispersed granulosa and luteal cells were prepared according to the method of Croze and Franchimont (1981).

The progesterone content of culture medium was assayed directly by radioimmunoassay according to the method of Orczyk *et al.* (1974). Oestradiol was measured in diethylether extracted aliquot of culture media by radioimmunoassay using the antiserum and the methods described by Dorrington and Armstrong (1975).

Production of Inhibin and Progesterone by
Bovine Granulosa and Luteal Cells

Luteal cells make 25 times more progesterone than granulosa cells over the first 24 h. During the next 24 h, progesterone production by granulosa cells rises, presumably as a consequence of luteinization while progesterone production by the luteal cells declines. Inhibin activity is undetectable in volumes of up to 50 μl of culture medium of luteal cells during the first and second days of culture. In contrast, inhibin secretion by granulosa cells is elevated in the first day culture medium and declines in the second day culture medium (Fig. 6).

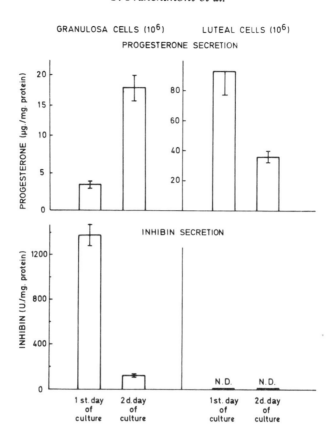

Fig. 6. Progesterone (upper pannel) and inhibin (lower pannel) secretion by granulosa (left parts) and luteal (right parts) cells during the first and the second day of culture. Results are expressed in μg for progesterone and in unit for inhibin per mg protein by measuring the total protein content of the cells remaining attached to the culture dish at the end of the culture.

The analysis of the results of several (four) experiments on bovine granulosa cell culture clearly demonstrates an inverse relationship between progesterone and inhibin secretion (Fig. 7).

Effect of 17 β-Oestradiol and Testosterone on Progesterone and Inhibin Secretion by Bovine Granulosa Cells

Oestradiol has a marked inhibitory effect on progesterone production particularly during the second 24 h of culture when both concentrations (0.1 and 1 μg/ml) are inhibitory (Fig. 8). Only one microgram of 17 β-oestradiol is inhibitory over the first 24 h. Both concentrations of 17 β-oestradiol do not modify the inhibin secretion by the granulosa cells whatever the day of the culture.

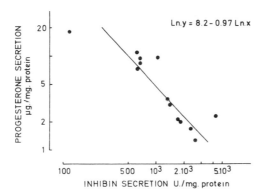

Fig. 7. Inverse relationship between progesterone and inhibin secretion by granulosa cells. Progesterone and inhibin secretions are respectively expressed in μg and unit per mg protein on log. scales. Coefficient of correlation (r) is 0.76.

Testosterone at the dose of 100 ng and 1 μg/ml of culture medium has no significant effect on progesterone production at either 24 h or 48 h of culture. In contrast, the addition of 1 μg of testosterone to granulosa cell culture medium significantly increases inhibin secretion during the first and the second day of culture.

Stimulation of Aromatization and Inhibin Secretion in Immature Rats

Secretion of progesterone, oestradiol and inhibin by gonadotrophin-induced granulosa and luteal cells (10^4 cells) was investigated for 4 days. The fourth day, PMSG 0.02 U/ml and testosterone $5 \cdot 10^{-7}$ M were added to some cultures in order to stimulate the aromatization of testosterone to oestrogens. Progesterone secretion by luteal cells is more elevated than that by granulosa cells whereas inhibin secretion is higher for granulosa than for luteal cells. Oestradiol remained low over the whole culture period for both cellular types. The fourth day of culture, no inhibin was detectable in the culture medium of granulosa and luteal cells. Oestradiol was at the limit of detection and progesterone secretion was still sustained for luteal cells. Addition of PMSG and T to some cultures significantly increased the secretion of oestradiol and inhibin by granulosa and luteal cells without modifying the levels of progesterone (Table I).

DISCUSSION

It is now possible to assay inhibin in biological fluids using an *in vitro* method consisting of the selective reduction of FSH secretion by dispersed anterior pituitary cells. Inhibition of LHRH-induced FSH secretion is, in our opinion, more precise and sensitive than the inhibition of basal FSH secretion. Criteria for the quality of a multiple parallel line bioassay are fulfilled. Thus, we con-

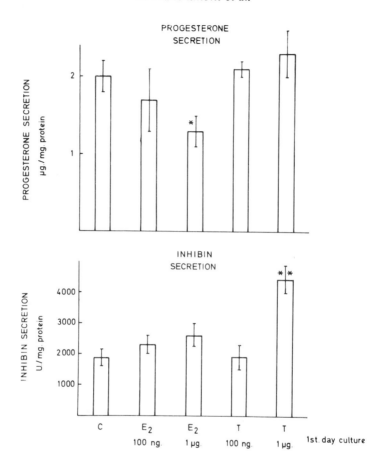

Fig. 8a. Effect of 0.1 and 1 µg of oestradiol (O₂) and testosterone (T) on progesterone and inhibin secretion by granulosa cells during the first day of culture. *P < 0.05; **P < 0.01.

firm the usefulness of dispersed pituitary cell culture as a method for assaying inhibin (De Jong *et al.,* 1979; Eddie *et al.,* 1979; Hudson *et al.,* 1979; Lee *et al.,* 1979).

Biological identity of inhibin preparation extracted from ram rete testes fluid and of inhibin present in follicular fluid or in lyophilized ovine testicular lymph is assessed by the parallelism of curves of reduction of FSH release into the culture medium. As already demonstrated (Franchimont *et al.,* 1979), inhibin contained in mare follicular fluid decreases both the synthesis and the release of FSH without modifying the synthesis of LH. Only high volumes of follicular fluid are capable of inhibiting the LH release induced by LHRH added to the culture medium.

An inverse relationship exists between progesterone and inhibin production. Thus, when bovine granulosa cells undergo luteinization and differentiate into

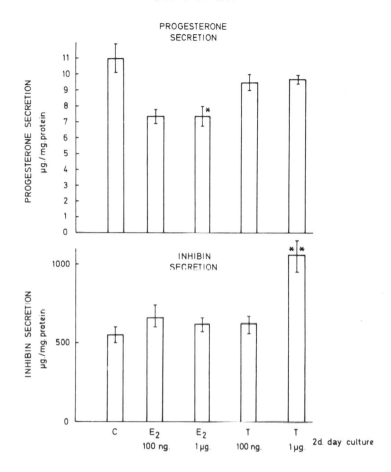

Fig. 8b. Effect of 0.1 and 1 μg of oestradiol (O₂) and testosterone (T) on progesterone and inhibin secretion by granulosa cells during the second day of culture. *P < 0.05; **P < 0.01.

luteal cells as indicated by histological changes and steadily increasing progesterone production, they progressively lose their capacity to make inhibin.

Luteal cells collected from bovine corpus luteum tissue have a very limited capacity, if any, to produce inhibin. Similarly, granulosa cells induced by injection of PMSG to immature female rats produce much more inhibin than PMSG-HCG-induced luteal cells in these animals.

Testosterone, but not oestradiol, stimulates inhibin production by granulosa cells. This positive effect of testosterone on inhibin secretion is concomitant with the stimulation of aromatization of androgens. This aromatization of exogenous androgens was clearly demonstrated by Henderson and Moon (1979) during the first 2 days of culture of large antral follicular cells. This positive effect on aromatization and on inhibin production does not require any exogenous FSH. Another demonstration of the association of androgen aromatization and inhibin pro-

Table I. Secretion of progesterone (P_4), 17 β-oestradiol (O_2) and inhibin (Inh.) on the 4th day of granulosa and luteal cell culture (10^4).

Treatment	Granulosa cells (10^4)			Luteal cells (10^4)		
	P_4 (ng)	O_2 (pg)	Inh. (mU)	P_4 (ng)	O_2 (pg)	Inh. (mU)
None (5)[c]	0.6 ± 0.09[a]	30 ± 12	0	4.5 ± 0.2	33 ± 10	0
PMSG : 0.02 U/ml + T5·10^{-7} M (5)[c]	0.82 ± 0.10	1.100 ± 89[b]	537 ± 45[b]	5.5 ± 0.6	670 ± 68[b]	262 ± 48[b]

[a] M ± SE; [b] $P < 0.01$ compared with the untreated culture; [c] ( ) number of culture.

duction is provided by cultures of gonadotrophin-induced granulosa and luteal cells in immature female rats. In control culture, no inhibin and very low amounts of oestradiol were detected after 4 days. In contrast, a significant increase of oestradiol and inhibin production was observed when PMSG and T were added to the culture.

It may be concluded that the principal source of inhibin is granulosa cells when they are capable of aromatizing testosterone into oestrogens and when they are non-luteinized. Luteinization of granulosa cells and subsequent luteal cell formation are associated with an increase of progesterone production and a loss in androgen aromatization and in inhibin production.

ACKNOWLEDGEMENTS

This work was supported by grants No. 74.039 of WHO, Geneva, and No. 3.4501.80 of Belgian Foundation for Medical Research (FRSH).

REFERENCES

Borth, R. (1976). *In* "Methods of Hormone Analysis" (H. Breuer, D. Hamel and H. L. Krüskemper Eds), 500–513. Georg Thieme Verlag, Stuttgart; John Wiley and Sons, New York.

Channing, C. P., Anderson, L. and Hodgen, G. D. (1980). *In* "VI International Congress of Endocrinology", Abst. no 178, 298, Melbourne.

Chappel, S. C., Acott, T. and Spies, H. G. (1979). *In* "Ovarian Follicular and Corpus Luteum Function" (C. P. Channing, J. Marsh and W. Sadler, Eds), 361. Plenum Press, New York.

Chari, S., Hopkinson, C. R. N., Daume, E. and Sturm, G. (1979). *Acta Endocrinologica* **90**, 157.

Croze, F. and Franchimont, P. (1981). In preparation.

De Jong, F. H. and Sharpe, R. M. (1976). *Nature* **263**, 71.

De Jong, F. H., Smith, S. D. and Van der Molen, H. J. (1979). *Journal of Endocrinology* **80**, 91.

De Paolo, L. V., Shander, D., Wise, P. M., Barraclough, C. A. and Channing, C. P. (1979). *Endocrinology* **105**, 647.

Dorrington, J. H. and Armstrong, D. T. (1975). *Proceedings of the National Academy of Sciences* **72**, 2677.

Dulbecco, R. and Freeman, G. (1959). *Virology* **8**, 396.

Eddie, L. W., Baker, H. W. G., Higginson, R. E. and Hudson, B. (1979). *Journal of Endocrinology* **81**, 49.

Erickson, G. F. and Hsueh, A. J. W. (1978). *Endocrinology* **103**, 1960.

Franchimont, P., Demoulin, A., Verstraelen–Proyard, J., Hazee–Hagelstein, M. T., Walton, J. S. and Waites, G.M.H. (1978). *International Journal of Andrology*, Suppl. 2, 69.

Franchimont, P., Demoulin, A., Verstraelen–Proyard, J., Hazee–Hagelstein, M. T. and Tunbridge, W.M.G. (1979a). *Journal of Reproduction and Fertility* Suppl. 26, 123.

Franchimont, P., Verstraelen–Proyard, J., Hazee–Hagelstein, M. T., Renard, Ch., Demoulin, A., Bourguignon, J. P. and Hustin, J. (1979b). *In* "Vitamins and Hormones", Vol. 37, 243.

Henderson, K. M. and Moon, Y. S. (1979). *Journal of Reproduction and Fertility* **56**, 89.

Hopkins, C. R. and Farquhar, M. G. (1973). *Journal of Cellular Biology* **59**, 276.

Hopkinson, C.R.H., Sturm, G., Daume, E., Fritze, E. and Hirschhauser, C. (1975). *International Research Communication System* **3**, 588.

Hopkinson, C.R.N., Daume, E., Sturm, G., Fritze, E., Kaiser, S. and Hirschhauser, C. (1977). *Journal of Reproduction and Fertility* **50**, 93.

Hudson, B., Baker, H. W. G., Eddie, L. W., Higginson, R. E., Burger, H. G., De Kretser, D. M., Dobos, M. and Lee, V. W. K. (1979). *Journal of Reproduction and Fertility* Suppl. 26, 17.

Lee, V. W. K., Scott, R. S., Dobos, M., Zachariah, E., De Kretser, D. M. and Burger, H. G. (1979). *In* "Recent Advances in Reproduction and Regulation of Fertility" (G. P. Talwar, Ed.) 241–252. Elsevier, North Holland, Biomedical Press.

Lorenzen, J. R., Channing, C. P. and Schwartz, H. B. (1978). *Biology of Reproduction* **19**, 635.

Marder, M. L., Channing, C. P. and Schwartz, N. B. (1977). *Endocrinology* **101**, 1639.

Orczyk, G. P., Hichens, M., Arth, G. and Behrman, H. R. (1974). *In* "Methods of Hormone Radioimmunoassay" (B. M. Jaffe and H. R. Behrman. Eds) 347–358. Academic Press, New York.

Welschen, R., Hermans, W. P., Dullaart, J. and De Jong, F. H. (1977). *Journal of Reproduction and Fertility* **50**, 129.

BIOLOGICAL ACTIONS OF INHIBIN IN
EXPERIMENTAL ANIMALS

G. Lugaro, M. M. Casellato, E. Manera, M. A. Bacigalupo, L. Riboni[1]
and G. Fachini[2]

Laboratorio di Chimica degli Ormoni, CNR, Via Mario Bianco, Milano; [1] *Istituto
di Patologia Generale dell'Università di Milano and* [2] *Laboratorio di Fisiologia
ed Anatomia, Istituto di Zootecnia, Università di Milano, Italy*

INTRODUCTION

The male and female germinal epithelium produces a water-soluble, non-steroidal factor, called inhibin* (McCullagh, 1932) or X-hormone (Klinefelter *et al.*, 1942), which partially and quite selectively regulates the peripheral concentration of the follicle stimulating hormone (FSH). Indeed, the presence of the dual stimulation of the testis by the pituitary FSH and the luteinizing hormone (LH) also suggests a dual hormonal secretion by male gonads. LH stimulates testosterone synthesis and secretion by the interstitial tissue (Leydig cells): then testosterone plasma concentration exerts a negative feedback control at hypothalamic level for pituitary LH release. FSH stimulates the seminiferous tubules (essentially Sertoli cells) and indirectly, the spermatogenic processes (Androgen Binding Protein synthesis, aromatizing enzymatic system activation, etc.).

Inhibin, a non-steroidal and non-androgenic factor, synthesized at tubular level (Sertoli cells, spermatogenetic cells?) would appear to be the negative feedback link for FSH secretion, which acts at pituitary or hypothalamic level. The

---

*We refer, therewith, to inhibin of testicular origin.

Serono Symposium No. 39, "The Menopause: Clinical, Endocrinological and Pathophysiological Aspects", edited by P. Fioretti, L. Martini, G. B. Melis and S. S. C. Yen, 1982. Academic Press, London and New York.

testicular androgens indeed cannot account for the full feedback control of FSH because a significant proportion of this control mechanism remains unexplained without the inhibin hypothesis. In fact, steroid hormone administration depresses FSH release, but only when LH release is already depressed (Setchell *et al.*, 1977). Bramble *et al.* (1975) assert that "testosterone plays no part in the control of FSH secretion within the physiological range" and that "FSH is normally controlled by inhibin alone".

Evidence for the existence of inhibin comes from various experiments in which germinal male tissue is selectively damaged, apparently without effect on testosterone synthesis. Local X-irradiation destroys dividing spermatogonia (this technique was already being used in 1923 by Mottram and Cramer, in demonstrating the existence of the second testicular hormone): an increased release of pituitary gonadotropins has been observed, with little or no effect on testosterone synthesis and secretion. In the same way, local heating (e.g., exposure of the testis at 43 °C for 30 min) causes a rise in plasma FSH level, and simultaneously a decrease in spermatid number (Main *et al.*, 1976). Experimentally cryptorchized animals also show a significant rise in plasma FSH and LH levels (Gupta *et al.*, 1975). Antispermatogenetic drgus induce changes in the pituitary hystological structure after more or less selective destruction of the germinal cells. For instance, cadmin salts, which produce severe necrosis of the testis (Gunn and Gould, 1975), diamines, which affect spermatid maturation and increase urinary excretion of gonadotropins (Moore *et al.*, 1962); alkylating agents, like busulfan[†], which induce a marked rise in plasma FSH and LH levels, with a reduction in spermatid number (Debeljuk *et al.*, 1973; Gomes *et al.*, 1973).

In men treated with cytotoxic drugs it has been demonstrated that the disappearance of germinal epithelium (and the following azospermia) were associated with a significant rise in plasma FSH levels (Van Thiel *et al.*, 1972). So there are clinical conditions in men where the plasma and urinary FSH contents are selectively increased, and which are associated with abnormality in the seminiferous tubules without involvement of the Leydig cells (Klinefelter syndrome), with oligospermia or azospermia, and with the Sertoli syndrome alone (Setchell *et al.*, 1977). Lastly, severe damage to the spermatogenic cells always induces a marked rise in serum FSH concentration, even if androgen secretion is unaffected or little affected.

The original concept of inhibin, dating back to late 1932, is not yet accepted by all endocrinologists. As matter of fact, some authors refer to inhibin as a possible artifact (de Jong, 1979) or as an endocrine enigme (Main and Davies, 1979), some admit that inhibin modulates FSH secretion against a background of predominant control by androgens; others maintain that inhibin is the only factor responsible for FSH control in the male. It is worth noting that inhibin or, at least, the impure preparations of testicular and ovarian tissue available at the present time, the so-called "inhibin-like" factors, are not specific in some cases for FSH inhibition, since some physiological effects on LH secretion also occur. In connection with this, we advance a theory (later on reported) containing the hypothesis that inhibin activity is only a manifestation of a wider spectrum of actions exerted by the peptide family (deprimerones; Hillar and Preyjemski, 1979) of a type

---

[†]Butane-1, 4-dimethane sulfonate.

which interfere with transcriptional processes and maybe with other intranuclear processes (Fachini *et al.*, 1980).

Inhibin-like activity, the correct expression to indicate inhibinic factors, has been associated with a number of different molecular weight proteins and polypeptides (values from about 1 500 to more thatn 100 000 M_a). The possibility of aggregation and dissociation of subunits, or of binding to a protein carrier is, to date, an unsolved problem. Morcover, the existence of different principles acting on different levels of the hypothalamus–pituitary–gonad axis is also suggested.

SOURCES OF INHIBIN-LIKE FACTORS

Inhibin-like activity has been detected, in the male, in both components of semen; spermatozoa (Fachini *et al.*, 1963; Lugaro *et al.*, 1969, 1973, 1974) and seminal plasma (Franchimont, 1972; Franchimont *et al.*, 1975a, b, c, 1977, 1978); in epididymal homogenates (Le Lannou and Chambon, 1977); in the total testicular tisue extracts (Lee *et al.*, 1974a; Keogh *et al.*, 1976; Moodhidri *et al.*, 1976; Nandini *et al.*, 1976), in rete testis fluid (Setchell and Sirinathsinghji, 1972; Setchell and Jacks, 1974; Davies *et al.*, 1976; Blanc *et al.*, 1978) and testicular lymph (Baker *et al.*, 1976); in testicular fluid obtained after ligation of the efferent ducts (Davies *et al.*, 1978) and in extracts of blood from the internal spermatic vein of bulls (Fachini and Ciaccolini, 1966).

The blood-testis barrier may limit the passage into the blood or lymph stream of the inhibin-like factor(s) very probably synthetized inside the seminiferous tubules. Setchell (1970) hypothesizes that inhibin-like factor(s) "could leave the germinal epithelium with the spermatozoa and rete testis fluid and pass into the epididymis for reabsorption": so rete testis fluid could be the origin of the inhibin-like activity demonstrated by Fachini and Ciaccolini (1966) in the testicular venous plasma. Inhibin-like non-steroidal factors, recently named folliculostatin, are also present in bovine, porcine and human ovarian follicular fluid (de Jong and Sharpe, 1976; Schwartz and Channing, 1977; Marder *et al.*, 1977; Welschen *et al.*, 1977). At the present time, it does not seem necessary to postulate that different inhibin-like principles are secreted from male and female gonads.

CHEMICAL NATURE OF INHIBIN-LIKE FACTORS

The protein structure of inhibin-like factors has been shown to partially or completely destroy their activity by means of some proteolytic enzymes, such as trypsin (Lugaro *et al.*, 1973; Hopkinson *et al.*, 1977), pronase (Lugaro *et al.*, 1973; Baker *et al.*, 1978), pepsin etc. Nevertheless, the activity is not diminished by extraction with steroid solvents or activated charcoal (Fachini *et al.*, 1963; Franchimont *et al.*, 1975a, b; Baker *et al.*, 1976; Keogh *et al.*, 1976; Nandini *et al.*, 1976). Inhibin-like activity has been associated with a number of different molecular weight proteins and polypeptides; most of these data are based on the behaviour of the inhibin-like factors on gel-filtration columns (Sephadex). Franchimont *et al.* (1978), by extracting inhibin-like factors from human seminal plasma and ovine rete testis fluid, after purification on Sephadex G-100 and G-25 columns, found the activity (assayed *in vitro* and *in vivo*) to be associated with protein fractions of low molecular weight (5 000 and less than 5 000 M_a). Moodbidri *et al.* (1976) isolated an inhibin-like substance from ram testis homogenate having a molecular weight less than 5 000 M_a (metaphosphoric acid deproteinization and gel filtration on Sephadex G-75); de Jong *et al.* (1979a), purifying bovine follicular fluid by dialysis equilibrium, ultrafiltration, ethanol precipitation and gel-filtration on Sephadex G-100 and G-75, found molecular weights of about 10 000 M_a; Davies *et al.* (1978), after gel-filtration on Sephadex G-200, G-100, G-75 and ion-exchange on DEAF-Sephadex of ovine rete testis fluid, obtained active fractions (*in vivo* and *in vitro*) having molecular weights of about 90 000, 20 000 and less than 5 000 M_a. Chari *et al.* (1978a, b) reported molecular weights of 19 000 M_a (purification from bull seminal plasma using ethanol precipitation, gel-filtration on Sephadex G-100 in urea and ion-exchange techniques) and of more than 25 000 M_a (extraction from human follicular fluid using ammonium sulphate salting out, gel-filtration on Sephadex G-100 and ion exchange chromatography).

Cahoreau *et al.* (1979) extracted an active protein (molecular weight of more than 100 000 M_a) from ovine rete testis fluid using ultrafiltration, ethanol fractionation and gel-filtration on Sephadex G-200. The widely assigned molecular weights suggest that inhibin-like factors so far purified could be oligomeric molecules or could be bound to protein carriers, i.e. the inhibin could be a small active polypeptide associated with one or more inactive proteins (Chari *et al.*, 1978b; Davies *et al.*, 1978; Franchimont *et al.*, 1978).

The "spread" of activity is generally found in fractions obtained using ion-exchange chromatography, where separation is based more on charge than on molecular weight. The inhibin-like factor, extracted from bull spermatozoa by Lugaro *et al.* (1969, 1973, 1974), appears on the contrary to be a small peptide. Furthermore, the active ninhydrin-positive spot present in the most purified fraction moves an appreciable distance from the origin during high voltage paper electrophoresis, suggesting that fairly small peptides are involved (molecular weight about 1 500 M_a).

BIOLOGICAL DETECTION OF INHIBIN-LIKE FACTORS

Since no purified inhibin preparations are available, it is not possible to exclude inhibin effects on LH secretion. However, to date, it seems reasonable to define inhibin as (a) water-soluble gonadal factor(s), which almost exert(s) an inhibiting effect on FSH release from the pituitary. Therefore the assays for inhibin-like activities depend on the measurement of the reduction in FSH secretion.

In Vivo Assays

Suppresion of Plasma FSH During
Intravenous Infusion
In castrated sheep, an i.v. or intracarotid infusion of testis extracts for 24 h has been shown to reduce plasma FSH levels from 40 to 60% (Keogh *et al.*, 1976; Blanc *et al.*, 1978). Similar results have been obtained in rabbits.

Prevention of the Postcastration Rise in
Plasma FSH in Rats

The greatest suppression of FSH (a reduction of 75% can be evidenced and a dose-response ratio has been demonstrated) was observed after administration of follicular fluid extracts to acutely unilaterally ovariectomized rats (Marder *et al.*, 1977; Welschen *et al.*, 1977). De Jong and Sharpe (1979) obtained an inhibition in plasma FSH levels of about 45% by administering follicular fluid extracts in acutely castrated adult male rats; reductions of 50–65% have been achieved by Nandini *et al.* (1976) using testis extracts in acutely castrated immature male rats. Setchell *et al.* (1977) assert that this technique is probably the simplest to use and will probably become the standard *in vivo* assay.

Suppression of Plasma FSH in Intact Rats

By treating intact adult male or female rats with testicular and follicular extracts, Franchimont *et al.* (1975a), Marder *et al.* (1977), Welschen *et al.* (1977) and de Jong *et al.* (1978) reported that the reduction in plasma FSH levels ranges from 20–40%.

Suppression of Plasma FSH in Long-term
Castrated Rats

Hopkinson *et al.* (1977) and Welschen *et al.* (1977) obtained a reduction in plasma FSH of about 40%, without any effect on plasma LH, by administering follicular fluid extracts in long-term ovariectomized rats. Using testicular and follicular extracts, Setchell and Jacks (1974), Franchimont *et al.* (1975a), Lee *et al.* (1977) and Hopkinson *et al.* (1977) achieved reductions in plasma FSH levels in long-term castrated adult male rats, with a variable inhibitory effect on LH levels.

Lugaro *et al.* (1974) demonstrated that the small peptide inhibin-like factor, extracted and partially purified from bull spermatozoa, reduces the plasma FSH levels in long-term castrated male rats by about 65%, without any effect on LH, when administered intraventricularly (Tables I and II). LH release is affected by this factor, only when injected i.v., i.p. and s.c. (Lugaro *et al.*, 1979; Lugaro, unpublished data). The same results have been reported by Le Lannou and Chambron (1977).

Reduction of the Uterine or Ovarian Response
to hCG in Immature Female Mice and Rats

This assay depends on the reduced sensitivity of the uterus and ovaries to hCG when the FSH in the plasma of the recipient animal is reduced (Chari *et al.*, 1976).

Parabiosis

This assay is based on the suppression of the weight of the uterus and ovaries in parabiotic pairs of immature female–mature castrated female rats (Fachini *et al.*, 1963; Lugaro *et al.*, 1969, 1973). This technique has the advantage of using a biological system for assaying the pituitary FSH secretion.

Prevention of the Prepuberal Rise in FSH in
Male Rats

The subcutaneous administration for 3 weeks of the inhibin-like spermato-

Table I. Effect of inhibin-like factor extracted from bull spermatozoa on serum FSH levels in long-term castrated male rats, when injected intraventricularly (Lugaro et al., 1974). Differences are highly significant ($P < 0.001$) between control (−30 min) and treated groups except for [b]

Dose (µg/rat)	No. animals	ng FSH/ml serum ± SE[a]			
		−30 min	+30 min	+60 min	+90 min
Saline	17	1079 ± 20	1125 ± 24	1121 ± 20	1091 ± 19
50	18	1091 ± 22	715 ± 25	548 ± 13	505 ± 9
10	18	1111 ± 27	538 ± 9	420 ± 12	827 ± 23
1	18	1122 ± 20	638 ± 21	410 ± 15	800 ± 10
0.1	12	1051 ± 33	779 ± 23	739 ± 26	894 ± 22[b]

[a]Daane and Parlow, 1971, in terms of NIAMDD–Rat–FSH–RP–I.

Table II. Effect of inhibin-like factor extracted from bull spermatozoa on serum LH levels in long-term castrated male rats, when injected intraventricularly (Lugaro et al., 1974).

Dose (μg/rat)	No. animals	ng LH/ml serum ± SE[a]			
		−30 min	+30 min	+60 min	+90 min
Saline	18	17.6 ± 0.5	16.7 ± 0.5	16.0 ± 0.6	15.2 ± 0.3
50	18	15.4 ± 0.4	16.1 ± 0.3	—	14.8 ± 0.5
10	17	16.4 ± 0.6	15.6 ± 0.6	14.6 ± 0.4	14.1 ± 0.5
1	18	15.0 ± 0.6	16.7 ± 0.7	16.4 ± 0.4	14.8 ± 0.5

[a]Niswender et al., 1968, in terms of NIH–LH–S–16.

zoan factor to immature male rats (20 days old) reduces plasma FSH levels by
about 60% (maximum 80%), and plasma LH levels by about 50% (Lugaro *et al.*,
1979; Table III).

In Vitro Assays

Several detection systems for the evaluation of inhibin-like activity are based
on the changes in the concentration of radioimmunoassayble gonadotropins in
the medium of cultured pituitary cells. Steinberger and Steinberger (1976)
observed a selective suppression in medium FSH levels of about 60-75% using a
Sertoli cells culture; similar results were obtained by de Jong *et al.* (1978, 1979b)
and Labrie *et al.* (1978) using follicular fluid extracts. Inhibition in medium
FSH levels of 60-75%, and in LH of 30-40%, has been reported by Baker *et al.*
(1978), de Jong *et al.* (1978, 1979a) and Labrie *et al.* (1978) in LH-RH treated
pituitary cells. In incubated pituitary halves, inhibin-like extracts slightly reduce
the basal release of FSH, but exert a marked effect (suppression of about 60%)
after LH-RH stimulation (Davies *et al.*, 1978). In these cases, LH release is also
inhibited, although at higher doses. Therefore, it might be concluded that the
specificity of the system is better defined when non-stimulated pituitary cells
are used.

MODE OF ACTION OF INHIBIN-LIKE FACTORS

At present, the mechanism of action of inhibin-like factors is not clear. They
may suppress the synthesis of FSH: indeed in cultured pituitary cells, both the
amount of FSH secreted and the FSH cellular content is decreased (de Jong
et al., 1979a). The inhibin-like factors may interfere with the metabolism of
pituitary cells (LH and FSH are synthetized in the same cells) or with phosphorila-
tion LH-RH regulated via C-AMP protein Kinase (de Jong, 1979).

The data (Tables IV and V) reported by Lugaro *et al.* (1974) and by Le Lannou
and Chambon (1977) indicate that the inhibition of pituitary FSH release might
be due to a highly-decreased concentration of a hypothetical FSH-RH (quite
distinct from LH-RH) at the hypothalamic level. We hypothesize that the spermatozoan inhibin-like factor acts by blocking FSH-RH synthesis, probably at
transcriptional level (cf. below). The finding of a factor that inhibits FSH release
in a highly specific fashion might help to answer the question of whether there
is a single or two releasing factors for FSH and LH.

SITE OF SYNTHESIS OF INHIBIN-LIKE FACTORS

It is most probable that all the inhibin-like factors isolated till now originate,
in the male, inside the seminiferous tubules, as clearly demonstrated in heat-
treated, drug-treated and X-irradiated rats (see above). In the female, the source
of inhibin-like activity might be the granulosa cells (de Jong and Sharpe, 1976;
Erickson and Hsueh, 1978). Some authors (Johnsen, 1964, 1970; Franchimont,
1972; Börsh *et al.*, 1973; Christiansen, 1975) have demonstrated a correlation

Table III. Effect of inhibin-like factor extracted from bull spermatozoa on immature male 20 day old rats (Lugaro *et al.*, 1980). Differences are highly significant ($P < 0.001$) between control and treated groups.

Measurement	Dose	Days			
		0	11	18	25
FSH (ng/ml)[a]	Control	562 ± 32	1056 ± 39	1320 ± 86	1329 ± 23
	T_1		753 ± 42	741 ± 31	758 ± 38
	T_2		508 ± 23	482 ± 31	513 ± 32
LH (ng/ml)[b]	Control	235 ± 54	278 ± 24	186 ± 26	224 ± 11
	T_1		107 ± 12	81 ± 7	140 ± 7
	T_2		123 ± 8	79 ± 7	132 ± 4

[a]Daane Parlow, 1971, in terms of NIAMDD–Rat–FSH–RP–1; [b]Daane Parlow, 1971, in terms of NIAMDD–Rat–LH–RP–1; T_1 = dose equivalent to 5×10^7 spermatozoa; T_2 = dose equivalent to 5×18^8 spermatozoa.

Table IV. Effect of hypothalamic extracts from long-term castrated male rats, intraventricularly treated with 10 μg of inhibin-like factor, on serum FSH levels of ovariectomized rats previously treated with oestradiol and progesterone (Lugaro *et al.*, 1974).

Treatment	No. animals	ng FSH/ml serum ± SE[a]	
		+20 min	+40 min
Saline	11	552 ± 15	517 ± 13
3/4 hypothalamus of male rat treated with saline	12	812 ± 24[b]	861 ± 15[b]
3/4 hypothalamus of male rat treated with 10 μg of inhibin-like factor	11	520 ± 16	507 ± 16

[a]In terms of NIAMDD–Rat–FSH–RP–1; [b] the differences from saline are highly significant (*P* < 0.001).

Table V. Effect of hypothalamic extracts from long-term castrated male rats, intraventricularly treated with 10 μg of inhibin-like factor, on serum LH levels of ovariectomized rats previously treated with oestradiol and progesterone (Lugaro *et al.*, 1974).

Treatment	No. animals	ng LH/ml serum ± SE[a]	
		+20 min	+40 min
Saline	12	5.8 ± 0.5	6.7 ± 0.5
3/4 hypothalamus of male rat treated with saline	11	14.5 ± 1.1[b]	8.7 ± 0.4[b]
3/4 hypothalamus of male rat treated with 10 μg of inhibin-like factor	11	16.7 ± 0.5[b]	10.5 ± 1.0[b]

[a] In terms of NIH–LH–S–16; [b] the differences from saline are highly significant ($P < 0.001$).

between elevated plasma and urine FSH levels and the decrease or absence of the late spermatids. The spermatogonial number in men was also significantly inversely correlated with plasma FSH level (de Kretser *et al.*, 1974; Baker *et al.*, 1976). In any case it is certain, and this is indeed the most important clinical observation, that "serum FSH level is *never* high when the late spermatid number is normal" (Setchell *et al.*, 1977).

Steinberger and Steinberger (1976) reported that pituitary cells showed a selective reduction in the output of FSH when cultured *in vitro* with isolated Sertoli cells. These data, and those reported by other authors (Rich and de Kretser, 1977; Labrie *et al.*, 1978; de Jong *et al.*, 1978, 1979b) suggested that the Sertoli cells could be the site of the production of inhibin-like factor(s), even if the possible role of spermatogenic cells, and particularly the later stages of spermatogenesis (de Jong and Sharpe, 1977; Hopkinson *et al.*, 1978) are not clear.

SITE OF ACTION OF INHIBIN-LIKE FACTORS

Inhibin-like factors, injected i.v. into castrated rats, block the effect of LH–RH on pituitary LH and FSH (Franchimont *et al.*, 1975a, b). The results obtained with cultured pituitary cells (Baker *et al.*, 1976; Davies *et al.*, 1976) demonstrate that inhibin-like factors block the stimulus of LH–RH on the pituitary. Lugaro *et al.* (1974) reported an effect on the hypothalamus of an inhibin-like factor extracted from bull spermatozoa: when injected into the cerebral ventricle, the content of FSH–RH in the hypothalamus of castrated male rats so treated was drastically reduced, while LH–RH was unaffected. It is possible that inhibin-like factors act on both the hypothalamus and the pituitary, according to the origin and/or the stage of purification of active extracts.

PHYSIOLOGICAL ROLE OF INHIBIN

The function of inhibin could be strictly correlated to the role of FSH in the control of spermatogenesis: increase in diameter of seminiferous tubules and in testis weight, synthesis of ABP, aromatizing enzymatic system activation, etc. Nevertheless, in adult male animals the role of FSH in the regulation of the testis is still little known. Setchell *et al.* (1977) assert that "if FSH has only a permissive effect on sperm production, the role of inhibin is probably to limit the rise in FSH which occurs at puberty" (Negro-Vilar *et al.*, 1973; Grumbach *et al.*, 1974; Lee *et al.*, 1974a, b; Gupta *et al.*, 1975; Baker *et al.*, 1976). This makes this importance of the presence of inhibin questionable. De Jong *et al.* (1978) reported that inhibin treatment lessens the development of spermatogenesis in immature males; Lugaro *et al.* (1979), on the contrary, demonstrated that in immature male rats, the suppression of FSH (about 65%) by chronic administration of an inhibin-like factor extracted from bull spermatozoa does not cause a delay in the morphological development of spermatogenesis. In the female, by regulating the peripheral concentration of FSH, follicular inhibin-like factors could modulate the development of ovarian follicles and consequently the secretion of oestrogen steroids.

CONCLUSIONS

De Jong (1979) states that, at the present time, the confusion concerning inhibin-like factors "is mainly caused by (1) differences in the definition of inhibin, (2) lack of a proper evaluation of many systems used for the assay and (3) the lack of a standard inhibin preparation". Last but not least, it is necessary to consider the paradox of a protein hormone secreted by a tissue of mesodermal origin. Main and Davies (1979) aptly said that it is possible that a new family of molecules involved in the control of germ cell differentiation is waiting to be discovered and that inhibin is one of these, being able to play a local role in the gonad itself. Therefore, we can summarize some considerations which arise from the fact that the inhibin-like factor extracted from bull spermatozoa shows regulatory effects on cellular kinetics, in all situations—such as castration, the climaterium and the peripuberal crisis—in which the cellular kinetics themselves appear to be altered. We also succeeded in demonstrating this activity, although with less intensity, in the water-soluble extracts of calf thymus. In this way, we were able to collect a considerable amount of results, which enabled us to supplement the data of the literature, and to propose a new interpretation of the data already known.

Amici and Gianfranceschi (1974), Amici *et al*. (1974, 1975, 1977) and Gianfranceschi *et al*. (1974) succeeded in showing that the pituitary-inhibiting extracts also exert their activity in many different conditions of altered cito-dynamics, completely outside the pituitary–gonad system. Fachini *et al*. (1977) believe, as was supposed by this author more than 20 years ago, that the inhibin-like activity at the level of the hyperactive pituitary in the castrate or immediately prepuberal animal, represents only one of the more general somatic responses. Namely, the experimental results seemed to confirm the presence in the inhibin-like extracts of a general type of biological non-gamic activities, that the gamete itself is capable of exerting, chiefly on the morphofunctional modifications of the senescene. Among the positive results obtained should be mentioned the research of Fachini and Pugliese (1961) on the capon and the photographic evidence of the clearing of the opacity of the crystalline lens in the senile cataract of the dog and rat (Fachini and Gianfranceschi, 1964), confirmed by Maselli *et al*. (1972) and more recently by Lugaro *et al*. (1980). Of particular interest is the highly significant stimulation of enzymatic induction in the liver of the senile rat (NADPH. oxydase, TAT, ALA-synthetase). This effect fails to appear in the young animal (Casellato *et al.*, 1980). All the effects described do not show any sex—or species—specificity. From this point of view, the inhibition of the hypothalamus–pituitary axis, usually referred to inhibin, could be intended as a particular event related to the peculiar sensitivity of the hypothalamic *relais*, in the more general phoenomenon of citodynamic homeostasis.

Our interpretative model of all the observed phenomena is based on the double activity of the active principle, both inhibitory and stimulatory, on the cellular dynamic and protein synthesis. We suppose a homeostatic intracellular type of activity, at the level of the dynamic of the information. Starting from this hypo-thesis, Gianfranceschi *et al.* (1975, 1976a, b; 1977) and Guglielmi *et al.* (1977) worked out a programme of control at biomolecular level, using peptide inhibin-like fraction(s) obtained from the calf thymus. They succeeded in confirming the hypothesis, showing that the proper point of impact of active principle(s) is transcriptional processes either in cell-free or cellular systems. More exactly, the inhibin-like factor(s) seem(s) to inhibit the initiation of m-RNA synthesis. The same activity, but much stronger, also appears using peptide fractions of gametic origin (spermatozoa and seminal plasma). So far, we cannot state whether the transcription–regulatory agent(s) can explain the complete biological activity, namely the stimulatory action, of the thymic and gametic extracts.

In conclusion, we can assert the following fundamental points. Active extracts obtained from spermatozoa are able to exert a temporary inhibition on the release of pituitary gonadotropins (mainly FSH) in any condition of exalted cellular functionality (castration, climaterium, peripuberal crisis, parabiosis). One of the target organs is probably the hypothalamus. The inhibin-like activity appears to be elicitable, chiefly but not exclusively, from gametic and para-gametic structures, without species–or sex–specificity. The active principle(s) seem(s) to be (a) non-hormonal and non-histonic peptide(s) of low molecular weight ($1\ 200\text{-}1\ 600\ M_a$), probably strongly bonded (hydrogen bonds?) to the spermatozoan DNA (bonded energy > 10 KCal/mole), and also present in the seminal plasma (from the spermatid?). The mechanism of action is probably to be referred to an effect of tonic inhibition of transcription. Inhibin, or at least some forms of inhibin, could be structurally similar or identical to depri-merones (Hillar and Przyjemski, 1979), a new family of low molecular weight peptides also strongly linked to spermatozoan DNA, which inhibit (or modulate) specific DNA-directed and chromatin-directed RNA-polymerase reactions.

REFERENCES

Amici, D. and Gianfranceschi, G. L. (1974). *Italian Journal of Biochemistry* **23**, 137–153.

Amici, D., Gianfranceschi, G. L., Marsili, G. and Michetti, L. (1974). *Experientia* **30**, 633–635.

Amici, D., Gianfranceschi, G. L. and Guglielmi, L. (1975). *Bollettino della Società Italiana di Biologia Sperimentale* **51**, 1497–1500.

Amici, D., Bossi, G. B., Cioé, L., Matarese, G. P., Dolei, A., Guglielmi, L. and Gianfranceschi, G. L. (1977). *Proceedings of National Academy of Science of USA* **74**, 3869–3873.

Baker, H. W. G., Bremner, W. J., Burger, H. G., de Kretser, D. M., Dulmanis, A., Eddie, L. H., Hudson, B., Keogh, E. J., Lee, V. W. K. and Rennie, G. C. (1976). *Recent Progress in Hormone Research* **32**, 429–469.

Baker, H. W. G., Burger, H. G., de Kretser, D. M., Eddie, L. W., Higginson, R. E. and Lee, V. W. K. (1978). *International Journal of Andrology* Suppl. 2, 115–124.

Blanc, M. R., Cahoreau, C., Courot, M., Dacheux, J. L., Hocheraude Reviers, M. T. and Pisselet, C. (1978). *International Journal of Andrology* Suppl. 2, 139–146.

Börsch, G., Hett, M., Mauss, J., Schach, H. and Scheidt, J. (1973). *Andrologie* **5**, 317–324.

Bramble, F. J., Broughton, A. C., Whittam, T. R., Eccles, S. S., Murray. M.A.F. and Jacobs, H. S. (1975). *Journal of Endocrinology* **65**, 11P.

Cahoreau, C., Blanc, M. R., Dacheux, J. L., Pisselet, C. and Courot, M. (1979). *Journal of Reproduction and Fertility* Suppl. 76, 97–116.

Casellato, M. M., Manera, E., Riboni, L., Comolli, R. and Lugaro, G. (1980). *Cancer Biochemie Biophysies* 4, (in press).

Chari, S., Duraiswami, S. and Franchimont, P. (1976). *Hormone Research* 7, 129–137.

Chari, S., Daume, E., Sturm, G. and Hopkinson, C. R. N. (1978a). *Acta Endocrinologica* (Copenhagen) Suppl. 215, 46.

Chari, S., Duraiswami, J. and Franchimont, P. (1978b). *Acta Endocrinologica* (Copenhagen) 87, 434–448.

Christiansen, P. (1975). *Acta Endocrinologica* (Copenhagen) 78, 192–208.

Daane, T. A. and Parlow, A. F. (1971). *Endocrinology* 88, 653–663.

Davies, R. V., Main, S. J., Young, M.G.W.L. and Setchell, B. P. (1976). *Journal of Endocrinologica* 68, 26P.

Davies, R. V., Main, S. J. and Setchell, B. P. (1978). *International Journal of Andrology* Suppl. 2, 102–114.

Debeljuk, L., Arimura, A. and Schally, A. V. (1973). *Endocrinology* 92, 48–54.

de Jong, F. H. (1979). *Molecular and Cellular Endocrinology* 13, 1–10.

de Jong, F. H. and Sharpe, R. M. (1976). *Nature* (London) 263, 71–72.

de Jong, F. H. and Sharpe, R. M. (1977). *Journal of Endocrinology* 75, 209–219.

de Jong, F. H., Welschen, R., Hermans, W. P., Smith, S. D. and van der Molen, H. J. (1978). *International Journal of Andrology* Suppl. 2, 125–138.

de Jong, F. H., Welschen, R., Hermans, W. P., Smith, S. D. and van der Molen, H. J. (1979a) *Journal of Reproduction and Fertility* Suppl. 76, 47–59.

de Jong, F. H., Smith, S. D. and van der Molen, H. J. (1979b). *Journal of Endocrinology* 80, 91–102.

de Kretser, D. M., Burger, H. G. and Hudson, B. (1974). *Journal of Clinical Endocrinology and Metabolism* 38, 787–793.

Erickson, G. F. and Hsueh, A. J. W. (1978). *Programe of the 60th Meeting of the American Endocrine Society* Abstract 540, p. 345.

Fachini, G. and Ciaccolini, C. (1966). *Endokrinologie* 50, 79–82.

Fachini, G. and Gianfranceschi, G. (1964). *Experientia* 20, 404–405.

Fachini, G. and Pugliese, A. (1961). *Atti della Società Italiana di Scienza Veterinaria XVth Meeting* 373–376.

Fachini, G., Toffoli, C., Gaudiano, A., Marabelli, M., Polizzi, M. and Mangili, G. (1963). *Nature* (London) 199, 195–196.

Fachini, G., Carrea, G., Gianfranceschi, G., Casellato, M. M. and Lugaro, G. (1977). *Revue roumene de Morphologie Embryologie Physiologie* 14, 193–205.

Fachini, G., Casellato, M. M., Manera, E., Bacigalupo, M. A., Riboni, L. and Lugaro, G. (1980). *9th International Congress on Animal Reproduction and AI* Madrid, (in press).

Franchimont, P. (1972). *Journal of Royal College of Physicians London* 6, 283–298.

Franchimont, P., Chari, S., Schellen, A. M. C. M. and Demoulin, A. (1975a). *Journal of Reproduction and Fertility* 44, 335–350.

Franchimont, P., Chari, S., Schellen, A.M.C.M. and Demoulin, A. (1975b). *Journal of Steroid Biochemistry* 6, 1037–1041.

Franchimont, P., Chari, S., Hagelstein, M. T. and Duraiswani, S. (1975c). *Nature* (London) 257, 402–404.

Franchimont, P., Chari, S., Hazee–Hagelstein, M. T., Debruche, M. L. and Duraiswani, S. (1977). *In* "The Testis in Normal and Infertile Man" (P. Troen and H. R. Naukin, Eds), 253–270. Raven Press, New York.

Franchimont, P., Demoulin, A., Verstraelen–Proyard, J., Hazee–Hagelstein, M. T., Walton, J. and Waites, G. (1978). *International Journal of Andrology* Suppl. 2, 69–80.

Gianfranceschi, G. L., Amici, D. and Guglielmi, L. (1974). *Experientia* **30**, 1049–1050.

Gianfranceschi, G. L., Amici, D. and Guglielmi, L. (1975). *Biochimica Biophysica Acta* **414**, 9–19.

Gianfranceschi, G. L., Amici, D. and Guglielmi, L. (1976a). *Nature* (London) **262**, 622–623.

Gianfranceschi, G. L., Amici, D. and Guglielmi, L. (1976b). *Molecular Biology Reproduction* **3**, 55–64.

Gianfranceschi, G. L., Guglielmi, L., Amici, D., Rossa, F., Barra, D. and Petruzzelli, R. (1977). *Molecular Biology Reproduction* **3**, 429–436.

Gomes, W. R., Hall, R. W., Jain, S. K. and Boots, D. R. (1973). *Endocrinology* **93**, 800–809.

Grumbach, M. M., Roth, J. C., Kaplan, S. L. and Kelck, R. P. (1974). *In* "Control of the Onset of Puberty" (M. M. Grumbach, G. D. Grave and F. E. Mayer, Eds), 115–181. Wiley, New York.

Guglielmi, L., Gianfranceschi, G. L., Venanzi, F., Polzonetti, A. and Amici, D. (1977). *Molecular Biology of Reproduction* **4**, 195–201.

Gunn, S. A. and Gould, T. C. (1975). *Handbook of Physiology* Section 7: *Endocrinology* **5**, 117–142.

Gupta, D., Rager, K., Zarzycki, J. and Eichner, M. (1975). *Journal of Endocrinology* **66**, 183–193.

Hillar, M. and Przyjemski, J. (1979). *Biochimica Biophysica Acta* **564**, 246–263.

Hopkinson, C. R. N., Daume, E., Sturm, G., Fritze, E., Kaiser, S. and Hirschhäuser, C. (1977). *Journal of Reproduction and Fertility* **50**, 93–96.

Hopkinson, C. R. N., Dulisch, B., Gauss, G., Hilscher, W. and Hirschhäuser, C. (1978). *Acta Endocrinologica* (Copenhagen) **87**, 413–423.

Johnsen, S. G. (1964). *Acta Endocrinologica* (Copenhagen) Suppl. 90, 99–124.

Johnsen, S. G. (1970). *Acta Endocrinologica* (Copenhagen) 64, 193–210.

Keogh, E. J., Lee, V. W. K., Rennie, G. C., Burger, H. G., Hudson, B. and de Kretser, D. M. (1976). *Endocrinology* **98**, 997–1004.

Klinefelter, H. F., Reifenstein, E. C. and Albright, F. (1942). *Journal of Clinical Endocrinology* **2**, 615–627.

Labrie, F., Lagacé, L., Ferland, L., Kelly, P. A., Drouin, J., Massicotte, J., Bonne, C., Raynaud, J. P. and Dorrington, J. H. (1978). *International Journal of Andrology* Suppl. 2, 203–318.

Lee, P. A., Jaffe, R. B. and Midgley, A. R. (1974a). *Journal of Clinical Endocrinology and Metabolising* **39**, 664–672.

Lee, V. W. K., Cumming, I. A., de Kretser, D. M., Findlay, J. K., Hudson, B. and Keogh, E. J. (1974b). *Journal of Reproduction and Fertility* **43**, 378–379.

Lee, V. W. K., Cumming, I. A., de Kretser, D. M. and Findlay, J. K. (1975). *Journal of Reproduction and Fertility* **46**, 494–495.

Lee, V. W. K., Pearce, P. T. and de Kretser, D. M. (1977). *In* "The Testis in Normal and Infertile Man" (P. Troen and H. R. Nankin, Eds) 293–303. Raven Press, New York.

Le Lannou, D. and Chambon, Y. (1977). *Comptes Rendus de la Société de Biologie* **171**, 636–638.

Lugaro, G., Giannattasio, G., Ciaccolini, C., Fachini, G. and Gianfranceschi, G. (1969). *Experientia* **25**, 147–148.

Lugaro, G., Carrea, G., Casellato, M. M., Mazzola, G. and Fachini, G. (1973). *Biochimica Biophysica Acta* **304**, 719–724.

Lugaro, G., Casellato, M. M., Mazzola, G., Fachini, G. and Carrea, G. (1974). *Neuroendocrinology* **15**, 62–68.

Lugaro, G., Casellato, M. M., Manera, E., Pasta, P., Bacigalupo, M. A. and Lauria, A. (1979). *Journal of Reproduction and Fertility* Suppl. 26, 193–196.

Lugaro, G., Casellato, M. M., Manera, E., Bacigalupo, M. A., Maselli, E. and Fachini, G. (1980). *British Journal of Ophthalmogic* 64, (in press).

Main, S. J. and Davies, R. V. (1979). *TIBS* 4, N128.

Main, S. J., Davies, R. V., Young, M. G. W. L. and Setchell, B. P. (1976). *Journal of Endocrinology* 69, 23P.

Marder, M. L., Channing, C. P. and Schwartz, N. B. (1977). *Endocrinology* 101, 1639–1642.

Maselli, E., Fachini, G. and Lugaro, G. (1972). *Atti LIV Congresso della Società Oftalmologica Italiana,* Roma.

McCullagh, D. R. (1932). *Science* 76, 19–20.

Moodbidri, S. B., Josji, L. R. and Sheth, A. R. (1976). *IRCS Medical Science* 4, 217.

Moore, D. J., Roscoe, R. T., Matson, L. J. and Heller, C. G. (1962). *Clinical Research* 10, 88 (Abstract only).

Mottram, J. C. and Cramer, W. (1923). *Quarterly Journal of Experimental Physiology* 13, 209–229.

Nandini, S. G., Lipner, H. and Moudgal, N. R. (1976). *Endocrinology* 98, 1460–1465.

Negro-Vilar, A., Krulich, L. and McCann, S. M. (1973). *Endocrinology* 93, 660–661.

Niswender, G. D., Midgley, A. R., Jr, Monroe, S. E. and Reichert, L. E., Jr (1968). *Proceedings of the Society Experimental Biology and Medicine* 128, 807–811.

Rich, K. A. and de Kretser, D. M. (1977). *Endocrinology* 101, 959–968.

Schwartz, N. B. and Channing, C. P. (1977). *Proceedings of the National Academy of Science (USA)* 74, 5721–5724.

Setchell, B. P. (1970). *In* "The Testis" (A. D. Johnson, W. R. Gomes and N. L. Van Demark, Eds), Vol. 1, 109–239. Academic Press, New York.

Setchell, B. P. and Jacks, F. (1974). *Journal of Endocrinology* 62, 675–676.

Setchell, B. P. and Sirinathsinghji, D. J. (1972). *Journal of Endocrinology* 53, lx–lxi.

Setchell, B. P., Davies, R. V. and Main, S. J. (1977). *In* "The Testis" (A. D. Johnson and W. R. Gomes, Eds), Vol. IV, 189–238. Academic Press, New York.

Steinberger, A. and Steinberger, E. (1976). *Endocrinology* 99, 918–921.

Van Thiel, D. H., Sherins, R. J., Myers, G. H., Jr and Da Vita, V. T. (1972). *Journal Clinical Investigation* 51, 1009–1019.

Welschen, R., Hermans, W. P., Dullaart, J. and de Jong, F. H. (1977). *Journal of Reproduction and Fertility* 50, 129–131.

OVARIAN STEROID PRODUCTION AND METABOLISM IN PRE- VERSUS POSTMENOPAUSAL WOMEN

J. P. Felber, M. Gasperi and G. Magrini

Division de Biochimie Clinique, Départment de Médicine, C.H.U.V., Lausanne, Switzerland

INTRODUCTION

During normal reproductive life virtually all 17β-oestradiol is secreted by the ovary (Baird, 1976). By the seventh day of the cycle, the preovulatory follicle is secreting over 90% of the 17β-oestradiol while in the luteal phase, almost all the oestradiol originates from the corpus luteum, as is the case for progesterone. Both oestrone and oestradiol derive from androgens as precursors and their biosynthesis is the result of the aromatization of androstenedione and testosterone. Oestrone is also a product from oestradiol metabolism through the mechanism of interconversion of these oestrogens.

At the menopause, the ovaries lose their cyclic secretory activity, as an inevitable consequence of the progressive atresia of the ovarian follicles. The ovaries however still retain some secretory activity, as shown by ovariectomy performed in postmenopausal women. After bilateral surgical removal of ovaries in postmenopausal women, no changes occur in oestrone and oestradiol, but a significant decrease in testosterone and androstenedione is observed, indicating that androgens are normally produced by postmenopausal ovaries (Judd *et al.*, 1974a; Vermeulen, 1976).

Serono Symposium No. 39, "The Menopause: Clinical, Endocrinological and Pathophysiological Aspects", edited by P. Fioretti, L. Martini, G. B. Melis and S. S. C. Yen, 1982. Academic Press, London and New York.

PERIMENOPAUSAL OESTROGEN PRODUCTION

With increasing age, the ovarian oestrogenic secretion significantly changes in character. In a group of five women, aged 40–41, Sherman and Korenman (1979) observed a shortened follicular phase but the hormone values did not differ significantly from those observed in younger subjects. In six premenopausal women, aged 46–51, the follicular phase was still shorter. 17β-oestradiol secretion was markedly diminished during both the late follicular and the mid-luteal phases. In all the cases under observation, FSH was persistantly high despite normal LH and progesterone levels. Thus the major change in plasma steroid concentration resulting from primary ovarian failure is a decline in peripheral oestradiol levels, even though some residual secretion is still present in the immediate years following menopause as shown by Vermeulen and Verdonck (1979). These authors demonstrated, in a study involving 100 postmenopausal women, that the oestradiol/oestrone ratio was higher in a group of 15 patients in the first 4 years within menopause than in another group of 55 women in whom the menopause had lasted for more than 4 years and up to 40 years.

POSTMENOPAUSAL OESTROGEN PRODUCTION

In late menopause, the ovary secretes only minimal amounts of oestrogens: in age matched ovariectomized women, the mean plasma oestrogen levels are not significantly different from values in women who had a natural menopause (Vermeulen, 1976). Similarly Barlow *et al.* (1969) were unable to show a decrease in oestradiol production following ovariectomy in postmenopausal women with breast cancer. In comparing data from the literature, the analytical difficulties existing in a precise evaluation of such extremely low levels of oestrogens must however be kept in mind. These data are also supported by results obtained directly in ovarian venous blood of postmenopausal women, even though data on blood flow are lacking. Judd *et al.* (1974b) showed only a two-fold increase in the ovarian vein blood oestradiol levels in comparison with the peripheral blood levels, in a group of nine women undergoing bilateral ovariectomy. This difference, although significant, is small compared with the differences reported in premenopausal patients by Lloyd *et al.* (1971) and would account only for minimal ovarian secretion in postmenopause. Evidence exists however for an extraglandular production of oestrogens after the menopause. As shown by Grodin *et al.* (1973), the principal oestrogen formed in postmenopausal women is oestrone, which is derived from androstenedione. Androstenedione is secreted mainly by the adrenals, with some participation of the ovaries. The aromatization of androstenedione seems to be almost entirely extraglandular. It occurs in part in adipose tissue (Schindler *et al.*, 1972). A significant correlation has been demonstrated by Vermeulen and Verdonck (1979) between obesity (fat mass) on the one side, and oestrone and oestradiol levels on the other side.

OESTROGENS AFTER MEDICAL ADRENALECTOMY

The problem of the aromatization of androstenedione into oestrone has been found to be of major interest in the endocrine treatment of metastatic or inoperable breast cancer. On the basis of *in vitro* experiments, aminoglutethimide (elipten) has been thought to have its main point of attack at the conversion of cholesterol to Δ5 pregnenolone, i.e. at the very beginning of the chain reaction that leads to the synthesis of adrenal cortical steroids. This is corroborated by the accumulation of cholesterol in the adrenal cortex following long-term treatment with aminoglutethimide. This leads to the use of the drug as an agent for "medical adrenalectomy". Treatment with aminoglutethimide resulted in objective remissions of both tumor and metastases in approximately one third of the treated patients (Lipton and Santen, 1974; Santen *et al.,* 1977a; Samojlik *et al.,* 1977). In postmenopausal women using a daily dose of 1000 mg of the drug combined with 2 to 3 mg dexamethasone or 20 to 60 mg cortisol to prevent ACTH rise resulting from decreased cortisol levels induced by the drug, Santen *et al.* (1977b) found, unexpectedly, an initial increase of androstenedione, followed by a slow decrease after 8 to 12 weeks of treatment. In contrast, the levels of oestrone and oestradiol fell precipitously within the first week and remained very low during the entire treatment period. This striking discrepancy suggests that aminoglutethimide might inhibit the aromatization of androstenedione and that this aromatization might perhaps already be influenced by low doses of the drug. In order to verify this hypothesis, a preliminary study was undertaken in a group of postmenopausal women after mastectomy for metastatic cancer of the breast from the Division of Oncology, Department of Medicine, CHUV, Lausanne (Dr L. Barrelet). A daily dose of 300 mg aminoglutethimide, together with 1.5 mg dexamethasone was given to the patients for a period of 10 days. The results of the first three patients treated with this low dose show in two cases a rapid and marked fall in both oestrone and oestradiol levels (Fig. 1). Oestrone dropped from 62 and 38 pg/ml before treatment to 8 and 8 pg/ml on day 3, and oestradiol from 19 and 21 pg/ml to 12 and 7 pg/ml at the same time. Thus, in these two cases, the oestrone and oestradiol values decreased to similarly low levels as found by Santen *et al.* (1977b) following treatment with a higher dose of aminoglutethimide. The changes in plasma androstenedione levels were not important, the levels decreasing from 380 to 150 pg/ml in one case and from 700 to 480 pg/ml in the other. This is in contrast to the results of Santen *et al.* (1977a) who found a temporary increase of plasma androstenedione during the first weeks of treatment with a higher dose of aminoglutethimide. Plasma ACTH remained below 20 pg/ml in both cases throughout the study. The third case (Fig. 2) presented hyperprolactinaemia with plasma prolactin values between 30 and 74 ng/ml, probably as a consequence of brain metastases. In this case, a decrease in oestrone and oestradiol was observed during the first 3 days, even though ACTH and androstenedione were rising during the same time. The treatment was well tolerated by all three patients, with no side effects except for a minor skin rash in one of them.

These preliminary results strongly suggest that the lowering effect of amino-

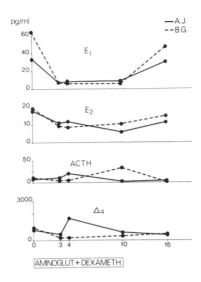

Fig. 1. Plasma oestrone (E1), oestradiol (E2), ACTH and androstenedione (Δ4) during treatment (from day 0 to day 10) with daily doses of 300 mg aminoglutethimide and 1.5 mg dexamethasone in two postmenopausal women.

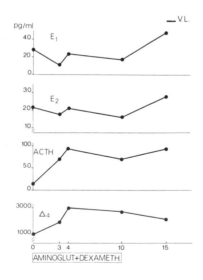

Fig. 2. Plasma oestrone (E1), oestradiol (E2), ACTH and androstenedione (Δ4) during treatment (from day 0 to day 10) with daily doses of 300 mg aminoglutethimide and 1.5 mg dexamethasone in a postmenopausal women with hyperprolactinemia.

glutethimide on oestrone and oestradiol results from a direct effect of the drug on the aromatization of androgens. Δ1-testololactone has also been reported to inhibit aromatization. Barone *et al.* (1979) showed that it causes a fall of oestrone, but however not of oestradiol. Another consequence of the gradual development of atresia of ovarian follicles in the menopause is the marked decrease in plasma progesterone. The low levels are almost exclusively of adrenal origin. Vermeulen (1976) has shown in postmenopausal women an increase by 500% in plasma progesterone levels after ACTH, a sharp decrease to almost undetectable levels after dexamethasone and no changes after HCG treatment.

PROGESTERONE AND ANDROGENS

Similarly, two metabolites of progesterone—the androgenic precursor 17α-hydroxyprogesterone and the progestin 20α-hydroxyprogesterone—are markedly decreased after the menopause. The low postmenopausal levels of 17α-hydroxyprogesterone are apparently exclusively of adrenal origin while 20α-hydroxyprogesterone become undetectable after the menopause (Abraham, 1974).

As far as the androgens are concerned, during the normal menstrual cycle, the ovary and the adrenal cortex seem to contribute roughly equally to peripheral testosterone, dihydrotestosterone and androstenedione, whereas DHEA–S originates predominantly from the adrenal cortex (Abraham, 1974). The *in vitro* studies of McNatty *et al.* (1979) have shown that granulosa cells from healthy follicles were producing large amounts of oestradiol, oestrone and progesterone. As the degenerative changes occurred, the granulosa cells dedifferenciated into androgen-producing cells since their capacity to produce androstenedione, testosterone and dihydrotestosterone was increasing with progressive follicular atresia. Eshkol and Lunenfeld (1977) have demonstrated that the response of the follicles to the LH surge in the normal cycle was dependent on the distribution of their LH and FSH receptors. Follicles not yet having LH receptors under the midcycle LH surge will produce thecal androgens in excess, which inhibit the binding of FSH, block the granulosa cells proliferation and promote progressive atresia. Follicular atresia may occur when the granulosa cells are locally deprived of FSH (McNatty *et al.*, 1979) or incapable of binding enough FSH (Lunenfeld and Insler, 1978) and is promoted by the local effects of an excess of ovarian androgens (Louvet *et al.*, 1975).

In postmenopausal women the ovary contributes to part of the total secretion of testosterone and androstenedione, as shown by stimulation–suppression studies, by comparison between ovariectomized and normal postmenopausal women and by direct ovarian samples obtained at the time for surgery from postmenopausal women undergoing bilateral ovariectomy (Vermeulen, 1976; Judd *et al.*, 1974b).

In conclusion, at the menopause, the progressive atresia of ovarian follicles ends in a loss of their cyclic activity. The ovaries lose almost completely their oestrogen and progesterone secretion, but maintain part of their androgen secretion through their relatively increased androgen contribution. Oestrone, and to a minor extent oestradiol, are still produced, essentially by aromatization in peripheral tissues of the androgens mostly of adrenal and to a lesser extent of ovarian origin.

Inhibition of aromatization can be achieved for therapeutical use by means of low doses of aminoglutethimide.

ACKNOWLEDGEMENTS

The authors should like to thank Dr F. Paesi, Ciba Geigy Co, Basle, for his help and support for part of this work.

REFERENCES

Abraham, G. E. (1974). *Journal of Clinical Endocrinology Metabolism* **39**, 340.

Abraham, G. E., Manlimos, F. S. and Garza, R. (1977). *In* "Handbook of Radioimmunoassay" (G. E. Abraham, Ed.), 591. Marcel Dekker Inc., New York, Basel.

Baird, D. T. (1976). *In* "The Endocrine Function of the Human Ovary" (V. H. T. James, M. Serio and G. Giusti, Eds), 125. Academic Press, London.

Barlow, J. J., Emerson, K. and Saxena, B. M. (1969). *New England Journal of Medicine* **280**, 633.

Barone, R. M., Shamonki, I. M., Siiteri, P. K. and Judd, H. L. (1979). *Journal of Clinical Endocrinology Metabolism* **49**, 672.

Eshkol, A. and Lunenfeld, B. (1977). *In* "Endocrinology" (V. H. T. James, Ed.), Vol. 1, 318. Excerpta Medica, Amsterdam.

Grodin, J. M., Siiteri, P. K. and MacDonald, P. C. (1973). *Journal of Clinical Endocrinology and Metabolism* **36**, 207.

Judd, H. L., Lucas, W. E. and Yen, S. C. C. (1974a). *American Journal of Obstetrics and Gynecology* **38**, 793.

Judd, H. L., Judd, G. E. and Lucas, W. E. (1974b). *Journal of Clinical Endocrinology and Metabolism* **39**, 1020.

Lipton, A. and Santen, R. J. (1974). *Cancer* **33**, 503.

Lloyd, C. W., Lobotsky, J., Baird, D. T., McCracken, J. A., Weisz, S., Pupkin, M., Zanartu, J. and Puga, J. (1971). *Journal of Clinical Endocrinology and Metabolism* **32**, 155.

Louvet, J. P., Harman, S. M., Schreiber, J. R. and Ross, J. T. (1975). *Endocrinology* **97**, 366.

Lunenfeld, B. and Insler, V. (1978). *In* "Diagnosis and Treatment of Functional Infertility". Grosse Verlag, Berlin.

McNatty, K. P., Makris, A., De Grazia, C., Osathanondh, R. and Ryan, K. J. (1979). *Journal of Steroid Biochemistry* **11**, 775.

Samojlik, E., Santen, R. J. and Wells, S. A. (1977). *Journal of Clinical Endocrinology Metabolism* **45**, 480.

Santen, R. J., Wells, S. A., Runic, S., Gupta, C., Kendall, J., Rudy, E. B. and Samojlik, E. (1977a). *Journal of Clinical Endocrinology and Metabolism* **45**, 469.

Santen, R. J., Samojlik, E., Lipton, A., Harvey, H., Ruby, E. B., Wells, S. A. and Kendall, J. (1977b). *Cancer* **39**, 2948.

Schindler, A. E., Ebert, A. and Friedrich, E. (1972). *Journal of Clinical Endocrinology and Metabolism* **35**, 627.

Sherman, B. M. and Korenman, S. G. (1979). *Journal of Clinical Investigation* **55**, 699.

Vermeulen, A. (1976). *Journal of Clinical Endocrinology and Metabolism* **42**, 247.

Vermeulen, A. and Verdonck, L. (1979). *Journal of Steroid Biochemistry* **11**, 899.

ADRENAL FUNCTION IN POSTMENOPAUSAL WOMEN

A. Vermeulen

*Department of Endocrinology and Metabolic diseases, Academic Hospital,
University of Ghent, Belgium*

INTRODUCTION

It is well known that, except for the immediate postmenopausal years, the
postmenopausal ovaries do not secrete any significant amount of oestrogens.
They do continue to secrete some testosterone (T) (Judd *et al.,* 1974; Vermeulen,
1976; Botella-Llusia *et al.,* 1980), but by far the most important source of sex
hormones are the adrenals. This is evident from the comparison of plasma sex
hormone levels between women in spontaneous menopause and women of similar
age, having undergone bilateral ovariectomy, the most significant difference
being a lower plasma T level in the latter group. If we compare, on the other
hand, the levels in spontaneous menopause to those in postmenopausal women
with adrenal cortical insufficiency, we observe that, except for only moderately
decreased plasma T levels, all sex hormone levels are extremely low in the latter
group, pointing towards the adrenals as the major source of the sex hormones.
Several factors may influence plasma sex hormone levels in postmenopausal
women. Besides pulsatile as well as nycthemeral variations in sex hormone levels,
making it necessary to take several plasma samples in order to obtain a mean
value which is representative for the situation prevailing over 24 h, other factors
appear to determine sex hormone levels in postmenopausal women.

STEROID METABOLISM AFTER MENOPAUSE

Age or years of postmenopause (YPM) was the first factor we studied. Plasma
levels of dehydroepiandrosterone (D) and its sulphate (DS) as well as of androst-

Serono Symposium No. 39, "The Menopause: Clinical, Endocrinological and Pathophysiological Aspects", edited by P. Fioretti, L. Martini, G. B. Melis and S. S. C. Yen, 1982. Academic
Press, London and New York.

5-ene-3β-17β diol (D5 diol) decrease significantly with YPM ($P < 0.05$), but neither androstenedione (A), estrone (E_1) nor estradiol (E_2) levels showed any significant relation with years of postmenopause (spontaneous MP). The E_1/A ratio, however, showed a borderline significant ($P < 0.05$) negative correlation with age (Vermeulen and Verdonck, 1978). As the metabolic clearance rate of neither DS nor D5 diol shows any age dependent increase, the decreased plasma levels reflect a decreased secretion rate and, as this age dependent decrease in D, DS and D5 diol levels was also observed in ovariectomized patients, it should be concluded that this decrease has an adrenal origin. As, on the other hand, cortisol secretion is largely age independent, the findings point towards changing biosynthetic pathways in the ageing adrenals.

It is remarkable that androstenedione levels apparently do not decrease with YPM and, although this might be fortuitous, we observed in ageing males a similar dissociation between an important decrease of D and DS levels on the one hand, and hardly decreasing androstenedione levels on the other hand.

We were therefore interested in the adrenal response upon stimulation with ACTH, 0.25 mg i.v.: D and D5 diol levels in postmenopausal women did increase, but the levels always remained below the values obtained after ACTH stimulation during reproductive life; A levels, on the other hand, increased to levels higher than those during reproductive life. Moreover, as in postmenopausal women we observed a lower response of 17-OH-Pregnenolone (17-OHP) levels, whereas the response of 17-OH-P and of progesterone (P) was even higher than during reproductive life, our data suggest an increased conversion of Δ-5 steroids to Δ-4 steroids in the ageing adrenals.

As to the factor(s) responsible for this age dependent decrease in Δ-5 steroids, it has been suggested that oestrogen deficiency might be responsible. This is however rather improbable, in view on the one hand of the fact that DS levels decrease with years of postmenopause, whereas after menopause oestrogen levels remain constant, and on the other hand that we observe the same phenomenon in the male, where, if anything, oestrogen levels increase with age. Moreover, oestrogen administration for 6 months did not change DS levels (Fig. 1). This is at variance

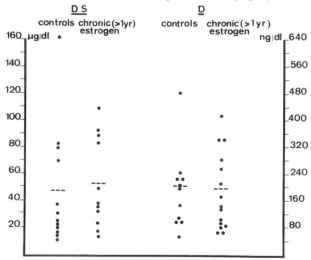

Fig. 1. Influence of oestrogens on D and DS levels in postmenopausal women.

with the results of Maroulis and Abraham (1976) who reported normalization of DS levels in women treated with oestrogen, but is in accordance with the results of Anderson and Yen (1976).

Another factor that should be considered for an aetiological role in the age dependent decrease in androgen levels is prolactin. It has been reported that in women with hyperprolactinaemia, mean androgen, especially DS, levels, are higher than in control group (Vermeulen and Ando, 1978). Hence, one might hypothesize that a decrease in plasma prolactin levels might play a role in the decreased androgen secretion. Although in postmenopausal women, prolactin levels are indeed lower than during reproductive life, it seems highly improbable that this is responsible for the decreased adrenal cortical function, as males, where prolactin levels are slightly increased in old age (Table I), show a similar decreased adrenal androgen secretion. A second factor we studied was *fat mass or overweight*. Obesity has been reported to be accompanied by an increased conversion rate of A into E_1. We observed a highly significant ($P < 0.001$) positive linear correlation between either fat mass or overweight and E_1 and E_2 levels as well as with E_1/A and E_2/T ratio levels. Neither E_2/E_1 nor T/A ratios were correlated with either fat mass or overweight however, in accordance with the data of MacDonald (1979), suggesting that the reduction in C17 steroids does not occur in the same sites as the aromatization.

Table I. Progressive decrease of plasma prolactin levels in postmenopausal women.

Women	
Reproductive life	14.3 ± 2.5 ng/ml (M ± SE)
< 4 YPM (N = 15)	12.4 ± 1.3 ng/ml
4 – 10 YPM (N = 15)	10.0 ± 1.5 ng/ml
10 – 20 YPM (N = 21)	9.0 + 1.5 ng/ml
20 – 30 YPM (N = 21)	8.1 ± 1.6 ng/ml

Men	
< 50 years (N = 93)	6.9 ± 0.4 ng/ml
> 50 years	8.2 ± 0.6 ng/ml

Much to our surprise however we found a significant negative correlation ($P < 0.05$) between fat mass and FSH (but not LH) levels as well as between E_1 and FSH levels ($P < 0.01$). In view of the multiple factors that influence the sex hormone levels in postmenopausal women, we performed an *analysis of covariance* to determine partial correlations.

As it has been reported that conversion of A into E_2 increases with age (Hemsell *et al.*, 1974), whereas we did not find such an influence of age, we first investigated whether variation in weight might have masked the influence of age: however, even after correcting for weight, no significant correlation ($r = 0.15$; n = 52) of E_1 levels with age was observed. On the other hand, the highly significant correlation of E_1 levels with either fat mass or overweight persisted after correction for influence of age. Both E_1 and fat mass are negatively correlated with FSH levels; however, when corrected for variations in plasma E_1 levels, the partial correlation between fat mass and FSH was no longer significant, whereas after correction for fat mass the partial negative correlation between E_1 and FSH was still statistically significant. A similar statistically significant ($P < 0.01$)

correlation was observed between E_2 and FSH levels. This would tend to suggest that, even in postmenopause, oestrogen levels exert a negative feedback on gonadotropin secretion.

As to the role of *precursor concentration* as a determinant of sex hormone levels in postmenopausal women, as expected E_2 and E_1 levels were significantly correlated ($P < 0.02$) as well as T and A levels, T and Dehydrotestosterone (DHT) levels and, finally, A and DHT levels. On the other hand, no significant correlation was observed between E_1 and A levels, which is rather surprising since A is the major precursor of plasma E_1. Marshall *et al.* (1977), in a study including postmenopausal women treated with corticosteroids (depressing adrenal function), observed an asymptotic curvilinear correlation between A and E_1 levels. These authors suggest the correlation between E_1 and A levels to be governed by Michaelis and Menten kinetics of the tissular aromatase, the latter being saturated at a concentration of $\pm$ 3 nMol of plasma A. This would give a negative curvilinear correlation between the E_1/A ratio and A levels, which indeed we observed. A similar correlation can also be observed if the product steroid has two precursors secreted independently of each other: for example E_2 has a precursor E_1, deriving largely (indirectly via A) from the adrenals, and T deriving for a non-negligible extent from the ovaries, which may explain the inverse curvilinear correlation between the E_2/E_1 ratio and E_1 levels. However A is the only important known precursor of plasma E_1 and moreover there is some direct evidence for increased conversion of A into E_1 at low A concentration (Poortman *et al.*, 1973).

CLINICAL SIGNIFICANCE OF POSTMENOPAUSAL STEROID METABOLISM

Two situations illustrate the clinical relevance of these observations. It is well known that obesity favours the development of endometrial (and mammary) cancer. As unopposed oestrogen stimulation is also a risk factor for these cancers, the link between obesity and endometrial cancer becomes clear. Moreover, as the source of these oestrogens is essentially the peripheral conversion of adrenal androgens, aromatase inhibition by aminogluthetimide, testolacton or 4 hydroxy androstenedione, is a logical approach to endocrine treatment of oestrogen responsive carcinoma.

Oesteoporosis with crush fractures occurs relatively frequently in postmenopausal women. Our data show the mean A and E_1 levels in these patients to be significantly lower than in a control group, whereas the T and D levels, although slightly decreased, were not significantly different from the control group. The correlation between E_1 plasma levels and fat mass remains, however, similar to the correlation in the control group, but it is striking that most postmenopausal women with crush fractures are underweight with, as a consequence, decreased conversion of androgen into oestrogen. Hence, there is evidence for oestrogen deficiency in pathological postmenopausal osteoporosis. Many authors have reported an arrest or at least a decrease in the rate of bone loss during oestrogen treatment of postmenopausal osteoporosis and recently a reduced calciuria during oestrogen treatment has been reported (Frumar *et al.* 1980).

On the other hand, it should be mentioned that Davidson *et al.* (1980), in 18 women with postmenopausal osteoporosis did not find significantly decreased A or E_1 levels and only marginally lower E_2 levels, whereas the cervical oestrogen receptor concentration was also comparable to a control group.

CONCLUSIONS

The two major determinants for plasma sex hormone levels in postmenopausal women are age (causing a decreased adrenal androgen secretion) and overweight, responsible for an increased conversion of androgens into oestrogens. There is some evidence for increased $\Delta 5$-isomerase activity in the ageing adrenal and for a persistence of a negative feedback of oestrogens, at physiological concentration, on gonadotropin secretion.

REFERENCES

Abraham, G. E. and Maroulis, G. B. (1975). *Obstetrics and Gynecology* **45**, 271.

Anderson, D. C. and Yen, S.S.C. (1976). *Journal of Clinical Endocrinology and Metabolism* **43**, 561.

Botella–Llusia, J., Oriol–Bosch, A., Sanchez–Garrido, F. and Jrerguerres, J.A.F. (1980). *Maturitas* **1**, 7.

Davidson, B. J., Riggs, B. L., Coulain, C. B. and Toft, D. O. (1980). *American Journal of Obstetrics and Gynecology* **136**, 480.

Frumar, A. M., McDrum, D. R., Geola, F., Shamonki, I. M., Tartaryn, I. V., Deftos, L. J. and Judd, H. L. (1980). *Journal of Clinical Endocrinology and Metabolism* **50**, 70.

Grodin, S. K., Siiteri, P. K. and MacDonald, P. C. (1973). *Journal of Clinical Endocrinology and Metabolism* **36**, 207.

Hemsell, D. L., Grodin, J. M., Brenner, P. F., Siiteri, P. K. and MacDonald, P. C. (1974). *Journal of Clinical Endocrinology and Metabolism* **38**, 476.

Judd, H. L., Judd, G. E., Lucas, E. E. and Yen, S.C.C. (1974). *Journal of Clinical Endocrinology and Metabolism* **39**, 1020.

MacDonald, P. C. (1979). *European Journal of Obstetric and Gynecological Reproductive Biology* **9**, 187.

MacDonald, P. C., Edmon, C. D., Hemsell, D. L., Porter, J. C. and Siiteri, P. R. (1978). *American Journal of Obstetrics and Gynecology* **130**, 448.

Maroulis, G. B. and Abraham, G. E. (1976). *Obstetrics and Gynecology* **48**, 150.

Marshall, D. H., Crilly, R. and Nordin, B.E.C. (1977). *British Medical Journal* **ii**, 1178.

Marshall, D. H., Crilly, R. and Nordin, B.E.C. (1978). *Clinical Endocrinology* **9**, 407.

Poortman, J., Thyssen, J. H. H. and Schwarz, C. (1973). *Journal of Clinical Endocrinology and Metabolism* **37**, 101.

Vermeulen, A. (1976). *Journal of Clinical Endocrinology and Metabolism* **42**, 247.

Vermeulen, A. (1980). *Maturitas* (in press).

Vermeulen, A. and Ando, J. (1978). *Clinical Endocrinology* **8**, 295.

Vermeulen, A. and Verdonck, L. (1978). *Clinical Endocrinology* **19**, 59.

POSTMENOPAUSAL LH PREFERENTIAL RELEASE:
TENTATIVE PATHOPHYSIOLOGICAL INTERPRETATION

S. Geller[1], I. Granier[2], K. Nahoul[2], C. Lemasson[1], J. N. Defosse[1],
J. R. Pasqualini[2] and R. Scholler[2]

[1] *Centre d'Exploration Fonctionelle et d'Etude de la Réproduction (CEFER),
Marseille, France,* [2] *Fondation de Recherche en Hormonologie, Paris, France*

INTRODUCTION

As is well known, the menopause is associated with a steep increase in pituitary gonadotropins. However, this rise affects essentially FSH, the production
of which, according to Coble *et al.* (1969), would be 14.1 fold increased over
the premenopausal period, whereas LH production would be only 3.2 fold greater
(Kohler *et al.,* 1968). It follows that in postmenopausal, unlike premenopausal
women, the FSH/LH ratio is generally >1 (Mahesh, 1976). Due to this preferential elevation in FSH basal level, following LH–RH, in postmenopausal, unlike
in premenopausal women, the FSH tracing is generally above the LH tracing
(Fig. 1, middle panel). The surface area S1, encompassed by FSH, is then larger
than the surface area S2, encompassed by LH, and the S2/S1 ratio is then <1.

In some cases however, in postmenopausal women, the LH tracing crosses
over the FSH tracing and comes up, as in premenopausal women, above the
FSH tracing; S2 becomes larger than S1, and the S2/S1 ratio becomes >1 (Fig. 1.,
right-hand panel). This peculiar pattern of FSH and LH tracings, following
LH–RH in postmenopausal women, was termed "Postmenopausal LH Preferential Release" (PM. LH. PR) (Geller and Schollar 1978a, 1980; Geller *et al.,*
1979). We were interested in this peculiar pattern and tried to further elucidate
its pathophysiology and significance and the S2/S1 ratio was investigated in a
variety of postmenopausal patients.

Serono Symposium No. 39, "The Menopause: Clinical, Endocrinological and Pathophysiological Aspects", edited by P. Fioretti, L. Martini, G. B. Melis and S. S. C. Yen, 1982. Academic
Press, London and New York.

LH · RH Test

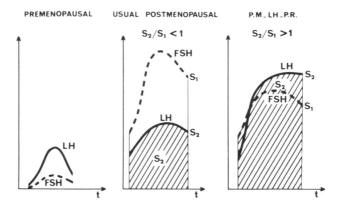

Fig. 1. FSH and LH response to LH–RH: in premenopausal women (left panel); usual response in postmenopausal women (middle panel); postmenopausal LH preferential release (right panel); (legend in text).

MATERIALS AND METHODS

The first group of patients selected for this study regards 89 "normal" post-menopausal women, namely with "natural" menopause that occurred at the usual time and was devoid of specific pathology. The menopausal state was considered as achieved when at least 1 complete year had elapsed since the last menstrual period. Patients were grouped in function of menopausal age (MA), as defined by the elapsed time since the last menstrual period, according to a classification adapted from Jaszmann *et al.* (1969): group I = MA < 2 years; group II = $2 \leqslant$ MA < 5 years; group III = $5 \leqslant$ MA < 10 years; group IV = MA $\geqslant$ 10 years. Fifty-five castrated patients (31 for fibroids, 24 for other gynaecological diseases) and 75 patients with breast cancer (49 postmenopausal, 26 castrated) were also investigated.

Fasting subjects were given a bolus i.v. injection of 100 μg of LH-RH. Plasma samples were taken 15 min before and 10, 20, 30, 45, 60 and 120 min after the injection. Venous blood was collected on EDTA (ethylenediamine tetraacetate) and immediately centrifuged. Plasma was then separated and frozen at $-20\,^{\circ}$C until the assays were carried out. FSH and LH were measured by radioimmunoassay, using a procedure previously described (Roger *et al.*, 1975).

Plasma oestradiol was measured by radioimmunoassay using a procedure previously reported (Castanier and Scholler, 1970).

FSH and LH total cumulative responses (TCR) following LH-RH, as defined by the surface area comprised between the tracing and the X axis, were calculated by planimetry, using the formula:

$$S = 10y'_{10} + 10y'_{20} + 12,5y'_{30} + 15y'_{45} + 37,5y'_{60} + 30y'_{120} + 10y_0$$

where $y' = y_i - y_0$, y_i being y value at t = i and y_0, y value at t = o. This formula which derived from the classical trapezium method, was computerized on a Hewlett-Packard 98.10 computer.

Statistical calculations were made using the classical Student's t test, Sukhatme's test (Morice and Chartier, 1954), Cochran's test (Cochran, 1964) and Welch and Aspin's test (Bennet and Franklin, 1954). In a number of patients sella turcica hypocycloidal tomograms were likewise carried out, according to Vezina and Sutton (1974). In a number of patients with breast cancer, mammary E_2 receptor assays have been carried out, using the techniques of Pasqualini *et al.* (1976).

RESULTS

Table I and Fig. 2 give the results obtained in normal postmenopausal patients. As can be seen, high S2/S1 values greater than 1 are found in the first age group, associated with substantial plasma E_2 levels. The S2/S1 ratios were further arbitrarily classified into three types: I S2/S1 < 0.8; II S2/S1 between 0.8 and I and III S2/S1 ⩾ 1. Table II gives the distribution of these three types of responses. As can be seen, the incidence of type II responses (i.e.: PM. LH. PR. pattern) is also maximal in the first age group and drops off thereafter with increasing menopausal age (Table II, line 3), whereas type I responses then become prevalent (Table II, line 1). Table III and Fig. 2 give the results in castrated patients. As can be seen, patients castrated for fibroids also display higher S2/S1 values in the first age group, although E_2 levels are significantly lower in these patients than in normal postmenopausal patients of the same age group (Fig. 2 and Table

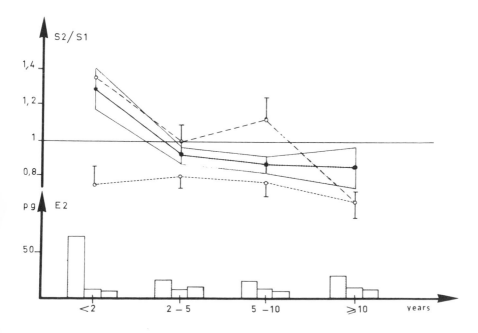

Fig. 2. S2/S1 (top panel) and plasma oestradiol (bottom panel) in 89 normal postmenopausal women (●—● and left bars), 31 patients castrated for fibroids (○—.—○ and middle bars), and 24 patients castrated for other gynaecological diseases (○ – – – ○ and right bars) in function of postmenopausal age.

Table I. FSH and LH, basal levels and total cumulative responses (TCR) following LH–RH, S2/S1 ratio and plasma oestradiol (E_2) in 89 normal postmenopausal women.

Group	N	Mean age (years)	Basal FSH mU/ml	Basal LH mU/ml	TCR–FSH (S1) mU/ml/sh <	TCR–LH (S2) mU/ml/sh	S2/S1	E_2 pg/ml
I M. A. [a] < 2 years	39	48.3	21.1 ± 1.5	13.3 ± 0.8	28.4 ± 2.1	39.9 ± 2.1	1.29 ± 0.11	72.7 ± 14.7
II 2 ≤ M. A. < 5 years	29	52.6	24.7 ± 1.6	13.8 ± 1.3	32.7 ± 2.6	28.1 ± 2.8[b]	0.92 ± 0.06[d]	20.8 ± 7.1[d]
III 5 ≤ M. A. < 10 years	13	54.4	30.0 ± 3.1[d]	16.4 ± 1.5[b]	34.1 ± 4.1	28.6 ± 3.0[b]	0.87 ± 0.06[d]	18.9 ± 4.2[d]
IV M. A. ≥ 10 years	8	67.7	23.5 ± 3.3	11.8 ± 1.2	30.3 ± 3.4	24.5 ± 3.9[b]	0.86 ± 0.12[c]	25 ± 9.5[d]

[a] M. A. = menopausal age; [b] non significant; [c] border line signification ($P < 0.05$); [d] highly significant ($P < 0.01$), as compared with group I.

Table II. Distribution of responses to LH-RH test in 89 normal postmenopausal patients and in 49 postmenopausal patients with breast cancer.

Patient group		MA[a] < 2 years		2 ≤ MA < 5 years		5 ≤ MA < 10 years		MA ≥ 10 years	
		N	%	N	%	N	%	N	%
Normal postmenopausal patients	I S2/S1 < 0.8	7	17.9	9	31	4	30.7	5	62.5
	II 0.8 ≤ S2/S1 < 1	17	43.6	15	51.7	8	61.5	2	25
	III S2/S1 ≥ 1	15	38.5	5	17.2	1	7.8	1	12.5
Postmenopausal patients with breast cancer	I S2/S1 < 0.8	1	12.5	6	46.2	3	37.5	7	35
	II 0.8 ≤ S2/S1 < 1	1	12.5	1	7.6	1	12.5	6	30
	III S2/S1 ≥ 1	6	75.0	6	46.2	4	50.0	7	35

[a]MA = menopausal age.

Table III. S2/S1 ratios and plasma oestradiol (E_2) levels in postmenopausal and castrated patients.

Patients group		< 2 years PM			2–5 years PM[a]			5–10 years PM			≥ 10 years PM		
		N	x	Sm	N	x	Sm	N	x	Sm	N	x	Sm
Normal postmenopausal	S2/S1	39	1.29	0.11	29	0.92	0.05	13	0.87	0.05	8	0.85	0.12
	E_2 (pg/ml)	31	72.7	14.7	25	20.8	7.1	12	18.2	4.3	5	25.2	9.5
Castrated for fibroids	S2/S1	9	1.36[b]	0.05	7	0.99	0.10	8	1.13	0.13	7	0.65	0.06
	E_2 (pg/ml)	7	10.1[d]	0.4	5	9.3	0.7	6	11.2	0.6	5	8.5	0.7
Castrated for other gynaecological conditions	S2/S1	6	0.74[d]	0.10	7	0.80	0.07	6	0.77	0.10	5	0.65	0.08
	E_2 (pg/ml)	5	9.3[d]	0.6	5	8.7	0.8	4	11.5	0.9	4	10.2	1.9
Postmenopausal and breast cancer	S2/S1	8	1.23[b]	0.18	13	1.16	0.17	8	1.17	0.18	20	1.10	0.12
	E_2 (pg/ml)	7	63.8[b]	17.9	10	18.3	9.4	9	21.5	6.8	16	15.3	5.3
Castrated for breast cancer	S2/S1	6	1.04[b]	0.07	8	1.15	0.20	8	1.43[d]	0.23	4	0.77	0.10
	E_2 (pg/ml)	5	9.2[d]	0.5	6	8.7	0.6	5	10.4	0.7	4	7.6	0.9

[a]PM = postmenopausal; [b] non-significant; [c]$P < 0.05$ (border line signification); [d]$P < 0.01$ (highly significant) as compared with the corresponding normal postmenopausal group.

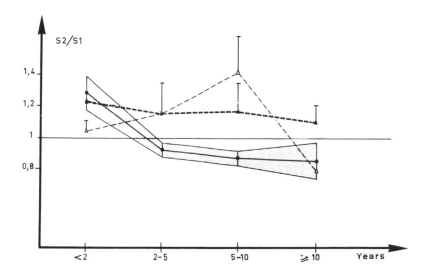

Fig. 3. S2/S1 in 89 normal postmenopausal women (•—•), 49 postmenopausal patients with breast cancer (▲- - -▲) and 26 castrated patients for breast cancer (△—.—△).

III, line 2). Patients castrated for other gynaecological conditions, in contrast, do not display such high values of S2/S1 ratio, even in the first age group (Fig. 2 and Table III, line 3).

Figure 3 and Table III give the results in patients with breast cancer. As can be seen, in postmenopausal patients with breast cancer, high S2/S1 values are maintained throughout the entire menopause, including the last age group (Fig. 3 and Table III, line 4). In these patients, the incidence of type III responses, i.e. PM. LH. PR. pattern, is significantly higher for each age group, than in normal postmenopausal patients of the same age group (Table II, line 6). In castrated patients with breast cancer, S2/S1 ratio, already high in the first age group, rises further in the following groups, the highest values of this ratio being reached in the third age group (Fig. 3 and Table III, line 5).

In patients with breast cancer, mammary E_2 receptor levels have been compared with S2/S1 ratios (Table IV). To make this comparison easier E_2 receptor (R. E_2) levels have been arbitrarily ranged into three types: I R. E_2 < 3 femtomoles; II R. E_2 between 3 and 10 femtomoles; III R. E_2 ≥ 10 femtomoles/mg protein. As can be seen, type III S2/S1 values, i.e. PM. LH. PR. pattern, are apparently associated with high or at least substantial mammary E2 receptor levels.

Sella turcica tomograms have been likewise carried out in a number of postmenopausal and castrated patients, with or without breast cancer. Radiological findings have been compared with S2/S1 values: for that purpose, radiological findings have also been ranged into three types: A normal, B disputable, C indisputable microenlargement. As can be seen (Table V), type III S2/S1 ratios are apparently associated with indisputable sella turcica microenlargements.

Table IV. Relationship between responses to LH–RH and mammary E_2 levels (RE_2) in 49 postmenopausal or castrated patients with breast cancer.

	Oestradiol Receptors (RE_2)			
Responses to LH–RH	I $RE_2 < 3$ fm	II $3 \leqslant RE_2 < 10$ fm	III $RE_2 \geqslant 10$ fm	Total
Type I S2/S1 < 0.8	6	4	4	14
Type II 0.8 ⩽ S2/S1 < 1	3	5	1	9
Type III S2/S1 ⩾ 1	2	3	21	26
				49

Table V. Relationship between LH response to LH–RH and radiological findings of sella turcica tomogram in 62 postmenopausal or castrated patients.

	Radiological findings			Total
	A Normal	B Disputable micro-enlargement	C Indisputable micro-enlargement	
Type I S2/S1 < 0.8	10	3	3	16
Type II 0.8 ≤ S2/S1 < 1	3	9	14	26
Type III S2/S1 ≥ 1	3	3	14	20
				62

Responses to LH–RH

DISCUSSION

Following LH-RH, a far higher LH than FSH release is observed in a rich oestrogen milieu, as in the case of the late follicular phase or the peri-ovulatory period (Nillius and Wide, 1971; Yen *et al.*, 1972; Jaffe and Keye, 1974; Hoff *et al.*, 1977; De Kretzer *et al.*, 1978). Conversely, higher FSH (versus LH) release is observed in a poor oestrogen milieu, as is the case in the early follicular phase, in early post partum and in the first stages of puberty in girls (Franchimont and Walcke, 1975). The statistical prevalence of PM. LH. PR. observed in the first age group of normal postmenopausal women may then be logically postulated to be related to the substantial plasma E_2 levels found in these patients. As shown by Yen *et al.* (1975), oestrogens are liable to augment the levels of LH-RH pituitary receptors in the gonadotroph cell. One can then fancy that the preferential LH release observed in a rich oestrogen milieu would be linked to the higher oestrogen-induced LH-RH receptor level. Such a mechanism has been put forward to account for the oestrogen-induced potentiation of TSH response to TRH (Labrie *et al.*, 1977), which is quite comparable, *mutatis mutandis*, to the oestrogen-induced augmentation of LH response to LH-RH. Anyhow, the statistical prevalence of PM. LH. PR. in the first age group, associated with substantial plasma E_2 levels and its disappearance thereafter, along with the lowering of estrogen levels, would be consistent with this interpretation.

High S2/S1 values found in patients castrated for fibroids, in spite of very low E_2 levels in these patients, look apparently at variance with this pathophysiological assumption. However, as is well known, fibroids and related lesions, such as polycystic ovaries, endometrial hyperplasia and endometriosis are admittedly associated with oestrogen excess. Thus, the main factor able to play a role in this effect might not be the present oestrogen status, but rather, the previous longstanding oestrogen stimulation (Geller and Scholler, 1978a). The high S2/S1 values found in these patients, as opposed to the low values of this ratio found in patients castrated for other gynaecological diseases are at any rate consonant with this hypothesis.

The persistence of high S2/S1 values in postmenopausal patients with breast cancer and the prevalence of PM. LH. PR. pattern in these patients, as compared with normal postmenopausal patients, suggests that such a mechanism may also be at play in these patients. Oestrogens have been shown to augment the level of their own receptors in their target cells (Sarff and Gorski, 1971). The longstanding oestrogen overstimulation, of which the PM. LH. PR. would be the witness, could then likewise, at least under certain conditions, allow the synthesis of a greater amount of E_2 receptors at the mammary gland target. This could thus account for the apparent relationship between PM. LH. PR. pattern and the high mammary E_2 receptors levels found in these patients.

This hypothesis would be in agreement with the pathophysiological model proposed by King *et al.* (1978), according to which longstanding oestrogen stimulation would play a leading role, via changes in the receptors, in the development of hyperplasia, and eventually cancer, of the endometrium, another oestrogen target. It would also be in agreement with the well known epidemiological data which emphasize the favourable role in this regard of early menarche and late menopause (Yusa and MacMahon, 1970; MacMahon and Cole, 1973; Henderson *et al.*, 1974). Anyhow, if this relationship between the PM. LH. PR. pattern and the mammary E_2 receptors level can be confirmed, PM. LH. PR. could then be considered as an additional index of hormonal sensitivity in breast cancer (Geller *et al.*, 1979).

Landolt (1978) has reported anterior pituitary proliferative lesions, so-called "focal hyperplasia". Unlike true adenomas, "focal hyperplasias" would still be hormone-dependent lesions, liable to regress to normal with the disappearance of the hormonal stimulus which had triggered them. Now, according to Landolt, such focal hyperplasias would be more frequent with increasing age and most frequently composed of gonadotropic cells, which, in contrast, are practically never encountered in true adenomas (Peillon *et al.*, 1978).

So, it is tempting to speculate that Landolt's focal hyperplasias would represent the anatomical substratum of the sella turcica microenlargements found in postmenopausal women with PM. LH. PR. pattern. This would account for the apparent relation between PM. LII. PR. pattern and sella turcica microenlargements in these patients. In premenopausal patients affected by what was termed "hyperovarism", a condition associating both oestrogen and LH hyperactivity, we previously reported sella turcica microenlargements for which the hypothesis of "LH microadenoma" had been put forward (Geller and Scholler, 1977). Sella turcica microenlargements found later in postmenopausal women with PM. LH. PR. were postulated to be the postclimateric form of the microenlargements previously found in premenopausal women with "hyperovarism" (Geller and Scholler, 1978b). In view of Landolt's data, these so-called "LH microadenomas" should be more rightly interpreted as "LH focal hyperplasias", liable to wane along with their hormonal inducer, namely the oestrogens. The peculiar outcome of PM. LH. PR. pattern (apparently associated with sella turcica microenlargements) statistically prevalent in the first age group of normal postmenopausal patients, associated with substantial E_2 levels, and its disappearance thereafter, along with the lowering of E_2 levels, is in agreement with this hypothesis.

CONCLUSIONS

The PM. LH. PR. pattern is essentially dependent on the amount and particularly the duration of the previous oestrogen stimulation, which would allow the synthesis of a higher amount of LH–RH receptors at the pituitary level (hence the PM. LH. PR. pattern, the development of focal hyperplasias and, possibly, sella turcica microenlargements) and also of E_2 receptors at the mammary gland site, according for the association which appears to exist between PM. LH. PR. pattern and the high mammary E_2 receptor levels in patients with breast cancer (Fig. 4). Oestradiol-induced receptors would then be the common pathophysiological link uniting the different, clinical, radiological and biological expressions of PM. LH. PR. Of course this is still only a working hypothesis and caution is in order. Other factors may well be at play, such as inhibin for instance, the existence of which has now been conclusively shown (Franchimont *et al.*, 1978) or the well known difference in FSH and LH half-lives. As far as E_2 receptors

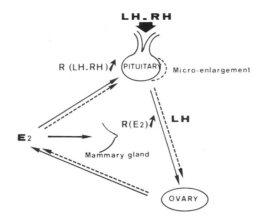

Fig. 4. Postmenopausal LH preferential release. Tentative pathophysiological interpretation; (legend in text).

are concerned, neither occupied and unoccupied sites in the cytosol, nor nuclear receptors have been considered. So the above assumptions should remain hypothetical. The famous french physiologist Claude Bernard used to say that "there are not true and false hypotheses, there are those which are fruitful and those which are not". To which the above hypothesis belongs, the future will decide.

REFERENCES

Bennet, C. A. and Franklin, N. L. (1954). "Statistical analysis, in chemistry and the clinical industry" p. 177. John Wiley and Sons, Inc. New-York.

Castanier, M. and Scholler, R. (1970). *Comptes Rendus Academie Science,* Paris, **271**, 1787.

Coble, Y. D., Kohler, P. O., Cargille, C. M. and Ross, G. T. (1969). *Journal of Clinical Investigation* **48**, 359.

Cochran, W. G. (1964). *Biometrics* **20**, 191.

De Kretzer, D. M., Burger, J. G. and Dumpys, R. (1978). *Journal of Clinical Endocrinology and Metabolism* **46**, 227.

Franchimont, P. and Walcke, J. C. (1975). *In* "La Fonction Gonadotrope", p. 139–155. Masson, Paris.

Franchimont, P., Demoulin, A., Verstraelen–Proyard, J., Hazee–Hagelstein, M. T., Walton, J. S. and Waites, G. M. H. (1978). *Journal International of Andrology* **2**, 69.

Geller, S. and Scholler, R. (1977). *VIth International Seminar on reproductive physiology and sexual endocrinology,* Brussells, May 1976. *Progressive Reproductive Biology* **2**, 176.

Geller, S. and Scholler, R. (1978a). *2nd International Congress on the menopause,* Jerusalem, June 1978.

Geller, S. and Scholler, R. (1978b). *International symposium on pituitary microadenomas,* Milan, 12–14 October, 1978. Serono Symposia Vol. 29 (G. Faglia, M. A. Giovanelli and R. M. MacLeod, Eds) p. 295–301, Academic Press, London.

Geller, S. and Scholler, R. (1980). *Maturitas* **2**, 45.
Geller, S., Ayme, Y., Amalric, R., Brandone, H., Spitalier, J. M., Pasqualini, J. R. and Scholler, R. (1979). *First International Congress on Hormones and Cancer,* Rome, October 3–6. Abstracts **63** (7), 1205.
Henderson, B. E., Powell, D. and Rosario, I. (1974). *Journal of National Cancer Institute* **53**, 609.
Hoff, J. D., Lasley, B. L., Wang, C. F. and Yen, S. S. C. (1977). *Journal of Clinical Endocrinology and Metabolism* **44**, 302.
Jaffe, R. B. and Keye, W. R., Jr (1974). *Journal of Clinical Endocrinology and Metabolism* **39**, 850.
Jaszmann, L., Van Lith, N. D. and Zaat, J. C. A. (1969). *Medicine Gynaecologie Sociale* **4**, 268.
King, R. J. B., Whitehead, M., Campbell, S. and Minardi, J. (1978). *Postgraduate Medical Journal* **54**, (suppl. 2), 65.
Kohler, P. O., Ross, G. T. and Odell, W. D. (1968). *Journal of Clinical Investigation* **47**, 38.
Labrie, F., Lagace, L., Drouin, J., Delean, A., Kelly, A. P., Ferland, L., Beaulieu, M., Raymond, V., Dupont, A. and Cusan, L. (1977). *In* "Les oestrogénes", pp. 3–23. Masson, Paris.
Landolt, A. M. (1978). *International Symposium on pituitary microadenomas,* Milan, 12–14 October 1978. Serono Symposia Vol. 29 (G. Faglia, M. A. Giovanelli and R. M. MacLeod, Eds.) pp. 107–122. Academic press, London.
MacMahon, B. and Cole, M. D. (1973). *Journal of National Cancer Institute* **50**, 21.
Mahesh, V. B. (1976). *In* "Consensus on Menopause Research" (P. A. Van Keep, R. B. Greenblatt and A. Albeaux–Fernet, Ed) pp. 11–18. M.T.P, Press Ltd., Lancaster.
Morice, E. and Chartier, F. (1954). *Methode statistique,* II Analyse statistique, pp. 204–238. Imprimerie Nationale, Paris.
Nillius, S. J. and Wide, L. (1971). *Journal of Obsteties and Gynecology of British Commonwealth* **79**, 862.
Pasqualini, J. R., Sumida, C., Gelly, C. and Nguyen, B. L. (1976). *Journal of Steroid Biochemistry* **7**, 1031.
Peillon, F., Racadot, J., Olivier, L. and Vila–Porcile, E. (1979). *International Symposium on pituitary microadenomas,* Milan, 12–14 October 1978. Serono Symposia Vol. 29 (G. Faglia, M. A. Giovanelli and R. M. MacLeod, Eds.) p. 91–106. Academic Press, London.
Roger, M., Veinante, A., Soldat, M. C., Tardy, J., Tribondeau, E. and Scholler, R. (1975). *Nouvelle Presse Médicol* **4**, 2173.
Sarff, M. and Gorski, J. (1971). *Biochemistry* **10**, 2557.
Vezina, J. L. and Sutton, T. J. (1974). *Annual Journal Roentgenology* **120**, 46.
Yen, S. S. C., Vandenberg, G., Rebar, R. and Ehara, J. (1972). *Journal of Clinical Endocrinology and Metabolism* **35**, 931.
Yen, S. S. C., Lasley, B. L., Wang, C. F., Leblanc, H. and Siler, T. M. (1975). *Recent Progress in Hormone Research* **31**, 321.
Yusa, S. and MacMahon, B. (1970). *Japan, Bulletin WHO* **42**, 185.

GONADOTROPIN RESERVE IN POSTMENOPAUSAL OLD WOMEN

[1]E. Pucci, [1]D. Silvestri, [1]G. P. Bernini, [3]G. Baggiani, [2]A. M. Paoletti, [2]M. Gambacciani, [4]F. Franchi and [1]M. Luisi

[1]*Postgraduate School of Endocrinology and* [2]*Institute of Obstetrics and Gynaecology, University of Pisa and* [3]*Geriatric Department, Santa Chiara Hospital of Pisa, Pisa, Italy*

Decline in ovarian function is shown by a decrease in peripheral plasma steroid levels and by a concomitant increase in gonadotropin output from the pituitary due to a reduced negative feedback by oestrogens (Bellamy, 1967; Bourne, 1978). However the hormonal reserve and dynamic patterns of pituitary secretion after the menopause are still unknown.

Gonadotropin responses to a constant infusion of luteinizing hormone-releasing hormone (LH-RH) (Debeliuk *et al.*, 1972) in very old women in postmenopause during the last 30 years are reported here.

MATERIALS AND METHODS

Six healthy women (over 75 years of age) were chosen for the present study: in spite of their age they were free from cardiovascular, hepatic and renal diseases. During the test hematocrit, heart rate and blood pressure were accurately assessed.

A preliminary evaluation of LH and FSH levels was carried out between 7.00 and 8.00 a.m. for 6 consecutive days. On the 7th day, the subjects were given an LH-RH infusion (12.5 μg/h for 48 h) via an indwelling catheter placed in an antecubital vein (Sherman *et al.*, 1976).

Serono Symposium No. 39, "The Menopause: Clinical, Endocrinological and Pathophysiological Aspects", edited by P. Fioretti, L. Martini, G. B. Melis and S. S. C. Yen, 1982. Academic Press, London and New York.

Before and during the infusion (from −2 to 48 h) plasma samples were collected: LH and FSH levels were determined at 1 h intervals and 17β-oestradiol and progesterone every 8 h. Hormone concentrations were measured by radioimmunoassay. Mean values and standard deviations were calculated for all times of assessment and Student's *t*-test was used for statistical analysis.

RESULTS

Mean basal levels of LH and FSH were found to be 42 ± 15 and 93 ± 19 mIU/ml, respectively (Fig. 1). LH–RH infusion caused a ready response of LH which, after 1 h, had already reached 160 mIU/ml. The increase continued and a significant peak (218 ± 18 mIU/ml) was obtained at the 5th hour. Subsequent values showed a plateau for the following 11 h; afterwards they decreased to levels of about 80 mIU/ml which were maintained till the end of infusion. All these values were always greater than basal ones.

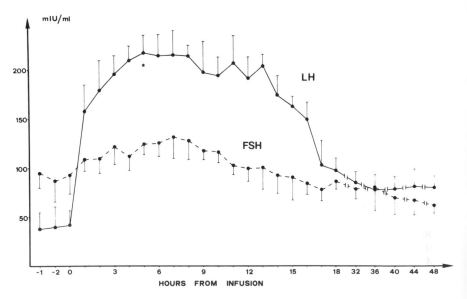

Fig. 1. LH and FSH levels during 48 h LH–RH infusion. *P < 0.001.

The FSH pattern was found to be very different: mean values rose slightly to a not significant peak of 132 ± 22 mIU/ml after 7 h, then returned to lower values than basal levels. In Fig. 2, the percentage increases of LH and FSH during LH–RH infusion are reported.

Though a pharmacological dose and a protracted infusion were used, 17β-oestradiol and progesterone values were low and didn't show any significant variation. No variations were observed in hematocrit, heart rate and blood pressure.

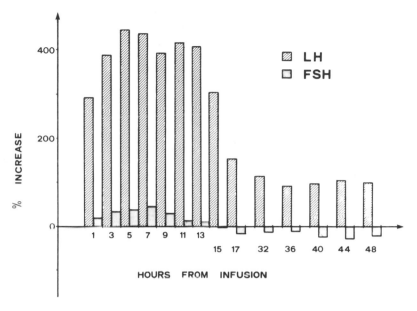

Fig. 2. Percentage increase of LH and FSII during 48 h LH–RH infusion.

CONCLUSIONS

It is well known that for several years after the menopause, plasma levels of FSH are always higher than those of LH (Blichert-Toft, 1975). Results obtained show that in very old women LH-RH infusion elicited a high, persistent LH response from the pituitary and a more limited FSH response. Therefore our experiments seem to demonstrate that, even after a prolonged absence of cyclic functions, the pituitary maintains its capacity to secrete gonadotropins in reponse to 48 h continuous stimulation.

This fact seems to suggest the hypothesis that a tonic effect on hypothalamic-hypophyseal structures may be due to the adrenals which still secrete oestrogens and their precursors, thus maintaining an LH pituitary reserve. Moreover a partially persisting function of the ovaries may be postulated (Franchimont, 1977).

However, this does not occur for FSH: the fact that hormone levels invariably declined after the initial stimulation, even though infusion continued at the same rate, is of particular interest. It may be supposed that the absence of folli-cular maturation leads to a shortage in inhibin secretion by granulosa cells. FSH, lacking in one of its most important control systems, is always produced and immediately secreted. For this reason, if pituitary is stimulated, no efficient reserve of FSH can be observed.

REFERENCES

Bellamy, D. (1967). *Society for Experimental Biology* **21**, 427.
Blichert–Toft, M. (1975). *Acta Endocrinologica* **78**, (Suppl. 195), 1.
Bourne, G. H. (1978). *Acta Endocrinologica* **89**, 48.
Debeliuk, L., Arimura, A. and Schally, A. V. (1972). *Endocrinology* **90**, 1499.
Franchimont, P. (1977). *Clinics in Endocrinology and Metabolism* **6**, 1.
Sherman, B. M., West, J. H. and Korenman, S. C. (1976). *Journal of Clinical Endocrinology and Metabolism* **42**, 629.

CIRCADIAN AMPLITUDE OF PROLACTIN, CORTISOL AND ALDOSTERONE IN HUMAN BLOOD SEVERAL DECADES AFTER MENOPAUSE

P. Cugini[1], D. Scavo[1], F. Halberg[2], A. Schramm[3], H. -J. Pusch[3] and H. Franke[3]

[1] I^ Patologia Medica, University of Rome, Italy [2] Chronobiology Laboratories, University of Minnesota, Minneapolis, USA [3] Medizinsche Poliklinik, University of Würzburg, West Germany

INTRODUCTION

Circadian, circatrigintan (about 30 day) and circannual variations have been concomitantly studied for the systemic venous concentrations of prolactin (PRL), cortisol (F) and aldosterone (A) (Halberg et al., 1980a). Moreover, in recent work carried out on Japanese and North American women of three age groups (adolescent, young and postmenopausal), an age dependent trend has been noted for the circadian amplitude of several hormones (LH, E_2, 17-OH progesterone, DHEA-S) (Haus et al., 1979; Nelson et al., 1980). Results were qualified twice. Firstly, multiple testing was carried out. Secondly, the postmenopausal women were younger than 60 years of age; it was emphasized that further study was required for PRL and A (preferably in older women). The present investigation complements in a broadening geographic context the knowledge on changes in rhythm characteristics for PRL, F and A at a relatively advanced age of 70 or more years.

MATERIALS AND METHODS

Nine menstrually-cycling (aged 23–29 years), and 10 postmenopausal, (aged 70–81 years), women, on a routine of diurnal activity and nocturnal rest, volun-

Serono Symposium No. 39, "The Menopause: Clinical, Endocrinological and Pathophysiological Aspects", edited by P. Fioretti, L. Martini, G. B. Melis and S. S. C. Yen, 1982. Academic Press, London and New York.

teered with informed consent for study in Würzburg, Federal Republic of Germany. Peripheral venous blood was drawn at 7 a.m., 10 a.m., 1 p.m., 4 p.m., 7 p.m. and 10 p.m. in December 1978 or January 1979 from the young women and between January and May 1979 from the postmenopausal women*. During these spans at the same circadian times young and old men were also sampled. After centrifugation, serum was stored frozen at −28 °C until it was radioimmunoassayed for PRL, F and A. Data were fitted by a 24-h cosine function and summarized by the population-mean cosinor method (Halberg *et al.*, 1967) and by a multivariate analysis of rhythm characteristics (by Hotelling's T^2).

RESULTS

The geometric mean systemic concentrations (± SE) of PRL, F and A are depicted in Fig. 1. By macroscopic inspection, consistent differences are apparent between results for young and old subjects. These differences are more prominent in women than in men, notably for hormone concentrations in the morning.

The rhythm characteristics (mesor, amplitude and acrophase[†]) obtained from microscopic by the mean-cosinor procedure and application of a Hotelling T^2 test for multivariate comparison are listed in Fig. 2.

The clearest effect of advanced age (at several decades after menopause) is a decrease in circadian amplitude for F and A. Such changes detected in women are not found in men. An amplitude decrease for PRL, in turn, is seen for both sexes in clinically healthy subjects 70 years of age or older.

DISCUSSION

Circadian rhythms of PRL (Nokin *et al.*, 1972; Sassin *et al.*, 1972), F (Halberg *et al.*, 1961; Hellman *et al.*, 1970; Krieger *et al.*, 1971; Weitzman *et al.*, 1971; de Lacerda *et al.*, 1973) and A (Bartter *et al.*, 1962; Michelakis and Horton, 1970; Vagnucci *et al.*, 1974; Katz *et al.*, 1975; Kowarski *et al.*, 1975) are by now well recognized. As a symposium volume on biorhythms and reproduction (Ferin *et al.*, 1964) among others, reveals, only limited data are available however for any comparison of rhythms with several frequencies in multiple hormones studied concurrently at different ages in groups of clinically healthy subjects. After such a study on North American (mostly Minnesotan) and Asiatic (mostly Kyushuan Japanese) women (Haus *et al.*, 1979; Halberg *et al.*, 1980a), the extension of the chronoepidemiologic work to a European (West German) population seems highly desirable as a follow-up on studies of PRL in Italy by Tarquini *et al.* (1979) and on the analyses of data presented here.

The present study shows a decrease in circadian amplitude for A in women

---

*The seasonal overlap of sampling spans notwithstanding, the failure to sample concomitantly pairs of young and old women, preferably with systematic distribution along the 1-year scale, consitutes a limitation of this study, among others mentioned in the text.

[†]Mesor: rhythm-adjusted mean; amplitude: half the total predictable extent of change; acrophase: lag from a reference time (here local midnight) of the crest time.

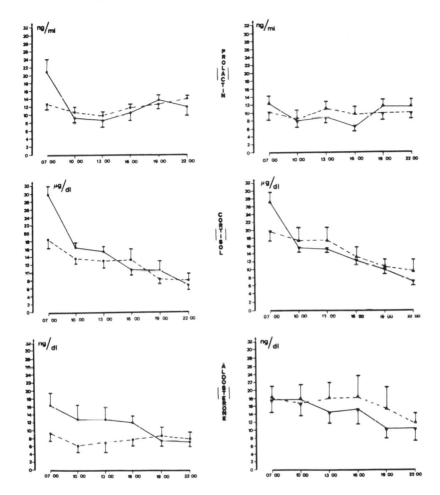

Fig. 1. Circadian variation in systemic venous concentration (mean ± SE) of prolactin, cortisol and aldosterone concomitantly assessed in menstrually-cycling (●—●) and post-menopausal women (●---●) as compared to age-matched groups of men (▲—▲ young men, ▲---▲ old men).

of central Europe, several decades after menopause. As far as the comparison allows, this finding is in keeping with the previous results obtained on Minnesotan and Japanese women in a wider geographic context and in a narrower age range. The foregoing qualifications also apply to the decrease in circadian amplitude of PRL and F which was not seen in the Minnesotan data. An added critical qualification of the data here presented is the lack of samples by night, yet this study did cover at least a 15 h time span (from 7 a.m. to 10 p.m.).

The effect of age on the circadian amplitude of West German women, 70 to 80 years of age, compared with women of 20 to 30 years of age, is statistically significant for prolactin in both sexes, whether it is analyzed in original values

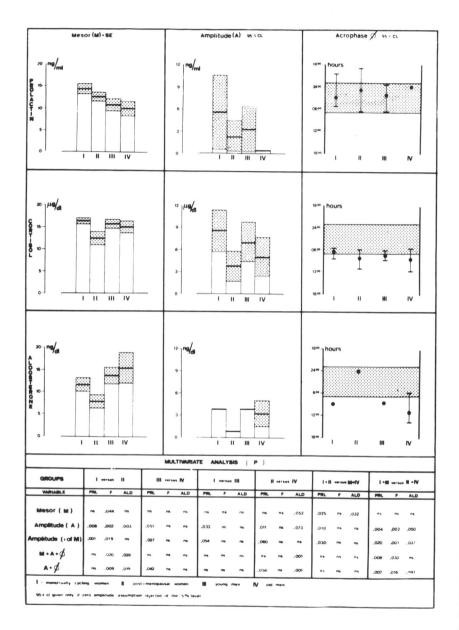

| Mesor (M) + SE | Amplitude (A) 95 × CL | Acrophase φ 95 × CL |

MULTIVARIATE ANALYSIS (P)

GROUPS	I versus II			III versus IV			I versus III			II versus IV			I+II versus III+IV			I+III versus II+IV		
VARIABLE	PRL	F	ALD	PRL	F	ALD	PRL	F	ALD	PRL	F	ALD	PRL	F	ALD	PRL	F	ALD
Mesor (M)	ns	.044	ns	ns	ns	ns	ns	ns	ns	ns	ns	.052	.025	ns	.032	ns	ns	ns
Amplitude (A)	.008	.002	.003	.051	ns	ns	.033	ns	ns	.011	ns	.073	.010	ns	ns	.004	.002	.050
Amplitude (·of M)	.001	.019	ns	.027	ns	ns	.054	ns	ns	.080	ns	ns	.030	ns	ns	.020	.001	.037
M+A+φ	ns	.020	.028	ns	ns	ns	ns	ns	ns	ns	ns	.001	ns	ns	ns	.008	.033	ns
A+φ	ns	.009	.019	.042	ns	ns	ns	ns	ns	.058	ns	.001	ns	ns	ns	.002	.016	.093

I = menstrually cycling women   II post-menopausal women   III young men   IV old men

95 ± cl given only if zero amplitude assumption rejected at the 5% level

Fig. 2. Rhythm characteristics for systemic venous concentration of prolactin, cortisol and aldosterone concomitantly assessed in menstrually-cycling (I) and postmenopausal (II) women as well as in young (III) and old (IV) men compared in a multivariate analysis by a T_2-test.

or values reexpressed as a percentage of the series mean. A similar effect was not detected for much younger postmenopausal women (less than 60 years of age) studied in Minnesota. Actually, in relative terms the amplitude of PRL is slightly greater in these postmenopausal Minnesotan women than in the menstrually cycling group. In Japanese women of ages similar to those studied in Minnesota, there is a possible postmenopausal decrease in the circadian amplitude of plasma PRL when considered in original values, but not when PRL is expressed as percentage of the series mean.

The same qualification applies to plasma cortisol, in that the effect found in West Germany for women over 70 years of age (as compared with 20 to 30 year olds) is not found in Japanese and Minnesotan women up to 60 years of age. In the case of plasma A, however, the pool of results from Minnesota and Japan reveals a decrease in both circadian mesor and amplitude—the latter is in keeping with the data from West Germany. A prominent observation in the present work is that an effect of advanced age upon the circadian amplitude of F and A is (female) sex-related, while the corresponding effects for PRL is seen in both sexes. Thus, the modifications in adrenocortical function more than the changes in pituitary secretion of PRL characterize the possibly sex-related effects on the circadian aspects of the endocrine system of ageing at several decades after menopause.

In addition to the physiological implications, the serial hormonal values obtained in this distribution of clinically healthy subjects may have practical utility; they constitute a step towards the construction of reference intervals for a European population (Halberg *et al.*, 1980a, b). Work on age-related maps for rhythm characteristics and chronodesms (90–90 tolerance intervals) for the interpretation of time-specified single samples, at least in some chronobiology laboratories of each country, notably for hormones, is overdue. Eventually, if such work should prove to be useful in designated test hospitals, least chronodesms may have to be established for each pertinent variable in each hospital.

REFERENCES

Bartter, F. C., Delea, C. S. and Halberg, F. (1962). *Annals of the New York Academy of Science* **98**, 969.

de Lacerda, L., Kowarski, A. and Migeon, C. J. (1973). *Journal of Clinical Endocrinology and Metabolism* **36**, 227.

Ferin, M., Halberg, F., Richart, R. M. and Cande Wiele, R. L. (Eds) (1964). *In* "Biorhythms and Human Reproduction" p. 665. John Wiley and Sons, New York.

Halberg, F., Frank, G., Harner, R., Matthews, J., Aaker, H., Gravem, H. and Melby, J. (1961). *Experientia* **17**, 282.

Halberg, F., Tong, Y. L. and Johnson, E. A. (1967). *In* "The Cellular Aspects of Biorhythms" (H. V. Mayersbach, Ed.) p. 20–48. Springer–Verlag, Berlin.

Halberg, F., Haus, E., Tarquini, B., Cagnoni, M., Cornelissen, G., Lakatua, D., Kawasaki, T., Wallach, L. A., Halberg, E. and Omae, T. (1980a). *In* "Internal Medicine, Proc. XIVth Int. Cong. Internal Med. ISM, Rome, Italy, October 5–19, 1978" (L. Condorelli, U. Teodori, M. Sangiorgi and R. Neri Serneri, Eds). Excerpta Medica, Amsterdam/Oxford (in press).

Halberg, F., Cornelissen, G., Sothern, R. B., Wallach, L. A., Halberg, E., Ahlgren, A., Kuzel, M., Radke, A., Barbosa, J. Goetz, F., Buckley, J., Mandel, J., Schuman, L., Haus, E., Lakatua, D., Sackett, L., Berg, H., Kawasaki, T., Ueno, M., Uezono, K., Matsuoka, M., Omae, T., Tarquini, B., Cagnoni, M., García Sainz, M., Griffiths, K., Wilson, D., Donati, L., Tatti, P., Vasta, P., Locatelli, I., Camagna, A., Lauro, R., Tritsch, G. and Wendt, H. (1980b). *In* "Neoplasms—Comparative pathology of Growth in Animals, Plants and Man" (H. Kaiser, Ed.) Williams and Wilkins, Baltimore. (in press).

Haus, E., Halber, F., Nelson, W., Lakatua, D. J., Kawasaki, T., Ueno, M., Uezono, K. and Omae, T. (1979). *Chronobiologia* **6**, 266 (abstract).

Hellman, L., Nakada, F., Curti, J., Weitzman, E. D., Kream, J., Roffwarg, H., Ellman, S., Fukushims, D. K. and Gallagher, T. F. (1970). *Journal of Clinical Endocrinology* **30**, 411.

Katz, F. H., Romfh, P. and Smith, J. A. (1975). *Journal of Clinical Endocrinology and Metabolism* **40**, 125.

Kawasaki, T., Wallach, L. A., Halberg, E. and Omae, T. (1980a). *In* "Internal crinology and Metabolism* **40**, 205.

Krieger, D. T., Allen, W., Rizzo, F. and Krieger, H. R. (1971). *Journal of Clinical Endocrinology and Metabolism* **32**, 266.

Michelakis, A. M. and Horton, R. (1970). *Circulation Research* XXVI-XXVII (Suppl. 1), 185.

Nelson, W., Bingham, C., Haus, E., Lakatua, D., Kawasaki, T. and Halberg, F. (1980). *Journal of Gerontology.* (in press).

Nokin, J., Vekemans, M., L'Hermite, M. and Robyn, C. (1972). *British Medical Journal* **3**, 561.

Sassin, J. F., Frantz, A. G., Weitzman, E. D. and Kapen, S. (1972). *Science* **177**, 1205.

Tarquini, B., Gheri, R., Romano, S., Costa, A., Cagnoni, M., Lee, J. K. and Halberg, F. (1979). *American Journal of Medicine* **66**, 229.

Vagnucci, A. H., McDonald, R. H., Drash, A. L. and Wong, A.K.C. (1974). *Journal of Clinical Endocrinology and Metabolism* **38**, 761.

Weitzman, E. D., Fukushima, D. K., Nogeire, C., Roffwarg, H., Gallagher, T. F. and Hellman, L. (1971). *Journal of Clinical Endocrinology and Metabolism* **33**, 14.

CHRONO-REGULATION OF CORTISOL SECRETION IN OLD WOMEN

E. Ferrari[1], P. A. Bossolo[1], B. M. Mandelli[1], R. Frajria[2], F. Agrimonti[2]

[1] *Clinica Medica I "A Ferrata", Università di Pavia, Italy and* [2] *Clinica Medica B, Università di Torino, Turin, Italy*

INTRODUCTION

The study of the circadian chrono-organization of the ACTH-secreting system of ageing is very interesting both from a pathophysiological and clinical point of view. In fact, even if the physiological significance of the circadian periodicity of ACTH and cortisol levels is still unclear, nevertheless the study of cortico-steroid circadian cycle represents a very useful tool for the functional evaluation of the hypothalamic–pituitary–adrenal axis. Furthermore, owing to the role played by the rhythm of the adrenocortical secretion as pace-maker for the rhythms of several biological functions (i.e. blood cells, enzyme levels, cell mitoses, electrolytes urinary excretion), the study of cortisol circadian periodicity may give some information about the temporal structure of the organism and the inherent changes related to ageing. The aim of this paper was to present the results concerning the study of the circadian rhythm of plasma and urinary gluco-corticoids as well as of the plasma Corticosteroid Binding Globulin or trascortin (CBG) binding capacity in old women. Under physiological conditions, plasma CBG is a very important modulator of the gluco-corticoid – receptor interactions (Munck and Leung, 1977; De Kloet *et al.*, 1977), by influencing all the steps of the hormonal biological activity, after the secretion of cortisol from adrenals.

Concerning the age-related changes of plasma transcortin levels in humans,

Serono Symposium No. 39, "The Menopause: Clinical, Endocrinological and Pathophysiological Aspects", edited by P. Fioretti, L. Martini, G. B. Melis and S. S. C. Yen, 1982. Academic Press, London and New York.

it is well established that CBG levels rise rapidly in the first months after birth (De Moor and Heyns, 1968; August *et al.*, 1969), are enhanced prior to puberty (De Moor *et al.*, 1966), and subsequently decrease to adult values (Angeli *et al.*, 1977b), remaining nearly constant throughout life. No significant changes in plasma CBG have been described in elderly subjects, apart from the data of Wagner (1978), who described a sharp rise in plasma CBG levels in men over 74 years of age. On the contrary, it is well established that plasma concentrations of other carrier proteins, such as Sex Hormone Binding Globulin (SHBG), increase with age (Kley *et al.*, 1974; Gaidano *et al.*, 1977; Wagner, 1978).

Plasma CBG binding capacity exhibits in normal subjects a circadian rhythmicity (Doe *et al.*, 1964; Angeli *et al.*, 1977b), with an acrophase in the early afternoon (from 12 a.m. to 4 p.m.), and a minimum during the night (from 12 p.m. to 4 a.m.), namely at the time of the circadian activation of the ACTH-secreting system (Angeli *et al.*, 1977b).

Even if the mechanisms regulating the circadian fluctuation on plasma transcortin are to date not completely known, it seems well established that cortisol rhythmicity represents a very important synchronizer of the circadian variation of its specific transport protein (Feldman, 1975; Munck and Leung, 1977; Angeli *et al.*, 1977b).

MATERIALS AND METHODS

Thirteen clinically healthy women, aged 65–88, were studied as in-patients, well synchronized to the hospital schedule (meals at 8 a.m., noon and 6 p.m., sleep in darkness from 9 p.m. to 6 a.m. approximately).

The study of urinary 17-hydroxy-corticosteroids (17-OHcs) circadian rhythm was performed during two consecutive days; urine was collected by an indwelling catheter every 4 h, beginning at midnight, and urinary 17-OHcs were measured as Porter–Silber chromogens (Schoeller *et al.*, 1962) in each urine sample, and expressed in mg/4h. During the sleep span, subjects were awakened at collection times. On the second day of the study, 12 of these subjects were also evaluated for the circadian rhythm of plasma cortisol and of plasma C.B.G., by means of blood samples which were drawn every 4 h for 24 h, together with urine collection. Plasma cortisol was measured by fluorimetric method (Mattingly, 1962).

The CBG, expressed as mcg cortisol bound/100 ml, was evaluated by an equilibrated procedure of gel-exchange with Sephadex G-25. This method (Angeli *et al.*, 1977b) allows calculation of the binding parameters under thermodinamically proper conditions. Ten young clinically healthy women (20–40 years), studied as in-patients during the follicular phase of the menstrual cycle, were chosen as controls.

The hormonal results were placed on punched cards and were analyzed by means of the least squares and the "mean cosinor" method (Halberg *et al.*, 1967). By this procedure, parameters of the circadian rhythm such as mesor M (a rhythm adjusted mean), amplitude A (measure of one half the extent of rhythmic changes in the cycle) and acrophase θ (measure of timing of the crest time in the function), were calculated with respective 95% confidence limits.

The chrono-sensitivity of the adrenal cortex to pulse stimulation by a micro-dose of synthetic corticotropin was studied in every subject. The test was performed by means of an i.v. injection of 2500 ng of $\beta1$ 24-corticotropin (Synacthen[®]) at 8.30 a.m. and 8.30 p.m. on different days. The lag between the two tests was always 36 h at least; the succession of the two tests changed randomly. In our experience (Ferrari *et al.*, 1977; Bossolo *et al.*, 1979) the dose of Synacthen[®] used is sufficient to give a significant release of cortisol from the adrenals, when the glands contain a sufficient amount of cortisol or of its pre-cursors. In every case blood samples for cortisol estimation were drawn through an indwelling polyethylene catheter inserted in the antecubital vein before the injection of corticotropin, and then at 5, 10, 15, 20, 30, 60 and 90 min after the injection. The adrenocortical response was evaluated by the absolute increase (Δ mcg/100 ml) and by the maximal percentage increase ($\Delta\%$) of plasma cortisol on the basal value (resulting from the mean of two samples collected at 10 min intervals).

The results of Synacthen tests in old women were compared with those of out-patients. The absolute increases in plasma cortisol after Synacthen injection were compared by a trifactorial analysis of variance (timing of the stimulation test, subjects, and time span after the injection). For the percentage variations of plasma cortisol in old and young women the Student's *t*-test was performed.

RESULTS

The circadian pattern of the three variables studied is summarized in Table I and plotted in Fig. 1. By "macroscopic" approach, the plasma and urinary steroid curves and that of plasma transcortin show the usual circadian pattern. The maximum of plasma cortisol occurs about 2 h before that of urinary 17-OHcs and about 6 h before that of plasma CBG. The urinary steroid flow curves of two consecutive days are quite overlapping.

Plasma levels of CBG binding capacity throughout the 24 h cycle do not

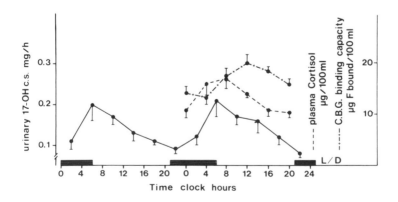

Fig. 1. Circadian pattern of several hormonal functions in old women (N = 13 for urinary 17-OHcs; N = 12 for plasma cortisol and CBG) ($\bar{X}$ ± SE).

Table I. Circadian pattern of plasma cortisol, plasma CBG binding capacity and urinary 17-hydroxy-corticoids ($\bar{x} \pm SE$).

Time	00^{00}	04^{00}	08^{00}	12^{00}	16^{00}	20^{00}
Old women (65–88 years)						
(A) pl. Cortisol (N = 12) mcg/100 ml	10.92 ± 1.48	16.04 ± 2.29	17.12 ± 1.99	14.01 ± 0.72	10.91 ± 1.17	10.36 ± 0.95
(B) pl. CBG (N = 12) mcg F bound/100 ml	14.17 ± 1.41	13.43 ± 1.40	17.60 ± 1.35	20.08 ± 1.71	18.56 ± 0.84	15.87 ± 1.01
Young women (20–40 years)						
(C) pl. Cortisol (N = 10) mcg/100 ml	7.35 ± 0.62	14.66 ± 1.56	22.20 ± 0.95	13.64 ± 1.05	11.99 ± 0.73	10.48 ± 1.07
(D) pl. CBG (N = 10) mcg F bound/100 ml	12.60 ± 0.86	10.52 ± 0.70	19.07 ± 1.26	20.29 ± 0.51	21.37 ± 0.91	16.36 ± 0.75
	00–04	04–08	08–12	12–16	16–20	20–24
Old women (65–88 years)						
(E) ur. 17-OHcs Ist day mg/h (N = 13)	0.11 ± 0.02	0.20 ± 0.04	0.17 ± 0.02	0.13 ± 0.01	0.11 ± 0.01	0.09 ± 0.01
(F) id. 2nd day	0.12 ± 0.02	0.21 ± 0.04	0.16 ± 0.02	0.15 ± 0.03	0.12 ± 0.02	0.08 ± 0.01
Young women (20–40 years)						
(G) ur. 17-OHcs mg/h (N = 10)	0.17 ± 0.01	0.30 ± 0.03	0.34 ± 0.03	0.26 ± 0.02	0.24 ± 0.03	0.19 ± 0.02
Student's t-test						
A vs C P	< 0.05	NS	< 0.05	NS	NS	NS
B vs D P	NS[a]	NS	NS	NS	< 0.05	NS
E vs F P	NS	NS	NS	NS	NS	NS
E vs G P	< 0.05	NS	< 0.001	< 0.001	< 0.001	< 0.001
F vs G P	< 0.05	NS	< 0.001	< 0.005	< 0.01	< 0.001

Table II. Mean cosinor analysis of circadian rhythm of plasma cortisol and plasma CBG binding capacity and urinary 17-hydroxy-corticoids.

Variable	N	P Rhythm detection	Mesor M ± SE	Amplitude A (95% confidence limits)	Acrophase θ [a] (95% confidence limits)
Old women					
pl. Cortisol mcg/100 ml	12	0.015	13.23 ± 1.06	3.669 (1.393 to 5.945)	−110.8° (− 80.4 to −161.5) h. 7.23 (5.22 to 10.46)
pl. CBG mcg F bound/100 ml	12	0.001	16.62 ± 1.13	3.264 (2.439 to 4.088)	−197.5° (−177.9 to −235.9) h. 13.10 (11.51 to 15.44)
ur. 17-OHcs (2nd day) mg/h	13	0.013	0.14 ± 0.02	0.049 (0.019 to 0.079)	−135.6° (−100.3 to −160.0) h. 9.02 (6.41 to 10.40)
Young women					
pl. Cortisol mcg/100 ml	14	0.001	13.80 ± 1.03	5.982 (5.788 to 6.176)	−127.1° (−110.3 to −156.4) h. 8.28(7.21 to 10.25)
pl. CBG mcg F bound/100 ml	10	0.001	16.80 ± 4.70	5.460 (4.040 to 6.880)	−204.0° (−189.0 to −222.0) h. 13.36 12.36 to 14.48)
ur. 17-OHcs mg/h	10	0.001	0.25 ± 0.02	0.074 (0.058 to 0.091)	−154.7° (−123.8 to −184.8) h. 10.19 (8.15 to 12.19)

360° = 24 h   15° = 1 h

[a] phase reference = local midnight.

Table III. Plasma Cortisol response to pulse stimulation by synthetic $\beta1$, 24-corticotropin (Synacthen® 2500 ng i.v.) at different times (mcg/100 ml) ($\bar{x} \pm$ SE).

Subjects	N	Baseline	5'	10'	15'	20'	30'	60'	90'	Peak mcg/100 ml	Time to peak
Old women											
test h. 8^{30}	13	14.50 ± 0.89	18.19 ± 1.27	22.19 ± 1.45	25.08 ± 1.55	26.03 ± 1.35	30.17 ± 1.79	21.23 ± 1.53	16.50 ± 1.51	32.06 ± 1.12	29.61 ± 2.91
test h. 20^{30}	13	9.79 ± 0.81	14.07 ± 0.45	18.70 ± 1.00	23.76 ± 1.15	26.56 ± 1.36	30.67 ± 1.35	22.19 ± 2.64	16.32 ± 2.29	32.98 ± 1.50	33.84 ± 5.60
Young women											
test h. 8^{30}	21	10.60 ± 0.45	13.40 ± 1.18	15.84 ± 1.18	18.40 ± 1.23	20.83 ± 1.23	21.44 ± 1.43	19.40 ± 1.48	15.34 ± 1.34	25.23 ± 1.16	30.71 ± 4.40
test h. 20^{30}	21	7.28 ± 0.48	11.19 ± 0.81	15.58 ± 1.06	18.63 ± 1.17	20.97 ± 1.31	23.99 ± 1.42	21.81 ± 1.92	16.72 ± 1.93	27.47 ± 1.67	43.09 ± 5.00

show any difference between old and young subjects. On the contrary, plasma cortisol levels of old women are greater at midnight and lower at 8 a.m. if compared with those of controls, the differences being highly significant at the Student's *t*-test. Likewise, the urinary gluco-corticoid excretion during the circadian cycle is always significantly smaller in all subjects than in controls.

Table II summarizes the results of the statistical analysis of the rhythms by the "mean cosinor" method (Halberg *et al.*, 1967). A statistically significant circadian rhythm was detected both for plasma CBG and for plasma and urinary steroids. The circadian acrophase occurs at 1 p.m. for plasma CBG, at 7 a.m. for plasma cortisol and at 9 a.m. for urinary 17-OHcs, without any significant differences in comparison with controls. The amplitude of the rhythms of the three variables studied is significantly reduced in old women, in comparison with young subjects; only for urinary steroids was a reduction in the mesor in old women observed, whereas for plasma cortisol and CBG binding capacity the mesor does not differ in old and young people.

The results of the adreno-cortical stimulation at different times of the day are summarized in Table III and Fig. 2. After pulse stimulation by a microdose

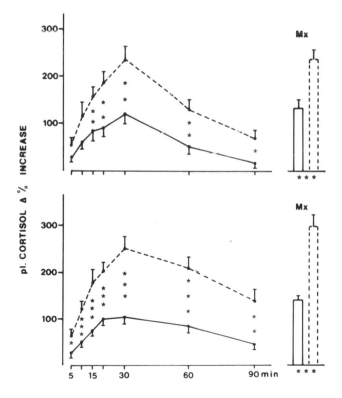

Fig. 2. ACTH-induced percentage increments of plasma cortisol related to the timing of the stimulation test. The top graph shows the results for old subjects (65–88 years; N = 13) and the bottom graph, for young subjects (20–45 years; N = 21). —— 8^{30}; – – – – 20^{30}; *$P < 0.05$; **$P < 0.01$; ***$P < 0.001$. $\bar{X} \pm$ SE.

Table IV. Trifactorial analysis of variance of cortisol increases (Δ mcg/100 ml) after Synacthen injection at different times. A = timing of the stimulation test. B = subjects. C = time span after the injection.

Cases	N	Significance of single factors and interactions (P)					
		A	B	C	A × B	B × C	A × C
Old women	13	0.0001	0.0001	0.0001	0.0036	0.0001	0.094 (NS)
Young women	21	0.0001	0.0001	0.0001	0.0001	0.0001	0.098 (NS)

of synthetic β1 24-corticotropin, the adrenocortical response in elderly patients does not significantly differ from that of young subjects, both from a qualitative and quantitative point of view; nevertheless, in old women we observe a more rapid decrease of plasma cortisol after the peak value, which usually occurs 30 min after injection. Besides, in old women, as well as in young controls, the adrenal responsiveness to exogenous corticotropin is significantly higher in the evening than in the morning. The chrono-dependence of the amplitude of cortisol increases after pulse stimulation by Synacthen was highly significant also at the analysis of variance, in spite of individual variability; the pattern of plasma cortisol after Synacthen injection does not differ in the two tests (cf. Table IV).

CONCLUSIONS

The results of this study prove the maintenance in old age of the circadian rhythmicity of gluco-corticoid function, both for its adrenal secretion and for the specific binding to the plasma carrier protein.

Plasma levels of CBG binding capacity throughout the circadian cycle are quite overlapping in old and young women, in agreement with previous data assessing the absence of transcortin changes related with ageing (De Moor *et al.*, 1962; Kley *et al.*, 1974). In comparison with young people, the amplitude of circadian rhythm of plasma and urinary steroids is significantly reduced in old women, and for urinary 17-OHcs only there is also a reduction in the mesor.

The lower extent of rhythmic changes of plasma cortisol and urinary 17-OHcs observed in old women do agree with other data concerning the reduction of the amplitude of some biological rhythms in ageing, both in animals (Halberg *et al.*, 1955; Yunis *et al.*, 1974) and humans (Descovich *et al.*, 1974; Scheving *et al.*, 1974). Besides, the reduction of the mesor of urinary corticoid circadian rhythm results from the decrease of cortisol secretion rate (Romanoff *et al.*, 1961) and the slower cortisol disposal rate (Samuels *et al.*, 1957; West *et al.*, 1961) in ageing. The most important differences in plasma and urinary steroid circadian pattern between old and young women are observed during the night and the early morning hours, namely at the moment of circadian activation of the ACTH-secreting system. In fact, both plasma and urinary gluco-corticoids exhibit in old women a smaller nocturnal increase, in comparison with young people. Since it is well known that the nocturnal increase of gluco-corticoids reflects the circadian release of CRH and consequently of ACTH, it is possible to infer that the nocturnal corticotropin secretion is lowered with age. This is in agreement with our data concerning the prevalent impairment of the ACTH-secreting system at the hypothalamic-pituitary level in old age (Ferrari and Bossolo, 1973). This functional behaviour of the ACTH-secreting system in old people could be related to the slower metabolism of cortisol in the liver (West *et al.*, 1961) and subsequently to the persistence of higher plasma levels of cortisol during the "critical" phase of the circadian activation of the pituitary-adrenal axis. Furthermore, the changes in the nocturnal phase of gluco-corticoid circadian rhythm observed in older subjects may be related to sleep disturbances often present in the elderly, as well as to some alterations in the rhythm of plasma GH (Williams, 1970; D'Agata *et al.*, 1974).

The adrenocortical responsiveness to pulse injection of a sub-maximal dose of synthetic corticotropin in old women is quantitatively normal and is greater in the evening than in the morning, as observed in healthy young subjects. In fact, the pituitary–adrenal axis exhibits in normal subjects a different sensitivity to specific stimuli, according to the timing of their administration (Haus and Halberg, 1960; Ungar and Halberg, 1962; Martin and Hellman, 1964; Ichikawa *et al.*, 1972; Angeli *et al.*, 1977a; Ferrari *et al.*, 1977). This behaviour seems in our opinion to be in some way related to the normal chrono-organization of the ACTH-secreting system, because no significant difference in cortisol's response, related to the timing of corticotrophic stimulation are observed in patients whose circadian rhythm of cortisol secretion is not detectable (Ferrari *et al.*, 1980).

REFERENCES

Angeli, A., Frayria, R., Fonzo, D., Bertello, P., Gaidano, G. P. and Ceresa, F. (1977a). Proc. XII Int. Conf. of Chronobiology, Washington 1975. 189. Il Ponte, Milano.

Angeli, A., Frayria, R., Richiardi, L., Agrimonti, F. and Gaidano, G. P. (1977b). *Clinical Chimica Acta* 77, 1.

August, G. P., Trachuk, M. and Grumbach, M. M. (1969). *Journal of Clinical Endocrinology and Metabolism* 29, 891.

Bossolo, P. A., Mandelli, B. M., Sironi, P. L., Pompeo, A., Solerte, S. B. and Ferrari, E. (1979). *Minerva Endocrinologica* 4, 69.

D'Agata, R., Vigneri, R. and Polosa, P. (1974). *In* "Chronobiology" (L. E. Scheving, F. Halberg and J. E. Pauly, Eds) p. 81. Igaku Shoin, Tokyo.

De Kloet, E. R., Burbach, P. and Mulder, G. H. (1977). *Molecular and Cellular Endocrinology* 7, 261.

De Moor, P. and Heyns, W. (1968). *Journal of Clinical Endocrinology and Metabolism* 28, 1281.

De Moor, P., Heirwegh, K., Heremans, J. F. and Declerck–Raskin, M. (1962). *Journal of Clinical Investigation* 41, 816.

De Moor, P., Steeno, O., Brosens, J. and Hendrix, A. (1966). *Journal of Clinical Endocrinology and Metabolism* 26, 71.

Descovich, G. C., Montalbetti, N., Kühl, J.F.W., Rimondi, S., Halberg, F. and Ceredi, C. (1974). *Chronobiologia* I, 163.

Doe, R. P., Fernandez, R. N. and Seal, U. S. (1964). *Journal of Clinical Endocrinology* 24, 1029.

Feldman, (1975). *Annales Internal Medicine* 26, 83.

Ferrari, E. and Bossolo, P. A. (1973). *In* "Les endocrines et le troisième âge" (H. P. Klotz, Ed.), pp. 227–267. Exp. Scient. Franç., Paris.

Ferrari, E., Bossolo, P. A., Rea, A., Vailati, A., Bertulessi, C., Martinelli, I., Tamborini, M. and De Matte, S. (1977). *In* "Giornate Endocrinologiche Pisane" (F. Menelini, Tebris and F. Treneletti, Eds), Vol. I, 431–443. Pacini, Pisa.

Ferrari, E., Bossolo, P. A., Mandelli, B. M., Vailati, A., Sironi, P. L., Solerte, S. B. and Romano, S. (1980). *Journal of Endocrinological Investigation* 3, suppl. 1, 86.

Gaidano, G. P., Frayria, R., Berta, L., Boccuzzi, G. and Angeli, A. (1977). *Giornale Italiano di Chimica Clinica* 8, 55.

Halberg, F., Bittner, J. J., Gully, R. J., Albrecht, P. G. and Brackney, E. L. (1955). *Proceedings of the Experimental Biology NY* 88, 169.

Halberg, F., Tong, Y. L. and Johnson, E. A. (1967). *In* "The Cellular aspects of biorhythms", pp. 20–48. Springer–Verlag, Berlin.

Haus, E. and Halberg, F. (1960). Proc. Ist. Int. Congr. Endocrinol., 219. Fuchs, Copenhagen.

Ichikawa, Y., Nishikai, M., Kawagoe, N., Yoshida, K. and Homma, M. (1972). *Journal of Clinical Endocrinology and Metabolism* **34**, 895.

Kley, H. K., Nieschlag, E., Bidlingmaier, F. and Krüskemper, H. L. (1974). *Hormone Metabolism Research* **6**, 213.

Martin, M. N. and Hellman, D. E. (1964). *Journal of Clinical Endocrinology* **24**, 253.

Mattingly, D. (1962). *Journal of Clinical Pathology* **15**, 374.

Munck, A. and Leung, K. Y. (1977). *In* "Receptors and mechanisms of action of steroid hormones" (J. R. Pasqualini, Ed.), pp. 311–397. Marcel Dekker, New York and Basel.

Romanoff, L. P., Morris, C. W., Welch, P., Rodriguez, R. M. and Pincus, G. (1961). *Journal of Clinical Endocrinology* **21**, 1413.

Samuels, L. T., Brown, H., Eik–Nes, K., Tyler, F. H. and Dominguez, O. V. (1957). *Ciba Found. Coll. Endocr.* **11**, 208.

Scheving, L. E., Roig, C., Halberg, F., Pauly, J. E. and Hand, E. A. (1974). *In* "Chronobiology" (L. E. Scheving, F. Halberg and J. E. Pauly, Eds), pp. 353–357. Igaku Shoin, Tokyo.

Scholler, R., Busigny, M. and Jayle, M. F. (1962). *In* "Analyse des stéroïdes hormonaux" (M. F. Jayle, Ed.) Vol. 2, 137. Masson, Paris.

Ungar, F. and Halberg, F. (1962). *Science* **137**, 1058.

Yunis, E. J., Fernandes, G., Nelson, W. and Halberg, F. (1974). *In* "Chronobiology" (L. E. Scheving, F. Halberg and J. E. Pauly, Eds), pp. 358–363. Igaku Shoin, Tokyo.

Wagner, R. K. (1978). *Acta Endocrinology* **88**, Suppl. 218.

West, C. D., Drown, H., Simons, E. L., Carter, D. B., Kumagai, L. F. and Englert, E. Jr (1961). *Journal of Clinical Endocrinology* **21**, 1197.

Williams, R. H. (1970). *Journal Clinical Endocrinology and Metabolism* **31**, 461.

MEDROXYPROGESTERONE ACTION ON GONADOTROPINS IN POSTMENOPAUSAL WOMEN

F. Iannotta, G. Pinotti and C. Pollini

Divisione "B" di Medicina Generale, Ospedale Regionale di Varese; Biometria,
Farmitalia Carlo Erba, Milan, Italy

INTRODUCTION

Medroxyprogesterone acetate (MAP or 17α acetoxy-6α methyl-pregn-4-ene-3, 20-dione), a progestational drug used for contraception and for the treatment of idiopathic precocious puberty, menopausal syndrome and hormone dependent tumours, has been attributed with a well-known action in inhibiting gonadotropin secretion. Nevertheless, the site of action (at hypothalamic and/or pituitary level) is still obscure. Conflicting results have been reported about MAP interactions with gonadotropin response to exogenous GnRH. Reiter *et al.* (1975) have shown a decrease of gonadotropin response to exogenous GnRH in four out of five subjects treated with MAP for idiopathic precocious puberty and they concluded that the drug could act at hypothalamic as well as at pituitary level, or both. In normally cycling and postmenopausal women, however, gonadotropin response to GnRH, after MAP treatment, was not different from the basal one (Franchimont and Legros, 1975; Perez-Lopez *et al.*, 1975; Franchimont, 1977; Mishell *et al.*, 1977; Toppozada *et al.*, 1978). These results could indicate that progestogen acts primarily at hypothalamic level. To clarify the action of MAP on gonadotropin release we studied the effects of i.m. administration of MAP on basal and stimulated secretion of FSH and LH, in postmenopausal women.

Serono Symposium No. 39, "The Menopause: Clinical, Endocrinological and Pathophysiological Aspects", edited by P. Fioretti, L. Martini, G. B. Melis and S. S. C. Yen, 1982. Academic Press, London and New York.

MATERIALS AND METHODS

Eight postmenopausal women, 52–59 years, without endocrine diseases and not taking drugs interfering with the hypothalamic–pituitary–ovarian axis, volunteered for GnRH tests before and after MAP administration (500 mg/day i.m. for 8 days). The subjects were injected i.v. with 100 γ GnRH at 9 a.m. after an overnight fast. Blood samples were collected 15 and 0 min before, and 20, 30, 60, 90 and 120 min after GnRH administration, through a catheter inserted in a forearm vein and kept open by slow infusion of normal saline. The first day MAP was administered i.m. after the basal GnRH test and the following 7 days at 8 a.m. On the 8th day, GnRH test was performed 1 h after MAP administration. FSH and LH serum levels were measured by RIA technique (Sorin Kits, Saluggia, Italy). Gonadotropin response to GnRH stimulation test was assessed by considering the FSH and LH absolute increment. Statistical analysis was performed using analysis of variance according to a split-plot design.

RESULTS

MAP administration induced a significant decrease in mean basal levels of both gonadotropins (Fig. 1, Table I) but FSH decrease was greater than LH decrease. Mean gonadotropin levels after GnRH administration were always significantly greater in comparison with mean basal values (Fig. 1, Table I).

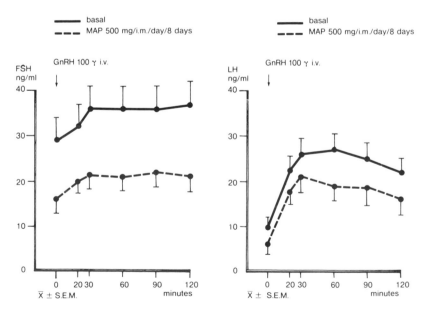

Fig. 1.   Serum FSH and LH levels following 100 γ GnRH injection, before and after MAP treatment (500 mg/day i.m. for 8 days) in eight postmenopausal women. The values are reported as mean ± SE.

Table I. Analysis of variance according to a spit-plot design.

	FSH ng/ml		LH ng/ml	
	d.f.	Variance	d.f.	Variance
Pre vs Post[a]	1	4778.21	1	687.05
Patients[a]	7	1344.82	7	718.05
error (a)	7	182.75	7	32.20
Times[a]	5	114.22	5	504.17
Times x pre vs post	5	6.68	5	9.49
error (b)	70	6.41	70	11.43

[a]$P < 0.01$.

After MAP administration, FSH and LH levels following GnRH administration were significantly lower in comparison with pretreatment values (Fig. 1, Table I). Nevertheless there was no statistically significant difference between gonadotropin response to GnRH before and after MAP administration (Table I), when absolute FSH and LH increment was considered.

DISCUSSION

MAP administration induced a statistically significant decrease in basal values of both FSH and LH. These data agree with those previously reported in menopausal women (Franchimont and Legros, 1975; Franchimont, 1977), in normally cycling women (Mishell, 1967; Perez–Lopez *et al.,* 1975), in castrated adults (Rifkind *et al.,* 1969), in idiopathic precocious puberty (Kaplan *et al.,* 1968; Kenny *et al.,* 1969; Kupperman and Epstein, 1962; Rifkind *et al.,* 1969; Schoen, 1966) and in gonadal dysgenesis (Laron *et al.,* 1963). However conflicting results have been reported in normally cycling women (Gaspard *et al.,* 1969; Goldzieher *et al.,* 1970), as well as in menopausal women (Bullock *et al.,* 1975) and in idiopathic precocious puberty (Lemli *et al.,* 1964; Richman *et al.,* 1971; Rifkind *et al.,* 1969).

Our data show that MAP administration induced a statistically significant decrease of gonadotropin peak after GnRH stimulation in comparison with pretreatment values. However gonadotropin response to GnRH was the same before and after MAP treatment, when absolute gonadotropin increment was considered. These results agree with those of Franchimont and Legros (1975), Perez–Lopez *et al.,* (1975), Mishell *et al.,* (1977) and Toppozada *et al.* (1978), showing a normal gonadotropin response to GnRH stimulation after MAP treatment.

The decrease of gonadotropin basal concentrations after MAP, without modifications of gonadotropin response to GnRH, could be interpreted as the effect of hypothalamic or suprahypothalamic action, decreasing gonadotropin release without affecting synthesis or storage. This interpretation is also supported by Mishell *et al.* (1977) who did not find a significant decrease of pituitary residual capacity for gonadotropin secretion after MAP treatment. Finally, Perez–Lopez *et al.* (1975) did not find a decrease of gonadotropin response to GnRH even after many years of MAP treatment.

REFERENCES

Bullock, J. L., Massey, F. M. and Don Gambrell, R. (1975). *Obstetrics and Gynecology* **46**, 165.
Franchimont, P. (1977). *Clinics in Endocrinology and Metabolism* **6**, 101.
Franchimont, P. and Legros, J. J. (1975). *In* "Hypothalamic Hormones" (M. Motta, P. G. Crosignani and L. Martini, Eds), pp. 311–324. Academic Press, London and New York.
Gaspard, U., Franchimont, P., Beco, G. and Legros, J. J. (1969). *Comptes Rendus Société Belge De Biologie* **163**, 2456.
Goldzieher, J. W., Kleber, J. W., Moses, L. E. and Rathmacher, R. P., (1970). *Contraception* **2**, 225.
Kaplan, S. A., Ling, S. M. and Irani, N. G. (1968). *American Journal Diseases of Children* **116**, 591.
Kenny, F. M., Midgley, A. R., Jaffe, R. B., Garces, L. Y., Vazques, A. and Taylor, F. H. (1969). *Journal of Clinical Endocrinology and Metabolism* **29**, 1272.
Kupperman, H. S. and Epstein, J. A. (1962). *Journal of Clinical Endocrinology* **22**, 456.
Laron, Z., Rumney, G., Rat, L. and Naji, N. (1963). *Acta Endocrinologica* (Kbh) **44**, 75.
Lemli, L., Aron, M. and Smith, D. W. (1964). *The Journal of Pediatrics* **65**, 888.
Mishell, D. R. (1967). *American Journal of Obstetrics and Gynecology* **99**, 86.
Mishell, D. R., Kletzky, O. A., Brenner, P. F., Roy, S. and Nicoloff, J. (1977). *American Journal of Obstetrics and Gynecology* **128**, 60.
Perez–Lopez, F. R., L'Hermite, M. and Robyn, C. (1975). *Clinical Endocrinology* **4**, 477.
Reiter, E. O., Kaplan, S. L., Conte, F. A. and Grumbach, M. M. (1975). *Pediatric Research* **9**, 111.
Richman, R. A., Underwood, L. E., French, F. S. and Van Wyk, J. J. (1971). *The Journal of Pediatrics* **79**, 963.
Rifkind, A. B., Kulin, H. E., Cargille, C. M., Rayford, P. C. and Ross, G. T. (1969). *Journal of Clinical Endocrinology* **29**, 506.
Schoen, E. J. (1966). *Journal of Clinical Endocrinology* **26**, 363.
Toppozada, M., Parmar, C. and Fotherby, K. (1978). *Fertility and Sterility* **30**, 545.

THYROID AND MENOPAUSE

L. Baschieri, E. Martino, S. Mariotti, F. Lippi, F. Monzani, E. Motz, G. Vaudagna and V. Aloisio

Cattedra di Patologia Medica 2, Univeristy of Pisa, Pisa, Italy

INTRODUCTION

The relationship between thyroid function and the female reproductive system has been extensively investigated (Burrow, 1978; De Groot, 1979; Burrow, 1980). It is well known that thyroid disorders are four to seven times more frequent in women than in men. Furthermore, pregnancy is associated with complex female reproductive physiological modifications and sex hormone metabolism.

Although thyroid disorders have long since been suspected to be associated with the menopause, to our knowledge no specific study has been carried out to clarify this problem. In the present report we shall review the link between menopause and thyroid function. In particular, we shall focus our attention on the incidence of different thyroid diseases in the menopausal period. Before discussing this topic, we shall summarize the data available on the influence of female sex hormones on thyroid function.

INFLUENCE OF FEMALE SEX HORMONES ON THYROID FUNCTION

Circulating Thyroid Hormones and Thyroxine-binding Globulin

Pregnancy and oestrogen administration are associated with clearly elevated serum thyroxine (T_4), triiodothyronine (T_3) and reverse T_3 as observed in mild hyperthyroidism (Schatz *et al.*, 1968; Man *et al.*, 1969a; Fisher *et al.*, 1970;

Serono Symposium No. 39, "The Menopause: Clinical, Endocrinological and Pathophysiological Aspects", edited by P. Fioretti, L. Martini, G. B. Melis and S. S. C. Yen, 1982. Academic Press, London and New York.

Rastogi *et al.*, 1974; Chopra and Crandal, 1975; Yamamoto *et al.*, 1979). These
alterations are due to increased serum thyroxine-binding globulin (TBG) concentration (Dowling *et al.*, 1960; Man *et al.*, 1969b; Gershengorn *et al.*, 1980),
which affects mainly the bound thyroid hormone levels, while the free thyroid
hormone concentrations remain unchanged (Oppenheimer *et al.*, 1963; Abuid
et al., 1973; Osathanondh *et al.*, 1976; Kurtz *et al.*, 1979; Pinchera *et al.*, 1979;
Chopra *et al.*, 1980). This concept remained controversial for many years, since
easy and precise methods of assessing free thyroid hormones in serum were not
available. Recently, using a simple method based on column chromatography
for separation of free from bound thyroid hormones, followed by radioimmunoassay of absorbed fractions (Romelli *et al.*, 1979), evidence has been provided
that in pregnancy the levels of free thyroid hormones are in the normal range
(Pinchera *et al.*, 1979). The high TBG levels observed in oestrogen-related con-
ditons are due to increased liver synthesis of this protein (Glinoer *et al.*, 1977).
Oestrogens are probably also important in the determination of higher serum
TBG levels observed in young adult women with respect to men of the same
age. However, as illustrated in Fig. 1, we recently showed that, in addition to
sex (Braverman *et al.*, 1976; Hesh *et al.*, 1977; Fisher *et al.*, 1977), the age appears
to be an important factor in the determination of serum TBG levels (Bigazzi
et al., 1980).

Thyrotropin and its Response to Thyrotropin-releasing Hormone

The administration of thyrotropin-releasing hormone (TRH) is followed by
a transient increase of serum thyrotropin (TSH), which is higher in females than
in males (Noel *et al.*, 1974; Pinchera *et al.*, 1980). Sanchez–Franco *et al.* (1973)
demonstrated that the higher TSH response to TRH in females is present only
during the oestrogen phases of the menstrual cycle, while during the luteal phase
no difference between females and males is observed.

Many reports indicate that in pregnancy serum immunoreactive TSH levels
are increased (Genazzani *et al.*, 1971), but other authors showed that the levels
were normal (Odell *et al.*, 1967; Fisher *et al.*, 1970) or even reduced (Braunstein
and Hershman, 1976). The reason for these discrepancies is probably due to the
cross-reactivity of human chorionic gonadotropin (HCG) with the anti-TSH
antiserum used in the radioimmunoassay. The pregnant serum also shows increased
TSH-like bioactivity (Hennen *et al.*, 1969; Nisula *et al.*, 1974): this phenomenon
is now explained on the basis of the demonstrated intrinsic thyroid-stimulating
activity of HCG (IU = 0.5 μU of human TSH) (Kenimer *et al.*, 1975).

The results obtained assaying TSH after TRH administration to pregnant
women show in general a normal response (Kannan *et al.*, 1973; Burrow *et al.*,
1975; Koutros *et al.*, 1978) even though augmented responses have been reported
(Ramey *et al.*, 1975). Thus, it is unclear if the hypothalamic–pituitary–thyroid
axis is altered during pregnancy. However, the observed increase in TSH responsiveness to TRH during pregnancy would militate against the possibility that hyperfunction of the thyroid gland is present during gestation, since elevation of serum
thyroid hormone concentration results in a reduced pituitary TSH response to

TRH. In conclusion, in spite of some controversial evidence of perturbation in hypothalamic–pituitary–thyroid axis, the normal pregnant woman is probably euthyroid.

INFLUENCE OF THYROID STATUS ON FEMALE REPRODUCTIVE PHYSIOLOGY

Hypothyroidism

Thyroid hormone deficiency affects the female reproductive physiology in several different ways. Hypothyroidism in children is sometimes followed by delayed puberty and in adults it is associated with spontaneous abortions, anovulatory cycles and menstrual abnormalities such as menorrhagia. In some patients with long-term hypothyroidism, ovarian failure with amenorrhoea due to pituitary disorders can be observed. These abnormalities can usually be reversed by thyroxine administration. Furthermore, thyroid hormone affects the meta-

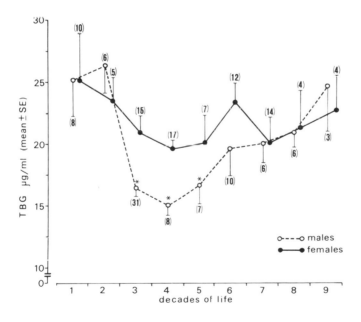

Fig. 1. Serum Thyroxine binding globulin (TBG) concentration (mean ± SE) versus age in 173 euthyroid subjects. In parentheses are reported the number of observations at a given point. The data obtained at various ages were compared to those observed in the first decade by means of the Student's *t*-test. In females no significant change in serum TBG was observed between different ages. In contrast, serum TBG levels were significantly reduced (*$P < 0.01$) in males aged 30–59 years. At this age range, serum TBG level in males was also lower (*$P < 0.01$) than that observed in females.

bolism and the serum transport of oestrogens. Hypothyroidism enhances the
16O-hydroxylation of 17-oestradiol leading to an increased oestriol formation
(Fishman *et al.*, 1965). The levels of sex-hormone-binding globulin (SHBG) are
decreased (Olivo *et al.*, 1970; Tulchinsky and Chopra, 1973) with reduction
of serum total oestrogen concentration, although the free hormone fraction is
increased. Finally, hypothyroidism is one of the risk factors for the development of endometrial cancer. As suggested by Casey and Madden (1976), hypo-
thyroid women should be submitted to endometrial screening, even in the absence
of significant symptoms.

Hyperthyroidism

Excess of thyroid hormones results in complex modifications of female reproductive physiology. In thyrotoxic women abnormalities such as oligomenorrhoea,
amenorrhoea and perhaps reduced fertility are frequently observed. Serum oestrogen and SHBG concentrations are higher in hyperthyroid than in euthyroid
women during all phases of the menstrual cycles (Akande and Hockaday, 1972a;
Tulchinsky and Chopra, 1973). Luteinizing hormone (LH) levels are also higher
in hyperthyroidism: however, in patients with scanty regular periods or with
amenorrhoea, blunted or absent LH ovulatory peaks are observed (Akande and
Hockaday, 1972b).

Table I. Comparison of most frequent signs and symptoms of hyperthyroids
and menopausal syndrome.

Sign or symptom	Hyperthyroidism	Menopause
Weight loss	++	−
Increased appetite	++	−
Diarrhoea	++	−
Polydipsia	++	−
Polyuria	++	−
Shortness of breath	++	++
Palpitations	+++	++
Tachycardia	++	+
Arrhythmias	++	−
Nervousness	++	++
Tremors	+++	+
Vertigo	−	+
Insomnia	++	++
Weakness	+	+
Increased sweating	+++	++
Heat intolerance	+++	++
Hot flushes	−	+++
Arthralgies	−	+
Paresthesiae	−	+
Goiter	++	−
Exophthalmos	+	−

THYROID PHYSIOLOGY AND MENOPAUSE

Serum T_4 and T_3 levels progressively decrease as age increases (Rubenstein *et al.*, 1973), but no difference has been observed between males and females, suggesting no effect of the menopause on circulating thyroid hormone levels. Serum TBG concentration in women does not show a clear age-related pattern, as observed in males (Fig. 1) (Bigazzi *et al.*, 1980).

Very few studies have been carried out on circulating TSH levels during the menopausal period. Yen (1977) reported no significant variation in basal TSH concentration in premenopausal women when compared to that observed in postmenopausal women.

Hayward *et al.* (1978) observed that serum TSH levels in menopausal Hawaiian women were significantly higher than those found in menopausal Japanese or British women. The significance of this observation has not yet been fully clarified. Snyder and Utiger (1972) studied the TSH response to TRH in subjects of both sexes aged between 20 and 79 years. The mean maximal incremental responses in females were virtually the same at all ages, in contrast, in males a decrease of

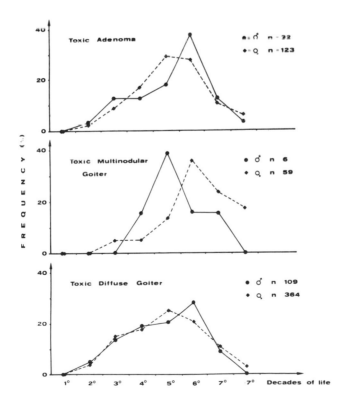

Fig. 2. Percentage frequency of non-toxic nodular goiter and non-toxic diffuse goiter in females and males during the different decades of life.

TSH response to TRH with ageing was observed. It is therefore conceivable that the menopause has poor, if any, influence on serum TSH and on its response to TRH.

THYROID DISEASE AND MENOPAUSE

In the past the presence of thyroid disorders, particularly hyperthyroidism, has been suspected on clinical grounds to be frequently associated with the menopausal syndrome. Actually, besides some overlapping, there are major differences in the clinical presentation of the two conditions. The differential diagnosis is listed in Table I.

The relationship between the menopausal period and the incidence of various thyroid disorders is not completely known as yet. In particular, no information is available on the incidence of thyroid disease in menopausal age in Italy or other Mediterranean countries. In order to clarify this problem we reviewed 2407 patients examined in the Thyroid Unit of the Patologia Medica 2, University of Pisa, during the last 7 years. As expected, thyroid disorders were more

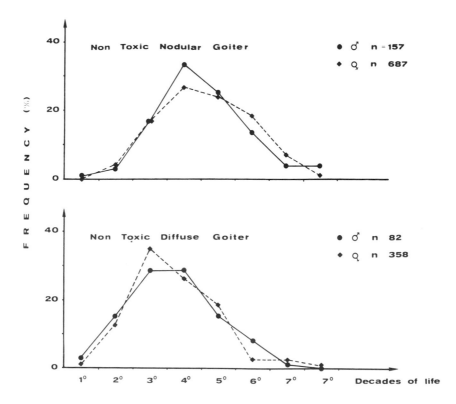

Fig. 3. Percentage frequency of hyperthyroidism due to toxic adenoma, toxic multinodular goiter and toxic diffuse goiter in females and males during the different decades of life.

frequent in women than in men. The ratio females/males was 5:1 in benign and 3:1 in malignant disease. In each category of patients the age of first diagnosis was recorded. Figure 2 shows the results obtained in 239 males and 1045 females with non-toxic diffuse or nodular goitre. The age of maximal incidence was earlier in diffuse than in nodular goiter, but no difference was observed between males and females at all the ages considered. Figure 3 shows the age- and sex-related incidence of different thyrotoxic conditions, such as toxic adenoma, toxic multinodular goiter and Graves' disease. No difference was found between males and females.

It is well known that in the normal population the incidence of detectable thyroid antibodies is higher in females and increases progressively with age (Doniach and Roitt, 1976). The frequency of clinically manifest thyroid autoimmune disease (Hashimoto's thyroiditis, idiopathic myxoedema and Graves' disease) in our series of patients is illustrated in Fig. 4. There was no difference between the two sexes in the prevalence of Hashimoto's thyroiditis. Women in the fifth decade of life had a slightly higher incidence of primary myxoedema but the relatively low number of patients calls for caution in the interpretation of these findings. Of 219 patients with thyroid cancer, 18 had undifferentiated, 56 folli-

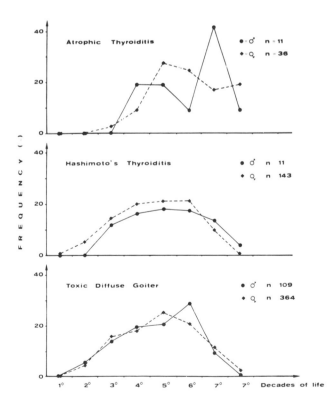

Fig. 4. Percentage frequency of autoimmune thyroid disorders, atrophic thyroidis, Hashimoto's thyroiditis and Graves' disease, in females and males during the different decades of life.

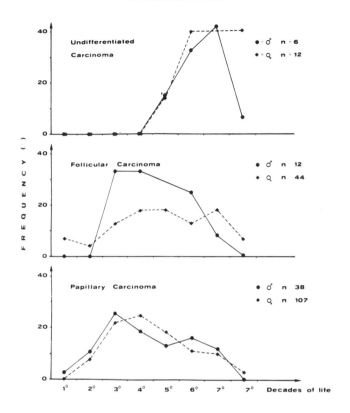

Fig. 5. Percentage frequency of undifferentiated and differentiated (follicular and papillary) thyroid carcinomas in females and males during the different decades of life.

cular and 145 papillary carcinomas. As illustrated in Fig. 5 the incidence of undifferentiated tumours was maximal over 50 years of age, while differentiated tumours occurred mainly in the third, fourth and fifth decades of life. Similar to that observed in benign disorders, the relative incidence of malignant tumours was similar in men and in women at all ages.

CONCLUSION

While pregnancy or oestrogen treatment affect different aspects of thyroid function and, in turn, alteration of thyroid activity may influence the female reproductive physiology, the menopause appears to be unrelated to thyroid function or to thyroid disease. As suggested by the comparative study on the incidence of thyroid disorders in males and females, the increased prevalence of some thyroid abnormalities during the fourth and fifth decades of life is probably not a consequence of menopause, but is an age-related phenomenon.

REFERENCES

Abuid, J., Stinson, D. A. and Larsen, P. R. (1973). *Journal of Clinical Investigation* **52**, 1195.

Akande, E. O. and Hockaday, T.R.D. (1972a). *Proceedings Royal Society of Medicine* **65**, 789.

Akande, E. O. and Hockaday, T.R.D. (1972b). *Journal of Endocrinology* **53**, 173.

Bigazzi, M., Sardano, G., Martino, E., Vaudagna, G., Ronga, G., Pinchera, A., Baschieri, L. (1980). *Journal of Endocrinological Investigation* **3**, 367.

Braunstein, G. D. and Hershman, J. M. (1976). *Journal of Clinical Endocrinology and Metabolism* **42**, 1123.

Braverman, L. E., Dawber, N. A. and Ingbar, S. H. (1976). *Journal of Clinical Investigation* **45**, 1273.

Burrow, G. N. (1978). *In* "Reproductive Endocrinology" (S.C.C. Yen and R. B. Jaffe, Eds), 373–387. Saunders Company, Philadelphia.

Burrow, G. N. (1980). *In* "The Thyroid Gland" (M. De Visscher, Ed.), 215–229. Raven Press, New York.

Burrow, G. N., Polackwich, R. and Donabedian, R. (1975). *In* "Perinatal Physiology and Disease" (D. A. Fischer and G. N. Burrow, Eds), 1–15. Raven Press, New York.

Casey, M. J. and Madden, T. J. (1976). *In* "Consensus on Menopause Research" (P. A. Van Keep, R. B. Gremblatt and M. Albeaux–Fernet, Eds), 139–151. M.T.P. Press.

Chopra, I. J. and Crandal, B. F. (1975). *New England Journal of Medicine* **293**, 740.

Chopra, I. J., Van Herle, A. J., Chuateco, G. N., Nguyen, A. H. (1980). *Journal of Clinical Endocrinology and Metabolism* **51**, 135.

De Groot, L. J. (1979). *In* "Endocrinology" (L. J. De Groot, Ed.), 377–378. Grune and Stratton, New York.

Doniach, D. and Roitt, I. (1976). *In* "Textbook of Immunopathology" (P. A. Miescher and H. J. Müller–Eberhard Eds), Vol 2, 715–735. Grune and Stratton, New York and London.

Dowling, J. T., Freinkel, N. and Ingbar, S. H. (1960). *Journal of Clinical Investigation* **39**, 1119.

Fisher, D. A., Hobel, C. J., Garza, R. and Pierce, C. A. (1970). *Pediatrics* **46**, 208.

Fisher, D. A., Sack, J., Oddie, T. N., Pekary, A. E., Hershman, J. N., Lam, R. W., Parlow, M. E. (1977). *Journal of Clinical Endocrinology and Metabolism* **45**, 191.

Fishman, J., Hellman, L., Zumoff, B. and Gallagher, T. F. (1965). *Journal of Clinical Endocrinology and Metabolism* **25**, 365.

Genazzani, A. R., Fioretti, P. and Lemarchand–Berand, T. (1971). *Journal of Obstetric and Gynecology* **78**, 117.

Gershengorn, M. C., Glinoer, D. and Robbins, J. (1980). *In* "The thyroid gland" (De Vischer, M. Ed), 81–121. Raven Press, New York.

Glinoer, D., Gershengorn, M. C., Dubois, A. and Robbins, J. (1977). *Endocrinology* **100**, 807.

Hayward, J. L., Greenwood, F. C., Glober, G., Stemmerman, G., Bulbrook, R. D., Wang, D. Y. and Kumaokas, S. (1978). *European Journal of Cancer* **14**, 1221.

Hennen, G., Pierce, J. C. and Freychet, P. (1969). *Journal of Clinical Endocrinology and Metabolism* **29**, 581.

Hesch, R. D., Gatz, J., Juppner, H. and Stubbe, P. (1977). *Hormone Metabolic Research* **9**, 141.

Kannan, V., Sinha, M. K., Devi, P. K. and Rastogy, G. K. (1973). *Obstetric and Gynecology* **42**, 547.

188 L. Baschieri et al.

Kenimer, J. G., Hershman, J. M. and Higgins, H. P. (1975). *Journal of Clinical Endocrinology and Metabolism* **40**, 482.

Koutros, D. A., Pharmakiotis, A. D., Koliopulos, N., Tsoukalos, J., Souvatzoplon, A. and Spontouris, J. (1978). *Journal of Endocrinological Investigation* **1**, 227.

Kurtz, A., Dwyzer, K. and Ekins, R. (1979). *British Medical Journal* **2**, 550.

Man, E. B., Reid, W. A., Hellegers, A. E. and Jones, W. S. (1969a). *American Journal of Obstetric and Gynecology* **103**, 328.

Man, E. B., Reid, W. A., Hellegers, A. E. and Jones, W. S. (1969b). *American Journal of Obstetric and Gynecology* **103**, 338.

Nisula, B. C., Morgan, F. J. and Canflied, R. E. (1974). *Biochemical Biophysical Research Communications* **59**, 86.

Noel, G. I., Dimond, R. C., Wartofsky, I., Earll, J. M. and Frantz, A. G. (1974). *Journal of Clinical Endocrinology and Metabolism* **39**, 6.

Odell, W. D., Rayford, P. L. and Ross, G. T. (1967). *Journal of Laboratory and Clinical Medicine* **70**, 972.

Olivo, J., Southren, A. L., Gordon, G. G. and Tochimoto, S. (1970). *Journal of Clinical Endocrinology and Metabolism* **31**, 579.

Oppenheimer, J. H., Scuef, R., Surks, M. I. and Haver, N. (1963). *Journal of Clinical Investigation* **42**, 1769.

Osathanondh, R., Tulchinsky, D. and Chopra, I. J. (1976). *Journal of Clinical Endocrinology and Metabolism* **42**, 98.

Pinchera, A., Sardano, G., Capiferri, R., Vaudagna, G. and Simonetti, S. (1979). *In* "Free Thyroid Hormoncs" (R. Ekins, G. Faglia, F. Pennisi and A. Pinchera, Eds), 208–220. Excerpta Medica, Amsterdam.

Pinchera, A., Martino, E., Sardano, G. and Chiovato, L. (1980). *Journal of Endocrinological Investigation,* Suppl. 3, 121.

Ramey, J. N., Burrow, G. N., Polackwich, R. J. and Donabedian, R. K. (1975). *Journal of Clinical Endocrinology and Metabolism* **40**, 712.

Rastogi, G. K., Sawhney, R. C., Sinha, M. K., Thomas, Z. and Devi, P. K. (1974). *Obstetrics and Gynecology* **44**, 176.

Romelli, P. B., Pennisi, F. and Vancher, L. (1979). *Journal of Endocrinological Investigation* **2**, 25.

Rubenstein, H. A., Butler, V. P., Jr and Werner, S. C. (1973). *Journal of Clinical Endocrinology and Metabolism* **37**, 247.

Sanchez–Franco, F., Garcia, M. D., Cacicedo, L., Martinez–Zurro, A. and Escobar del Rey, F. (1973). *Journal of Clinical Endocrinology and Metabolism* **37**, 736.

Schatz, D. L., Palter, C. N. and Russel, C. S. (1968). *Canadian Medical Association Journal* **99**, 882.

Snyder, P. J. and Utiger, R. D. (1972). *Journal of Clinical Endocrinology and Metabolism* **34**, 1096.

Tulchinsky, D. and Chopra, I. J. (1973). *Journal of Clinical Endocrinology and Metabolism* **37**, 873.

Yamamoto, T., Amino, N., Tanizawa, D., Doi, K., Ichinara, K., Azukizawa, M. and Miyai, K. (1979). *Clinical Endocrinology (Oxford)* **10**, 459.

Yen, S.S.C. (1977). *Journal of Reproductive Medicine* **18**, 287.

SECTION III
MORPHOLOGY OF THE AGEING OVARY

MORPHOLOGICAL FEATURES OF THE HUMAN OVARY DURING THE MENOPAUSE

G. C. Balboni

Institute of Human Anatomy, University of Florence, Florence, Italy

INTRODUCTION

If, from a clinical point of view, the menopause may be considered as corresponding to the definitive ending of menstruation, much more difficult is to establish the moment when the ovary really ceases its activity and to ascertain the morphological patterns that characterize the progressive involution of the organ.

Classically, in the first phase (premenopausal or perimenopausal period) the morphological changes of the human ovary are described essentially as a progressive disappearance of the evolutive gametogenic follicles and functioning corpora lutea, an increase of atretic follicles and corpora fibrosa or albicantia, vascular alterations and fibrosis.

In the second phase (postmenopausal period, advanced menopause) a general sclerosis of the organ with a sharp decrease in its volume are considered the main indications. These morphological patterns seem to match well the functional events that, according to the classical theory of Zondek (1935), have been considered as typical of the menopause and have been represented by a succession of three phases: the hypoluteal–hyperoestrogenic, the hypo–oestrogenic and the hypergonadotropic phases. However, this nice picture does not always correspond to the reality because of the remarkable variability of both morphological and functional events that occur during the course of the menopause (Trevoux *et al.*, 1979).

Serono Symposium No. 39, "The Menopause: Clinical, Endocrinological and Pathophysiological Aspects", edited by P. Fioretti, L. Martini, G. B. Melis and S. S. C. Yen, 1982. Academic Press, London and New York.

The more recent investigations on the endocrine activity of the menopausal ovary, based mainly on the radioimmunological methods as well as on histochemical procedures, have demonstrated that in the advanced menopause the organ is still able to produce some amount of hormones, particularly androgens (Novak *et al.*, 1965; Mattingly and Huang, 1969; Judd *et al.*, 1974; Vermeulen, 1976).

It seems well established that the production of progesterone decreases in the early phases of the premenopause in relation to the lack of functioning corpora lutea (anovulatory cycles), but according to Ingiulla and Gasparri (1965), in many cases the cycles in this period, are ovulatory and a true corpus luteum may be formed. However, on the basis of their observations, these authors believe that corpor lutea could have, in this period, a prevalent oestrogenic activity probably because of an alteration in their steroid metabolism. In any case, the plasma levels of progesterone, are generally attributed in the advanced menopause to adrenal activity (Vermeulen, 1976).

As for oestrogens, no general agreement exists. A real hyperoestrogenic phase in the perimenopausal period is not generally ascertained (Papanicolau *et al.*, 1969; Adamopoulos *et al.*, 1971) and when it exists it may be attributed to the activity of both the theca cells of atretic follicles and the cells (theca lutein cells) of regressing corpora lutea.

On the other hand, a possibility of follicular maturation with ovulation and oestrogen production is admitted by some authors in the advanced menopause (Trevoux *et al.*, 1979) and the morphological data may account for this possibility (Block, 1952; Costoff and Mahesh, 1975). However, as a rule, the ovary stops producing oestrogens in the advanced menopause and the majority of these hormones derive in this period, from the peripheral conversion (at the level of the liver, skin and adipose tissue) of androstenedione of adrenal origin (Vermeulen, 1976).

The ovarian production of androgens is generally believed to be due to the stroma cells (Rice and Savard, 1966; Lemaire *et al.*, 1968; Channing, 1969). *In vivo* studies on steroid concentrations in ovarian venous plasma (De Jong *et al.*, 1974; Serio *et al.*, 1976) confirm the androgenic activity of the human ovary. As noted previously, this androgenic activity persists during the menopause and represents in this period the main endocrine function of the organ and an important contribution to the total plasma pool of steroid precursors available for peripheral aromatization.

According to Vermeulen (1976), testosterone, dihydrotestosterone and androstenedione plasma levels in postmenopausal women are significantly lower than the mean values observed during the cycle, but comparable to values in the early follicular phase. The ovaries would contribute to about 50% of the testosterone and to 1/3 of the androstenedione level, the main source of androgens being the adrenal cortex.

To what extent can the histology contribute to the knowledge of the endocrine activity of the ovary in the course of the menopause and to the understanding of the mechanisms involved in determining the "aging" of the ovary? The same difficulties encountered in the functional investigations exist for the morphological ones; the extreme individual variability and the consequent dangers in generalizing the obtained data is the main limitation. In addition, the difficulty in evaluating the true functional significance of the structures observed and the role that they may play in the general behaviour of the organ must be considered.

Our observations are based on more than 100 human ovaries of subjects aged from 37 to 62 years, studied at the light microscopy (LM) with the usual histological and histochemical methods and at the electronic microscopy (EM). These observations confirm, generally speaking, findings of previous reports, but, in our opinion, they allow for some remarks on the morphological aspects of the endocrine function of the three compartments of the ovary: the follicle, the corpus luteum and the stroma, during the course of the menopause.

MORPHOLOGICAL ASPECTS OF PERIMENOPAUSAL FOLLICLE

As far as follicles are concerned, the first fact to be pointed out is that the number of evolutive follicles is already very low in the early premenopausal period. Some primordial or primary follicles may be found in some cases in the advanced menopause too. Evolutive follicles are very rarely encountered in the ovary of women over 50 years of age; however, in such cases, the ultrastructural and histochemical findings testify a normal activity of both granulosa and theca cells.

The sharp decrease of primordial and growing follicles in premenopausal women was statistically documented by Block (1952). In any case, the follicular atresia is the most prominent finding in this period. As is well known (Balboni, 1976), the atretic process evolves in two fundamental ways: obliterans atresia and cystic atresia.

In the first case, the small and medium sized cavitary follicles are affected and a vigorous connective tissue proliferation fills the follicular cavity, whereas the oocyte and the granulosa cells are degenerating. At first, the theca layer undergoes a sharp hypertrophy and its cells show the histological and histochemical appearances of active steroidogenic cells. The hypertrophic theca interna layer of atretic follicles is considered the main source of the ovarian oestrogens (Dubreuil, 1953; Balboni, 1976). The persistence in time of an active theca layer is difficult to determine; generally, the fibrotic process goes on and at a certain moment the theca is overwhelmed.

The cystic atresia affects the large cavitary follicles and gives rise to cystic cavities with a fibrous wall, where the theca cells are not so well represented and tend to disappear very soon. The presence of many cystic follicles in the premenopausal ovary is a frequent finding. However, it is not always so easy to distinguish cystic formations derived from follicles or from the superficial epithelium or from the rete ovarii (Centaro, 1965).

An attempt to classify different morphological types of ovaries in the premenopause may be found in the exhaustive work of Ingiulla and Gasparri (1965). Four types have been described: polyfollicular ovary, normal ovary, paucifollicular ovary and atrophic-senile ovary. The frequency increases in that order. According to the same authors, in the postmenopause the ovary is involuting without any luteo-follicular structure. As noted previously, in our experience, some primordial or initially growing follicles may be seen.

If the first step in the menopausal involution of the ovary is represented by the incapacity of follicles to reach their maturation with the consequence of anovulatory cycles and no formation of true corpora lutea, an attempt must be made to identify the possible mechanisms involved in determining this situation.

Without entering into the still yet unresolved problem of the genesis of the menopause (genetic, endocrine, vegetative, central nervous influences, etc.), attention can be payed to the relationships existing between the three components (oocyte, granulosa and theca cells) of the growing follicles. Some facts may be pointed out:

(1) Normally, the oocytes of growing follicles are arrested in the prophase of the first meiotic division and resume meiosis under the influence of LH surge shortly before ovulation. Since in cultured oocytes nuclear maturation occurs spontaneously, even in the absence of the hormone, it is evident that the follicle exerts an inhibitory influence on the oocyte (Foote and Thibault, 1969). Granulosa cells are believed to exert this inhibitory influence upon meiosis by secretion of a chemical message in the follicular fluid (Tsafriri and Channing, 1975). Granulosa cells from large porcine follicles luteinize spontaneously in culture, but in a particularly evident way in the presence of HCG (Balboni and Zecchi, 1978). According to Channing (1970), granulosa cells of large follicles are primed *in vivo* by endogenous gonadotropins, which reduce their ability to bring about inhibition of oocyte maturation. In fact, *in vitro* experiments demonstrated that inhibition of rat oocyte maturation by follicular fluid (FFl) and purified follicular fluid (PFFl) is overcome by LH, but the maturation changes are delayed even in the presence of LH in comparison with control oocytes cultured without inhibitor (Tsafriri *et al.*, 1977).

On the other hand, follicular fluid from small porcine follicles inhibits luteinization and LH-induced cyclic AMP production by granulosa cells of large follicles (Ledwitz-Rigby *et al.*, 1973). Furthermore, it was found that the human follicular fluid, besides preventing oocyte maturation *in vitro*, inhibits progesterone secretion by the cumulus cells surrounding the cultured oocytes (Hillensjo *et al.*, 1978).

The oocyte maturation inhibition (OMI) of FFl is not species specific, as the porcine FFl can act on rat oocytes (Tsafriri *et al.*, 1977) and the human FFl or a purified fraction of it acts on the porcine oocyte maturation (Hillensjo *et al.*, 1978). Both the porcine and the bovine FFl inhibitors appear to be small polypeptides with molecular weight between 1000 and 10 000 (Gawtkin and Andersen, 1976; Tsafriri *et al.*, 1976).

(2) In the first stages of organogenesis of the human ovary, two cell types, one dark and the other clear, may be identified in the common blastema and encircle the oocytes as follicular cells (Balboni, 1977). The dark cells are suspected of being responsible for the meiotic inhibitory effect, whereas the clear cells would be responsible for an unascertained meiosis inducing effect (Wartemberg, 1977).

(3) Preliminary data to be verified (Balboni and Zecchi, 1978) also seems to indicate the existence in the adult ovary of two different types of granulosa cells, probably playing a different role in the activity of the follicle.

(4) Our recent research (Zecchi and Balboni, 1980) has demonstrated that the appearance of a theca layer begins at the follicular pole corresponding to the cumulus oophorus and that at this site the theca layer of evolutive follicles is generally thicker than in the remainder of the follicular circumference.

(5)   It is general opinion that in oestrogen production by evolutive follicles a sort of cooperation exists between the granulosa and the theca cells (Balboni, 1962, 1973, 1976). The above mentioned data demonstrate a close functional relationship between the three components of the follicles and suggest the possibility that the failure of one of these components may break the harmony of the whole organelle and determine its regression. The oocyte is more suspect, its lifespan being probably genetically predetermined. Of course, further more difficult investigations are needed for a complete knowledge of the mechanisms of follicular regression in the menopause.

MORPHOLOGICAL ASPECTS OF PERIMENOPAUSAL CORPORA LUTEA

The finding of true functioning corpora lutea decreases progressively from the early premenopause. In our cases, no true corpora lutea were found in the ovaries of women with ascertained clinical signs of advanced menopause (more than 2 years without menstruation), also some cases are described in the literature (Trevoux *et al.*, 1979). On the other hand, corpora lutea in different stages of involution may be found easily.

From a morphological point of view, the characteristics of these involutive corpora lutea are well known. The luteal cells undergo vacuolization due to pigmented lipids accumulation. According to Guraya (1968), the involutive luteal cells accumulate deeply sudanophilic droplets consisting mainly of triglycerides, cholesterol and/or its oesters and some phospholipids. This accumulation suggests a storage of hormone precursors because of the inability of the cells to utilize them in hormone synthesis.

The regression of the luteal cells is accompanied by a proliferation of the interstitial connective tissue, that brings about the formation of a corpus fibrosum; that can evolve afterwards into a jaline body (Balboni, 1956).

The presence of several so called corpora lutea atretica is one of the more striking features of the menopausal ovary. These structures derive from large follicles that were unable to attain complete maturation and ovulation. They are initially characterized by a sharp hypertrophy of the theca interna cells and by an initial luteinization of the granulosa cells. Their fate is regression and formation of corpora fibrosa or albicantia, whose aspect is practically indistinguishable from that of the same structures derived from true corpora lutea.

Recently, Guraya (1976 a, b) has made an histochemical study on these corpora lutea atretica in the human postmenopausal ovary and has demonstrated that both the theca interna and granulosa cells develop the histochemical features of well established actively secreting steroid cells, i.e. abundant diffuse sudanophilic lipoproteins and some lipid granules composed mainly of phospholipids. Of course, these histochemical findings do not permit us to establish the nature of the steroid produced. However, it might be that theca cells continue to produce oestrogens and contribute to oestrogen levels during the postmenopause.

According to the same author, these cellular characteristics may be due to an LH activity of the human menopausal gonadotropin (HMG). With the onset of degenerative changes (accumulation of coarse lipid droplets, consisting of triglycerides, cholesterol and/or its oesters, pigments etc.), these cells become refractory to gonatropic stimulation. Some residual theca cells filled with pigmented lipids may persist in the periphery of the corpus fibrosus or albicans derived from this regression.

In the advanced menopause (more than 5 years after the cessation of menstruation), in the majority of cases, the ovary is a sclerotic organ, where only fibrous or jaline structures, derived from follicular, luteal or vascular regression, are present. However, some groups of cells of different origin may be found near the involutive remainders or scattered in the stroma, displaying histological features of endocrine cells. This problem will be discussed presently in relation to the ovarian stroma.

MORPHOLOGICAL ASPECTS OF OVARIAN STROMA

As has already been stated, the ovarian stroma is generally believed to be the source of ovarian androgens during both active sexual life and the postmenopause. From a morphological point of view the problem exists as to what cellular type in the stroma this androgenic activity can be attributed.

The persistence of residual cells derived from the theca cells of atretic follicle and regressing corpora lutea is a common finding especially in the menopausal ovaries. These cells are generally arranged at the periphery of corpora fibrosa or albicantia. Isolated small groups of cells may be found embedded in the undifferentiated cortical stroma. The appearance of these cells at the LM is characteristic; polyhedral in shape, they show a clear or condensed nucleus and a cytoplasm filled with pigmented lipids. A positive reaction for the 3-ol-hydroxysteroid dehydrogenase (HSD) may be present, but generally it is weak or absent, while an important lipids content is well demonstrable.

At the EM the majority of these cells do not present the typical ultrastructural pattern of active steroidogenic cells, i.e. well developed smooth endoplasmatic reticulum and Golgi apparatus, mitochondria with vescicular cristae and lipid droplets. On the contrary, their cytoplasm appears very poor in organelles and is filled with large vacuoles of extracted lipids, essentially tryglicerides in nature. To what extent these cells may be involved in steroidogenesis is difficult to say and a quantitative evaluation of the cells exibiting an as yet well conserved cellular machinery might solve the question.

On the other hand, it is necessary to admit that this stromal endocrine component (theca cells of regressing follicles and corpora lutea), may secrete oestrogens or androgens in relation to different gonadotropic as well as nervous influences in the various phases of the cycle, pregnancy and menopause (Balboni, 1976). These influences might act by blocking the cellular steroidogenesis prior to the final aromatisation. Furthermore, androgen production might be accomplished by specialized cells such as the hilus cells. These cells which are so similar to the interstitial cells of the testicle (Berger, 1922; Kohn, 1928; Stemberg, 1949; Stemberg *et al.*, 1953; Dohn, 1955a), are thought to increase in number during the menopause (Stemberg, 1949).

According to Poliak *et al.* (1968), a marked hyperplasia of hilar cells and an infiltration of the stroma by nets and cords of "hilus type cells" occurs in post-menopausal ovaries stimulated with human chorionic gonadotropin (HCG). In our experience, some particularly well developed clusters of hilus-like cells can be found in rare cases in menopausal ovaries. According to some authors (Ingiulla and Gasparri, 1965; Mattingly and Huang, 1969), a cortical stroma hyperplasia with some focal areas of so-called "luteinization" can occur in the menopausal ovaries, probably as a response to high levels of circulating gonadotropins.

In our experience, great prudence is necessary in evaluating the true endocrine value of this stroma transformation. Guraya (1976a, b) studied the histochemical changes of the stroma and blood vessels of the human ovary with advancing age and observed a fatty metamorphosis of the stroma progressively increasing from the third decade until the sixth decade. A similar lipid change also occurs in the blood vessel wall of ovarian medulla. The author suggests that a close relationship may exist between the alteration of primordial follicles that he observed (Guraya, 1970) occuring with ageing and that of the ovarian stroma and blood vessels.

Our findings at the EM confirm that many stroma cells during menopause undergo a fatty change, characterized by the appearance in the cytoplasm of many vacuoles of different size, containing partially extracted lipids. These cells do not present any signs of steroidogenic activity, and if they are at the LM, they can easily be misinterpreted. On the other hand, in some cases, during both fertile life and menopause, isolated cells, directly deriving from mesenchymal cells of the ovarian stroma, may develop into steroidogenic cells (Balboni, 1970, 1973). At the EM, I was able to observe the different phases of this evolution that proceeds through a so-called "blastic phase", during which the cells develop an abundant RER devoted to building up the organelles (i.e. SER) and the enzymes necessary for steroidogenesis. The development of these cells is probably regulated by hormonal influences and continously balanced by their regression, as some ultra-structural pictures seem to demonstrate (Balboni, 1973, 1976).

All these facts confirm once more the great functional adaptability of the human ovarian stroma (Dubreuil, 1946; Balboni, 1973), as demonstrated, during active sexual life, by its ability to undergo changes in the different phases of the cycle (Duke, 1947; Catchpole *et al.*, 1950; Balboni, 1959, 1962) and to give rise to endocrine cells.

With the advancing menopause, the ovarian stroma also tends to grow old and its responsiveness to gonadotropic stimulation becomes restricted to relatively few cells. As noted previously, the majority of stroma cells begin to develop involutive changes, while the extracellular component of the stroma tends to fibrosis and jaline regression. Many factors may be involved in the ageing process of ovarian stroma as well of all the other structures in the organ: the progressive loss of cellular receptors to gonadotropins is certainly an important one. However, it is possible that nervous influences also play a role (Ingiulla and Gasparri, 1965; Unsiker, 1970; Fink and Schofield, 1971; Balboni, 1976). In any case, the fact that, according to the mordern view on gonadal development (Groop and Ohno, 1966), all the ovarian steroidogenic cells have the same origin from the so-called "common blastem" (Balboni, 1977), may explain the general decrease of their activity that occurs in the menopause.

THE VASCULAR APPARATUS OF THE POSTMENOPAUSAL OVARY

The vascular alterations in the menopausal ovaries are long since well known. Ovarian vessels were thought to be under oestrogen control so the decrease in the hormone in the menopause was responsible for the vascular alterations, especially at the level of the spiral arteries (Netter *et al.*, 1956). However, no general agreement exists on the subject (Ingiulla and Gasparri, 1965).

In our studies, very often the regressive changes of medullary vessels were dramatic, consisting of a sharp thickening of the arterial wall with partial or complete obliteration of the lumen, evident fibrosis of the subendothelial layer, degeneration and jalinosis of the tonaca media. According to Guraya (1976a, b) an extensive lipid deposition occurs in the wall of ovarian vessels in the advancing menopause. Many vascular corpora albicantia may develop as a consequence of these degenerative phenomena.

In our EM research (Balboni and Tedde, 1973), we also observed important changes in the capillary bed. When ovarian structures (theca interna of atretic follicles, corpora lutea etc.) are undergoing regression, capillaries also give evidence of alteration. The endothelial cells lose their normal appearance and structure and are represented by clear and dark cells very irregular in shape, poor in organelles and vacuolated. The capillary basal lamina becomes thicker and perycytes also present some regressive changes.

Niswander *et al.* (1976), on the other hand, have demonstrated that a close correlation exists between the blood flow to the corpus luteum and progesterone synthesis. As corpus luteum regresses, the blood flow declines dramatically and arterial–venous shunts develop within the corpus luteum, which shunt blood away from the capillary network (Niswander *et al.*, 1976).

CONCLUSIONS

All the above mentioned data permit a general outline of the morphology of the human ovary during the menopause, but, at the same time, offer clear evidence for the remarkable individual variability in the behaviour of the organ and demonstrate the existence of many unresolved problems concerning ovarian histophysiology.

REFERENCES

Adamopoulos, D. A., Dove, G. A. and Loraine, J. A. (1971). *Journal of Obstetrics and Gynaecology of the British Commonwealth* **78**, 62.
Balboni, G. C. (1956). *Archivio italiano d' Anatomia e Embriologia* **61**, 373.
Balboni, G. C. (1959). *Archivio italiano d' Anatomia e Embriologia* **64**, 40.
Balboni, G. C. (1962). "Scritti in onore del Prof. E. Maurizio" Saga, Genova, **1**, 201.
Balboni, G. C. (1970). *Bulletin de l' Association des Anatomistes* **147**, 106.
Balboni, G. C. (1973). *Archivio italiano d' Anatomia e Embriologia* **78**, 37.
Balboni, G. C. (1976). *In* "The endocrine function of the human ovary" (V. H. T. James, M. Serio and G. Giusti, Eds). Academic Press, London and New York.

Balboni, G. C. (1977). *Folia Morphologica Cekoslovaeca* **25**, 46.
Balboni, G. C. and Tedde, G. (1973). *Bulletin de l' Association des Anatomistes* **156**, 41.
Balboni, G. C. and Zecchi, S. (1978). *Bulletin de l'Association des Anatomistes* **177**, 159.
Berger, L. (1922). *C. R. Academy de Science (Paris)* **175**, 907.
Block, E. (1952). *Acta Anatomica* **14**, 108.
Catchpole, H. R., Gersh, I. and Pan, C. (1950). *Journal of Endocrinology* **6**, 227.
Centaro, A. Quoted from Ingiulla, W. and Gasparri, F. (1965).
Channing, C. P. (1969). *Journal of Endocrinology* **45**, 297.
Channing, C. P. (1970). *Endocrinology* **87**, 156.
Costoff, A. and Mahesh, V. B. (1975). *Journal American Geriatric Society,* **3**

Costoff, A. and Mahesh, V. B. (1975). *Journal American Geriatric Society,* **23**, 193.
De Jong, F. H., Baird, D. T. and Van der Molen, H. J. (1974). *Acta Endocrologica (Copenhagen),* **77**, 575.
Dohn, G. (1955a). *Zeitscrhift fur Geburtshulfe und Gynakologie* **142**, 182.
Dohn, G. (1955b) *Zeitscrhift fur Geburtshulfe und Gynakologie* **142**, 289.
Dubreuil, G. (1946). *Bulletin de Histologie applique* **23**, 17.
Dubreuil, G. (1953). *C. R. Association des Anatomistes* 40e Réun. Bordeaux, 1–27.
Duke, K. L. (1947). *Anatomic Records* **98**, 507.
Fink, G. and Schofield, G. C. (1971). *Journal of Anatomic* **109**, 115.
Foote, W. D. and Thibault, C. (1969). *Annales des Biologie Animale, Biochimique Biophysique* **9**, 329.
Gawtkin, R. B. L. and Andersen, O. F. (1976). *Life Science* **19**, 527.
Groop, A. and Ohno, S. (1966). *Zeitschaift Zellforschung* **74**, 505.
Guraya, S. S. (1968). *American Journal of Obstetrics and Gynecology* **101**, 448.
Guraya, S. S. (1970). *Acta Anatomica* **77**, 617.
Guraya, S. S. (1976a). *Archivio Italiano di Anatomia e Embriologia* **81/3**, 189.
Guraya, S. S. (1976b). *Archivio Italiano di Anatomia e Embriologia* **81/1**, 61.
Hillensjo, T., Batta, S. K., Schwartz-Kripner, A., Wentz, A. C., Sulewski, J. and Channing, C. P. (1978). *Journal Clinical Endocrinology and Metabolism* **47**, 1332.
Ingiulla, W. and Gasparri, F. (1965). *In* "La sindrome menopausale". Atti Congresso Soc. It. Ost. e Ginec., Torino.
Judd, H. L., Judd, G. E. and Lucas, W. E. (1974). *Journal Clinical Endocrinology and Metabolism* **39**, 1020.
Kohn, A. (1928). *Endocrinology* **1**, 3.
Ledwitz-Rigby, F. Stetson, M. and Channing, C. P. (1973). *Biology of Reproduction* **9**, 94 (Abstract 85).
Lemaire, W. J., Rice, B. F. and Savard, K. (1968). *Journal Clinical Endocrinology* **28**, 1249.
Mattingly, R. F. and Huang, W. Y. (1969). *American Journal of Obstetrics and Gynecology* **103**, 679.
Nagy, T. and Kovasc Nagy, S. Quoted from Ingiulla, W. and Gasparri, F. (1965).
Netter, A., Yaneva, H., Salomon, J. and de Lestrade, F. (1956). *In* "Physiologie de la ménopause". "Assises Franç. Gin." Nice, Deshons, Colombes.
Niswander, G. D., Akbar, A. M. and Nett, T. M. (1976). *In* "The endocrine function of the human ovary". (V. H. T. James, M. Serio and G. Giusti, Eds.) pp. 71. Academic Press, London and New York.
Novak, E. R., Goldberg, B., Jones, G. E. S. and O'Toole, R. V. (1965). *American Journal of Obstetrics and Gynecology* **93**, 669.

Papanicolau, A. D., Loraine, J. A. and Dove, G. A. (1969). *Journal of Obstetrics and Gynecology of British Commonwealth* **76**, 308.
Poliak, A., Jones, G. E., Goldberg, B., Solomon, D. and Woodruff, J. D. (1968). *American Journal of Obstetrics and Gynecology* **101**, 731.
Rice, B. F. and Savard, D. (1966). *Journal of Clinical Endocrinology* **26**, 593.
Serio, M., Dell' Acqua, S., Calabresi, E., Fiorelli, G., Forti, G., Cattaneo, S., Lucisano, A., Lombardi, G., Pazzagli, M. and Borrelli, D. (1976). *In* "The endocrine function of the human ovary" (V. H. T. James, M. Serio and G. Giusti, Eds). 471. Academic Press, London and New York.
Stemberg, W. H. (1949). *American Journal of Pathology* **25**, 493.
Stemberg, W. H., Segaloff, A. and Gaskill, C. J. (1953). *Journal of Clinical Endocrinology* **13**, 139.
Trevoux, R., De Bryx, J., Grenier, J., Roger, M., Bailleul, S. and Scholler, R. (1979). *Journal de Gynecology, Obstetrique et Biologie d' la Reproduction* **8**, 13.
Tsafriri, A. and Channing, C. P. (1975). *Endocrinology* **96**, 922.
Tsafriri, A., Pomerantz, S. H. and Channing, C. P. (1976). *Biology of Reproduction* **14**, 511.
Tsafriri, A., Channing, C. P., Pomerantz, S. H. and Linder, H. R. (1977). *Journal of Endocrinology* **75**, 285.
Unsiker, K. (1970). *Zeitschrift Zellforschung* **109**, 46–54.
Vermeulen, A. (1976). *In* "The endocrine function of the human ovary" (V. H. T. James, M. Serio and G. Giusti, Eds). pp. 237. Academic Press.
Wartenberg, H. (1977). *Acta Anatomica* **99**, 346. (abstract 389).
Zecchi, S. and Balboni, G. C. (1980). *Verhandlungen der Anatomischen Gesellschaft* (in press).
Zondek, B. (1935). *In* "Hormone des Ovariums und des Hypophysenvorderlappens. Springer, Wien.

SCANNING ELECTRON MICROSCOPY OF FEMALE REPRODUCTIVE ORGANS DURING MENOPAUSE AND RELATED PATHOLOGIES

E. S. E. Hafez

Department of Gynecology and Obstetrics, C. S. Mott Center for Human Growth and Development, Wayne State University School of Medicine, Detroit, Michigan, USA

INTRODUCTION

Age-related changes in the female reproductive organs which accompany the menopause occur at a relatively earlier age than changes in other systems of the body. Ultrastructural changes of the reproductive system associated with menopause are related to the well-defined changes of the hormonal output of the endocrine glands, reduced estrogen stimulation and the inherent changes of tissue aging. The menopausal years are characterized by a stage of hypoestrogenism whereas the postmenopausal years are characterized by complete absence of ovarian estrogens.

Recently, scanning electron microscopy has been used extensively to study the surface ultrastructure of the female reproductive organs (Patek *et al.*, 1972; Hafez, 1973; Patek and Nilsson, 1973; Ferenczy and Richart, 1974; Hafez *et al.*, 1975; Ludwig and Metzger, 1976). This chapter deals with the surface ultrastructral characteristics of the ovarian surface epithelium, granulosa cells, oviductal epithelium, endometrial surface, endometrial glands, surface of cervical crypts, vaginal epithelium and the vulva in menopausal and postmenopausal women (20–30 years after the initiation of clinical menopause). The pathophysiological and ultrastructural characteristics of the postmenopausal reproductive organs will be also evaluated.

Serono Symposium No. 39, "The Menopause: Clinical, Endocrinological and Pathophysiological Aspects", edited by P. Fioretti, L. Martini, G. B. Melis and S. S. C. Yen, 1982. Academic Press, London and New York.

OVARY

Extensive investigations have been conducted on scanning and electron microscopy of the ovary (Hafez, 1973; Ferenczy and Richart, 1974; Hafez *et al.*, 1975;
Hafez and Makabe, 1979). Little has been done on the postmenopausal ovary.

In women and probably some species of non-human primates, the cessation
of reproductive capacity is quite well defined by the termination of menstrual
periods. In other mammalian species cessation of reproductive life is less predictable, since the ovaries of these species contain oocytes into old age, whereas
the postmenopausal human ovary contains very few normal appearing oocytes.
The aging of the human ovary is a very complex process because of its dual role
as a source of gametes and of steroid hormones. All ovarian functions decline
but the rate of decline is not the same for each function, nor is it the same in
the different menopausal women.

Postmenopausal changes of the female reproductive tract begin with loss of
the ovarian sensitivity to gonadotropins. About the menopause, the concentration of gonadotropins in plasma is high and it is not before late menopause that
the gonadotropin level returns to normal and finally to subnormal values. There
are only a few follicles in the deeper layers of the postmenopausal ovary. The
hilus cells may be proliferated and the vessels of the hilus and medulla undergo
severe arteriosclerosis. Age changes are not confined to oocytes, follicles, and
corpora lutea, but also involve epithelial, stromal, and interstitial elements. Some
of these change are degenerative in nature, but others consist of hyperplasia of
specific tissues.

The medullary portion of the ovary of postmenopausal women is characterised
by the accumulation of corpora albicantia, the sclerosis of the walls of blood
vessels, and hyalinisation of collagen elements. Proliferative changes in the superficial epithelium include papillomatous outgrowths from the surface of the
ovary and duct-like ingrowths into the ovarian cortex. These changes seem to be
transitory and of little physiological or clinical significance.

OVIDUCT

During **reproductive life** the epithelium consists of ciliated cells, non-ciliated
(secretory) cells, intercalary or peg cells and indifferent cells. Ciliated cells,
present at all ages in various frequencies are about 30 μm high and 12 μm wide
(Figs 1 and 2). The cilia are up to 4 μm high and 0.2 μm wide. Up to 80 cilia
may arise from a single cell. Ciliated cells occur most frequently in the ampulla
and are less frequent in the isthmus and interstitial part. The oviductal epithelium
undergoes cyclical changes in the size of ciliated cells and, more importantly, in
the different secretory activity of the secretory cells (Ferenzcy *et al.*, 1972).
During the premenstrual and late luteal phase, there is full restoration of non-
ciliated cells which become flattened, exposing distinct polygonal boundaries.

The oviductal epithelium during early menopause looks quite similar to that
of the postmenstrual and premenstrual phases. The secretory cells are covered by
densely arranged erect microvilli. The boundaries of the non-ciliated cells are

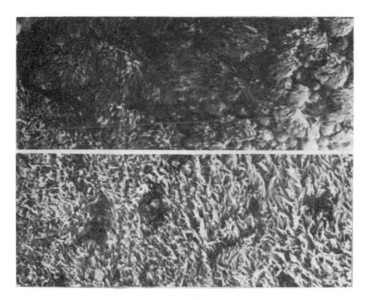

Fig. 1. Closely packed ciliated cells in human fimbriae.

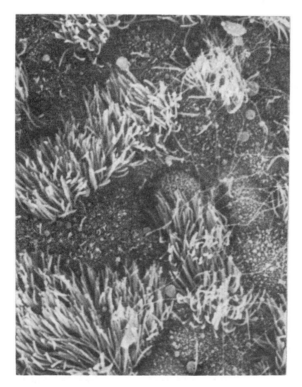

Fig. 2. Ciliated cells in the ampulla at ovulatory phase.

smooth compared to the premenstrual stage. In the ampulla, the ciliated cells are found singly alternating with clusters of ciliated cells which appear as long tracts. The possible physiological significance of this cell pattern is unknown.

The oviductal epithelium shows a decrease in the secretory function in all segments of the tube and atrophy of all cell types. During early postmenopausal life, there is little ultrastructural change in the cilia and microvilli. During 20 to 30 years postmenopause, abundant cilia are still visible in the infundibulum and ampulla, whereas the isthmus has areas of flattened cells denuded of cilia and secretion, with areas of fibrous-appearing hexagonal cells (Patek et al., 1972). However, Ferenczy et al. (1972) reported that during menopause rare tufts of oviductal cilia are noted while most cells are covered with fine microvilli that may be interrupted by areas of flattened cells in scattered areas. The cells have a hexagonal pattern with prominent terminal bar attachments resembling those found in mesothelia (Soriero, 1978).

Although the oviductal epithelium remains unaffected for a long period of time after the cessation of menstruation, there is remarkable deciliation during postmenopausal stages (Fredricsson and Bjorkman, 1973; Patek and Nilsson, 1973). This response is primarily hormonal rather than age related. In aged ovarectomised monkeys, the administration of exogenous estrogen stimulates ciliogenesis, whereas exogenous progesterone inhibits it. Menopause is also associated with the gradual decrease and subsequent cessation of the secretory activity of the secretory cells, which are under hormonal control.

During the postmenopausal period (20–30 years after onset of menopause), the oviductal epithelium is flattened and the cells are hexagonal in appearance. The epithelium of the fimbriae shows atrophic changes and the flat-surfaced cells are in cobblestone arrangement and covered by short and sparse microvilli, indicating absence of apocrine secretory activity. The broad mucosal folds of the ampulla exhibit a different appearance due to dome-shaped non-ciliated cells, which may be transformed into giant cells. The cells are variable in size and are demarcated by intercellular deep clefts. The borders of the non-ciliated cells are elevated even above the level of the tips of the adjacent ciliated cell. Their microvilli are variable in length and extend parallel to the cell surface.

There are large denuded epithelial areas with flat hexagonal cells, and no secretory activity. During postmenopausal stages, the ciliated cells are present in scattered patches whereas the secretory cells have very few microvilli. The postmenopausal oviduct has a decreased length and thickness. Smooth muscle cells are replaced by connective tissue. The folds of the oviductal mucosa are flattened or absent. The height of the epithelium, however, is only about 10 μm as compared with 20–30 μm at the height of proliferation.

There is a remarkable decrease in the number of ciliated cells, particularly in the infundibulum. There are fewer cilia per cell and they are shorter. There is also apparent sloughing off of epithelial cells, both secretory and ciliated, in localised areas, particularly in older patients (Gaddum-Rosse et al., 1975).

The ciliated and secretory cells, which are the predominant cells in the epithelium, do not atrophy for several years after the menopuase, and there is little evidence of secretion (Novak and Everett, 1928). After 60, there is lessening in the height of the epithelium and gradual loss of cilia, but these atrophic changes do not progress uniformly in different portions of the oviduct (Talbert, 1977).

Twenty to thirty years after the menopause, there are large areas of flattened epithelium with no cilia or indication of secretion in the isthmus (Patek *et al.*, 1972). At postmenopausal age, there is little or no evidence of deciliation in the ampullary or infundibular regions.

It would appear that estrogens play a physiological role in both ciliogenesis and maintenance of the ciliated cells in the oviduct and the endometrium (Schueller, 1973; Gaddum-Rosse *et al.*, 1975). Long-, but not short-term estrogen therapy in postmenopausal women causes normal ciliation of the infundibular epithelium, and more effective ciliary activity. In the rabbit and rhesus monkey, ciliogenesis and maintenance of the ciliated cells are dependent on estrogen, where as progesterone induces deciliation and dedifferentiation in the oviductal epithelium of the rhesus monkey (Brenner and Anderson, 1973; Rumery and Eddy, 1974). During childbearing age, low-dose gestogen causes the oviductal epithelium to have a similar appearance to that in the late secretory phase, whereas long-acting progestin given to a woman 25 years after the menopause causes extensive deciliation in the oviduct (Patek, 1974).

In postmenopausal patients with ovarian carcinoma (possibly hormone active) the oviductal epithelium shows swelling of the secretory cells, distinct polyhedral cell shapes, and cells devoid of their apical membrane, and with no signs of ciliary degeneration.

In patients with acute salpingitis, the ciliated cells remain intact but there is an abundance of polymorphonuclear cells in the lamina propria and a predominantly limphocytic permeation of the oviductal epithelium and muscularis. In patients with subacute salpingitis, the oviductal epithelium becomes compressed or degenerated. The epithelial basal lamina appears intact. Little is known about the inflammation-associated intraepithelial lymphocytes. The immunologic defense mechanism seems to be related to delayed sensitivity to foreign proteins, rather than to the formation of circulating antibodies (Dustin, 1966). The ultrastructural characteristics of the oviductal epithelium that are not degenerating are not altered with respect to the distribution, number and height of secretory and ciliated cells.

UTEROTUBAL JUNCTION

The epithelium of the interstitial endosalphinx (Fig. 3) made of ciliated and secretory (non-ciliated) cells, has morphologic and functional similarities to the endometrium. The epithelium shows cyclic changes that are comparable, but quantitatively much less than those occurring in the endometrium.

Ciliated cells comprise 5% and 10% of the cell population in the cornual endometrium and interstitial endosalpinx, respectively. Endometrial glands are present in the cornual endometrium (Fadel, 1978). Ciliated cells increase the number around the opening of the endometrial glands.

The transitional area between the endosalpinx and endometrium is characterized by: (a) a remarkable increase in the frequency of ciliated cells—the ratios between ciliated and non-ciliated cells become 1:2 or 1:1; and (b) the secretory cells tend to be flattened and assume a polygonal elongated shape (Fadel, 1978). Both changes increased in both the endometrial and oviductal cells with proximity to the transitional area. The abundance of ciliated cells in uterotubal junc-

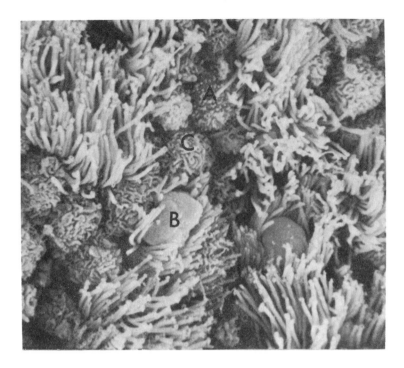

Fig. 3. Interstitial endosalpinx: secretory phase. Secretory cells in different stages of activity. Some are seen with secretory protrusions (A); others are exhausted/degenerated "peg" cells (B); still others have prominent microvilli and microridges (C); (Reproduced by permission from *Fertility and Sterility* **17**: 1176, 1976).

tion and especially in the transitional area suggests the presence of fluid currents which are probably important in the transport of the spermatozoa into the oviduct and/or the ova into the uterine cavity.

Early during the menopause (Fig. 4), the secretory cells of both the cornual endometrium and interstitial endosalpinx become lower and more flattened, but there is no atrophy, degeneration, or desquamation. The cells in the interstitial portion are characterised by flattened polygonal rather than rounded shape, increased and distinct intercellular spaces, reduced secretory activity and apparent widening of the openings of the endometrial glands (probably due to flattening of surrounding epithelium) (Fadel, 1978).

ENDOMETRIUM

The endometrial mucosa consists of two zones: the inactive basalis and the overlying functionalis (spongiosa and compacta). The endometrial glands open onto the epithelial surface and are supported in their course through the endometrium by endometrial stromal cells. The endometrial surface consists of a layer of simple columnar epithelium which is continuous with endometrial glands in the underlying connective tissue stroma. The glands, as well as the

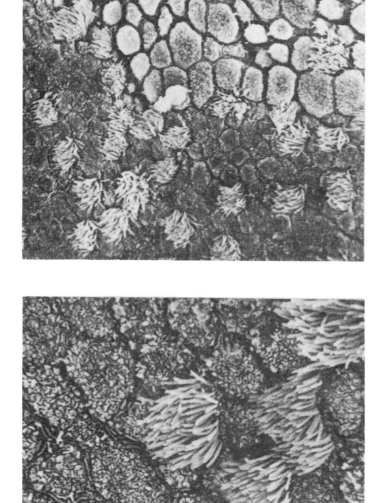

Fig. 4. (a) Cornual endometrium: postmenopause. The secretory (non-ciliated) cells are flattened, but still their surfaces are covered with regular, evenly distributed, rounded, prominent microvilli. The ciliated cells are also well developed with no signs of degeneration or atrophy. (b) Transitional area: postmenopause. There is a relative increase in the number of ciliated cells. The non-ciliated cells are flattened, polygonal and widely separated from each other (Fadel, 1978).

surface epithelium, are lined by a single layer of columnar epithelium, composed of secretory and ciliated cells. Degenerating peg cells and reserve cells are also noted, especially in the surface epithelium. The endometrium undergoes quantitative ultrastructural changes in response to cyclical fluctuations in ovarian hormones. Thus, surface ultrastructural changes are noted in the proliferative, secretory and postmenopausal phases. Cyclical changes during the menstrual cycle also affect the structure of the endometrial glands, the stroma and the endometrial vascular apparatus.

A few years preceding and following clinical menopause, cessation of ovarian steroidogenesis causes inactive resting endometrium. The thin flattened endometrial epithelium appears low cuboidal with abundant non-ciliated cells covered with abundant and short microvilli and scattered ciliated cells. The intercellular matrix appears loosely arranged due to low collagen production. These cytological features are associated with a decline in the ergastoplasm (Borell *et al.*, 1959) and in the cytoplasmic RNA and apical alkaline phosphatase (Dallenbach-Hellweg, 1971).

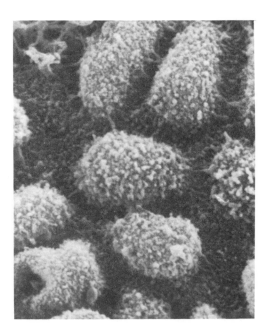

Fig. 5. Pathological changes of human endometrium: menopausal atrophic changes.

The endometrium is the most sensitive indicator of hormonal stimulation. Aging occurs in every menstrual cycle either at the end of an ovulatory or anovulatory cycle. Near the end of the reproductive phase anovulatory cycles predominate in frequency and bleeding is not of the withdrawal but rather of the breakthrough type. Before menopause there are prolonged periods of estrogen stimulation unopposed by progesterone. During late menopause there is only minimal estrogen secretion, which is insufficient for the development of the endometrium.

Several types of postmenopausal endometrium are noted: (a) a thin and atrophic mucosa in most cases; (b) a mucosa of varying thickness with Swiss cheese type of hyperplasia without proliferation; (c) active hyperplasia, either diffuse or in scattered patches, sometimes polypoid (Kuppe *et al.*, 1976).

The ultrastructural characteristics of the postmenopausal endometrium are extremely variable due to variability in the functional integrity of the ovary (Fig. 5). In an extensive study of curretage samples from 1521 postmenopausal women with no irregular menstrual bleeding, 31% had simple atrophy and 41% showed inactive cystic endometrial glands (McBride, 1954). Active hyperplasia was noted during the first 5 years after the menopause, whereas only 1% showed some secretory activity of the endometrial glands indicating progresterone stimulations.

One year after menopause there is distinct glandular proliferation and dense stroma in the endometrium whereas 7 years after menopause the inactive endometrium becomes thin with isolated cystic glands and fibrous stroma (Witt, 1963). The surface is made of flattened cuboidal cells devoid of microvilli with rupture of the apical membrane of some fragile cells. In the atrophic postmenopausal endometrium the ciliated cells are extremely rare and when present have a smaller number of short ciliary shafts (Sirtori and Morano, 1963). They are uniformly absent in the advanced postmenopausal stages. There is a remarkable decrease in the number and height of the surface microvilli in the superficial senile endometrium (Ferenczy and Richart, 1973). There are no epithelial collars around the openings of endometrial glands as noted during the post-menstrual stage characterised by the re-epithelisation of the endometrial cavity.

The ultrastructural characteristics of the postmenopausal endometrium depend upon whether ovulatory or anovulatory cycles preceded menopause. Ovulatory cycles are associated with cystic atrophy whereas anovulatory cycles are associated with glandular cystic hyperplasia. The presence of polyps is related to the local sensitivity or refractoriness to hormonal stimulation. In the endometrium with cystic atrophy the functional layer is low and clearly demarcated from the basal layer. Endometrial glands are narrow and the epithelial cells flatten taking a cuboid shape instead of a columnar appearance. The ciliated cells decrease in number and the cilia themselves become shorter or missing (Kuppe *et al.*, 1976). Some endometrial glands lined by a single layer show moderate cystic dilation.

Glandular cystic hyperplasia is characterised by an increase in size of the epithelial and stromal cells. Endometrial glands are wider in size. The larger glands are lined by a single layer of large columnar cells whereas the smaller glands may show some stratifications. Glandular cystic hyperplasia may be difficult to differentiate from the beginning of adenocarcinoma of the endometrium.

Hyperestrogenic, anovulatory cycles are characterised by clusters of well-developed ciliated cells, wrinkled non-ciliated cells and persistent proliferative endometrium, which is similar to normal proliferative endometrium (Ancla and de Brux, 1965). In cystic glandular hyperplasia, an hyperestrogenic state associated with abnormally high estrone levels or exogeneous estrogen administration, there are more ciliated cells and microvillous projections than are found in normal proliferative endometrium (Ferenczy and Richart, 1973). The number of ciliated cells and microvillous projections decline in the highly dilated cystic glands whereas reciliation is not uncommon.

Long-term progestogen administration, as in the treatment of pelvic endometriosis, cause glandular atrophy, massive pseudodecidual reaction, decreased
epithelial ciliogenesis and microvilli and increased secretory activity (Ferenczy
and Richart, 1974). The remarkable response of hyperplastic endometria to
progesterone may be due to high progesterone binding capacity associated hyperplastic endometrial tissues (Haukkamaa *et al.*, 1971).

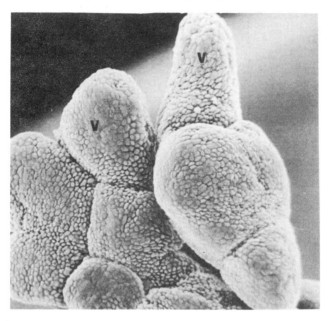

Fig. 6. Columnar epithelium from the human cervix with numerous finger-like villi: v = villi
(Allen and Jordan, 1978).

CERVIX UTERI

The internal and external cervix is covered with three types of epithelium:
original columnar, original squamous and metaplastic squamous: (a) columnar
epithelium (Fig. 6) lining the endocervical canal and continuous with the
endometrium; (b) squamous epithelium of the ectocervix is continuous in the
vaginal epithelium; (c) a well-defined junction between the columnar and
squamous located within the cervical canal, may undergo "squamous metaplasia", whereby columnar epithelium that has been everted onto the ectocervix
is replaced by squamous epithelium (Coppleson and Reid, 1967). In fact it has
been postulated that cervical neoplasia may be initiated during the process of
metaplasia (Fig. 7).

The cervical crypts are made of finger-like structures and ridges separated by
deep clefts which are oriented obliquely towards the cervical canal and the
external os. The elongated columnar cells (about 4 μm in diameter, closely packed
in a cobblestone-like arrangement) are types of secretory cells and ciliated cells.
The secretory columnar cells are covered by numerous microvilli, which are about

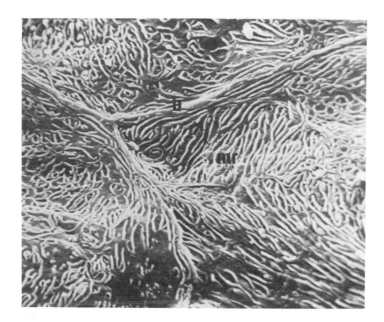

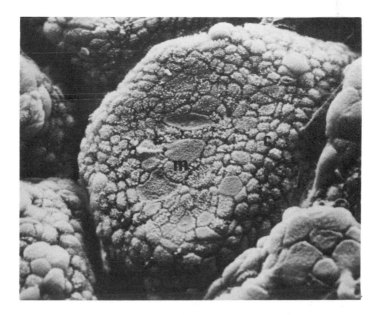

Fig. 7. (a) The junction of three cells with prominent cell boundaries and surface micro-ridges: b = cell boundary; mr = microridges (reproduced by permission from Cancer Research). (b) Columnar villous from the human cervix showing the early stages of meta-plasia, where larger more flattened cells are visible among the columnar cells: m = meta-plastic cells; c = columnar cells (Allen and Jordan, 1978).

2 μm in length, with no intercellular junctions between the cells, interspersed with the secretory cells. The ciliated columnar cells seem to be involved in the movement of cervical mucus produced by the secretory cells.

The squamo-columnar junction lies within the endocervical canal during childhood, on the ectocervix in reproductive years and within the endocervical canal during menopause. The position of the junctional zone is determined by the volume of the cervical stroma which in turn depends on hormonal stimulation leading to a different electrolyte and fluid content. Depending upon the age and the degree of the reproductive functions, the ecto–endocervical boundary varies in its topographical location: it descends during pregnancy towards the ectocervical area, but ascends in postmenopausal women (Ludwig and Metzger, 1976). The shrinkage of the connective tissue of the cervical stroma leads to a decrease in volume, and the lack of hormonal stimulation enhances this process (Kuppe *et al.*, 1976). The postmenopausal ectocervix is flattened and does protrude into the vaginal vault. Menopause is associated with sclerosis of the cervical stroma. The columnar epithelium of the endocervix becomes flat, similar to the squamous epithelium of the ectocervix. At the squamo-columnar junction, there is distinct demarcation between columnar and squamous epithelium without proliferation. The epithelial cells become flattened and hexagonal, with sharp boundaries. The cells are reduced in volume and the microvilli become slender.

The squamo-columnar junction is important because virtually all cervical neoplasia begins in the squamous epithelium at this junction. The transformation zone is of some clinical significance since cervical intra-epithelial neoplasia spreads onto the portio within the transformation zone, and its limits are those of this zone (Richart, 1968).

The preclinical stages of squamous carcinoma have been extensively studied (Coppleson and Reid, 1967; Shingleton *et al.*, 1968; Shingleton and Lawrence, 1976). In cervical metaplasia the columnar epithelium is transformed into squamous epithelium. Colposcopy (Coppleson and Reid, 1967), and scanning electron microscopy (Williams *et al.*, 1973) have been used to identify the stages of tissue transformation: (1) early stages of metaplasia are characterised by a shortening of the columnar cells at the tips of the columnar villi, the presence of a cuboidal-type cell, and the appearance of larger cells among the regular columnar cells at the tips of the columnar villi (Fig. 8). The surfaces of these cells are covered with short, closely packed microvilli without terminal bars; (2) in advanced stages of metaplasia, the new squamous epithelium consists of mature cells with a microridge surface structure.

Carcinoma *in situ* (CIS) is quite different from the appearance of normal epithelium. Under low magnification, the epithelium has a disorganised appearance with an uneven surface, by contrast to the appearance of normal squamous epithelium. The cells are rounded and of irregular shape and size, have no well-defined intercellular junction, and are covered with numerous microvilli, which are about 0.15 μm in diameter (Allen and Jordan, 1978). The presence of these microvilli in addition to the rounded shape of the cells may inhibit interdigitation of adjacent surfaces, thus leading to the increased exfoliation of these cells.

The vagina undergoes considerable shrinkage so that the organ is shorter and the caliber of the lumen smaller, primarily due to loss of elasticity which

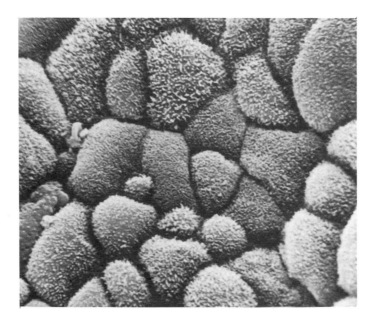

Fig. 8. Carcinoma *in situ* in human cervical epithelium, with a disorganised appearance due to the irregular shape and size of the cells.

may be related to fragmentation of elastic fibers in the tunica propria (Toth and Gimes, 1964; Lang and Aponte, 1967). The vaginal rugae disappear as estrogen levels diminish. The epithelial cells frequently contain pycnotic nuclei and show increased beta glucuronidase, acid phosphatase, and non-specific esterase activity.

The postmenopausal vagina undergoes atrophic changes without any hyperplasia. The vaginal rugae disappear and flatten and the vaginal epithelium becomes thin. Due to increased vulnerability of the thinned vaginal epithelium, there may be some bleeding spots that have been compared with flea-bites or referred to as "senile colpitis', representing the vessels entering the papillae of the fragile epithelium (Kuppe *et al.*, 1976).

Microscopically there are only three to four layers of epithelial cells instead of the eight to ten at the height of proliferation (Thomsen and Humke, 1972). The superficial cells no longer contain glycogen due to insufficient estrogenic stimulation. Cell volume seems to decrease with increasing age during the postmenopausal period. The cytoplasmic microridges become flattened and irregular There is a tendency towards fragmentation of superficial cells. Exfoliation of single superficial cells continues.

Estrogen originating from ovarian tumors or from topical or oral exogenous replacement not only restores the thickness and glycogen content of the vaginal epithelium but partially restores the surface ultrastructural appearance. However, the pattern of microridge distribution is somewhat different from that noted in premenopausal women and not all cells are completely covered with microridges. The functional significance of these changes is not known but may represent an abnormal differentiation of parabasal and intermediate cells into superficial cells.

VULVA

The senile vulva ("craurosis" vulvae) is thin and atrophic due to the hyperplastic and hyperkeratotic skin alternation (Kraus, 1967; Dougherty, 1968; Laszlo and Gaal, 1969). The vulvar folds are flattened in some places and thickened in others, with white patches in uneven distribution. The parchmentlike skin appeared cracked with some superficial ulceration.

The menopausal vulva is characterised by hyperkeratosis and acanthosis of the epidermis with an infiltration of lymphocytes and plasma cells in the subepithelial layer (Kuppe *et al.*, 1976).

In postmenopausal women epidermoid carcinoma of the vulva primarily in the labia majora accounts for about 3% of all genital cancers (Ferenczy and Richart, 1974). Perineal extension and lymphatic metastases are associated with cervical and vaginal neoplasia. In rodents, riboflavin deficiency causes epidermal atrophy associated with decreased tritiated thymidine uptake, hyperkeratosis and hyperplasia (Wynder and Klein, 1965; Wynder and Chan, 1970). Temporary riboflavin deficiency in young mice enhances chemically induced skin carcinogenesis (Wynder and Chan, 1970).

The invasive neoplastic squamous cells show a disorganised pattern whereas the well-differentiated cancer cells contain cytoplasmic microridges, stubby microvilli and keratin pearls which appear as concentric masses of multilamellated horney cells (Ferenczy and Richart, 1974).

CONCLUDING REMARKS

Ultrastructural changes of the reproductive system associated with menopause are related to the well-defined changes of the hormonal output of the endocrine glands, reduced estrogen stimulation and the inherent changes of aging tissue.

Age changes in the ovary are not confined to oocytes, follicles, and corpora lutea, but also involve epithelial, stromal, and interstitial elements. Some of these changes are degenerative in nature, but others consist of hyperplasia of specific tissues. Proliferative changes in the superficial epithelium include papillomatous outgrowths from the surface of the ovary and duct-like ingrowths into the ovarian cortex. These changes seem to be transitory and of little physiological or clinical significance. The epithelium of the fimbriae shows atrophic changes and the flat-surfaced cells are in cobblestone arrangement and covered by short and sparse microvilli, indicating absence of apocrine secretory activity. The broad mucosal folds of the ampulla exhibit a different appearance due to dome-shaped non-ciliated cells, which may be transformed into giant cells. The oviductal cells are variable in size and are demarcated by intercellular deep clefts. The borders of the non-ciliated cells are elevated even above the level of the tips of the adjacent ciliated cells. Their microvilli are variable in length and extend parallel to the cell surface. There are large denuded epithelial areas with flat hexagonal cells, and no secretory activity.

During postmenopausal stages, the ciliated cells are present in scattered patches whereas the secretory cells have very few microvilli. There are also fewer cilia per cell and cilia seem shorter. There is also apparent sloughing off of epithelial cells, both secretory and ciliated, in localised areas, particularly in older patients. After 60, there is gradual loss of cilia, but these atrophic changes do not progress uniformly in different portions of the oviduct.

Early during the menopause, the secretory cells of both the cornual endometrium and intersitial endosalpinx become lower and more flattened, but there is no atrophy, degeneration, or desquamation. The cells in the interstitial portion are characterised by a flattened polygonal rather than a rounded shape, increased and distinct-intercellular spaces, reduced secretory activity and apparent widening of the openings of the endometrial glands.

Several types of postmenopausal endometrium are noted: (a) a thin and atrophic mucosa in most cases; (b) a mucosa of varying thickness with Swiss cheese type of hyperplasia without proliferation; (c) active hyperplasia, either diffuse or in scattered patches, sometimes polypoid. In the atrophic postmenopausal endometrium the ciliated cells are extremely rare and when present have a smaller number of short-ciliary shafts. They are absent in the postmenopausal advanced stages. There is a remarkable decrease in the number and height of the surface microvilli in the superficial senile endometrium.

The columnar epithelium of the endocervix becomes flat, similar to the squamous epithelium of the ectocervix. At the squamo-columnar junction, there is distinct demarcation between columnar and squamous epithelium without proliferation. The epithelial cells become flattened and hexagonal, with sharp boundaries. The cells are reduced in volume and the microvilli become slender.

The postmenopausal vagina undergoes atrophic changes without any hyperplasia. The vaginal rugae disappear and flatten and the vaginal epithelium becomes thin. Due to increased vulnerability of the thinned vaginal epithelium, there may be some bleeding spots. Cell volume seems to decrease with increasing age during the postmenopausal period. The cytoplasmic microridges become flattened and irregular. There is a tendency towards fragmentation of superficial cells. Exfoliation of single superficial cells continues. Estrogen originating from ovarian tumors or from topical or oral exogenous replacement not only restores the thickness and glycogen content of the vaginal epithelium but partially restores the surface ultrastructural appearance. However, the pattern of microridge distribution is somewhat different from that noted in premenopausal women and not all cells are completely covered with microridges. The functional significance of these changes is not known but may represent an abnormal differentiation of parabasal and intermediate cells into superficial cells. The menopausal vulva is characterised by hyperkeratosis and acanthosis of the epidermis.

REFERENCES

Allen, J. and Jordan, J. A. (1978). *In* "The Cervix Uteri: Scanning Electron Microscopy of Human Reproduction" (E. S. E. Hafez, Ed.). Ann Arbor Science, Ann Arbor.

Ancla, M. and de Brux, J. (1965). *Obstetrics and Gynecology*, **26**, 23.

Borell, U., Nilsson, O. and Westman, A. (1959). *Acta Obstetrics and Gynecology of Scandinavica* **38**, 364.

Brenner, R. M. and Anderson, R. G. W. (1973). *In* "Handbook of Physiology: Endocrine Control of Ciliogenesis in the Primate Oviduct" (R. O. Greep and E. B. Astwood, Eds), Vol. 2, 123–140. American Physiological Society, Washington, DC.

Coppleson, M. and Reid, M. (1967). *In* "Pre-clinical Carcinoma of the Cervix Uteri". Pergamon Press, London.

Dallenbach-Hellweg, G. (1971). *In* "Histopathology of the Endometrium". Springer-Verlag, New York.

Dougherty, C. M. (1968). *In* "Surgical Pathology of Gynecologic Disease". Harper and Row, New York.

Dustin, P. (1966). *In* "Lecons d'Anatomie Pathologique Générale" (P. Dustin, Ed.), pp. 293–341. Presses Académiques Européennes, Brussels, Belgium. Belgium.

Fadel, H. E. (1978). *In* "Scanning Electron Microscopy of Human Reproduction" (E. S. E. Hafez, Ed.). Ann Arbor Science, Ann Arbor.

Ferenczy, A. and Richart, R. M. (1973). *American Journal of Obstetrics and Gynecology* **155**, 151, 151.

Ferenczy, A. and Richart, R. M. (1974). *New York State Journal of Medicine* **74**, 794.

Ferenczy, A., Richart, R. M., Agate, J. R. Jr, Purkerson, M. L. and Dempsey, E. W. (1972). *Fertility and Sterility* **23**, 515.

Fredricsson, B. and Bjorkman, N. (1973). *Fertility and Sterility* **24**, 19.

Gaddum-Rosse, P., Rumery, R. E., Blandau, R. J. and Thiersch, J. B. (1975). *Fertility and Sterility* **26**, 951.

Hafez, E. S. E. (1973). *In* "Handbook of Physiology: Anatomy and Physiology of the Mammalian Uterotubal Junction" (R. O. Greep and E. B. Astwood, Eds), Vol. 2, 87–96. American Physiological Society, Washington, DC.

Hafez, E. S. E. and Makabe, S. (1979). *In* "Scanning Electron Microscopy of Ovulation in Human Ovulation" (E. S. E. Hafez, Ed.). Elsevier-North/Holland, Amsterdam.

Hafez, E. S. E., Ludwig, H. and Metzger, H. (1975). *American Journal of Obstetrics and Gynecology* **122**, 929.

Haukkamaa, M., Karjalainen, O. and Luukkainen, T. (1971). *American Journal of Obstetrics and Gynecology* **3**, 205.

Kraus, F. T. (1967). *In* "Gynecologic Pathology" (F. T. Kraus, Ed.). C. V. Mosby, St. Louis.

Kuppe, G., Metzger, H. and Ludwig, H. (1976). *In* "Aging and Reproductive Physiology" (E. S. E. Hafez, Ed.). Ann Arbor Science, Ann Arbor.

Lang, W. R. and Aponte, E. C. (1967). *Clinical Obstetrics and Gynecology* **10**, 454.

Laszlo, P. and Gaal, T. (1969). *In* "Gynecologic Pathology". Akademiai Kiado, Budapest.

Ludwig, H. and Metzger, H. (1976). *In* "The Human Female Reproductive Tract: a scanning electron microscopic atals". Springer-Verlag, New York.

McBride, J. M. (1954). *Journal of Obstetrics and Gynecology of the British Empire* **61**, 691.

Motta, P. and Hafez, E. S. E. (1980). *In* "Biology of the Ovary" (P. Motta and E. S. E. Hafez, Eds.). Martinus-Niejhoff, The Hague, The Netherlands.

Novak, E. and Everett, H. S. (1928). *American Journal of Obstetrics and Gynecology* **16**, 499.

Patek, E. (1974). *Acta Obstetrics and Gynecology of Scandinavia* **53**, Suppl. 31.

Patek, E. and Nilsson, L. (1973). *Fertility and Sterility* **24**, 819.

Patek, E., Nilsson, L. and Johannisson, E. (1972). *Fertility and Sterility* **23**, 459.
Richart, R. M. (1968). *Clinical Obstetrics and Gynecology* **5**, 748.
Rumery, R. E. and Eddy, E. M. (1974). *Anatomical Record* **178**, 83.
Schueller, E. F. (1973). *Obstetrics and Gynecology* **41**, 188.
Shingleton, H. M. and Lawrence, D. (1976). *In* "The Cervix" (J. A. Jordan and A. Singer, Eds). W. B. Saunders, London.
Shingleton, H. M., Richard, R. M., Weiner, J. and Spires, D. (1968). *Cancer Research*.
Sirtori, C. and Morano, E. (1963). *In* "Cancer of the Uterus, from Gross Appearance to Ultrastructure" (C. Sirtori and E. Morano, Eds), pp. 321–329. Charles C. Thomas, Springfield, Illinois.
Soriero, A. A. (1978). *In* "The Aging Reproductive System" (E. L. Schneider, Ed.), Vol. 4, 85–118. Raven Press, New York.
Talbert, G. B. (1977). *In* "Handbook of the Biology of Aging, Aging of the Reproductive System" (C. E. Finch and L. Hayflick, Eds). Van Nostrand Reinhold, New York.
Thomsen, K. and Humke, W. (1972). *In* "Gynaekologie und Geburtshilfe". Thieme Verlag, Stuttgart.
Toth, F. and Gimes, R. (1964). *Acta Morphologica Hungarica* **12**, 301.
Williams, A. E., Jordan, J. A., Allen, J. M. and Murphy, J. F. (1973). *Cancer Research* **33**, 504.
Witt, II-J. (1963). *In* "The Normal Human Endometrium" (H. Schmidt-Matthiesen, Ed.), pp. 24–64. McGraw-Hill, New York.
Wynder, E. L. and Chan, P. C. (1970). *Cancer* **26**, 1221.
Wynder, E. L. and Klein, U. E. (1965). *Cancer* **18**, 167.
Wynn, R. M. and Woolley, R. S. (1967). *Fertility and Sterility* **18**, 721.

LAPAROSCOPY IN NORMAL AND
PATHOLOGICAL CLIMATERIUM

N. Garcea, A. Caruso, S. Campo, P. Siccardi, R. Dargenio and M. Lenci

Catholic University, Department of Obstetrics and Gynaecology, Largo A. Gemelli, Rome, Italy

INTRODUCTION

Laparoscopy is one of the most important investigations in diagnostic gynaecology. It is used at any age, but mainly at the reproductive age, since one of its most frequent indications is sterility (Garcea *et al.*, 1975; Garcea *et al.*, 1976; Phillips, 1977; Semm, 1977; Garcea *et al.*, 1978a; Garcea *et al.*, 1978b; Caruso *et al.*, 1979; Garcea *et al.*, 1979). Nevertheless laparoscopy "at climaterium" is useful in studying gynaecological pathology and in particular, ovarian pathology.

CASES STUDIED

We carried out laparoscopy in a group of 2327 women, we named this group "at any age". Of these, 103 were women over 40, we called this group "at climaterium". The indications for these two groups are reported in Table I.

It is evident that women who have had laparoscopy "at climaterium" are a small minority in respect to the others, with a percentage of between 2% and 7%. The relative frequency of the different indications is reported in Fig. 1. "At climaterium" laparoscopy was done by us for pelvic pain or tumefactions, then for menstrual irregularities, and lastly for pelvic tumours. These indications were respectively 33% more frequent, and 37% less frequent in comparison with the

Serono Symposium No. 39, "The Menopause: Clinical, Endocrinological and Pathophysiological Aspects", edited by P. Fioretti, L. Martini, G. B. Melis and S. S. C. Yen, 1982. Academic Press, London and New York.

Table I. Indications of the laparoscopy.

Indications	Pelvic pains or pelvic tumefactions	Menstrual irregularity	Sterility	Tumours	Other	Tota
In any age	689	814	814	= =	181	232'
In climaterium (age 40 years)	40	23	11	15	14	10:

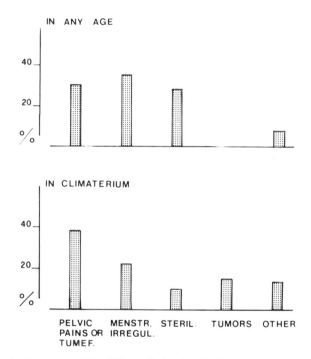

Fig. 1. Relative frequency of the different indications for laparoscopy "in climaterium" and "in any age".

same indications in the "at any age" group. The patients "at climaterium" were rarely examined by laparoscopy for sterility. They were 74% less frequent in comparison with those in the "at any age" group. The laparoscopic findings in women "at climaterium" examined for pelvic pains or tumefactions are reported in Table II. Figure 2 shows the relative percentage frequency of the different pathologies.

In the "at climaterium" group, in comparison with women "at any age" there is a greater frequency of normal findings (20%), mainly of uterine (100%) and ovarian (48%) pathology. Tubarian pathology and other findings are less frequent (41% and 44%).

Table III reports the laparoscopic findings on patients with menstrual irregularities. It consists of 23 women over 40, in which hormone dosages and gynaeco-

Table II. Laparoscopic findings in patients with pelvic pains or pelvic tumefactions.

Indications	Findings						
	Normal	Uterine pathology	Ovarian pathology	Adhesions or tubal pathclogy	Extrauterine pregnancy	Other	Total
Pelvic pains or pelvic tumefactions In any age	236	32	60	197	46	118	689
In climaterium	20	4	5	7	= =	4	40

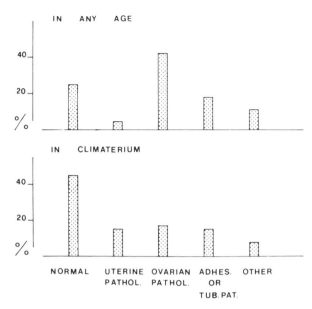

Fig. 2. Relative percentage frequency of the different pathologies in women "in climaterium" and "in any age" affected by pelvic pain and tumefactions.

logical examination together were not able to give a precise diagnosis. In these cases, we prefer to carry out a laparoscopy for the possible risk inherent because of their age. In this group of patients, in comparison with all the others, we verified a large frequency of normal findings (350%), mainly of uterine pathology (1350%) but also of tubarian pathology or adhesions (400%). Ovarian pathology, that in the group of women "at any age" represents the greatest part, is very low in women "at climaterium" (Fig. 3).

Table IV gives us the laparoscopic findings of patients with sterility problems. There are only 11 women over 40. Usually after 40 we dissuade against investigation for sterility. These represent a few particular cases in patients highly motivated, with favourable family history of late menopause, with short-term sterility, with cycles normally preserved, without partner pathology, etc... For these particular reasons, in these women we did not apply the normal principle. In this case we have included in the "ovarian pathology" group three patients whose ovarian ageing aspect was practically normal. This is because these physiological ageing aspects are the reasons for the actual pathology which results in sterility. In the final analysis, reported in Tables V and VI and in Fig. 5, these cases are included in the normal group.

In women over 40 investigated by laparoscopy for sterility problems, normal findings were 47% less than those in women "at any age". Uterine and ovarian pathology is greater, 51% and 96% respectively (Fig. 4). The total laparoscopic findings are reported in Table V. It is possible to verify that "at climaterium" women, in comparison with women "at any age", show normal findings and uterine pathology 80% and 375% higher respectively. The ovarian pathology and tubal pathology or adhesions are 60% and 15% less (Fig. 5).

Table III. Laparoscopic findings in patients with menstrual irregularities.

Indications	Normal	Uterine pathology	Ovarian pathology	Tubal pathology or adhesions	Other	Total
			Findings			
Menstrual irregularity In any age	84	6	671	14	39	814
In climaterium	8	6	5	2	2	23

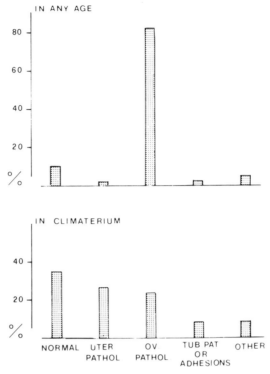

Fig. 3. Relative percentage frequency of the different pathologies in women "in climaterium" and "in any age" affected by menstrual irregularities.

The analytical findings "at climaterium" can be seen in Table IV. It is evident that it deals with predominantly benign pathology. Also in ovarian pathology we found mostly benign ovarian cysts, but in two patients, with pelvic tumefactions, there were two malignant ovarian tumours instead. Malignant ovarian tumours were found to be 15% of the ovarian pathology and 2% of all the laparoscopies carried out "at climaterium".

Besides these occasional findings, malignant ovarian tumours represent a precise indication for laparoscopy. Table VII reports our experience for the years 1979 and 1980 (until April). The first two cases reported as "first look" are two tumours found by chance, referred to in the previous table. The other cases were suspicious or "second look" laparoscopies, according to the therapeutic diagnosis reported in Fig. 6.

Laparoscopy, alone or together with biopsy or cytology has always allowed us a precise and secure diagnostic approach. As a matter of fact, in case No. 2 of the "second look" group, biopsy was even less exact than the laparoscopic view, probably because it was carried out in a marginal area.

In menopausal pathology it is suitable to include premature ovarian failure. Table VIII shows our experience in recent years. It consists of seven women between the ages of 24 and 37 affected by secondary amenorrhoea. The laparoscopic findings almost constantly showed "hypoplastic ovaries". In two cases

Table IV. Laparoscopic findings in patients with sterility.

Indications	Findings					
	Normal	Uterine pathology	Ovarian pathology	Tubal pathology or adhesions	Other	Total
Sterility In any age	218	35	180	178	32	643
In climaterium	2	1	6	2	= =	11

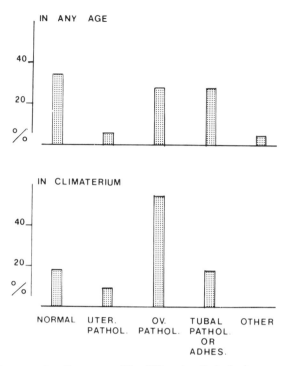

Fig. 4. Relative percentage frequency of the different pathologies in women "in climaterium" and "in any age" affected by sterility.

the ovary even had a "streak-like" aspect. It was probably a transitory situation between "gonadal disgenesya" and "ovarian hypoplasia". In fact, the patients had little menstrual flow and the ovaries were depleted. In addition to the reduced ovarian volume, we often find the appearance of a consumed ovary with many scars: therefore showing a "cerebral aspect". This appearance is present in 50% of cases. Ovarian biopsy was not done on all patients because, until a few years ago, before the identification of the "resistant ovary syndrome", it was not thought to be necessary. Presently it is done in every case.

DISCUSSION AND CONCLUSION

The use of laparoscopy is still indicated in women over 40. But the use of this method is less significant in these women than in younger women where laparoscopic indications are more uniformly represented. In climateric women the most frequent indications for laparoscopy are pelvic pains and pelvic tumefactions which represent about 40%. Other indications are less frequent.

Among "climateric women" undergoing laparoscopy for pelvic pains or tumefactions, 50% are normal, while in "at any age" women, in the same conditions, 30% are normal. This higher frequency of normal findings "at climaterium" could be explained by psychosomatic reasons, such as anziety and anguish,

Table V. Laparoscopic findings.

	Normal	Uterine pathology	Ovarian pathology	Tubal pathology or adhesions	Other	Total
In any age	538	73	911	389	235	2146
In climaterium	33	11	13	11	6	74

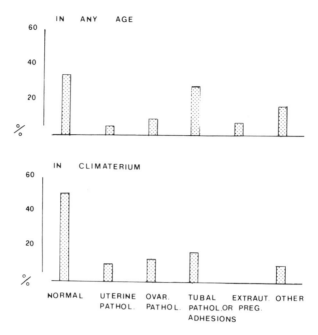

Fig. 5. Relative frequency between different findings of laparoscopy carried out on women "in climaterium" or "in any age".

which often affect women of this age. In this same group of patients, the uterine pathology is much more frequent. Of the climateric patients undergoing laparoscopy for menstrual irregularities 30% are apparently normal. This normality is probably only morphological, not functional. In fact, in women "at any age" with menstrual irregularities, normal findings are rare, while we almost always find ovarian pathology. In a few women over 40 who have had laparoscopy for sterility, ovarian pathology is almost always present, as expected. Considering all women "at climaterium" who had laparoscopy for different reasons, 45% were normal. This normality is about twice that found in women "at any age". Uterine pathology, instead, is four times more frequent. They are uterine "miomata" or widespread uterine fibrosis. This is understandable, dealing with women over 40, who often have had more than one child. The ovarian pathology in these women is about a third of that found in women "at any age". This should be a positive statistic, but unfortunately, 15% of this ovarian pathology are represented by malignant ovarian tumours. In these cases, laparoscopy has been of great importance, in the diagnostic stage or in future time. Laparoscopy is often used for malignant ovarian tumours. A few years ago, in operated ovarian tumours which were then treated by chemio-therapy or by radiation, the "second look" was often only laparoscopic. At present laparoscopy is used between the "first and second look". In fact, the "second look" (and also the "third look") eventually together with laparoscopy, are preferably made by laparotomy. This is justified by the seriousness of the illness and of the possible presence of adhesions that limit the diagnostic possibility of laparoscopy. On the other hand, only laparo-

Table VI. Analysis of pathology findings in climateric women.

Laparoscopic findings	Pelvic pains or tumefactions	Menstrual irregularity	Sterility	Total
Uterine pathology	2 miomata 2 uterine fibrosis	4 miomata 2 uterine fibrosis	1 uterine fibrosis	6 miomata 5 uterine fibrosis 11
Ovarian pathology	3 cystis 2 malignant tumours	5 cystis	2 cystis 1 P.C.O. (3 too cons. ovary)	10 cystis 1 P.C.O. 2 malignant tumours 13
Tubal pathology or adhesions	1 sactosalpinx 6 adhesions	2 adhesions	2 sactosalpinx	3 sactosalpinx 8 adhesions 11
Other	1 endometriosis 1 bleeding corpus luteus 1 uterine modification 1 disont. cyst	2 endometriosis		6
Normal	20	8	2	30 (+3)
Total	40	23	11	74

Table VII. Laparoscopy in patients with malignant tumours.

First look n° 4	Indications	Laparoscopy findings	Peritoneal metastasis	Biopsy and/or citology
	(1) Pelvic tumefactions	Malignant tumour or left ovary		
	(2) Pelvic tumefactions	Malignant tumour of left and right ovaries		
	(3) Prob. OV. Mal. Tumor	Peritoneal carcinosis	+++	
	(4) Prob. HEP. Mal. Tumor	Peritoneal carcinosis	+++	

Second look n° 13	Indications	Pelvic relapse	Peritoneal metastasis	Biopsy and/or citology
	(1) Malignant ovarian tumour	−	++	+
	(2) Malignant ovarian tumour	−	+	−
	(3) Malignant ovarian tumour	+	−	−
	(4) Malignant ovarian tumour	−	++	
	(5) Malignant ovarian tumour	−	++	
	(6) Malignant ovarian tumour	−	−	+
	(7) Malignant ovarian tumour	−	−	
	(8) Malignant ovarian tumour	−	−	
	(9) Malignant portio tumour	−	−	
	(10) Malignant portio tumour	−	−	
	(11) Gastric tumour	−	+++	+
	(12) Intestine tumour	−	+++	
	(13) Medio-sternal tumour	−		

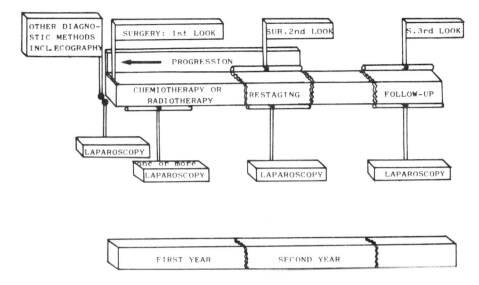

Fig. 6. Treatment plan for ovarian malignant tumours.

scopy gives us the possibility to investigate the areas which are difficult to reach (Bagley *et al.*, 1973; Piven *et al.*, 1977; Mangioni *et al.*, 1979). The recent development of echography should be very promising in this field (Cochrone and Thomas, 1974; Levi and Delvol, 1976; De Land *et al.*, 1979; Mastrantonio *et al.*, 1979; Spinelli *et al.*, 1979). Nevertheless, for a precise view of even small metastasis and also in areas difficult to control using other methods (for example under diaphragm metastasis) and for the possibility of carrying out an exactly pointed biopsy or "washing", laparoscopy finds a precise place in the "management" of malignant ovarian tumours. In patients with premature ovarian failure, the role of laparoscopy has gained, in recent years, much importance. Some years ago it was useful in a few cases in which the endocrinological assays were doubtful. Now, after the identification of the "resistant ovary syndrome" laparoscopic investigation has become indispensable in distinguishing, together with biopsy, one or the other pathology.

The "cerebral" appearance of the ovary, which we found in 50% of women with premature ovarian failure, seems to be typical of this alteration. In fact we have found up till not three cases of "resistant ovary syndrome" and in all these three cases the ovaries were small, very small, but never with the "wrinkled" appearance of premature ovarian failure. Therefore, the finding of very small ovaries, depleted, even "streak-like", in all the patients with premature ovarian failure, suggests that a peripheral source of the alteration can be suspected.

ACKNOWLEDGEMENTS

This work has been partially supported by the "Ministero della Pubblica Istruzione", Rome.

Table VIII. Premature ovarian failure.

Patient	Age	Symptomatology	Laparoscopic ovaric findings	Biopsy	Other
(1) C. A.	37	Sec. am.	Streak-like ovaries (2 cm × 0.2 cm)	No	- - - -
(2) D'A. G.	27	Sec. am.	Streak-life ovaries (2 cm × 0.2 cm)	No	- - - -
(3) D. M.	33	Sec. am.	Very small ovaries (2.5 cm × 0.5 cm)	Yes: without follicles	With many scars
(4) G. M.	24	Sec. am.	Very small ovaries (2.5 cm × 0.5 cm)	No	With many scars
(5) F. M.	34	Sec. am.	Very small ovaries (2.5 cm × 0.5 cm)	No	With many scars
(6) F. F.	35	Sec. am.	Very small ovaries (2.5 cm × 0.5 cm)	Yes: without follicles	With many scars
(7) A. A.	30	Sec. am.	Very small ovaries (2.5 cm × 0.5 cm)	Yes: without follicles	Rare scars

REFERENCES

Bagley, C. M., Young, R. C., Schein, P. S., Chambner, B. A. and De Vita, V. (1973). *American Journal of Obstetrics and Gynaecology* **116**, 397.

Caruso, A., Garcea, N., Campo, S., Siccardi, P. and Sgreccia, M. (1979). *In* "Atti del X^ Congresso Nazionale della Società Italiana di Fertilità e Sterilità" Roma 24–25/XI/1979.

Cochronc, W. I. and Thomas, M. A. (1974). *Radiology* **110**, 649.

De Land, M., Fried, A., Van Nogell, J. R. and Donaldson, E. S. (1979). *Surgery Gynecology and Obstetrics* **148**, 346.

Garcea, N., Caruso, A., Campo, S and Bompiani, A. (1975). *In* "VIII^ Congresso Nazionale della Società Italiana di Fertilità e Sterilità. Salsomaggiore, Giugno 1975.

Garcea, N., Caruso, A., Micchia, T. and Morace, E. (1976). *Minerva Ginecologica* **28**, 124.

Garcea, N., Caruso, A., Campo, S. and Siccardi, P. (1978a). *In* "Atti del XVII^ Congresso della Società Italiana di Endocrinologia." Saint–Vincent 17/V/1978.

Garcea, N., Caruso, A. and Campo, S. (1978b). *In* "Proceedings of V^ ESCO Venice 2–6/X/1978.

Garcea, N., Caruso, A., Campo, S., Siccardi, P. and Panetta, V. (1979). *In* "Proceedings of IX^ Meeting of International Study Group for Steroid Hormones." Rome 5–7/XII/1979.

Levi, S. and Delvol, R. (1976). *Acta Obstetica et Gynaecologica Scandinavica* **55**, 261.

Mangioni, C., Bolis, G., Molteni, P., Belloni, C. (1979). *Gynaecological Oncology* **7**, 47.

Mastrantonio, P., De Placido, G., Tinelli, F. G., Tolino, A., Di Meglio, A. and Nappi, C. (1979). *Rivista di Oncologia* **6**, 367.

Phillips, J. M. (1977). "Laparoscopy". The William and Wilkins Company, Baltimore, Maryland, USA.

Piven, M. S., Lopy, R. G., Xynos, F. and Barlow, J. J. (1977). *American Journal of Obstetrics and Gynaecology* **127**, 288.

Semm, K. (1977). *In* "Gynecologic laparascopy and Hysteroscopy". (L. S. Borow, Ed.). W. B. Saunders Company, Philadelphia, USA.

Spinelli, P., Pilotti, S., Luini, A., Spotti, G. B., Pizzetti, B. and De Paolo, G. (1979). *Tumori* **65**, 601.

PELVISCOPIC OVARIAN SURGERY

K. Semm

*Department of Gynaecology and Obstetrics,
University of Kiel and Michaelis-Midwifery School,
Kiel, West Germany*

INTRODUCTION

Until recently surgical interventions on the ovary were limited to ovarian biopsy and puncture of benign ovarian cysts during pelviscopy/laparoscopy. Today ovarian surgery is performed during endoscopic-intraabdominal-surgery (Table I) because of the development of the endocoagulation technique and the ROEDER-loop with an adequate haemostasis. The prerequisites for this intervention are: education in ovarian surgery per laparotomy; optimal training in diagnostic and surgical pelviscopy; modern pelviscopic equipment (Table II).

EDUCATION IN OVARIAN SURGERY PER LAPAROTOMY

The monocular diagnostic judgement of the ovary presupposes many years of experience in surgical interventions per laparotomy on the female adnexa. Although endoscopic ovarian surgery represents a great advantage for the patient as far as the physical stress and the hospitalization are concerned, we should never forget the danger of a false judgement of an ovarian tumour, especially in relation to its malignancy. As many as 6232 pelviscopies were carried out in the Department of Gynaecology at the University of Kiel, without there being one wrong judgement with consequent damage for the patient. On the contrary, the

Serono Symposium No. 39, "The Menopause: Clinical, Endocrinological and Pathophysiological Aspects", edited by P. Fioretti, L. Martini, G. B. Melis and S. S. C. Yen, 1982. Academic Press, London and New York.

Table I.   Pelviscopic ovarian surgery.

---

(1)   Biopsy
(2)   Cyst punction
(3)   Total cyst enucleation (e.g. Chocolate cyst, Dermoid)
(4)   Ovariolysis–Mobilization
(5)   Resection
(6)   Ovariectomy with or without salpingectomy

Table II.   Preconditions for endoscopic ovarian surgery.

---

(1)   Full trained surgeon in adnexa by laparatomy
(2)   Full trained pelviscopic gynaecologist
(3)   High modern pelviscopic equipment such as:

    (a)   Cold–Light optics
    (b) CO_2–Pneu–electronic
    (c)   Haemostasis apparatus:
       –Endocoagulator
       –ROEDER–Loop
    (d)   Complete endoscopic instrument set

---

advantage of pelviscopy is shown by the fact that pelviscopy is performed rather than laparotomy in order to verify the findings of the ovarian manual examination.

OPTIMAL TRAINING IN DIAGNOSTIC AND SURGICAL PELVISCOPY

The prerequisite for the undertaking of ovarian surgery is a complete training in gynaecological pelviscopy. The one-eyed or monocular observation of the ovary should only take place when, after an extended optical training, the proportions and the structure of the ovarian surface etc. can be judged thoroughly. Furthermore, the endoscopic surgeon, compared to the classic surgeon, will easily recognize small morphological structures under magnification, such as the papillomatosis structure of a small ovarian cyst.

Furthermore, the gynaecological endoscopist must be perfectly trained. He can perform a second, third and fourth incision to manipulate the female adnexa without bleeding. The best way to acquire the necessary ability to handle pelviscopic instruments is by open abdomen during multiple laparotomies, by handling them in a "pelviscopic manner"

MODERN PELVISCOPIC EQUIPMENT

Cold–light Optic

The cold–light optics for the endoscopic interabdominal observation and the endoscopic photo (proximal flash) are technically mature, above all because of the

HOPKINS-Optic. As the top of the Optic does not heat up, there is no danger of bowel-burns, for example when the bowels are touched in cases of extended adhesiolysis in the abdominal cavity.

CO_2-Pneu-electronic

The CO_2-Pneu, developed by myself 20 years ago, was only produced for diagnostic pelviscopy and is inadequate for interabdominal surgery: the surgeon should not have to face any mechanical incidents, such as a big loss of gas or gas-bladders of various sizes. Therefore we developed an electronically controlled CO_2-Pneu, which will regulate automatically all gas-filling problems. The simultaneous filling of the interabdominal wall and the measurement of the static intraabdominal pressure are performed with a single insufflation tube. With this the gas-flow can be monitored. Before surgery, the size of the gas-bladders will be preselected according to the desired static pressure. If necessary this pressure can be changed during surgery. Electronically monitored digital light indicators are combined to conventional manometers. This guarantees absolute security of the patient in cases of electronic disturbances. In summary, continuous endoscopic abdominal surgery became possible with the CO_2-Pneu-electronic. With the traditional CO_2-Pneu, endoscopic intraabdominal surgery is performed under extremely difficult conditions.

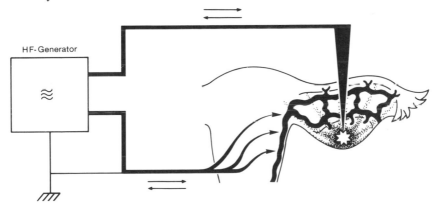

Fig. 1. Scheme of the coagulation of blood after ovarian biopsy with high frequency current: the whole ovary and the uterine vessels are heated up to an unknown and uncontrollable degree.

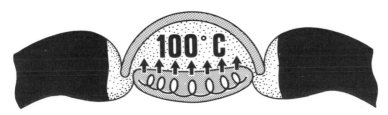

Fig. 2. Scheme of the 100°C haemostasis for the coagulation of proteins (like the boiling of a chicken egg).

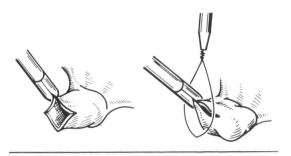

Fig. 3. Adaptation of the sound walls of the ovary after enucleation of an ovarian cyst – pelviscopic ovarial suture.

Haemostasis

A high frequency current enables haemostasis after a surgical intervention on the ovaries only in a very limited manner. At the same time the use of a high frequency current for coagulation purposes leads to uncontrollable increases of temperature in the whole ovary (Fig. 1) and in the vessels leading to it. These vessels conduct the high frequency current through the electrolytic poor mesovarium which results in the thermic destruction of ovarian tissue or its vessels (Rubinstein *et al.*, 1976, 1979; Rioux, 1977; Liebermann *et al.*, 1978).

At present the endocoagulator (according to Semm, 1977, 1978, 1979) is used. With this apparatus haemostasis is obtained by heating up the tissue (Fig. 2) to a maximum of $100°C$. This blood coagulation can be compared to the coagulation of the egg-white when boiling a chicken egg. The coagulation instruments are the Crocodile Forceps and the Point-Coagulator.

When enucleating carefully chocolate cystis, dermoids, etc., there are gaping wounds on the ovary. These can easily be adapted with the ROEDER-loop (Fig. 3). Subsequent periovarian adherences can be avoided. The very poor bleeding in all endoscopic interventions on the ovaries should be emphasized especially if compared with interventions per laparotomy: a phenomenon which has not yet been explained.

The complete endoscopic instrument set

The prime condition for intraabdominal endoscopic surgery is the availability of a complete set of instruments. To maintain the frequency of laparotomy within a limit of $1-2°/oo$, it is also necessary to have instruments which are rarely required.

POSSIBLE INTERVENTIONS ON THE OVARY

If we have the prerequisites, we can perform an important number of surgical interventions (Table I) which were in former times an indication for laparotomy.

The Ovarian Biopsy

This is performed with biopsy forceps having two teeth to fix the ovary. Up to now no biopsy forceps could cut the ovarian tissue. This is the reason why we perform the ovarian biopsy according to the technique shown in Fig. 4. After grasping and closing the biopsy forceps, we pull down the trocar sheath over the forceps with rotating movements and punch out a big specimen of ovarian tissue. If necessary we repeat this procedure. Haemostasis is performed with the Point-Coagulator: the instrument is put into the wound and coagulation takes place at a temperature of $120°-130°C$ for 20–40 s.

Ovarian Cyst

A puncture is performed to collect the cyst contents: rather small cysts are aspirated with the Syringe-Aspirator and bigger cysts with the Aquapurator (Fig. 5).

The contents of the cysts are caught separately in order to judge their colour and consistence (clear, mucinous, contents of chocolate cysts or dermoids) and to forward them to the Cytology Department. A single puncture alone is no therapy. The endoscopist should act like the laparotomist: in both cases a cyst enucleation is added to the ovarian puncture.

Full Enucleation of Cysts

After the puncture, the wall of the ovarian cyst is opened with the Hook-form Scissors; (Fig. 6). Examination of the endothelial structure follows. Laparotomy with two or a maximum of three incisions. This enucleation is not as problematic of malignant growth.

Benign cysts (e.g. chocolate cysts or dermoids) are enucleated as in laparotomy with two or a maximum of three incisions. This enucleation is not as problematic as in laparotomy because of the minor haemorrhage. A close approach to the Radix ovarii or the Mesosalpinx must be avoided. After cyst enucleation or cyst wall resection, the remaining wound edge is coagulated with the Point Coagulator or with the Crocodile Forceps. If the wound is gaping too much, the wound edges are adapted with the ROEDER-loop (Ethi-ligator, see Fig. 3). At the end, and in the course of the intervention, the lower pelvis is purged carefully from remaining cyst contents or blood.

Ovariolysis

This is very important in sterility cases. One should never forget that 20% of all endometriotic foci of the lower pelvis are retro-ovarial. Therefore after a second and third incision, the ovary must be elevated and the retro-ovarial area carefully inspected. Ovariolysis is performed after coagulation with the Crocodile Forceps or the Point Coagulator. Among other things, the pelviscopic ovariolysis is an important prerequisite for egg recovery in extracorporal fertilization.

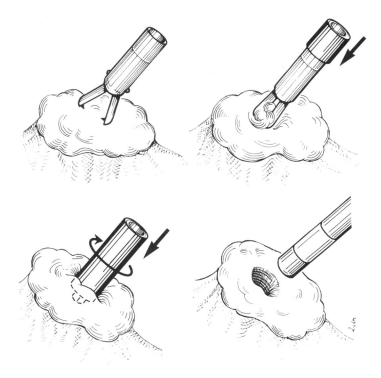

Fig. 4. Technique of ovarian biopsy.

The Partial Ovary Resection

As mentioned above regarding cystectomies, this is possible. At present, the resections, which in former times were carried out with the sharp high frequency current scissors, are easier to perform with the hook-formed scissors. The desired portion of the ovary is removed with accuracy and haemostasis is performed with the Point Coagulator or the Crocodile Forceps. The Ethi-ligator closes the wound.

Endoscopic Ovariectomy

Figure 7 shows the different stages of ovariectomy: First, ligation of the Radix ovarii, for more security with three Ethi-ligators. Then, ovary resection with the aid of the hook-formed scissors. Coagulation of the tissue stump with the Point Coagulator to prevent later adhesions. Technically it is easier to perform an adnectomy than an ovariectomy: with three Ethi-ligators the Fallopian tube is ligated together with the Mesovarium. The binding of the Fallopian tube into the vessel-stump guarantees a secure ligation. This ligation technique is identical to the one used in vaginal procedures for adnectomy and therefore is not an innovation in Gynaecology. Under adnectomy three, five and six the ovarian tissue is morcellated. If the cyst walls are thick, they are cut into longitudinal strips by scissors kicks and taken out *in toto* through an 11 mm φ trocar sheath. For this

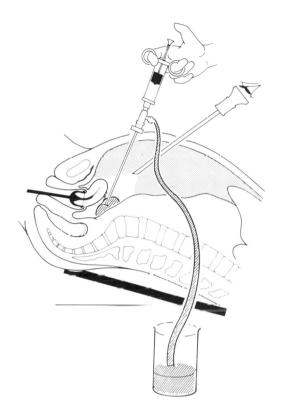

Fig. 5. Puncture of an ovarian cyst with collection of the contents.

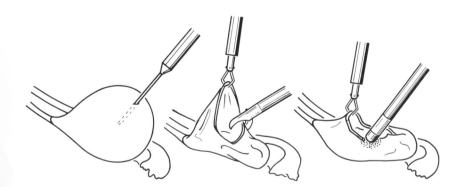

Fig. 6. Resection of an ovarian cyst after puncture with the hook-formed scissors and following endocoagulation of the bleeding wall.

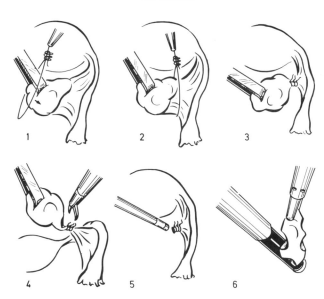

Fig. 7. Ovariectomy by pelviscopy: schematic drawing of the technique for ovariectomy by laparascopy. (1) Grasping of the ovary with the big forceps (11 mm ϕ) and pulling it through the ROEDER–loop (Ethi–ligator). (2) Slipping loop round the infundibulum ovary for ligation. (3) The infundibulum ovary is ligated three times for reasons of safety. (4) Under slight retraction the ovary is separated with the hook-shaped scissors. (5) The remaining tissue-stump must be coagulated with the point coagulator to prevent later adhesions. (6) Morcellation of the ovary with the tissue puncher.

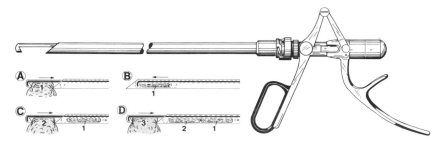

Fig. 8. Tissue puncher according to Semm (1977, 1978, 1979), for morcellation of fibromas, ovaries, etc. (A) the tissue is grasped; (B) the cut tissue is moved into the instrument-cannula; (C) the second cut procedure is shown; (D) after a movement like B the tissue puncher is ready for the third cut f.f.

reason it is necessary to dilate with the 5 mm ϕ trocar sheath to 11 mm. This dilation is safer and easier for the patient than a new incision with an 11 mm ϕ trocar. The morcellation of strong morphological tissue is performed with the tissue puncher (Fig. 8). This instrument morcellates the tissue into 1 cm^3 portions. These are accumulated in the centre of the tissue puncher and removed *in toto* through the 11 mm ϕ trocar sheath. After morcellation, the lower pelvis is cleaned with the Aquapurator and with approximately 1000 to 2000 ml physiological saline solution, so that at the end of the operation the lower pelvis is perfectly clean.

Table III. Survey of pelviscopic activity (1971–1979) in the Department of Obstetrics and Gynaecology at the University of Kiel.

		%
Diagnostical	2129	34.2
Diagnostical–Surgical	457	7.3
Surgical–Therapeutic	3646	58.5
	6232	100.0
Complications	52	0.8
Therefore Laparotomies	6	0.1

CONCLUSIONS

In summary, today 80% of laparotomies for ovarian surgery are avoided. Endoscopic ovarian surgery, (performed up till 1980 more than 3212 times), at the University of Kiel, Department of Obstetrics and Gynaecology, lowers the physical strain on the patient to a minimum. This strain is identical to that of a sterilization of the Fallopian tubes. Hospitalization is shortened, for example to 5–6 days after adnectomy. Table III gives a short survey of our pelviscopic activity from 1971 to 1979, and shows a different kind of pelviscopy, in connection with complications which make a laparotomy necessary. The combination of CO_2-Pneu-electronic, cold-light-optic, haemostasis-instruments (Semm, 1977, 1978, 1979), with a new endoscopic surgical technique, opens up new avenues for the diagnosis and therapy of the ovary in operative gynaecology.

REFERENCES

Liebermann, B. A., Belsey, E., Gordon, A. G., Wright, C. S. W., Letchworth, A. T., Noble, A. D. and Niven, P. A. R. (1978). *British Journal of Obstetrics and Gynaecology* **85**, 376.
Rioux, J. E. (1977). *Journal of Reproductive Medicine* **19**, 329.
Rubinstein, L. M., Lebherz, T. B. and Kleinkopf, V. (1976). *Contraception* **13**, 631.
Rubinstein, L. M., Benjamin, L. and Klinkopf, V. (1979). *Contraception* **31**, 641.
Semm, K. (1977). *International Journal of Medicine* **22**, 238.
Semm, K. (1978). *Endoscopy* **10**, 119.
Semm, K. (1979). *Endoscopy* **2**, 101.

SECTION IV
BREAST DISEASES IN PREMENOPAUSAL AND POSTMENOPAUSAL AGE

CLINICAL AND ENDOCRINOLOGICAL FEATURES OF
BENIGN BREAST DISEASE

G. B. Melis, G. Guarnieri, A. M. Paoletti, V. Mais, F. Strigini, N. Cappelli,
M. Selli[1], A. Ruju[2] and P. Fioretti

*Clinica Ostetrica e Ginecologica; Clinica Chirurgica dell 'Università[1] ; and
2^ Divisione Radiologica OORR[2] , Pisa, Italy*

INTRODUCTION

As is well known, mammary gland cells respond to a great number of hormonal
stimuli. From foetal life to adulthood, corticosteroids (Lockwood *et al.*, 1967),
thyroid hormones (Vanderhaar and Greco, 1979), gonadal steroids (Lasfargues,
1960; Van Bogaert, 1978), androgens (Elger and Neumann, 1966; Van Bogaert,
1978) prolactin (PRL) (Dilley, 1971; Dilley and Kister, 1975), insulin (Elias,
1962) and growth hormone (GH) (Meites, 1965) exert their influence on the
development of the mammary gland.

From *in vitro* and *in vivo* studies, it has been shown that 17-β Estradiol (E_2)
stimulates epithelial cell mitosis and duct growth, whereas progesterone (P) acts
on the breast as a modulatory agent by complementing and inhibiting oestrogen
effects on glandular and perilobular tissues; moreover, progesterone induces
the development of acini (Lyons *et al.*, 1958; Porter, 1974). Nevertheless, synergic
actions of prolactin, insulin and gluco-corticoids are also necessary for the definitive lobulo–alveolar development (Lockwood *et al.*, 1967). Recent *in vitro* studies
have shown that addition of insulin or gluco-corticoids to culture medium increases
mitotic activity in human breast specimens (Ichinose and Nandi, 1966). Subsequent addition of human prolactin induces a further significant increase in
mitotic activity (Dilley and Krister, 1975).

Hormonal effects on target tissue as well as on mammary glands are regulated

Serono Symposium No. 39, "The Menopause: Clinical, Endocrinological and Pathophysiological Aspects", edited by P. Fioretti, L. Martini, G. B. Melis and S. S. C. Yen, 1982. Academic
Press, London and New York.

by specific binding sites. Really, normal breasts and many experimental or spontaneous mammary tumours have specific binding sites for oestrogens (Leclercq *et al.*, 1973) and prolactin (Turkington, 1970; Posner *et al.*, 1974), whereas an influence on receptor concentration is also exerted by gluco-corticoids and insulin (Sakai *et al.*, 1979).

From these observations, it is evident that when functional, displastic or neoplastic pathologies of the breast take place, hormonal alterations may be involved. As a direct extension of this, research has long been carried out for evidence that some displastic or neoplastic breast diseases occur in given patients because their hormonal environment is different from that of other women (Kirschner, 1977). If such observations were true, it should be possible to identify those hormonal differences and, what is better, the hormonal differences could be corrected.

Benign breast diseases (BBD) is a vague term to define a great number of breast non-neoplastic alterations with a series of different clinical as well as anatomical and hystological aspects so that their classification requires great attention. Out of all BBD, two forms seem to have the greatest clinical interest either for their frequency or for their direct relationships with neoplasms: the fibrocystic mastopathy and the breast gross cystic disease.

Fibrocystic mastopathy may be very frequently found in young women as an isolated element or as a part of complex reproductive pathologies (Azzopardi, 1979). Epidemiological studies have shown that these patients have a two-fold greater risk for developing breast cancer than normal women (Kodlin *et al.*, 1977). Breast gross cystic disease affects a great number (10%) of women between the 4th and 5th decades of life (Haagensen, 1975). There is a great correlation between this pathology and the onset of breast cancer, since epidemiological studies have demonstrated that patients with breast gross cystic disease present a four-fold higher risk of cancer than normal subjects of the same age group (Haagensen, 1975).

By investigating the endocrine function of subjects with displastic illness of the breast for evaluating the presence of hypothalamic–pituitary–ovarian axis alterations, it was seen that either normal hormonal patterns (Sitruk–Ware *et al.*, 1979) or a series of anomalies such as anovulatory cycles, luteal insufficiency (Sitruk–Ware *et al.*, 1977), hyperoestrogenism (Mauvais–Jarvis and Kutten, 1975) and hyperprolactinaemia (Cole *et al.*, 1977), may be found in subjects with fibrocystic mastopathy. On the other hand, the hormonal pattern of subjects with breast gross cystic disease has been poorly studied (Cole *et al.*, 1977). The aim of this paper was therefore to evaluate pituitary–gonadal function in patients affected by BBD.

SUBJECTS, MATERIALS AND METHODS

Out of 93 women (15–53 years of age) suffering from BBD, 83 subjects were seen to have fibrocystic mastopathy. Women with clinical and echographic findings of fibroadenoma or benign disease of mammary nipple and ducts were excluded. Bioptic specimens were obtained as useful. Seventy-one were suffering from mastodynia and breast pain during the whole menstrual cycle or during the

second part of the cycle. Ninety had spontaneous menses with minor alterations of bleeding rhytmicity or quantity, whereas three were in postmenopausal
age. None of the patients were given active hormone preparations for at least
6 months before the study. Their pathology was first defined from a clinical
point of view; thereafter, the diagnosis was confirmed by xeromammographies
which showed the wellknown radiological heterogeneity of these pathologies:
there was one group of patients with a diffuse micronodular mastopathy, whereas
some presented with either macronodular mastopathy or isolated non-neoplastic
breast alterations, or signs of calcifications. Doubtful cases were further investigated by means of echography (Fig. 1). Using the same methods, out of 93
subjects, 10 were seen to have breast gross cystic disease.

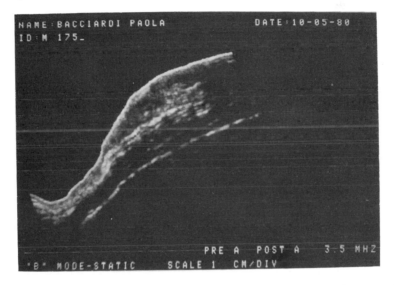

Fig. 1. Mammary echography of the patient P. B. (23 years) showing isolated macronodular
alteration.

Starting from spontaneous or induced menstrual bleedings, morning heparinized
blood samples were collected on the 4th, 10th, 14th, 20th and 24th days from
the last period. In each sample plasma concentrations of LH, FSH, PRL, E_2 and
P were measured by radioimmunoassay (RIA); GH plasma levels were only assayed
on the 10th and 20th day of the cycle.

From patients with breast gross cystic disease, cyst fluid was obtained by
needle aspiration. In seven women with a normal menstrual cycle the aspiration
was performed during the early follicular phase of the cycle, whereas in three
postmenopausal subjects no paticular days were selected.

Just before breast cyst fluid aspiration, blood samples were also collected.
According to the Papanicolau technique, staining was immediately obtained:
no malignant cells were found. After centrifugation at 30 000 r.p.m. for 15 min,
cyst fluid was kept frozen until assayed by RIA.

Circulating and cyst fluid levels of gonadotropins, PRL, GH, human chorionic
gonadotropin (HCG), E_2, estrone (E_1), dihydroepiandrosterone (DHA) and its

sulphate (DHA–S), androstenedione (A), testosterone (T) and dihydrotestosterone (DHT) were measured by specific RIA methods. While proteic hormones were directly assayed in the plasma and cyst fluid using the previously described RIA methods (Fioretti *et al.*, 1978; Melis *et al.*, 1977), E_2 and P were measured after plasma and cyst fluid extraction with diethylether (Fioretti *et al.*, 1974). The other steroid hormones were assayed by RIA after purification by means of a celite chromatography as previously described (Facchinetti and Genazzani, 1978).

RESULTS

Our sample method for monitoring patients affected by fibrocystic mastopathy have demonstrated some defects in their cycle. The endocrine balance which has been found is reported in Fig. 2.

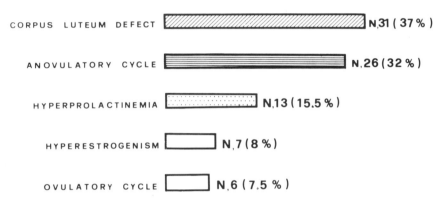

CORPUS LUTEUM DEFECT   N.31 (37 %)

ANOVULATORY CYCLE   N.26 (32 %)

HYPERPROLACTINEMIA   N.13 (15.5 %)

HYPERESTROGENISM   N.7 (8 %)

OVULATORY CYCLE   N.6 (7.5 %)

Fig. 2. Percentage of menstrual disorders found in 83 subjects with fibrocystic mastopathy examined by evaluating circulating levels of prolactin (PRL), LH, FSH, 17-β estradiol (E_2) and progesterone (P) during the menstrual cycle. The values are reported as mean ± standard error (M ± SE).

Evident alterations were immediately seen in only eight patients (9.5%), who showed pathological high levels of plasma PRL (mean values of 32 ± 4 ng/ml on the 4th day of cycle) (Fig. 3) during the early follicular phase of the cycle. The other subjects showed normal levels of PRL. When the hormone secretion during the menstrual cycle was considered, plasma PRL levels higher than normal were found in five other subjects during the luteal phase (mean values were 40 ± 2 ng/ml on the 20th day of the cycle) (Fig. 4). Thus, hyperprolactinaemia could be considered to affect 13 subjects (15.5%) with fibrocystic mastopathy of this series (Fig. 2). The majority of patients with fibrocystic mastopathy however had alterations in their ovarian cyclical function, in contrast with normal follicular phase values of the hormones under study. P levels in particular, were altered in many cases during luteal phase (Fig. 2). Thirty-one patients (37%) showed corpus luteum defects (Fig. 5) in the sense that either constant low levels of P or short length of P secretion were found according to the method of Fioretti

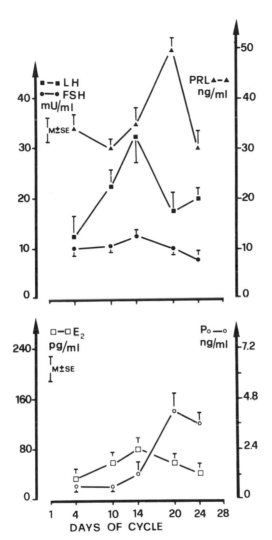

Fig. 3. Increased basal levels of plasma PRL in eight patients with fibrocystic mastopathy. The values are reported as mean ± standard error (M ± SE).

et al. (1978). With the same criteria, 26 subjects (32%) also showed an absence of P increase during the second part of the cycle (Fig. 6), since the P levels were constantly lower than 2 ng/ml in the sample collected after midcycle. Another group of seven subjects (8%) showed a higher than normal cyclical E_2 secretion (Fig. 7). The other six subjects, out of 83 patients with fibrocystic mastopathy, had a normal ovulatory cycle with the normal ratio between P and E_2 (Fig. 8).

In the same patients further analysis of basal levels of different proteic and steroid hormones showed that most parameters had normal levels with the exception of T and DHT values, which were slightly higher, and DHEA-S which was

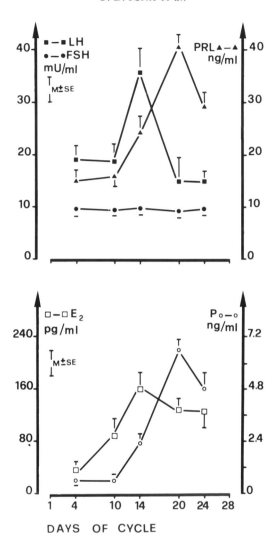

Fig. 4. Elevated levels of plasma PRL during the luteal phase in five subjects with fibro-cystic mastopathy. The values are reported as mean ± standard error (M ± SE).

slightly lower in comparison with the normal range (Fig. 9). However, when PRL and GH levels were considered in this last group of six subjects (Fig. 10), slightly elevated values of both hormones were seen in the luteal phase of the cycle in comparison with control subjects without breast diseases. With regard to patients with gross breast cystic disease, either slightly hyperprolactinaemia or a short luteal phase were observed in premenopausal patients, whereas the other three subjects showed the typical hormonal pattern of postmenopausal age. Also, considering the age of the subjects (35–53 years), these results seem to indicate that also in this series, the alterations of E_2/P ratio represent the main finding concerning subjects with breast pathology.

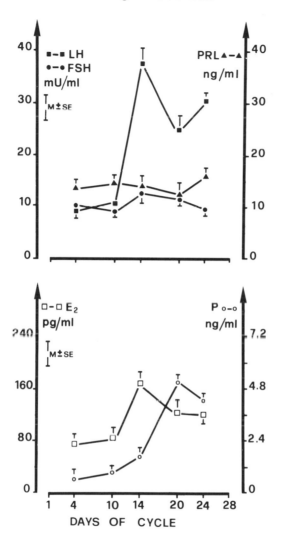

Fig. 5. Hormonal menstrual pattern in 31 subjects affected by fibrocystic mastopathy. The mean (± SE) levels of P during the second part of the cycle were lower than corresponding values measured during normal ovulatory cycles. The graph reports patients with either true luteal insufficiency or short luteal phase.

Relative to hormone contents in the fluid of breast cysts (Fig. 11), high levels of HCH and LH were detected, while PRL, GH, FSH and steroid levels were within or below the range of peripheral blood concentrations.

DISCUSSION

The present data have shown that only a few subjects with BBD have a normal function of the pituitary–ovarian axis, whereas many patients in our series had either altered basal PRL levels or an altered ratio between E_2 and P.

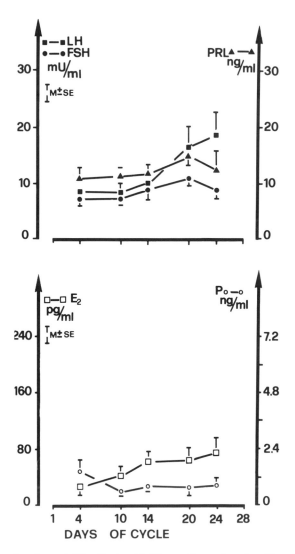

Fig. 6. Hormonal pattern of 26 patients with fibrocystic mastopathy. Mean (± SE) P levels measured during the second part of the cycle failed to show any increase.

PRL has been shown to act as a physiological stimulator of breast function (Tyson, 1977). It has been also demonstrated that this hormone, besides insulin and gluco-corticoids, is necessary for lobular–alveolar development as well as for mammary gland differentiation and growth (Bassler, 1970; Lockwood *et al.*, 1967). The addition of PRL to culture medium for breast specimens is able to increase the mitotic activity of cells (Dilley and Krister, 1975). Both normal breast tissue and spontaneous or experimental mammary tumours show specific binding sites for PRL (Posner *et al.*, 1974). Owing to all these observations, it appears that PRL plays an important role in the control of mammary gland

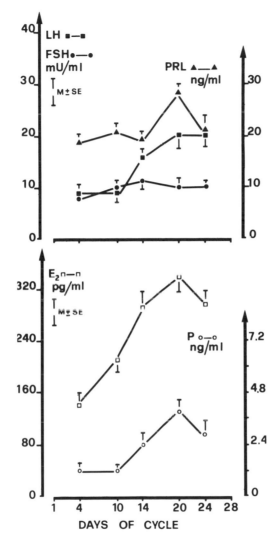

Fig. 7. Slight elevated mean (± SE) values of E_2 in patients affected by fibrocystic masto-pathy.

function and, as a consequence, alterations of PRL secretion could represent an aetiological factor for BBD and breast tumour onset. In our patients, blood PRL levels were pathologically higher in a great number of subjects. In addition, PRL response to Sulpiride stimulation tests and PRL 24 h pattern were altered in more than 80% of the same patients with BBD (Melis *et al.*, unpublished data).

These data agree with those of other authors, who have shown that premeno-pausal patients with breast tumours had a significant increase either in basal levels or in nocturnal PRL concentrations, when compared to normal subjects of the same age group (Sheth *et al.*, 1975; Ohgo *et al.*, 1976; Malarkey *et al.*,

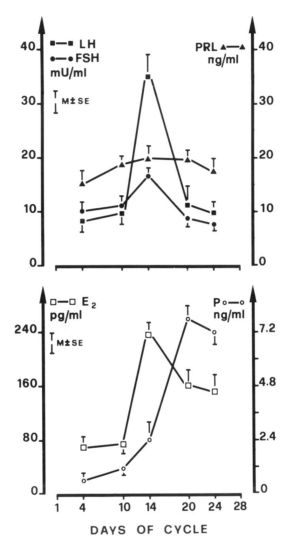

Fig. 8. Hormonal menstrual pattern of six subjects with fibrocystic mastopathy and normal ovulatory cycle.

1977). On the other hand, plasma PRL response to TRH stimulation tests in breast tumour or BBD patients seems to be prompter and greater than in normal subjects (Ohgo *et al.*, 1976). In turn, the treatment of BBD with the dopaminergic agent bromocriptine, which is known to decrease PRL levels, seems to improve breast pathology (Mussa and Dogliotti, 1979; Paoletti *et al.*, 1980). From all those observations and from the results of the endocrine study of patients with BBD, PRL levels seem to play a critical role in either the development of and/or the progression of female breast pathology. Further evidence of this view is represented by the fact that also in patients with normal PRL levels and an

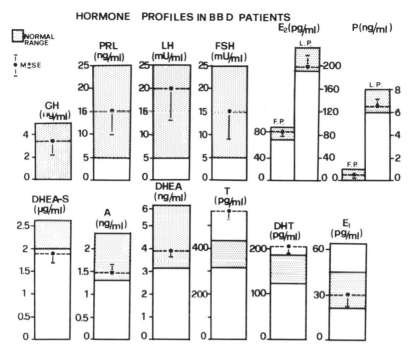

Fig. 9. Basal levels of proteic and steroidal hormones in six subjects (see Fig. 14) with fibrocystic mastopathy and ovulatory menstrual cycle. Slightly elevated levels of testosterone (T) and dihydrotestosterone (DHT) were found whereas Dihydroepiandrosterone sulphate (DHEAS) was slightly decreased.

anovulatory cycle, the cumulative PRL secretion either during the luteal phase or during the follicular phase, was larger than in normal subjects (Fig. 10). This last finding seemingly represents the explanation of the positive effect of bromocriptine treatment in BBD patients without altered basal levels of PRL. In the same patients, increased GH secretion during the luteal phase was also observed (Fig. 10). These data agree with the findings of Carter *et al.* (1975), who have shown that glucose ingestion, paradoxically, stimulates rather than suppresses GH secretion in patients with mammary cancer.

More than 60% of subjects with both fibrocystic mastopathy and gross cyst breast disease had anovulatory cycles, corpus luteum defect or high levels of oestrogens. All these findings are characterized by a discrepancy between P and E_2 secretion through the menstrual cycle with a relative or absolute hyperoestrogenism. It has been demonstrated that oestrogens have specific binding sites in normal and tumoral mammary tissues (Leclercq *et al.,* 1973). Oestrogens are able to stimulate epithelial cell mitosis and ductal growth, while progesterone induces the development of acini and also counteracts the mesenchimal actions of oestrogens (Bassler, 1970; Porter, 1974). Moreover, the continuous administration of oestrogens without progesterone supplementation to castrated animals was shown to induce proliferation of tubular system, dilatation of ducts, formation of cysts and, also, stimulation of connective tissue with histological features

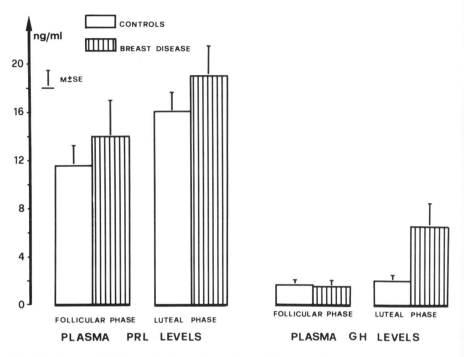

Fig. 10. Mean (± SE) plasma levels of PRL and growth hormone (GH) during follicular and luteal phase in patients with fibrocystic mastopathy and normal ovulatory cycles. Slight elevated levels of both hormones were found, particularly during the second part of the cycle.

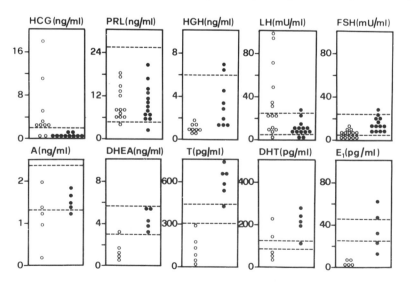

Fig. 11. Mean (± SE) plasma levels of proteic and steroidal hormones simultaneously evaluated both in blood and in cyst fluids of patients with breast gross cyst disease. - - - - normal range; ○ cyst fluid levels; ● plasma levels.

comparable with fibrocystic mastopathy of human pathology (Eisein, 1942; Bassler, 1970). Previous studies (Sherman and Korenman, 1974; Sitruk-Ware *et al.,* 1977, 1979) have pointed out that subjects with BBD had inadequate corpus luteum function characterized by normal secretion of oestradiol contrasting with abnormally low secretion of progesterone.

Our data represent a direct extension of the findings of the above-mentioned authors. However, an important difference seems to be represented by the finding that, besides corpus luteum defects, patients with fibrocystic mastopathy of our series also present absolute high levels of oestradiol and anovulatory cycles. The presence of high E_2 levels confirms the previous *in vitro* findings of Cortes-Gallegos *et al.* (1975) who found that the breast tissues of patients with benign mastopathies show a higher estradiol concentration than that of normal women.

On the other hand, anovulation is also effective on the target tissues as a factor of hyperoestrogenism, since like inadequate corpus luteum function, the protective effect of progesterone is absent, confirming that the imbalance between oestrogens and progesterone production, could represent the main aetiological factor of fibrocystic mastopathy. The same altered P/E_2 ratio, together with the above said pathological changes of menstrual cycles, can be also observed in women with breast gross cystic disease.

With regard to other steroid hormones, it has been shown that patients with breast benign and malignant pathology show reduced levels of androgens and reduced excretion of their metabolites (Bulbrook *et al.,* 1971). In an attempt to further elucidate the role of androgens in the onset or maintenance of breast pathology, many authors have made in depth studies on the metabolism of androstenedione that represents the major source of oestrone and testosterone in females (Kirschner and Bardin, 1972). In the same way, the roles of DHEA and its sulphate (Poortman *et al.,* 1975), of testosterone and dihydrotestosterone (Persijn *et al.,* 1975), have also been investigated in view of the presence of androgen receptors in breast tissue (Poortman *et al.,* 1975). However the results so far obtained are conflicting: some of them being favourable and some unfavourable for an involvement of androgens in the inducion of breast pathology (Wilson *et al.,* 1967; Kumaoka *et al.,* 1968; Kirschner, 1977). Our data seem to exclude the importance of androgens in inducing human fibrocystic mastopathy, since no variation of androgen levels was found during the follicular phase (Fig. 10). However, our investigation has been limited to a few patients: thus our data are not definitive and require further investigations.

Relative to the content of cyst fluids, many investigators have shown the presence of different steroid and proteic hormones (Raju *et al.,* 1977; Srivastava *et al.,* 1977; Bradlow *et al.,* 1979; Haagensen *et al.,* 1979). Cyst fluid may represent the trasudate from the blood supplied to the breast or an exudate from the near tissue. Moreover, Haagensen *et al.* (1979) have shown that cyst fluids contain a major component protein, not found in plasma. Furthermore, Bradlow *et al.* (1979) have demonstrated high levels of HCG and PRL in cyst fluids which do not relate to circulating levels. Thus, in some way, cyst fluid contents could represent the secretion of epithelial cells surrounding breast cyst. As reported above, in the samples obtained from our patients, high levels of HCG and PRL have been found, whereas the other hormones were always at lower levels than corresponding blood concentrations (Fig. 11).

Ectopic production of proteic substances and particularly of HCG, has been reported to be produced by trophoblastic and non-trophoblastic tumours (Braunstein *et al.*, 1973; Vaitukaitis, 1974). Since the relationship between breast gross cystic disease and mammary tumours is well defined, the findings of high HCG levels in cyst fluids may be speculative for a greater malignancy of some breast cysts than another.

In conclusion, various reproductive functions are altered in patients with BBD, so treatment should be predicted on the patient's endocrinological profile. In addition, the assay of HCG or other proteins performed on the fluid obtained from the breast cysts could represent an adjunctive factor to select those mammary cysts at risk for developing breast cancer. Comparative histopathological and biochemical studies are necessary in this view.

REFERENCES

Azzopardi, J. G. (1979). *In* "Problems in breast pathology" (J. L. Bennington, Ed.) 11, 57. W. B. Saunders, London and Philadelphia.

Bassler, R. (1970). *Current Topics Pathology* 53, 1.

Bradlow, H. L., Schwartz, M. K., Fleicher, M., Nisselbaum, J. S., Boyar, R., O'Connor, J. and Fukushima, D. K. (1979). *Journal of Clinical Endocrinology and Metabolism* 49, 778.

Braunstein, G. D., Vaitukaitis, J. L., Carbone, P. P. and Ross, G. T. (1973). *Annals Internal Medicine* 78, 39.

Bulbrook, R. D., Havward, J. L. and Spicer, C. C. (1971). *Lancet* ii, 395.

Carter, A. C., Lefkon, B. W., Farlin, M. and Feldman, E. B. (1975). *Journal of Clinical Endocrinology and Metabolism* 40, 260.

Cole, E. N., Sellwood, R. A., England, P. C. and Griffiths, K. (1977). *European Journal of Cancer* 13, 597.

Cortes–Gallegos, V., Gallegos, A. J. and Basurto, C. (1975). *Journal Steroid Biochemistry* 6, 15.

Dilley, W. G. (1971). *Endocrinology* 88, 514.

Dilley, W. G. and Krister, S. J. (1975). *Journal of National Cancer Institute* 55, 35.

Eisein, M. J. (1942). *Cancer Research* 2, 632.

Elger, W. and Neumann, F. (1966). *Proceedings of Society of Experimental Biology* 123, 637.

Elias, J. J. (1962). *Experimental Cell Biology* 27, 601.

Facchinetti, F. and Genazzani, A. R. (1978). *Journal Nuclear Medicine Allied Sciences* 22, 419.

Fioretti, P., Genazzani, A. R., Facchinetti, F., Nasi, A., Melis, G. B. and Paoletti, A. M. (1974). *In* "Atti LVIˆCongresso Nazionale Società Italiana di Ostetricia e Ginecologia". 637.

Fioretti, P., Melis, G. B., Paoletti, A. M., Parodo, G., Caminiti, F., Corsini, G. U. and Martini, L. (1978). *Journal of Clinical Endocrinology and Metabolism* 47, 1336.

Haagensen, C. D. (1975). *In* "Diseases of the breast" (2nd edition) p. 195. W. B. Saunders Company, Philadelphia.

Haagensen, D. E., Mazoujian, G., Dilley, W. G., Pedersen, C. E., Kister, S. J. and Wells, S. A. (1979). *Journal National Cancer Institute* 62, 239.

Ichinose, R. R. and Nandi, S. (1966). *Journal of Endocrinology* 35, 331.

Kirschner, M. A. (1977). *Cancer* 39, 2716.

Kirschner, M. A. and Bardin, C. W. (1972). *Metabolism* **21**, 667.
Kodlin, D., Winger, E. E., Morgerstern, N. L. and Chen, U. (1977). *Cancer* **39**, 2603.
Kumaoka, S., Sakauchi, N. and Abe, N. (1968). *Journal of Clinical Endocrinology* **28**, 667.
Lasfargues, E. Y. (1960). *Comptes rendus des séances de la société de biologie et de ses filiales (Paris)* **154**, 1720.
Leclercq, G., Henson, J. C., Schoenfeld, R., Mattheiem, W. H. and Tagnon, H. J. (1973). *European Journal of Cancer* **9**, 665.
Lockwood, D. H., Stockdale, F. E. and Topper, Y. J. (1967). *Science* **156**, 945.
Lyons, W. R., Li, C. H. and Johnson, R. E. (1958). *Recent Progress in Hormone Research* **14**, 219.
Malarkey, W. B., Schroeder, L. L., Stevens, V. C., James, A. G. and Lanese, R. R. (1977). *Cancer Research* **37**, 4650.
Mauvais–Jarvis, P. and Kutten, F. (1975). *Nouvelle Presse Médicale* **4**, 323.
Meites, J. (1965). *Endocrinology* **76**, 1220.
Melis, G. B., Mameli, M., Cardia, S., Genazzani, A. R., Milia, A., Nasi, A., Paoletti, A. M., Puddu, R. and Fioretti, P. (1977). *Acta Europea Fertilitatis* **8**, 283.
Mussa, A. and Dogliotti, L. (1979). *Journal of Endocrinological Investigation* **2**, 87.
Ohgo, S., Kato, Y., Chichara, K. and Imura, H. (1976). *Cancer* **37**, 1412.
Paoletti, A. M., Murru, S., Guarnieri, G., Gargiulo, T., Melis, G. B., Madrigali, E. and Fioretti, P. (1980). *Journal of Endocrinological Investigation* (in press).
Persijn, R. P., Korsten, C. B. and Engelsman, E. (1975). *British Medical Journal* **4**, 503.
Poortman, J., Prenen, J. A. C., Schwarz, F. and Thijssen, J. H. H. (1975). *Journal of Clinical Endocrinology and Metabolism* **40**, 373.
Porter, J. C. (1974). *Journal Investigation Dermatology* **63**, 85.
Posner, B. I., Kelly, P. A. and Friesur, H. G. (1974). *Proceedings of the National Academy of Sciences USA* **71**, 2407.
Raju, U., Ganguly, M. and Lewitz, M. (1977). *Journal of Clinical Endocrinology and Metabolism* **45**, 429.
Sakai, S., Bowman, P. D., Young, J., McCormick, K. and Nandi, S. (1979). *Endocrinology* **104**, 1447.
Sherman, B. M. and Korenman, S. G. (1974). *Cancer* **33**, 1306.
Sheth, N. A., Ranadive, K. J., Suraiya, J. N. and Sheth, A. R. (1975). *British Journal of Cancer* **32**, 160.
Sitruk–Ware, L. R., Sterkers, N., Mouszowicz, I. and Mauvais–Jarvis, P. (1977). *Journal of Clinical Endocrinology and Metabolism* **44**, 771.
Sitruk–Ware, L. R., Sterkers, N. and Mauvais–Jarvis, P. (1979). *Obstetrics and Gynaecology* **53**, 457.
Srivastava, L. S., Pescovitz, H., Singh, R. D., Perisutti, G. and Knowlesh, C. (1977). *Experientia* **33**, 1659.
Turkington, R. W. (1970). *Biochemical and Biophysical Research Communications* **41**, 1362.
Tyson, J. E. (1977). *In* "Prolactin and Human Reproduction" (Crosignani, P. G. and Robyn, C., Eds), p. 67. Academic Press, London, New York and San Francisco.
Vaitukaitis, J. L. (1974). *Annals of Clinical and Laboratory Science* **4**, 276.
Van Bogaert, L. J. (1978). *Hormone Metabolism Research* **10**, 337.
Vanderhaar, B. K. and Greco, A. E. (1979). *Endocrinology* **104**, 409.
Wilson, R. E., Crocker, D. W. and Fairgrieve, J. (1967). *JAMA* **199**, 474.

GLUCO-CORTICOID BINDING ACTIVITIES IN HUMAN BREAST CYST FLUID

R. Frairia, M. Casulini, A. M. Fazzari, S. Del Bello, V. Aimone[1] and A. Angeli

Clinica Medica Generale e Terapia Medica B, Università degli Studi, Turin and Ente Ospedaliero S. Anna, Turin[1] Via Genova 3, 10126 Turin, Italy

INTRODUCTION

Patients with fibrocystic lesions constitute a population with a higher than normal risk of cancer, evaluated by various authors as being two to five times that of normal women (Davis *et al.*, 1964; Haagensen, 1971; Donnelly *et al.*, 1975). On this basis, it has been suggested that benign and malignant breast disease could have common factors, such as patterns of hormone metabolization and protein synthesis.

Gross cystic breast disease (GCD) is a common condition in premenopausal women, appearing after the age of 25 years and disappearing at menopause. Pathologically, cysts are amorphous fluid-filled structures lined with a single layer of epithelium or connective tissue (epithelial layer sloughed). Various subsidiary pathological changes are frequently associated, including abnormal epithelial proliferation and secretion.

The agents responsible for these changes are at present unknown, but hormonal stimulation admittedly plays an important role. Very little has been published regarding the hormonal composition and the biochemistry of the breast cyst fluid (BCF), even though it is admitted that such studies may shed light on the mechanisms underlying the disease.

Chemical components of breast cyst fluid that have been studied include electrolytes and trace elements (Fleisher *et al.*, 1974; Schwarts, 1976; Gatzy

Serono Symposium No. 39, "The Menopause: Clinical, Endocrinological and Pathophysiological Aspects", edited by P. Fioretti, L. Martini, G. B. Melis and S. S. C. Yen, 1982. Academic Press, London and New York.

et al., 1979), tumour-associated antigens (Fleisher *et al.*, 1974; Schwartz, 1976; Haagensen *et al.*, 1977; Dufour *et al.*, 1978), steroid hormones (Schwartz, 1976; Bradlow *et al.*, 1976; Levitz *et al.*, 1977; Bradlow *et al.*, 1979), enzymes (Fleisher *et al.*, 1974; Binkley *et al.*, 1975; Schwartz, 1976) and proteins, which have been described as being present in relatively high concentrations (Pearlman *et al.*, 1973; Fleisher *et al.*, 1974; Pearlman *et al.*, 1977).

A progesterone-binding protein of the fluid has been described by Pearlman *et al.* (1973). These authors analyzed fluid from GCD by acrylamide gel electrophoresis and found significant differences in GCD fluid compared to normal human serum.

Haagensen Jr. *et al.* (1979) analyzed GCD fluid by sodium dodecyl-sulphate-acrylamide gel electrophoresis and identified four major proteins. One of these had progesterone-binding activity and, immunologically, it was identical to a component of human plasma. To our knowledge, information is not available on other steroid-recognizing components.

In the present study we tested the occurrence of gluco-corticoid-binding activities in BCF using as the ligands tritiated cortisol, corticosterone, progesterone and dexamethasone. The gluco-corticoid-binding properties of BCF were then compared to those of a normal human mammary secretion, i.e., *post partum* milk and to those of human plasma.

MATERIALS AND METHODS

Clinical Material

Seventy seven breast GCD fluids were obtained by needle aspiration from 73 women (aged 25–47 years) under treatment GCD at the Ospedale Ostetrico Ginecologico S. Anna, Turin. Four cyst fluid samples were aspirated from different cysts in the same patients. Initial processing consisted of ultracentrifugation at 105 000 x g at 4°C for 1 h; specimens were stored at −20°C until analysis. Peripheral blood serum was obtained from healthy non-pregnant women from our laboratory staff and stored at −20°C until analysis.

Milk (7–10 days *post partum*) was obtained from lactating women at the Ospedale Ostetrico Ginecologico S. Anna, Turin. Specimens were centrifuged in cellulose nitrate tubes at 105 000 x g for 30 min at 4°C. The tubes were then pierced with a syringe needle to remove the clear fluid, i.e. the whey, lying between the casein sediment and the floating lipid layer.

Steroids

The following labeled steroids were obtained from The Radiochemical Center, Amersham: 1,2-^{3}H cortisol, 44 Ci per mmol; 1,2-^{3}H corticosterone, 57 Ci per mmole; 1,2,6,7-^{3}H progesterone, 93 Ci per mmole; 1,2(n)-^{3}H dexamethasone, 25 Ci per mmole. Unlabeled steroids were obtained from Ikapharm. Ramat Gan, Israel.

RIA Determinations

The concentrations of the following steroids were assayed using radioimmuno-assay procedures routinely performed in our laboratory to measure plasma levels; cortisol, progesterone, aldosterone, dehydroepiandrosterone sulphate; radio-immunoassayable prolactin was also measured.

Protein Determination

The protein concentration in BCF, milk whey and plasma was determined by the method of Lowry *et al.* (1951), employing bovine serum albumin as a standard protein.

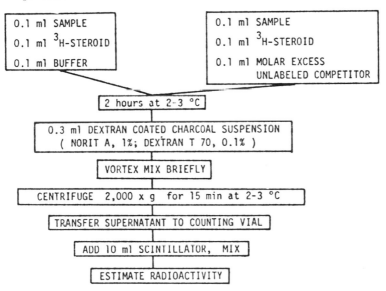

Fig. 1. Flow diagram of the method for evaluating specific binding activities for cortisol, corticosterone, progesterone and dexamethasone in BCF specimens.

Evaluation of Glucocorticoid Binding

Specific binding activities for cortisol, corticosterone, progesterone, and dexamethasone were tested according to the procedure described by Fazekas and MacFarlane (1977) with some modifications. Aliquots of BCF (50 μl/tube) were incubated at 2-3°C for 2 h with tritiated ligand (0.833 pmoles/tube). Non-specific binding was accounted for by performing the same incubations in the presence of a 250-fold molar excess of non-radioactive steroid. Figure 1 outlines the subsequent procedure. Radioactivity was counted by liquid scintillation spectrometry in 10 ml of scintillation fluid (120 g naphtalene, 4 g PPO, 0.05 g POPOP in 1000 ml 1,4-dioxan). Counts were corrected for quenching and systematically converted to moles of steroid using an external standard system of calibration.

Table I. Specific binding for different steroid molecules observed in BCF examined.

	Total No. assayed	No. positive	%	Range fmoles bound/ml
Cortisol	77	21	27.3	124–6128
Corticosterone	36	9	25	775–6948
Progesterone	25	6	24	184–1060
Dexamethasone	70	6	8.6	44–370

Table II. Mean ± SE hormonal concentrations and total protein content (Prot.) observed in BCF assayed. Abbreviations are as follows: F = cortisol; P = progesterone; PRL = prolactin; A = aldosterone; E_2 = estradiol-17β; DHA-S = dehydroepiandrosterone-sulphate; Prot. = total protein content.

	Breast cyst fluid		
	No. assayed	Mean	± SE
F (μg/dl)	70	2.85	0.27
P (pg/ml)	38	6737	681
PRL (ng/ml)	42	6.47	0.46
A (pg/ml)	20	89.4	10.85
E_2 (pg/ml)	35	16.7	5.4
DHA-S (μg/dl)	29	2696	569
Prot. (mg/ml)	77	28.7	1.53

Specific binding was calculated as the difference between the results in the absence and presence of unlabeled competitor. Non-specific binding was represented by the results obtained in the presence of an unlabeled competitor.

RESULTS

Macromolecular Binding of Gluco-corticoid Molecules

Screening of 77 BCF revealed significant amounts of specific binding for cortisol, corticosterone and progesterone in about 25% of these specimens. Specific binding for dexamethasone was found in only six samples. Quantitatively, the range of the binding activity was ample for each considered steroid. Data are presented in Table I. Due to the reduced amount of BCF aspirated in some cases, it was not possible to evaluate the entire pattern of gluco-corticoid-binding activities in all samples.

By examining individual data, no case was found presenting "positive" binding for corticosterone or progesterone and "negative" binding for cortisol. No correlation was found between values of cortisol-binding activity and steroid concentrations in BCF. Our data on the hormonal levels determined in our series are presented in Table II.

Scatchard Analyses

Scatchard plots of the results obtained in the presence of increasing concentrations of ^{3}H labeled steroids were used to define gluco-corticoid binding characteristics of BCF as compared to plasma and milk. For these studies three pools of each medium were treated with Norit-A in a manner similar to that described by Heyns *et al.* (1967) for removing endogenous steroids, since these steroids conceivably may compete with the radioactive steroid for the binding to the same site.

Two series of experiments were performed, using ^{3}H-cortisol and ^{3}H-progesterone, respectively. Mean data obtained at equilibrium in our conditions are presented in Figs 2–4. Calculation of apparent equilibrium association constant (K_a) and apparent equilibrium dissociation constant (K_d) gave mean data presented in Table III.

Effect of Unlabeled Competitors on Specific ^{3}H-cortisol Binding

In these experiments the specific binding for ^{3}H-cortisol was evaluated in the presence of increasing amounts of unlabeled competitors, in order to compare patterns of displacement in BCF, plasma and milk, respectively. The following steroid molecules were considered: cortisol, corticosterone, cortisone, 11-deoxycortisol, progesterone, prednisolone, aldosterone, dexamethasone. Molar excess ranged from 10 to 100 000. As shown in Figs 5–7 and in Tables IV and V, differences between the considered media were of minor entity. The general pattern that emerged from these experiments was compatible with the existence in BCF and in milk of a component similar to serum transcortin.

DISCUSSION

The present study has demonstrated that a corticosteroid-binding component may be present in breast cyst fluid. This component, which we found in about 25% of examined BCF samples, shows high affinity and low capacity for different steroid molecules, including both natural and synthetic gluco-corticoids and progesterone.

Data obtained in ligand competition experiments for different steroid molecules suggest the similarity with the plasma corticosteroid-binding globulin (CBG, transcortin) and especially with the corticosteroid-binding component detected in the whey of the human milk.

The human "milk CBG", first reported by Khan *et al.* (1975), has been demonstrated to be antigenically different from serum CBG, yet sharing the steroid binding properties of the circulating protein (Payne *et al.*, 1976).

It is still debated whether CBG enters the mammary epithelial cells from the peripheral circulation and in some way modifies its physicochemical properties in the milk or a specific CBG is synthesized *de novo* in the mammary gland. Biochemical analysis of BCF has provided evidence of fluid component proteins clearly secreted in this medium from breast epithelial cells (Pearlman *et al.*, 1977; Haagensen Jr *et al.*, 1979). Moreover, most recently, a cortisol binding globulin has been identified and isolated from porcine ovarian follicular fluid (Mahajan *et al.*, 1980). On these grounds, one can assume that CBG-like proteins may have

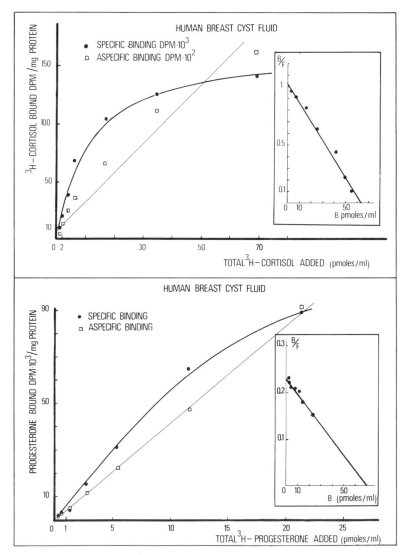

Fig. 2. Equilibrium binding of ³H-cortisol and ³H-progesterone to the gluco-corticoid-binding component in pooled BCF. Aliquots of samples were equilibrated at 2°C with a range of concentrations of ³H-cortisol or ³H-progesterone, either alone or in the presence of 250-fold molar excess of unlabeled steroid. Saturable binding, calculated as the difference between the results in the presence and absence of a 250-fold molar excess of unlabeled steroid, is represented by the method of Scatchard (1949), in the inset. Each point represents the mean of three pools

a physiological role in secretory fluids of different hormone-sensitive structures. In the light of this discussion it is conceivable that the gluco-corticoid binding component plays a role within the cysts in controlling kinetics of transport from the blood and the effective levels of cortisol and progesterone, generally regarded to be the unbound form (Westphal, 1971).

In our assay condition, no evidence was seen for an exclusive progesterone-

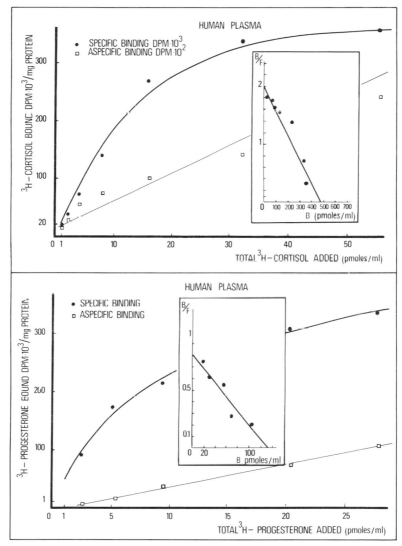

Fig. 3. Equilibrium binding of ^{3}H-cortisol and ^{3}H-progesterone to the gluco-corticoid-binding globulin in pooled sera collected from healthy non-pregnant women. Data are presented as in Fig. 2. Each point represents the mean of three pools.

binding component. Pearlman *et al.* (1973, 1977) have described a progesterone-binding glycoprotein peculiar of BCF; more recently, Haagensen Jr *et al.* (1979) have identified this protein with the GCDFP-24 component immunologically identical to a human plasma protein present in Cohn fraction VI. The binding constant for progesterone has been calculated to be approximately 1×10^6 litres/mole, which admittedly is not sufficient to classify this component as a specific steroid-recognizing protein. Finally, no conclusion can be drawn from the present study on the real occurrence in some BCF of a dexamethasone-binding component possibly indicating the cellular release of soluble gluco-corticoid receptors.

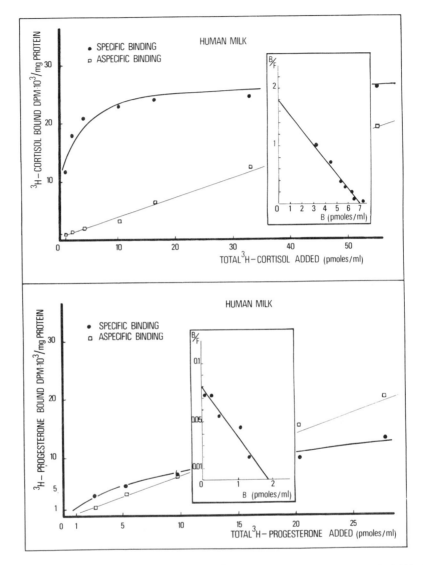

Fig. 4. Equilibrium binding of ³H-cortisol and ³H-progesterone to the gluco-corticoid-binding globulin in pooled milk samples collected 7–10 days *post partum*. Data are presented as in Fig. 2. Each point represents the mean of three pools.

ACKNOWLEDGEMENTS

This work has been supported by a grant of the Consiglio Nazionale delle Ricerche (CNR), Rome, Italy; Pzogetto Finalizzato: Controllo della czeseita neoplastica.

Table III. Mean values of the apparent equilibrium association constant (K_a) and of the apparent equilibrium dissociation constant (K_d) for cortisol and progesterone binding in BCF, plasma collected from healthy non-pregnant women and milk collected 7–10 days *post partum*. Data were calculated from Scatchard representations of binding curves (1949) constructed over a range of ^{3}H-steroid concentrations and corrected for low affinity binding by subtractions of values for ^{3}H-steroid binding in the presence of a 250-fold molar excess of unlabeled steroid.

	Apparent K_a	Apparent K_d (nM)	r, Scatchard analysis
	Cortisol		
BCF	$1.03 \cdot 10^9$ M^{-1}	0.97	-0.99
Plasma	$1.06 \cdot 10^9$ M^{-1}	0.94	-0.91
Milk	$2.01 \cdot 10^9$ M^{-1}	0.50	-0.97
	Progesterone		
BCF	$2.06 \cdot 10^8$ M^{-1}	4.86	-0.92
Plasma	$1.63 \cdot 10^9$ M^{-1}	0.61	-0.95
Milk	$2.38 \cdot 10^8$ M^{-1}	4.2	-0.91

Table IV. Amounts (molar excess) which produce equal displacement of labeled cortisol in our system assay. Abbreviations are as follows: F = cortisol; Prog. = progesterone; B = corticosterone; Dex = dexamethasone; Predn = prednisolone; Ald = aldosterone; E = cortisone; S = 11-deoxycortisol.

	F	Prog	B	Dex	Predn	Ald	E	S
				Steroid compound added				
BCF	250	2500	600	> 5000	5000	> 5000	> 5000	5000
Milk	250	1000	1000	> 5000	> 5000	> 5000	> 5000	> 5000
Plasma	250	1000	450	> 5000	5000	> 5000	> 5000	5000

Table V. Relative potency (%) of steroids as measured by integrated areas of displacement defined by competition curves. Abbreviations are as follows F = cortisol; Prog = progesterone; B = corticosterone; Dex = dexamethasone; Predn = prednisolone; Ald = aldosterone; E = cortisone; S = 11-deoxycortisol.

	F	Prog	B	Dex	Predn	Ald	E	S
				Steroid compound added				
BCF	100	63.1	91.7	7.2	67.4	22.3	27.8	76.2
Milk	100	93.5	98.2	6.7	56.9	14.9	26.5	62
Plasma	100	69.7	94.9	0	75	18.9	28.9	86.7

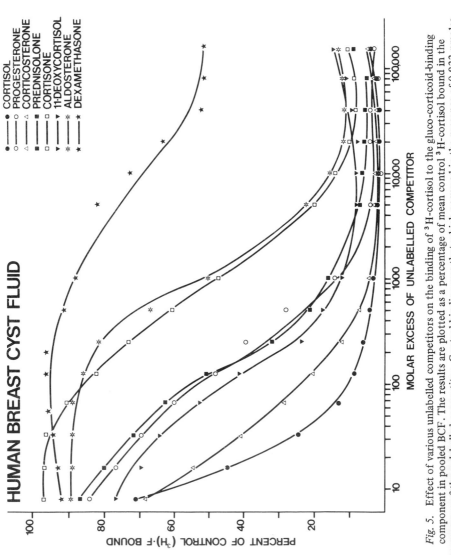

Fig. 5. Effect of various unlabelled competitors on the binding of ^{3}H-cortisol to the gluco-corticoid-binding component in pooled BCF. The results are plotted as a percentage of mean control ^{3}H-cortisol bound in the presence of the unlabelled competitor. Control binding was that which occurred in the presence of 0.833 pmoles

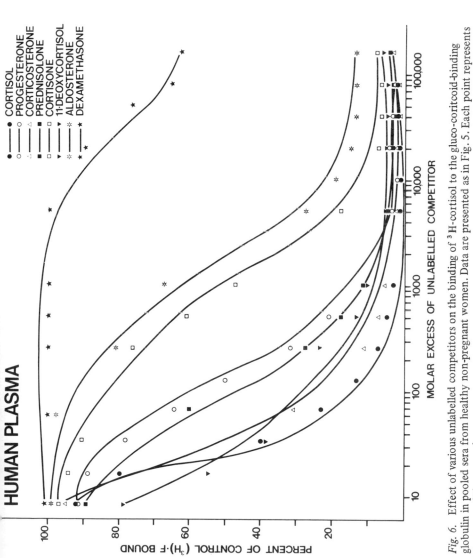

HUMAN PLASMA

- ● CORTISOL
- ○ PROGESTERONE
- △ CORTICOSTERONE
- ■ PREDNISOLONE
- □ CORTISONE
- ▶ 11-DEOXYCORTISOL
- ☆ ALDOSTERONE
- ★ DEXAMETHASONE

PERCENT OF CONTROL (³H)·F BOUND

MOLAR EXCESS OF UNLABELLED COMPETITOR

Fig. 6. Effect of various unlabelled competitors on the binding of ³H-cortisol to the gluco-coritcoid-binding globulin in pooled sera from healthy non-pregnant women. Data are presented as in Fig. 5. Each point represents the mean of three people.

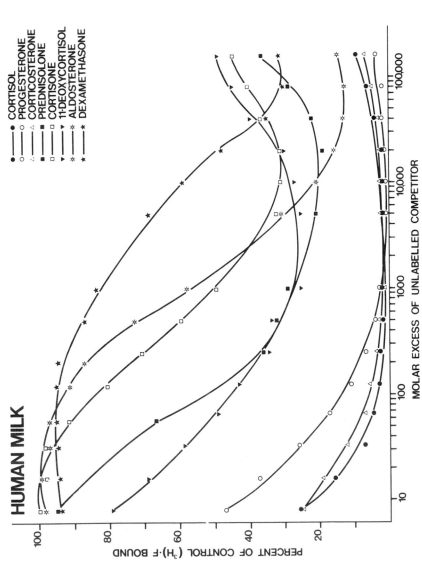

Fig. 7. Effect of various unlabelled competitors on the binding of ^{3}H-cortisol to the gluco-corticoid-binding globulin in pooled milk samples collected 7–10 days *post partum*. Data are presented as in Fig. 5. Each point is the mean of three pools.

REFERENCES

Binkley, F., Wiesman, M. L., Groth, D. P. and Powell, R. W. (1975). *FEBS Letters* **51**, 168–170.

Bradlow, H. L., Fukushima, D. K., Rosenfeld, R. S., Boyar, R. M., Kream, J., Fleisher, M. and Schwartz, M. K. (1976). *Clinical Chemistry* **22**, 1213.

Bradlow, H. L., Schwartz, M. K., Fleisher, M., Nisselbaum, J. S., Boyar, R., O'Connor, J. and Fukushima, D. K. (1979). *Journal of Clinical Endocrinology and Metabolism* **49**, 778–782.

Davis, H., Simons, M. and Davis, J. (1964). *Cancer* **29**, 338–349.

Donnelly, P. K., Baker, K. W., Carney, J. A. and Fallon, W. O. (1975). *Mayo Clinic Proceedings* **50**, 650–656.

Dufour, D., Page, M., Gauvin, L. and Gagnon, P. M. (1978). *Journal of Main Medical Association* **69**, 22–25.

Fazekas, A. G. and MacFarlane, J. K. (1977). *Cancer Research* **37**, 640–645.

Fleisher, M., Robbins, G. F., Breed, C. N., Fracchia, A. A., Urban, J. A. and Schwartz, M. K. (1974). *Memorial Sloan-Kettering Center Clinical Bulletin* **3**, 94–97.

Gatzy, J. T., Zaytoun, M. P., Gaskins, K. and Pearlman, W. H. (1979). *Clinical Chemistry* **25**, 745–748.

Haagensen, C. D. (1971). *In* "Diseases of the Breast" (2nd edition), pp. 155–176. W. B. Saunders Co., Philadelphia, PA.

Haagensen, D. E. Jr, Mazoujian, G., Holder, W. D. Jr, Kisler, S. J. and Wells, S. A. (1977). *Annals of Surgery* **185**, 279–285.

Haagensen, D. E. Jr, Mazoujian, G., Dilley, W. G., Pedersen, C. E., Kister, S. J. and Wells, S. A. Jr (1979). *Journal of National Cancer Institute* **62**, 239–244.

Heyns, W., Van Baelen, H. and De Moor, P. (1967). *Clinica Chimica Acta* **18**, 361–366.

Khan, M. S., Beers, P. C., Awan, T. and Rosner, W. (1975). *Endocrinology* **96**, (Suppl.), Abstr. 19.

Levitz, M., Weiss, G. and Raju, U. (1977). *Journal of Clinical Endocrinology and Metabolism* **45**, 429–434.

Lowry, D. H., Rosebrough, N. J., Farr, A. L. and Randall, R. J. (1951). *Journal of Biological Chemistry* **193**, 265–275.

Mahajan, D. K., Billiar, R. B. and Little, A. B. (1980). *Journal of Steroid Biochemistry* **13**, 67–71.

Payne, D. W., Peng, L., Pearlman, W. H. and Talbert, L. M. (1976). *Journal of Biological Chemistry* **251**, 5272–5279.

Pearlman, W. H., Guériguian, J. L. and Sawyer, M. E. (1973). *Journal of Biological Chemistry* **248**, 5736–5741.

Pearlman, W. H., Peng, L. H., Mazoujian, G., Haagensen, D. E. Jr, Wells, S. A. Jr and Kisler, S. K. (1977). *Journal of Endocrinology* **75**, 19P–20P.

Scatchard, G. (1949). *Annals of New York Academy of Sciences* **51**, 660–672.

Schwartz, M. K. (1976). *National Cancer Institute Breast Cancer Task Force INTERCOM* **5**, 11–13.

Westphal, U. (1971). "Steroid Protein Interactions". Springer Verlag, New York.

ESTRIOL AND BREAST CANCER; ANTI-ESTRADIOL EFFECT OR BIOCHEMICAL MARKER OF ALTERED ESTRADIOL METABOLISM?

H. M. Lemon

Division of Oncology, Department of Internal Medicine, University of Nebraska, Omaha, USA

INTRODUCTION

Cancer of the female breast constitutes an unsolved public health problem of enormous dimensions and complexity in both Europe and North America, striking as it does so many millions of women in the middle years of life. Current American Cancer Society estimates are that one out of every 11 United States females, or over 13 000 000 women, will develop this disease, with the majority succumbing to its ravages. There has been little emphasis upon breast cancer prevention in current research activities of most national cancer institutes, although considerable scientific data have now been obtained indicating the feasibility if not the practicality of several types of prophylactic approaches that might be subjects for prospective randomized clinical trials.

The incidence rate of breast cancer increases during the years of the menopause and continues to rise at a slower pace in the postmenopause in all North American and European nations with diets containing considerable amounts of fat. While the dietary relationship to breast cancer incidence rates has not been clarified, considerable biochemical and epidemiological research indicates a protective function of pregnancy, provided that pregnancy initially occurred prior to the age of 20-25 years (MacMahon *et al.*, 1973). The 2000-3000 fold

Serono Symposium No. 39, "The Menopause: Clinical, Endocrinological and Pathophysiological Aspects", edited by P. Fioretti, L. Martini, G. B. Melis and S. S. C. Yen, 1982. Academic Press, London and New York.

increase in endogenous estriol production in the pregnant human female, followed by a continuation of increased estriol production *post partum* for an unknown period of time, but at least for 2–3 years in many women (Cole *et al.,* 1976), has provided the biochemical basis for the epidemiologic observations of protective activity of pregnancy. Estriol has long been recognized as a physiologic antagonist of estrone and estradiol uterotropic functions (Hisaw *et al.,* 1954; Huggins and Jensen, 1955), but only in recent years has it been possible to pinpoint the locus of this antagonism to the estrogen receptor proteins of uterine cytosols, which estriol competes for with estrone or estradiol as well as 2–OH estrogens (Clark *et al.,* 1977a,b; Katzenellenbogen *et al.,* 1979).

The pathologic inception of breast cancer in many women occurs early in reproductive life, quite probably as a result of accumulation of dietary and environmental carcinogens in the non-lactating virginal mammary tissues, where mutagenesis occurs. Whether clinical breast cancer develops 20–40 years later largely depends upon the co-carcinogenic stimulus provided by the estrogenic mixture derived from ovarian function, extra-ovarian estrone biosynthesis from delta-4 androstenedione and from estrogenic metabolites capable of competing significantly with estradiol or estrone for uterine or mammary receptor proteins. It has now been experimentally proven that alteration of this co-carcinogenic stimulus either by castration or by modifying intermittently the mixture of estrogens competing for mammary estrogen receptors will prevent 50% or more of chemically induced breast cancers for the natural lifetime of the experimental host (Feinlieb, 1968; Chan and Cohen, 1974; Bern *et al.,* 1975; Lemon, 1975, 1978; Katzenellenbogen *et al.,* 1979). Herein may lie our chief hope for future breast cancer prevention. Thus far, all of the human epidemiologic investigations that have been reported indicate an inverse correlation between the incidence of mammary cancer in human populations and the mean ratio of estriol/estrone + estradiol excreted by premenopausal healthy women sampled from those populations (Lemon, 1980). The few reported observations of the estriol excretion ratio of premenopausal women with benign breast disease also indicate that 70% of these women are estriol deficient (Lemon, 1972). By the time breast cancer has appeared clinically decades later, the abnormality of the estriol excretion ratio may not be identified, as a result of occult hypothryoidism, obesity, menopause-related reductions in estradiol secretion, or the effect of stress (Lemon, 1980).

ESTRIOL EXCRETION AS A MARKER OF ALTERED ESTRADIOL METABOLISM

Nearly all epidemiologic investigations have emphasized the increased risk of breast cancer compared to nulliparous women, if pregnancy is delayed beyond 30 years of age (MacMahon *et al.,* 1973). In two recent population-based studies in Canada and Sweden, the protective effect of pregnancy was not identified (Adami *et al.,* 1978; Choi *et al.,* 1978). It is probable that such population-based studies fail to recognize a breast cancer resistant group in the population, diluting out risk factors. Many of these women are relatively infertile, as a result of anovulatory cycles, which provide mammary tissues with continuous estrogenic stimulation without a periodic progestational component to reduce the receptor content of the mammary tissue (Korenman, 1980). Hormonal therapy of these women with estrogens like estrone or estradiol during and after the menopause may be especially hazardous, by further continuation of unopposed estrogenic stimulation of DNA synthesis and cell growth of previously carcinogenically transformed duct epithelial cells.

Longcope (1971) has observed that the urinary fractional estrogen excretion studies, which have been correlated with breast cancer risk in epidemiologic studies, do not accurately represent endogenous biosynthetic ratios of estrone, estradiol 17β or estriol in the non-pregnant female, but rather peripheral metabolic changes affecting the excretion of these hormones, including conjugation (Longcope and Pratt, 1977; Pratt and Longcope, 1978). However, their own reports of the ratios of the blood production rates for estrone, estradiol and estriol in healthy pre- and postmenopausal Caucasian women and women with breast carcinoma, indicate that the postmenopausal women developing breast cancer have a much low median ratio of $E_3/E_1 + E_2$ production, than healthy postmenopausal women (Lemon, 1980). Addition research is urgently needed to confirm or refute their results. If their work is taken at face value, urinary estriol excretion ratios reported thus far may indicate that estriol may only be a *marker* of 15–30% of healthy premenopausal women who have a relative estrogen 16 alpha hydroxylase deficiency, or a glucuronide conjugation deficiency for estriol, which lacks any significant etiologic relationship to breast cancer clinical pathogenesis (Table I).

ESTRIOL AS A PHYSIOLOGIC ESTRADIOL ANTAGONIST ALTERING MAMMARY AND ENDOMETRIAL CELLULAR GROWTH RESPONSES

Nearly all epidemiological investigations derived either from hospital-based or population-based cases, indicate that nulliparous women are at a higher risk of breast carcinogenesis that parous women (MacMahon *et al.*, 1973). The death rate from breast cancer in the United States census registration of 1960 was up to 40% higher in nulliparous women compared to married, ever-married, widowed or divorced women. During pregnancy, the human breast is subjected to a 100-fold increase in endogenous estrone and estradiol production, along with a markedly increased serum prolactin, but in spite of these tremendous hormonal stimuli, abnormal breast growth occurs extremely rarely. The restraining influences upon mammary growth during pregnancy are probably either progestational in origin or result from the extremely high plasma concentrations of estriol conjugates which develop (Loriaux *et al.*, 1972). Following menopause, progestational activity disappears and estriol production and excretion continue in varying degrees throughout the remainder of a woman's life (Longcope and Pratt, 1977; Pratt and Longcope, 1978). Estrone production from extra-ovarian sources continues chiefly as a reflection of the level of adrenocortical secretion of androstenedione and the mass of adipose and muscle tissue capable of its conversion to estrone (Longcope, 1971). Thus in the normal postmenopausal woman, estrone and estriol are chiefly present to maintain mammary duct epithelial or endometrial tissues. Replacement therapy in estrogen-deficient

Table I.   Role of estriol in human mammary and endometrial carcinogenesis.

Biochemical marker of endogenous production rate of estriol:	Natural estradiol antagonist interfering with estrogen-induced proliferation in breast and uterus:
Urinary estriol is a reliable index of estriol production only in pregnancy.	Estriol co-administered with estrone or estradiol 17β partly blocks the uterotropic action of the latter estrogens (Hisaw *et al.*, 1954; Huggins and Jensen, 1955).
Increased urinary estriol excretion rates after full-term pregnancy may reflect peripheral conjugation, metabolism or entero-hepatic cycling (Cole *et al.*, 1976; Longcope and Pratt, 1977; Pratt and Longcope, 1978).	Estriol co-administered with estradiol 17β blocks DNA synthesis in adult virgin female mammary glands *in vivo*, as it does in the uterus.
Lack of correlation between endogenous estriol production rate and urinary estriol/estrone + estradiol ratios (Longcope and Pratt, 1977; Pratt and Longcope, 1978).	Inverse correlation between breast cancer risk and urinary estriol/estrone + estradiol excretion in healthy pre- or postmenopause populations (Lemon, 1980).
Similar urinary estriol excretion ratios between breast cancer subjects and controls in many studies (Lemon, 1980).	Nulliparity or rate onset of first full-term pregnancy (after 30 years) increases breast cancer risk (MacMahon, 1973).
	Intermittent therapy with estriol prevents 50% of chemically induced breast cancer, for rat natural lifespan (Lemon, 1975, 1978, 1980).

women using conjugated equine estrogens may add a third female sex hormone, equilin, which by virtue of its slow excretion rate from the body provides a continuous stimulation to growth and high affinity for cytosol estrogen receptors (Korenman, 1969), even when low doses are used in a cyclic manner (Whittaker *et al.*, 1980). Equilin is a highly uterotropic estrogen comparable to estrone and in the form of equilenin has demonstrated no significant anti-mammary carcinogenic activity (Lemon, 1975, 1978). Significant increased risk of both mammary and endometrial carcinoma has now been observed with prolonged conjugated equine estrogen therapy on American postmenopausal women (Rose *et al.*, 1980). In the most significant population-based investigation yet reported, limited only to postmenopausal women living in large retirement communities, a 2.5 increase in breast cancer incidence occurred in women with intact ovaries who had consumed more than 1500 mg of conjugated equine estrogen. Prior oophorectomy was noted to prevent any risk from conjugated equine estrogen use as might be anticipated, but the numbers of such cases at risk were small. Other investigations of the relationship of estrogenic hormone therapy and breast cancer risk did not find any increased risk, which relatively young largely premenopausal cases were evaluated from a hospitalized population of surgical cases (Sartwell *et al.,* 1977). In this investigation, only about 15% of the cases (under 50 in total) had significant hormonal exposure to postmenopausal estrogens. Estriol therapy of postmenopausal patients has not yet been reported to be associated with a higher risk either of endometrial or breast carcinomas (Salmi, 1979) and hence appears to be the safest form of estrogen therapy in this period of life.

INVESTIGATIONS OF ESTRIOL ANTAGONISM OF ESTRADIOL ACTION IN MAMMARY GLANDS

Although the role of estriol as a natural estradiol antagonist has been partially substantiated by recent experimental studies of its role in altering uterotropic response to estradiol, under conditions of pulse dose as well as continuous dosage (Hisaw *et al.*, 1954; Huggins and Jensen, 1955; Clark *et al.*, 1977a,b, 1978; Katzenellenbogen *et al.*, 1979), similar data have not yet been reported for mammary tissues. The anti-mammary carcinogenic activity of intermittent prophylactic estriol therapy in intact virgin Sprague–Dawley female rats exposed to two of the most potent chemical mammary carcinogens known (7, 12 dimethylbenzanthracene and procarbazine) who were followed for their natural life span has been postulated to be related to its role as an estradiol antagonist (Lemon, 1975, 1978, 1980). We have therefore investigated the early mammary events associated with multiple estrogenic stimulation to the mammary gland fat pad in these virgin adult females, to identify the mechanism of the estriol prophylactic activity.

Mammary fat pad DNA synthesis by equimolar concentrations of estriol or estradiol 17β

Female intact virgin Sprague–Dawley rats from the same breeding stock used for all of our investigations were randomized at 45–50 days of age into four groups. One group was not treated, the second group received 300–360 mcg of estradiol in NaCl pellets, the third group received an equivalent amount of estriol in pellets, and the fourth group received pellets containing mixtures of both estrogens, in varying proportions. The animals were sacrificed at 1–21 days after implantation of the pellets, which in the case of estriol took 1–2 weeks to be completely absorbed (Lemon, 1978). In one set of experiments, after sacrifice the mammary gland fat pads were removed from the animals, cut into 1–3 mm pieces and incubated for 1 h in Hank's solution containing 80×10^6 d.p.m. of ^{3}H-thymidine under hyperbaric oxygen (Meyer, 1976; Meyer and Bauer, 1975). In later experiments, ^{3}H-thymidine was injected i.p. in NaCl 3–4 h before sacrifice, to affect *in vivo* labelling. The uteri were also resected and counted. In either procedure the pre-weighted tissues from each set of four mammary glands per rat were then added to 10 ml Liquifluor and counted in a Unilux II scintillation spectrometer for 10 min. The tissues were then recovered and total DNA determined by the method of Burton (1956).

In histologic specimens from both estriol- and estradiol-treated females, marked development of breast ducts and terminal lobules was noted, with estradiol appearing to stimulate the growth of the latter more profusely. Mitotic labelling indices in autoradiographs of the glands showed some terminal lobules with 30–40% of the cells undergoing active DNA synthesis and ^{3}H-thymidine incorporation. Equimolar doses of estriol yielded one-third the total increase in DNA/mg of tissue as estradiol during the 1st week after implantation.

During the 2nd week the median DNA concentrations plateaued in the estradiol-treated and fell in the estriol-treated, but still remained above the normal variation seen in either untreated controls or controls receiving DMBA (Fig. 1). When both estriol and estradiol were simultaneously inplanted, there was a lesser increment in DNA synthesis during the first 2 weeks of exposure than in the females exposed to either estradiol or estriol alone.

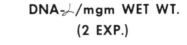

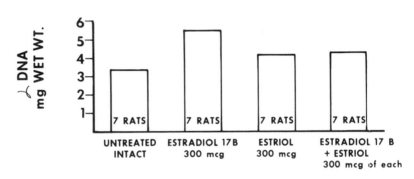

Fig. 1. DNA concentration in mammary gland fat pads of intact virgin female rats during the first week after estrogen implantation.

Incorporation of Tritiated Thymidine into the Virgin Rat Mammary Gland Fat Pad after Estrogenic Stimulation

Individually administered estriol and estradiol in equimolar dosage increased tritiated thymidine incorporation into mammary gland fat pads per unit wet weight during the first 2 weeks of treatment. The response was dose dependent with about a 30% increase noted with estradiol implants averaging ± 300 mcg and nearly a 100% increase noted with 600 mcg implants (Fig. 2). When the thymidine was administered *in vivo* 3.5 h before sacrifice (Fig. 2, upper panel), estriol induced an equivalent increase in tissue uptake of thymidine as estradiol, probably because the high circulating plasma concentrations of estriol maintained the cytoplasmic and nuclear estriol-receptor complexes in the breast at optimal levels for mitotic activity (Clark *et al.,* 1977; Katzenellenbogen *et al.,* 1979). When the rats were sacrificed, and the excised mammary fat pads incubated for one hour at 37°C in Hanks solution containing ^{3}H-thymidine under hyperbaric conditions, estriol induced less than 50% the thymidine incorporation

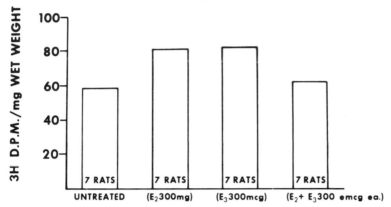

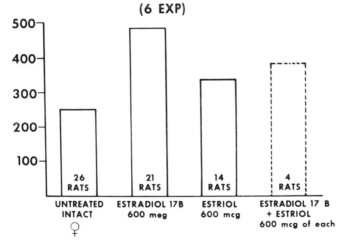

Fig. 2. Incorporation of tritiated thymidine into mammary gland fat pads during the first two weeks after estrogen implantation.

as estradiol, consistently in each of six experiments (Fig. 2, lower panel). Such a result might be anticipated from the rapid loss of nuclear bound estriol-receptor complexes of the excised tissues during incubation in the absence of a continued supply of additional estriol.

When the ^{3}H-thymidine was incorporated *in vitro* or *in vivo* into the mammary gland fat pads conditioned by simultaneous exposure to high plasma blood concentrations of both estriol and estradiol, thymidine incorporation was reduced compared to the estradiol treated groups and closely approximated the estriol response in the *in vitro* studies and the untreated controls in the *in vivo* studies (Fig. 2).

Table II. Molecular requirements for anti-mammary carcinogenic activity of steroid hormones in relation to nuclear receptor finding.

Molecular requirement for breast cancer prophylaxis	Uterine nuclear receptor complex and chromatin binding
Estra 1, 3, 5 (10) -triene 3 , 16a, 17β triol (estriol)	Less than 4–6 h binding reduces duration of estradiol-receptor complex binding when present and DNA synthesis in breast, uterus (Clark *et al.*, 1977a; Clark, 1978; Katzenellenbogen, 1979).
Estra 1, 3, 5 (10) triene 3–0 methyl 16a 17β diol (estriol 3 methyl ether)	No cytosol binding, unless demethylation occurs *in vivo* (Korenman, 1969; Hahnel and Twaddle, 1974).
Estra 1, 3, 5 (10) -triene 3 , 17β-ol, 6-one (6 oxo-estradiol 17β)	Unknown, but binds to uterine cytosol competitively with estradiol 17β (Clark *et al.*, 1977b).
Tri-phenyl-ethylene synthetic anti-estrogens (Nafoxidine, Tamoxifen, etc.)	24–48 h nuclear binding without replenishment of cytosol receptor (Clark *et al.*, 1977b; Katzenellenbogen *et al.*, 1979).
Ineffective steroids for breast cancer prophylaxis	
Estra 1, 3, 5 (10) -triene-2, 3, 17β, -16a-tetra-ol (2–OH estriol)	Unknown, but mammary DNA synthesis not stimulated (King and Mainwaring, 1974; Clark *et al.*, 1977b).

Compound	Binding
Estra 1, 3, 5 (10)-triene 3B, 16a-diol, 17a ethynyl (17a ethynyl estriol)	More than 24 h binding to chromatin (Katzenellenbogen, 1979), highly uterotropic.
Estra 1, 3, 5 (10)-triene 3-0-cyclo-pentyl 16a-ol 17a ethynyl (17a ethynyl estriol-3-cyclopentyl ether)	
Estra 1, 3, 5 (10)-triene 2, 3, 17B tri-ol (2-OH estradiol 17B)	Less than 4-6 h binding to chromatin (Abul-Hajj, 1980)
Estra 1, 3, 5 (10)-triene, 2B, 16a diol 17-one (16a-OH estrone)	Unknown
Estra 1, 3, 5 (10)-triene 3, 16, 17β triol (16 epi-estriol)	[a]Less than 4-6 h binding to chromatin (King and Mainwaring, 1974; Korenman, 1969).
Estra 1, 3, 5 (10)-triene 3B, 17a-ol (17a estradiol)	May augment 17β estradiol uptake into cytosol (King and Mainwaring, 1974; Korenman, 1969).
Estra 1, 3, 5 (10)-triene 3, 17β diol 16-one (16 keto-estradiol)	Minimal cytosol binding (Korenman, 1969).
Hexestrol	3-5x binding to cytosol as estradiol (17β) (Korenman, 1969).
Diethylstilbestrol	6-24 h nuclear binding (Clark et al., 1977b).
Testosterone	Do not bind to cytosol
Dehydroepiandrosterone Corticosterone Progesterone	Do not bind to cytosol (Clark et al., 1977a; Korenman, 1969; Gardner and Wittliff, 1973; Auricchio et al., 1976).

Further investigations are being carried out on the relative concentrations of thymidine in the isolated DNA from these mammary gland preparations. Although 80–90% of the tissue is fibrous-adipose tissue only the mammary tissues appear to account for most of these rapid changes in DNA metabolism during the first 2 weeks following estrogenic stimulation.

CONCLUSIONS

These preliminary observations suggest that the mammary gland responds like the uterus to simultaneous stimulation with two slightly different estrogens with varying affinity in receptor-complex form for the chromatin binding sites of the nucleus, resulting in a restriction of proliferative activity. Possibly a similar mechanism accounts for the antagonism of DNA synthesis by the mixture of estriol and estradiol receptor complexes at mammary nuclear chromatin binding sites that Clark and his associates have shown for the uterus; a more rapid "wash-out" occurred of estradiol complexes along with the less well bound estriol complexes with a lesser growth response induced as a result (Clark et al., 1978).

The dynamics of estrogen binding as receptor complexes to nuclear chromatin affinity sites are of critical importance in antagonizing mammary carcinogenesis (Table II).

In the doses employed in our previous studies using androgens, progestagens or adrenal corticoids, steroids which do not bind to any significant extent to uterine estrogen cytosol receptors, do not alter the incidence of chemically induced breast cancers. Tested hormones included testosterone, corticosterone, dehydro-epiandrosterone and progesterone. Estriol which has been most intensively investigated by repetitive intermittent administration over the natural rat lifespan binds as a receptor complex to uterine chromatin with less avidity than estradiol, and the complex is retained for less than 4 h after a pulse dose (Clark et al., 1977a; Clark et al., 1978; Katzenellenbogen et al., 1979).

Estriol 3 methyl ether should be inactive in binding to uterine cytosol receptors (King and Mainwaring, 1974), but after absorption in vivo is probably partly or wholly demethylated, accounting for its anti-mammary carcinogenic activity. The anti-mammary carcinogenic activity of 6-oxo-estradiol, another "impeded" estrogen, possessing anti-uterotropic activity in prior investigations, may result from its active competition against estradiol for cytosol estrogen receptors (Clark et al., 1977b); there is little data on its receptor metabolism. Catechol estrogens such as 2-OH-estriol and 2-OH-estradiol bind less durably to uterine cytosols, and although they are uterotropic, 2-OH-estriol has not been found active in stimulating thymidine uptake in the rodent breast (Yanai and Nagasawa, 1979). Very long-acting derivatives of estriol, such as ethynyl-estriol and ethynyl-estriol-3-cyclopentyl-ether are highly uterotropic as a result of the prolonged steroid complex binding to nuclear receptor sites (Katzenellenbogen et al., 1979), but these compounds do not interfere with carcinogenesis, acting as they do like estradiol. None of the estriol epimers, such as 16-epiestriol, which probably resemble estriol in their brevity of uterine nuclear binding, have shown anti-mammary carcinogenic activity thus far in our hands.

On the other hand, synthetic anti-estrogens derived from triphenylethylenes, which have a prolonged nuclear residence similar to the long-acting estriol deriva-tives, have anti-mammary carcinogenic activity superior to estriol although much higher dosages are necessary. As a class, these compounds translocate 90% of oestrogen receptor proteins into the nucleus, leaving only about 10% remaining in the cytoplasm, which is not replenished, thereby leading to a refractory state to further estrogen stimulation (Katzenellenbogen *et al.*, 1979). Another similar compound—chlorotrianisene—with greater estrogenic agonistic effect, also suppres-ses breast carcinogenesis (Kellen, 1973).

It is likely that several factors account for the rather unique role of estriol in modulating the response of the breast to estrogenic stimulation involved in co-carcinogenesis, which include not only duration of nuclear binding, but most importantly, the ability to interfere with estradiol—receptor complex binding to the DNA of the nucleus. It is likely that estriol epimers do not share in this latter activity, or other tri-hydroxy metabolites of estradiol, but further exten-sion of our investigations will be needed to clarify these and other aspects of the anti-mammary carcinogenic activity that has been found. It is our belief that the gradual clarification of the mechanism of this anti-mammary carcino-genic effect will add to our understanding of the protective action of early pregnancy on risk of mammary carcinoma and to emphasize that estriol (along with other possible estradiol metabolites) is more than just a marker of abnormal estrogen metabolism. In appropriate ratios to endogenous estrone or estradiol, it modulates both uterotropic and mammatropic activity, thereby lessening the risk of cancer development in both of these organs. As such, estriol appears to have valuable properties for the relief of menopausal symptoms, in that risk of adverse carcinogenic activity is indeed minimal.

REFERENCES

Abul–Hajj, Y. J. (1980). *Journal of Steroid Biochemistry* **13**, 83.
Adami, H. O., Rimsten, A., Stenkvist, B. and Vegelius, J. (1978). *Cancer* **41**, 747.
Auricchio, F., Rotondi, A. and Bresciani, F. (1976). *Molecular and Cellular Endocrinology* **4**, 60.
Bern, H. A., Jones, L. A., Mori, T. and Young, P. N. (1975). *Journal of Steroid Biochemistry* **6**, 673.
Burton, K. (1956). *Biochemistry Journal* **62**, 315.
Chan, P. -C. and Cohen, L. A. (1974). *Journal of the National Cancer Institute* **52**, 25.
Choi, N. W., Howe, G. R., Miller, A. B., Mathews, V. *et al* (1978). *American Journal of Epidemiology* **107**, 510.
Clark, E. R., Omar, A. M. E. and Prestwich, G. (1977a). *Journal of Medicinal Chemistry* **20**, 1096.
Clark, J. H., Paszco, Z. and Peck, E. J. (1977b). *Endocrinology* **100**, 91.
Clark, J. H. H., Peck, E. J., Hardin, J. W. and Eriksson, H. (1978). *In* "Receptors and Hormone Action" (B. W. O'Malley and L. Birnbinner, Ed.), Vol. II, Chapter 1, pp. 1–32. Academic Press, New York.
Cole, P., Brown, J. B. and MacMahon, B. (1976). *Lancet* **II**, 596.
Feinlieb, M. (1968). *Journal of the National Cancer Institute* **41**, 315.
Gardner, D. G. and Wittliff, J. L. (1973). *Biochemistry* **12**, 3090.
Hahnel, R. and Twaddle, E. (1974). *Journal of Steroid Biochemistry* **5**, 119.

Hisaw, F. L., Verlardo, J. T. and Goolsby, C. M. (1954). *Journal of Clinical Endocrinology and Metabolism* **14**, 1134.
Huggins, C. and Jensen, E. V. (1955). *Journal of Experimental Medicine* **102**, 335.
Katzenellenbogen, B. S., Bhakoo, H. S., Ferguson, E. R., Lan, N. C., Tatee, T., Tsai, T. -L. and Katzenellenbogen, J. A. (1979). *Recent Progress in Hormone Research* **35**, 259.
Kellen, J. A. (1973). *Krebsforschung* **79**, 75.
King, R. J. B. and Mainwaring, W. I. P. (1974). "Steroid–Cell Interactions". University Park Press, Baltimore.
Korenman, S. G. (1969). *Steroids* **13**, 163.
Korenman, S. G. (1980). *Lancet* **I**, 700.
Lemon, H. M. (1972). *Journal of Surgical Oncology* **3**, 255.
Lemon, H. M. (1975). *Cancer Research* **35**, 1341.
Lemon, H. M. (1978). *Frontiers of Hormone Research* **5**, 155.
Lemon, H. M. (1980). *Acta Endocrinologica* (Copenhagen). (in Press).
Longcope, C. (1971). *American Journal of Obstetrics and Gynecology* **111**, 778.
Longcope, C. and Pratt, J. H. (1977). *Steroids* **29**, 483.
Loriaux, D. L., Ruder, H. J., Knab, D. R. and Lipsett, M. B. (1972). *Journal of Clinical Endocrinology and Metabolism* **35**, 887.
MacMahon, B., Cole, P. and Brown, J. B. (1973). *Journal of the National Cancer Institute* **50**, 21.
Meyer, J. S. (1976). *Journal of Surgical Oncology* **8**, 165.
Meyer, J. S. and Bauer, W. C. (1975). *Cancer* **36**, 1374.
Pratt, J. H. and Longcope, C. (1978). *Journal of Clinical Endocrinology and Metabolism* **46**, 44.
Rose, R. K., Paganini–Hill, A., Gerkins, V. R., Mack, T. M., Pfeffer, R., Arthur, M. and Henderson, B. E. (1980). *Journal of the American Medical Association* **243**, 1635.
Salmi, T. (1979). *Lancet* **II**, 360.
Sartwell, P. E., Arthes, F. G., Tonascia, J. A. (1977). *Journal of the National Cancer Institute* **59**, 1589.
Whittaker, P. G., Morgan, M. R. A. and Cameron, E. W. D. (1980). *Lancet* **I**, 14.
Yanai, R. and Nagasawa, H. (1979). *Journal of Endocrinology* **82**, 131.

PLASMA OESTROGEN PROFILE AND SEX HORMONE BINDING GLOBULIN (SHBG) BINDING CAPACITY IN POSTMENOPAUSAL BREAST CANCER

L. Berta, C. Valenzano, C. Navello, E. Rovero, L. Todros and G. Gaidano

Istituto di Medicina Interna dell'Università di Torino
Cattedra di Patologia Speciale Medica B, Turin, Italy

INTRODUCTION

Sex hormones have long been suggested as playing a role in promoting breast cancer development (Bulbrook *et al.*, 1960; Zumoff *et al.*, 1975; Hill *et al.*, 1976). Experimental data have shown a direct relationship between growth of breast neoplasia and oestrogen concentration (MacKenzie, 1955; Cole and MacMahon, 1969). In premenopausal women plasma and urine oestrogen have been studied and the altered oestrogen ratio ($E_3/E_1 + E_2$) has been considered as risk factor for breast cancer (Lemon *et al.*, 1966; MacMahon *et al.*, 1974). Both in pre- and in post-menopause a significant increase in androgenic activity has been found and hypothesized as interfering in the ethiology of the mammary neoplasia (Grattarola, 1967; Grattarola *et al.*, 1974). In postmenopausal patients the role of sex hormone metabolism is as yet controversial. Oestrogens seem to originate from peripheral conversion of androgens, which is related to the menopause, to weight and to fat mass (Poortman *et al.*, 1973; Vermeulen and Verdonck, 1978; Kirschner *et al.*, 1978).

Plasma Sex Hormone Binding Globulin (SHBG) which modulates hormone biological activity (Anderson, 1974), has been demonstrated to modify its binding

Serono Symposium No. 39, "The Menopause: Clinical, Endocrinological and Pathophysiological Aspects", edited by P. Fioretti, L. Martini, G. B. Melis and S. S. C. Yen, 1982. Academic Press, London and New York.

capacity in premenopausal women with breast cancer (Murayama et al., 1978; Gaidano et al., 1979): interference of this glycoprotein cannot be excluded in this neoplasia.

In the present work plasma total oestrogens, oestrone (E_1) and oestradiol 17β (E_2), and SHBG binding capacity have been investigated in postmenopausal breast cancer women.

MATERIALS AND METHODS

Fourteen women with breast cancer were studied and compared with 18 healthy women as a control group. Age varied between 60 and 72 years and only women of more than 6 years post-natural menopause were retained for this study. All the women examined had never suffered from diabetes or endocrinological disease and did not receive any steroid treatment. The patients did not show metastasis and were hospitalized for surgical treatment. Neoplasia had been discovered from 1 to 3 months previous.

Blood samples were collected in each subject between 8.00 and 9.00 a.m.; plasma was immediately separated by centrifugation at $+4°C$ and stored at $-20°C$ until assayed.

Sex Hormone Binding Globulin (SHBG) binding capacity evaluation was performed by an equilibrated two-phase system (Dextran DT 40/Polyethilenglycole, PEG, 6000), according to Shanbhag et al. (1973), with some modifications (Gaidano et al., 1977). Specific plasma binding capacity was expressed as μg of dihydrotestosterone (DHT) bound/100 ml plasma.

Total oestrogens, oestrone and oestradiol 17β, were measured by radioimmunoassay (Sigma Chemicals antiserum against oestrone-3HS-BSA and Sorin Biomedica antiserum against oestradiol-17β-17-6CMO-BSA) and expressed as pg/ml.

Plasma oestrone and oestradiol assay was performed on seven breast cancer patients and 10 controls, provided with previous chromatography on celite 524 column (7 x 90mm), according to Facchinetti and Genazzani (1978), (Fig. 1). For each sample a low constant aliquot of labelled oestrogen was used for the recovery with results ranging from 70–85%.

RESULTS

Plasma mean values (± SD) of oestrone and oestradiol 17β were 64 ± 17 pg/ml and 16 ± 5 pg/ml in breast cancer women and, respectively, 60 ± 20 pg/ml and 12 ± 5 pg/ml in normal controls (Fig. 2).

No significant difference was found between the groups for each considered steroid, neither total oestrogen mean values (± SD) were different in breast cancer (69 ± 24 pg/ml) with respect to the normal clinical conditions (77 ± 14 pg/ml) (Fig. 2).

Mean values (± SD) of plasma SHBG binding capacity were 2.03 ± 1.04 μg DHT bound/100 ml plasma in breast cancer women, not different from those found in normal controls, 2.44 ± 1.32 (Fig. 3).

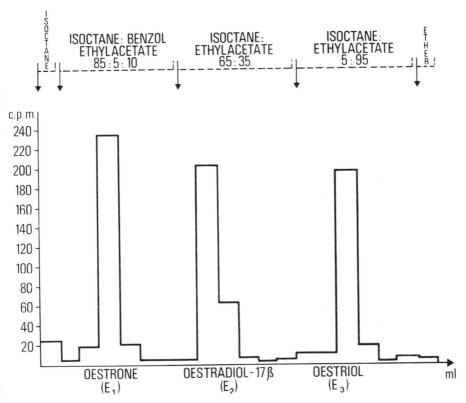

Fig. 1. Solvent systems of oestrogen chromatography on celite 524 column (7 × 90 mm) according to Facchinetti and Genazzani (1978).

DISCUSSION

In premenopausal women a direct influence of oestrogens has been documented. The clinical response to castration in premenopausal cancer patients and the decreased risk of mamary cancer which follows early surgically induced menopause are known (West *et al.*, 1952; Feinleib, 1968).

In postmenopause, oestrogen plasma levels are derived from peripheral androgen conversion, lacking ovarian secretion (Poortman *et al.*, 1973; Kirschner *et al.*, 1978). Androstenedione is considered as the major source of plasma oestrone and oestradiol-17β levels.

Our data have not demonstrated any significant difference in the plasma oestrogen profile of breast cancer women with respect to normal controls, according to other authors (Poortman *et al.*, 1973; Kirschner *et al.*, 1978). These results may suggest that in the postmenopause oestrogen plasma levels do not affect breast cancer development.

Sex Hormone Binding Globulin has been recognized to play a role in premenopausal breast cancer. In the patients with neoplasia this protein showed plasma binding capacity levels lower than those observed in normal controls (Gaidano *et al.*, 1979). In postmenopausal breast cancer patients, SHBG binding capacity did

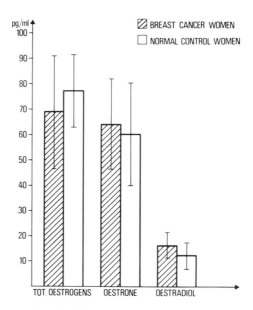

Fig. 2. Oestrogen mean values (± SD) in plasma of breast cancer patients and of normal controls (total oestrogens, oestrone (E_1), oestradiol 17β (E_2),).

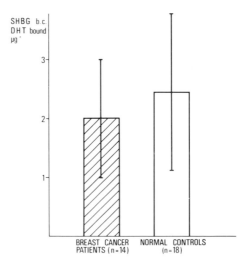

Fig. 3. Plasma SHBG binding capacity mean values (± SD) in breast cancer patients and in normal controls..

not show different plasma mean values from normal controls, according to Kirschner *et al.*, (1978).

Present data supported the hypothesis that breast neoplasia is conditioned, etiologically, by different factors in pre- and postmenopausal women, respectively. Further studies are in progress to clarify sex hormone interferences in postmeno-pausal breast cancer.

REFERENCES

Anderson, C. D. (1974). *Clinical Endocrinology* **3**, 68.

Bulbrook, R. D., Greenwood, F. C. and Hayward, J. L. (1960). *Lancet* **1**, 1154.

Cole, B. and MacMahon, B. (1969). *Lancet* **1**, 604.

Facchinetti, F. and Genazzani, A. R. (1978). *Journal Nuclear Medicine Allied Sciences* **22**, 419.

Feinleib, M. (1968). *Journal National Cancer Institute* **41**, 315.

Gaidano, G. P., Frajria, R., Berta, L., Boccuzzi, G. and Angeli, A. (1977). *Giornale Italiano di Chimica Clinica* **2**, 55.

Gaidano, G. P., Berta, L., Boccuzzi, G., Rovero, E., Todros, L. and Valenzano, C. (1979). *Cancer Treatment Reports* **63**, 1213.

Grattarola, R. (1967). *Journal of Endocrinology* **38**, 77.

Grattarola, R., Secreto, G., Recchione, C. and Castellini, W. (1974). *American Journal of Obstetrics and Gynaecology* **118**, 173.

Hill, P., Wynder, E. L., Helman, P., Hickman, R. and Rona, G. (1976). *Cancer Research* **36**, 1883.

Kirschner, M. A., Cohen, F. B. and Ryan, C. (1978). *Cancer Research* **38**, 4029.

Lemon, H. M., Wotiz, H. H., Parsons, L. and Mozden, P. J. (1966). *Journal of American Medicine Association* **196**, 112.

MacMahon, B., Cole, P., Brown, J. B., Aoki, K., Lin, T. M., Morgan, R. W. and Woo, N. C. (1974). *International Journal of Cancer* **14**, 161.

MacKenzie, I. (1955). *British Journal of Cancer* **9**, 284.

Murayama, Y., Sakuma, T., Udagawa, H., Utsunomiya, Y., Okamoto, K., and Asano, K. (1978). *Journal of Clinical Endocrinology and Metabolism* **46**, 998.

Poortman, J., Thijssen, J. H. H. and Schwarz, F. (1973). *Journal of Clinical Endocrinology and Metabolism* **37**, 101.

Shanbhag, V. P., Soedergard, R., Carstensen, H. and Albertsson, S. A. (1973). *Journal Steroid Biochemistry* **4**, 537.

Vermeulen, A. and Verdonck, L. (1978). *Clinical Endocrinology* **9**, 59.

West, C. D., Hollander, V. P., Whitmore, W. F., Randal, H. T. and Pearson, O. H. (1952). *Cancer* **5**, 1009.

Zumoff, B., Fishman, J., Bradlow, H. L. and Helman, L. (1975). *Cancer Research* **35**, 3365.

SECTION V
GENITAL DISEASES, HORMONES AND MENOPAUSE

NEW TOOLS OF POTENTIAL VALUE FOR PREDICTING HORMONE RESPONSIVENESS IN HUMAN ENDOMETRIAL CANCER

S. Iacobelli, P. Longo, V. Natoli, G. Sica[1], E. Bartoccioni, P. Marchetti and G. Scambia

Laboratorio di Endocrinologia Molecolare, Università Cattolica S. Cuore, Via della Pineta Sacchetti, Rome, Italy, Istituto di Istologia ed Embriologia Generale, Università Cattolica S. Cuore, Via della Pineta Sacchetti, Rome, Italy[1]

INTRODUCTION

Within the framework of the relationships between hormones and tumours, a place of primary importance concerns hormone therapy in cases of tumours precisely defined as hormone-dependent or hormone-sensitive. The advantage that hormone therapy offers (whether it is based on hormone deprival or on hormone interference) with respect to other types of treatment are quite evident; an elevated level of cancer-killing activity is reached with hardly any toxicity to normal tissues. Under the heading of objective results, it has been shown that treatment of advanced stage mammary carcinoma with high doses of medroxy-progesterone acetate (MPA) resulted in remissions in about 45% of the patients while only 26% of those who underwent treatment had progressive disease (Pannuti *et al.*, 1979). In the case of endometrial carcinoma, progestin treatment used alone eliminated the carcinoma *in situ* in 62% of cases (Steiner *et al.*, 1965; Nielsen and Kolstad, 1973), and resulted in a signficant remission (reduction of at least half of the tumour mass) in about 53% of a group of 106 advanced or

Serono Symposium No. 39, "The Menopause: Clinical, Endocrinological and Pathophysiological Aspects", edited by P. Fioretti, L. Martini, G. B. Melis and S. S. C. Yen, 1982. Academic Press, London and New York.

recurrent adenocarcinoma patients (Bonte, 1972, 1973, 1974; Bonte *et al.*, 1978). In addition, there were the following subjective results: an overall improvement in the general state in a high percentage (70%) of patients (Rendina and Iacobelli, 1979), regression of leucorrhea and bleeding and an increase in radiosensitivity (with combined hormone/radiation therapy objective remissions were achieved in about 80% of the cases) (Bonte *et al.*, 1978). From these facts and from the evidence that the selection of patients to undergo hormone therapy is still largely empirical, the importance of establishing tests which can indicate tumours' *in vitro* responsiveness to hormone therapy clearly emerges. The establishement of such tests would therefore permit the immediate initiation of a suitable treatment and, in cases of definitely deficient responsiveness, the avoidance of many months of useless treatment. In cases of mammary tumours, for example, the measurement of hormone receptors already represents an indispensable diagnostic tool in directing the choice of treatment either towards hormone therapy or towards cytotoxic chemotherapy or immunotherapy, despite the fact that 5–10% of patients with "negative" tests respond positively and 35% of those with "positive" tests respond negatively (Pannuti *et al.*, 1979).

In this article we will try to illustrate those tests which at the present time seem to be the most promising indicators of hormone responsiveness in cases of carcinoma of the endometrium.

HISTOLOGICAL GRADING

To determine a tumour's responsiveness to progestin treatment, an accurate histological examination of the tumour and the metastases seems most important. Generally, it can be stated that the higher the degree of differentiation of the carcinoma, the greater the probability of a positive response to the hormone therapy. However, in data furnished by various authors, numerous cases of poorly differentiated carcinomas showed positive responses to the hormone therapy and vice versa, well differentiated tumours had negative responses. Malkasian *et al.* (1971) obtained an objective response in 11 out of 37 well differentiated carcinomas (stages 1 and 2) and in three out of 28 poorly differentiated (stages 3 and 4). Geisler (1973) found four positive responses in a group of six carcinomas classified as well differentiated (stage 1) and one positive response (stage 3) in a group of 11 poorly differentiated carcinomas (stages 3 and 4). Furthermore, according to Rozier and Underwood (1974), three out of 12 carcinomas classified as well differentiated cases had progression of the disease while nine out of 15 poorly differentiated cases showed sensitivity to the progestin therapy (six arrests and three remissions). These facts, associated with the great histological heterogeneity of endometrial carcinoma (and therefore with the difficulty of a precise histological grading) make it doubtful that a responsiveness test could be based solely on the degree of differentiation, the determination of which, however, could certainly be a valid complement for other types of tests.

17-β-HYDROXY STEROID DEHYDROGENASE ACTIVITY

The starting point for this type of test was provided by observations performed on normal endometrial fragments obtained in various phases of the menstrual cycle. It has been proven that, during the cycle, with the increased progesterone levels in the serum and the endometrium (in the case of progesterone the two values are practically equivalent), there is a significant decrease in the quantity of oestrogen receptors and an approximately 10-fold increase in 17-β-hydroxy steroid dehydrogenase (17-β-HSD) activity (enzyme present only in glandular epithelium and not in the stroma) (Tseng and Gurpide, 1972a,b; 1974). In addition, the same variations of these parameters were obtained by administering progesterone to women in the follicular phase and confirmation was also seen in experiments conducted *in vitro* (Schmidt-Gollwitzer *et al.*, 1978). Therefore, it was thought that the concentration of oestrogen receptors and the level of 17-β-HSD activity might be possible indicators of responsiveness to progestins. In results obtained by Gurpide *et al.* (1977, 1978) in the cases of 10 endometrial carcinoma patients submitted to MPA treatment (60 mg/day) after an initial assay of oestrogen receptors and enzyme activity, for a period of 2–10 days, only one case of a completely negative response was reported in a tumour that had been classified as well differentiated. In three other patients the absence of variations in the two parameters can be explained by the incidence of glandular destruction (therefore the test has to be considered positive) and this fact demonstrates the importance, in this type of test, of histological examination after therapy. In the other cases, variations (almost always greater than 50%) in the oestrogen receptor levels and the 17-β-HSD activity, accompanied by secretive histological modifications or by no type of change (denoting the increased sensitivity of biochemical tests), were always obtained. The data which would allow a correlation between the short-term responsiveness to progestins and the effectiveness of the therapy and which would therefore give an indication of the real clinical value of these dynamic tests, are still missing.

PROGESTERONE RECEPTORS AND *IN VITRO* HORMONE SENSITIVITY

Another possible indicator for determining a tumour's responsiveness to hormone therapy seems to be furnished by the number of progesterone receptors and by the *in vitro* response to MPA. This type of test is not conceptually linked to the hypothesis that hormone action on cancer cells is necessarily mediated by receptor–hormone interaction (however this mechanism does operate under physiological conditions in normal tissues). In fact the presence of progesterone receptors could simply represent a biochemical indicator of the cells' sensitivity to progestin therapy (phenotypical expression of their genetic trait) and only as such be correlated to hormone therapy. In other words, in cases of pharmacological doses of hormone, it cannot be said that since the cell produces the receptors it therefore responds, but it could be that it has as its characteristics (for the most part these characteristics are associated) both the "responsiveness" and the "production of receptors" (the only link could be the degree of cell differentiation). In any case, the correlation between the presence of progesterone receptors, the *in vitro* sensitivity to progestins (measured by the inhibition of DNA and protein synthesis), and the percentage of response to treatment clearly emerges from the results presented herein. This correlation itself seems sufficient to justify the use of this type of test. It should be added that using the measurement of progesterone receptors alone, it is possible to have falsely positive results and this could be due either to a defect in some mechanism following receptor-

hormone interaction or the abovementioned independence of the two phenotypical characteristics (the cell has the "receptor-synthesis" gene and doesn't have
the "sensitivity" gene).

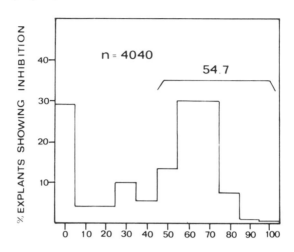

Fig. 1. Overall effect of MPA (1×10^{-6} M) on macromolecular synthesis (RNA, DNA, protein)
in explants of human endometrial carcinoma.

We have determined the progesterone receptor concentration in 18 carcinomas
obtained at hysterectomy from previously untreated patients (for methodological
aspects, see Iacobelli *et al.*, 1978 and Iacobelli *et al.*, 1981). The results, shown
in Table I, indicate that progesterone receptors are demonstrable in 11 endometria
(61%) with an average concentration of 188.78 fmoles/mg cytosol protein (range =
25–899 fmoles/mg cytosol protein). The results are analogous with those obtained
by other investigators (Janne *et al.*, 1979; Martin *et al.*, 1979; Rodriguez *et al.*,
1979). Among the 11 receptor-positive carcinomas, seven proved to be sensitive to
MPA *in vitro*, while for the other four despite the presence of appreciable quantities of receptors, there was no corresponding decrease of macromolecular
synthesis. All seven carcinomas without receptors proved to be insensitive to the
inhibitory effect of MPA on the incorporation of labelled precursors. Figure 1
shows that, assuming a reduction of macromolecular synthesis of at least 50% as
significant, the percentage of explants classifiable as positive (out of 4040) is
about 55%. This value is sufficiently close to the percentage of carcinomas which
effectively respond to MPA treatment. The facts stated above definitely show that
the level of progesterone receptors in combination with the determination of the
in vitro effect of MPA on carcinoma culture could represent a considerably
reliable test in evaluating a tumour's responsiveness to progestin therapy. Also to
be considered is that an *in vitro* test of this type offers the important advantage of
eliminating systemic factors and endocrine feedback mechanisms which could
inevitably influence the results of evaluations obtained *in vivo*.

Table I. Pr concentrations in human endometrial carcinoma

Tissue	PR (Fmoles/mg protein)	K_D (nM)
1	nd[a]	–
2	nd	–
3	25	1.85
4	44	2.91
5	nd	–
6	85	1.35
7	nd	–
8	99	3.05
9	101	2.09
10	nd	–
11	140	1.98
12	285	4.12
13	320	3.22
14	680	2.50
15	720	3.61
16	899	5.05
17	nd	–
18	nd	–

[a] = not detectable.

CONCLUSION

Finally, a new approach to the identification of the hormone dependency of tumour derives from the recent discovery that oestrogens can induce specific protein synthesis in target cells. In rat uterus the rapid (within 30–45 min) induction of a particular protein (IP, induced protein, molecular weight 45000, isoelectric point 4.7) by oestrogens is already an established fact. The development of a radioimmunoassay technique has allowed the quantification of IP in different stages of the oestrous cycle and in mammary tumours induced by carcinogens (Kaye *et al.*, 1980). Philogenetic considerations and recent evidence (Kaye, unpublished results) lead to the postulation of the presence of protein(s) specifically induced by oestrogens even in the human endometrium; regarding this, it is also interesting to note the observations of Shapiro and Forbes (1978) concerning a protein induced by progresterone in the endometrium (molecular weight 51000) and of Westley and Rochefort (1979) on the estrogen induction of secreted glycoproteins (molecular weight 46000) in the medium of cells derived from human mammary carcinoma (MCF-7 and ZR75-1). It is evident that the identification and characterization of such proteins will enable us to determine more precisely the hormone sensitivity of a carcinoma. This would again represent a dynamic test based on the possibility of inducing, *in vito* or *in vitro*, an increase in protein synthesis by means of hormone treatment.

In conclusion, we believe that, even though a definitive solution to the problem of identifying the hormone sensitivity of a tumour has not yet been found, some of the tests described herein already represent not only an indispensable diagnostic tool but also a successful starting point for further progress.

REFERENCES

Bonte, J. (1972). *Acta Obstetricia et Gynecologica Scandinavica*, Suppl. 19, 21.
Bonte, J. (1973). *In* "Symposium on Endometrial Cancer" (M. G. Brush, R. W. Taylor and D. C. Williams Eds) pp. 203–211. Heinemann, London.
Bonte, J. (1974). *Medical Hypotheses* 1107, 1106.
Bonte, J., De Coster, J. M., Ide, P. and Billiet, G. (1978). *In* "Endometrial Cancer" (M. G. Brush, R. J. B. King and R. W. Taylor. Eds) pp. 192–205. Baillière Tindall, London.
Geisler, H. E. (1973). *Gynecological Oncology* 1, 340.
Gurpide, E. and Tseng, L. (1978). *In* "Endometrial Cancer" (M. G. Brush, R. J. B. King and R. W. Taylor, Eds) pp. 252–257. Baillière Tindall, London.
Gurpide, E., Tseng, L. and Gusberg, S. B. (1977). American Journal of Obstetrics and Gynecology 129, 809.
Iacobelli, S., Paparatti, L. and Bompiani, A. (1973). *Febs Letters* 32, 199.
Iacobelli, S., Sica, G. Ranelletti, F. and Barile, G. (1978). *European Journal of Cancer* 14, 931.
Iacobelli, S., Longo, P., Scambia, G., Natoli, V. and Sacco, F. (1981). *In* "Role of Medroxyprogesterone in Endocrine-Related Tumors" (S. Iacobelli and A. DiMarco. Eds). Raven Press, New York, (In press).
Janne, O., Kuppilla, A., Kontula, K., Syryala, P. and Vihko, R. (1979). *International Journal of Cancer* 24, 545.
Kaye, A. M., Reiss, N., Iacobelli, S., Bartoccioni, E. and Marchetti, P. (1980) *In* "Hormones and Cancer" (S. Iacobelli, R. J. King, H. R. Linder and Lippmann, Eds) pp. 41–51. Raven Press, New York.
Malkasian, G. D., Decker, D. G., Mussey, E. and Johnson, C. E. (1971). *American Journal of Obstetrics and Gynecology* 110, 15.
Martin, P. M., Rolland, P. H., Germerre, M. Serment, H. and Toga, M. (1979). *International Journal of Cancer* 23, 321.
Nielsen, P. A. and Kolstad, P. (1973). *In* "Symposium on endometrial Cancer" (M. G. Brush, R. W. Taylor and D. C. Williams, Eds) pp. 115–125. Heinemann, London.
Notides, A. and Gorski, J. (1966). *Proceedings of the National Academy of Science of the United State of America* 56, 230.
Pannuti, F. Martoni, A., Piana, E., Fruet, F., Di Marco, A. R., Burroni, P. and Strocchi, E. (1979). *In* "Ormoni Recettori e Cancro" (S. Iacobelli. Ed.), pp. 165–189. Società Editrice Universo, Roma.
Rendina, G. M. and Iacobelli, S. (1979). *In* "Ormoni, Recettori et Cancro" (S. Iacobelli Ed.) 215–238. Società Editrice Universo, Roma.
Rodriguez, J., Sen, K. K., Seski, J. C., Menon, M., Johnson, T. R. and Menon, K. M. J. (1979). *American Journal of Obstetrics and Gynecology* 61, 660.
Rozier, J. C. and Underwood, P. B. (1974). *Obstetrics and Gynecology*, NY 44, 60.
Schmidt-Gollwitzer, M., Genz, T., Schmidt-Gollwitzer, K., Pollow, B. and Pollow, K. (1978). *In* "Endometrial Cancer" (M. G. Brush, R. J. B. King and R. W. Taylor. Eds), pp. 227–241. Baillière Tindall, London.
Shapiro, S. S. and Forbes, S. H. (1978). *Fertility and Sterility* 30, 175.

Steiner, G. J., Kistner, R. W. and Craig, J. M. (1965). *Metabolism Clinical and Experimental* **14**, 356.

Tseng, L. and Gurpide, E. (1972a). *American Journal of Obstetrics and Gynecology* **114**, 995.

Tseng, L. and Gurpide, E. (1972b). *American Journal of Obstetrics and Gynecology* **114**, 1002.

Tseng, L. and Gurpide, E. (1974). *Endocrinology* **94**, 419.

Westley, B. and Rochefort, H. (1979). *Biochemical and Biophysical Research Communication.* **90**, 410.

DOSE-DEPENDENT EFFECTS OF PROGESTINS ON THE OESTROGENIZED POSTMENOPAUSAL ENDOMETRIUM

P. T. Townsend[1], R. J. B. King[2], N. C. Siddle[1] and M. I. Whitehead[1]

Department of Obstetrics and Gynaecology, King's College Hospital Medical School, University of London, Denmark Hill, London, UK[1]; and Hormone Biochemistry Department, Imperial Cancer Research Fund Laboratories, Lincoln's Inn Fields, London, UK[2]

INTRODUCTION

From histological studies of postmenopausal women, unopposed oestrogen therapy has been associated with an increased risk of endometrial carcinoma (Cramer and Knapp, 1979) and with a high incidence of endometrial hyperplasia (Whitehead *et al.*, 1979). The addition of a progestin to oestrogen therapy has been shown to reduce both the incidence of endometrial carcinoma (Gambrell, 1977) and hyperplasia (Whitehead *et al.*, 1979). Biochemical studies have helped elucidate the mechanisms whereby progestins protect against excessive oestrogenic stimulation and we have reported previously on their ability to modify intracellular oestrogen concentrations (King *et al.*, 1980a; Whitehead *et al.*, 1980), receptor machinery (King and Whitehead, 1980; King *et al.*, 1979) and enzymatic activity (King and Whitehead, 1980; King *et al.*, 1980b).

Progestins *per se* can result in unwanted side-effects (Nelson, 1971) and have been associated with adverse changes in plasma HDL–cholesterol concentrations (Bradley *et al.*, 1978; Larsson-Cohn *et al.*, 1979). Therefore, it is important to determine the minimum monthly duration of progestin therapy and the minimum effective daily dosage necessary to completely protect against the development of

Serono Symposium No. 39, "The Menopause: Clinical, Endocrinological and Pathophysiological Aspects", edited by P. Fioretti, L. Martini, G. B. Melis and S. S. C. Yen, 1982. Academic Press, London and New York.

endometrial hyperplasia. Histological and biochemical studies indicate that progestins will have to be given for at least 10 and most probably 12 days each calendar month if this desired effect is to be achieved (Studd *et al.*, 1980; Whitehead *et al.*, 1980). The present chapter describes biochemical experiments aimed at determining the minimum effective daily dosage. In addition, these data have provided information on the interrelationship between receptor machinery and enzymatic activity with rates of DNA synthesis in glandular and stromal tissue. Their significance is discussed.

PATIENTS AND METHODS

The clinical methodology has been published in detail elsewhere (Whitehead, 1978; Whitehead and Campbell, 1978) and is only summarized here. All patients were postmenopausal and were receiving conjugated oestrogens (Premarin®; Ayerst Laboratories) 1.25 mg daily continuously. For 7 days each calendar month they took in addition either 2.5, 5 or 10 mg daily of norethisterone (Primolut N®; Schering Chemicals). Biopsy samples were obtained during oestrogen therapy alone and also on the 6th day of progestin administration by which time the progestational stimulus is maximal (Townsend *et al.*, 1980). Dependent upon the biochemical analyses to be performed, the samples were either frozen until assayed or placed in Dulbecco's modified Eagle's medium (DMEM) at room temperature and used within 4 h of collection.

The biochemical activities measured in the endometrium were of the oestrogen binding of the nuclei (oestrogen receptor; REN); oestradiol 17β dehydrogenase activity and the rates of DNA synthesis in epithelial and stromal cells. REN is related to biological effect and was determined as described previously (King *et al.*, 1979); oestradiol 17β dehydrogenase is a progestin-sensitive enzyme intimately related in mediating protective actions as it preferentially converts oestradiol to oestrone, thereby lowering the potency of the oestrogenic stimulus (King *et al.*, 1980a; Whitehead *et al.*, 1980). The activity was measured as previously described (King *et al.*, 1979). The rate of DNA synthesis represents cell proliferative activity and the autoradiographic techniques have been published elsewhere (King *et al.*, 1980c).

Statistical analyses were performed using Student's *t*-test or the Mann-Whitney *u*-test depending upon the number of observations and the distribution of values.

RESULTS

Data for REN, oestradiol 17β dehydrogenase activity and the rates of DNA synthesis in epithelial and stromal cells during the premenopausal proliferative and secretory phases are included for comparison. As for nuclear oestrogen receptors (Fig. 1) in postmenopausal women during oestrogen therapy, the mean content alone, 1.96 ± 0.33 pmol/mg DNA, was significantly higher than that observed in the premenopausal proliferative phase (1.25 ± 0.17 pmol/mg DNA; $P < 0.05$). Administration of all dosages of norethisterone was associated with a significant reduction of REN values ($P < 0.001$). The lowest values, (0.22 ± 0.02 pmol/mg

DNA) were observed with 5 mg daily and were significantly lower than the secretory phase range (0.50 ± 0.07 pmol/mg DNA; $P < 0.01$) whereas the values with 2.5 mg daily (0.38 ± 0.09 pmol/mg DNA) and 10 mg daily (0.52 ± 0.31 pmol/mg DNA) were within this range. The levels with norethisterone 5 mg daily were significantly lower than those with 2.5 mg daily ($P < 0.05$).

As for oestradiol 17β dehydrogenase (Fig. 1) no activity was detectable during oestrogen therapy alone (< 0.3 nmol/oestrone/mg protein/h). All dosages of norethisterone were associated with a significant elevation in enzymatic activity ($P < 0.001$). Maximal values (29.5 ± 6.4 nmol/oestrone/mg protein/h) were observed with 5 mg daily and were significantly elevated above the secretory phase range (11.3 ± 2.3 nmol/oestrone/mg protein/h; $P < 0.01$) whereas the activities with 2.5 mg daily (17.4 ± 3.1 nmol/oestrone/mg protein/h) and 10 mg daily (23.1 ± 6.8 nmol/oestrone/mg protein/h) were within this range. The levels with 5 mg daily were significantly higher than those with 2.5 mg daily ($P < 0.05$).

DNA synthesis in glandular epithelium (Fig. 2) was also different. During oestrogen therapy alone the rate of DNA synthesis (4.1 ± 1.2 labelled cells/100 epithelial cells) was within the premenopausal proliferative phase range (6.6 ± 1.9 labelled cells/100 epithelial cells). The rates of synthesis were significantly reduced during the administration of norethisterone 2.5 mg daily (< 0.2 labelled cells/100 epithelial cells; $P < 0.01$) and 5 mg daily (0.37 ± 0.11 labelled cells/100 epithelial cells; $P < 0.02$) to within the secretory phase range (0.92 ± 0.67 labelled cells/100 epithelial cells). The reduction during norethisterone 10 mg daily (2.25 ± 1.54 labelled cells/100 epithelial cells) was less marked and not significant ($P > 0.05$).

The rate of synthesis of DNA in stromal cells during oestrogen therapy alone (9.35 ± 3.22 labelled cells/microscope field) was within the proliferative phase range (4.08 ± 1.54 labelled cells/microscope field). There was a significant reduction in the rate of synthesis with norethisterone 2.5 mg daily (0.74 ± 0.26

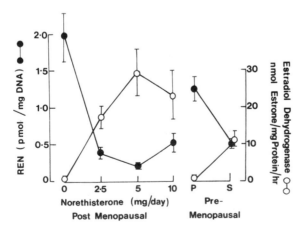

Fig. 1. Mean ± SE nuclear oestrogen receptor and oestradiol 17β dehydrogenase activity in postmenopausal women receiving oestrogen therapy alone (0 mg norethisterone) and the stated daily dosages of norethisterone; and during the premenopausal proliferative (P) and secretory (S) phases.

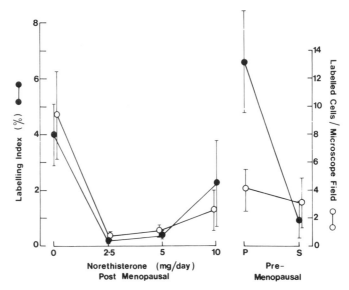

Fig. 2. Mean ± SE rates of DNA synthesis in epithelial and stromal cells in postmenopausal women receiving oestrogen therapy alone (0 mg norethisterone) and the stated daily dosages of norethisterone; and during the premenopausal proliferative (P) and secretory (S) phases.

labelled cells/microscope field; $P < 0.05$) and 5 mg daily (1.01 ± 0.46 labelled cells/microscope field; $P < 0.05$). With 10 mg daily (2.55 ± 1.44 labelled cells/ microscope field) this reduction was not significant ($P > 0.05$) but was to within the secretory phase range (3.12 ± 1.76 labelled cells/microscope field).

DISCUSSION

During oestrogen therapy alone the nuclear receptor level was above and the rates of DNA synthesis were within the premenopausal proliferative phase ranges. These observations provide further evidence to add to the histological and biological data presented (Sturdee *et al.*, 1978; Whitehead *et al.*, 1979; King *et al.*, 1979) that with unopposed oestrogens the stimulus being applied to the endometrium is potent. Norethisterone opposed oestrogenic stimulation and 2.5 mg daily resulted in a significant reduction in REN and glandular and stromal cell DNA synthesis to levels within the premenopausal secretory phase range. Norethisterone 5 mg daily further reduced REN content but no associated increase in suppression of DNA synthesis was observed. This is not surprising as the rates of synthesis with norethisterone 2.5 mg daily were already negligible (Fig. 2). Increasing the dose of norethisterone 10 mg daily resulted in a rise in REN content and DNA synthesis clearly indicating a lessening of progestogenic action (Figs 1 and 2). Similar effects were observed on the activity of oestradiol 17β dehydrogenase. Norethisterone 2.5 mg daily significantly increased dehydrogenase activity to within the secretory phase range and a further significant rise to levels above this range was observed with 5 mg daily. However, norethisterone 10 mg daily failed to enhance this biological effect further and resulted in a small decline in activity (Fig. 1). Daily dosages of 2.5 mg and 5 mg of norethisterone thus achieve maximal biochemical effects and are likely to provide optimal protection to the endometrium.

Increasing the dosage above this range, to 10 mg daily, was of no greater benefit as it failed to exert more potent anti-oestrogenic activity and is potentially more hazardous as the adverse effects of progestins on plasma HDL-cholesterol concentrations appear to be dose-dependent (Larsson-Cohn *et al.*, 1979). The paradox, whereby an increase in dose to 10 mg daily is associated with a reduction in activity, has a logical explanation. Receptor protein is required to transfer any steroid to its site of action within the cell nucleus and therefore absence of cytosol receptor is associated with tissue unresponsiveness. Progestins decrease the formation of their own receptor (King *et al.*, 1979) and in our opinion norethister-one 10 mg daily most probably reduced cytosol progesterone receptor content so much that tissue unresponsiveness resulted. With loss of opposing progestogenic effect oestrogenic stimulation increased and REN content and DNA synthesis rose. A cause and effect association between dehydrogenase activity and REN is suggested by the dose-dependent, inverse relationship shown in Fig. 1. These data provide further evidence that one of the mechanisms whereby progestogens affect endometrial cell function is by increasing oestradiol metabolism through the induction of oestradiol 17β dehydrogenase activity. Nuclear oestradiol mass correlates with REN content (King *et al.*, 1980a; Whitehead *et al.*, 1980) and the dehydrogenase enhances oestradiol metabolism by preferential conversion to the less active oestrone. The overall oestrogenic stimulus is thus reduced and REN content falls. We have reported previously that this protective, intracellular mechanism appears to be "amplified" as small increases in dehydrogenase activity result in large reductions in REN content (King and Whitehead, 1980; King *et al.*, 1980a). Although concentrated in glandular epithelium, dehydrogenase activity is also present in stromal cells (King *et al.*, 1980c) and the suppression of DNA synthesis in both glandular and stromal tissues observed in these studies may be related to progestin-induced acceleration of oestradiol metabolism.

ACKNOWLEDGEMENT

The clinical studies were performed in the Menopause Clinics at King's College Hospital, London, SE5 and the Chelsea Hospital for Women, London, SW3. The assistance of Jane Minardi and Osyth Young in collecting the endometrial samples is gratefully acknowledged as is the financial assistance of Ayerst International to PTT.

The biochemical studies were performed at, and financed by, the Imperial Cancer Research Laboratories. The assistance of Susan Leach and Rosemary Jeffery with the autoradiographic techniques is gratefully acknowledged and the secretarial help of Mrs J. Thow is greatly appreciated.

REFERENCES

Bradley, D. D., Wingerd, J., Petitti, D. B., Krauss, R. M. and Ramcharan, S. (1978). *New England Journal of Medicine* **299**, 17.

Cramer, D. W. and Knapp, R. C. (1979). *Obstetrics and Gynecology* **54**, 521.

Gambrell, R. D. Jr (1977). *Journal of Reproductive Medicine* **18**, 301.

King, R. J. B. and Whitehead, M. I. (1980). *In* "Prospective Steroid Receptor Research" (S. Bresciani, Ed.) Raven Press, New York (in press).

King, R. J. B., Whitehead, M. I., Campbell, S. and Minardi, J. (1979). *Cancer Research* **39**, 1094.

King, R. J. B., Dyer, G., Collins, W. P. and Whitehead, M. I. (1980a). *Journal of Steroid Biochemistry* **13**, 377.

King, R. J. B., Townsend, P. T. and Whitehead, M. I. (1980b). *In* "Menopause and Postmenopause" (N. Pasetto, R. Paoletti and J. L. Ambrus, Eds), p. 221. MTP Press, Lancaster.

King, R. J. B., Townsend, P. T. and Whitehead, M. I. (1980c). Submitted for Publication.

Larsson-Cohn, U., Wallentin, L. and Zador, G. (1979). *Hormone and Metabolic Research* **11**, 415.

Nelson, J. H. (1971). *Journal of Reproductive Medicine* **6**, 43.

Studd, J. W. W., Thom, M. H., Paterson, M. E. L. and Wade-Evans, T. (1980). *In* "Menopause and Postmenopause" (N. Pasetto, R. Paoletti and J. L. Ambrus, Eds), p. 127. MTP Press, Lancaster.

Sturdee, D. W., Wade-Evans, T., Paterson, M. E. L., Thom, M. H. and Studd, J. W. W. (1978). *British Medical Journal* **1**, 1575.

Townsend, P. T., King, R. J. B. and Whitehead, M. I., (1980). (In preparation.)

Whitehead, M. I. (1978). *Maturitas* **1**, 87.

Whitehead, M. I. and Campbell, S. (1978). *In* "Endometrial Cancer" (M. J. Brush, R. W. Taylor and R. J. B. King, Eds), p. 65. Baillière Tindall, London.

Whitehead, M. I., King, R. J. B., McQueen, J. and Campbell, S. (1979). *Journal of the Royal Society of Medicine* **72**, 322.

Whitehead, M. I., King, R. J. B. and Campbell, S. (1980). *In* "Proceedings of the Ninth World Congress of Obstetrics and Gynaecology", p. 61. Excerpta Medica, Amsterdam.

THE UPTAKE OF OESTRADIOL AND OESTRONE *IN VIVO* BY POSTMENOPAUSAL UTERINE TISSUES AND ENDOMETRIAL CANCER

M. A. H. M. Wiegerinck[1], G. H. Donker[2], J. Poortman[2] and J. H. H. Thijssen[2]

Department of Obstetrics and Gynaecology[1] and Department of Endocrinology[2], University Hospital, Utrecht, The Netherlands

INTRODUCTION

Oestradiol (E_2) is the prevalent oestrogen in blood during the menstrual cycle. After the menopause, oestrone (E_1) becomes the major circulating oestrogen, whereas the concentration of E_2 in the blood is low. A relatively high E_1 level in the blood, at the postmenopausal period or in infertility due to ovarian failure, is associated with an increased risk for the development of endometrial carcinoma. It has been well established that steroids have to bind to specific receptor proteins in the target cells as an obligatory step in a chain of intracellular events to effectuate the so-called oestrogenic effects. As a consequence the tissue levels of oestrogens will provide a better insight into the real activity of E_2 and E_1 than their levels in the blood. In other words the meaning of the concentrations of both steroids in blood is questionable in interpreting biological phenomena due to oestrogenic stimulation.

We studied the uptake of E_2 and E_1 *in vivo* by normal postmenopausal endometrium, myometrium and endometrial carcinoma and their intracellular distribution in relation to the plasma concentrations of these oestrogens.

Serono Symposium No. 39, "The Menopause: Clinical, Endocrinological and Pathophysiological Aspects", edited by P. Fioretti, L. Martini, G. B. Melis and S. S. C. Yen, 1982. Academic Press, London and New York.

PATIENTS AND METHODS

Thirteen women, admitted to the Department of Gynaecology of the University Hospital Utrecht, participated in the study after informed consent. In five women the diagnosis of endometrial carcinoma had been made on specimen obtained by curettage. The other eight women were postmenopausal (with the exception of patient BR whose gonadotropin levels showed premenopausal values); they had received no hormonal medication; the liver and kidney function tests were unimpaired; they had a normal glucose tolerance and normal thyroid function. These patients were scheduled for hysterectomy for non-oncological reasons such as vaginal prolapse. Radioactive tracers were infused. A ^{3}H-E$_1$ infusion was administered to five of these women and a ^{3}H-E$_2$ infusion to the other three. The patients with endometrial carcinoma received a ^{3}H-E$_1$ infusion. All infusions were started at least 10 h before hysterectomy. They were given i.v. via a Braun infusion pump at a constant rate. The dose of the administered oestrogen was 1-5% of the endogenous production of the infused oestrogen during the infusion period. Three blood samples were taken at intervals of 30 min prior to hysterectomy from the cubital vein contralateral to the infusion site. Immediately after hysterectomy the uterus was transported in ice to the department of pathology. Endometrium was obtained by abrasion or by slicing, endometrial carcinoma tissue was carefully excised. The adjacent parts of endometrium and myometrium were subjected to histological examination. The tissues were immediately processed according to the scheme shown in Fig. 1. The concentrations of ^{2}H-E$_1$ and ^{3}H-E$_2$ in plasma were determined using previously described methods (Poortman *et al.*, 1973).

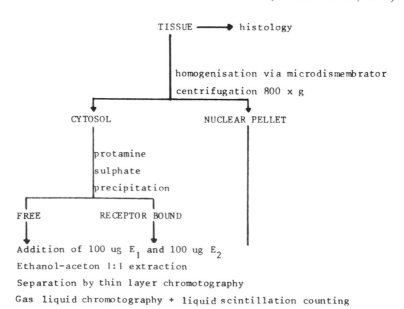

Fig. 1. Method used to measure and characterize the subcellular fractions of oestrogens in uterine tissues.

RESULTS

An equilibrium between ^{3}H-E$_1$ and ^{3}H-E$_2$ in plasma was found after the infusions of both radioactive oestrogens. The concentration in plasma of unconjugated ^{3}H-E$_2$ after ^{3}H-E$_1$ infusion was about 10% of the ^{3}H-E$_2$ concentration in plasma, similarly the plasma concentration of ^{3}H-E$_1$ after ^{3}H-E$_2$ infusion amounted to about 30% of the plasma ^{3}H-E$_1$ level. Figure 2 shows the concentrations of ^{3}H-E$_1$ and ^{3}H-E$_2$ in endometrium, myometrium and in plasma expressed according to the plasma concentration of ^{3}H-E$_2$ (= 1 as reference value) after ^{3}H-E$_1$ infusion or after ^{3}H-E$_2$ infusion. The activity in plasma was expressed in d/min/ml, the tissue activity in d/min/g wet weight. The mean values ± SE are shown. The tissue/plasma gradient of ^{3}H-E$_2$ in endometrium and myometrium is more than 10 after ^{3}H-E$_1$ infusion and even higher after ^{3}H-E$_2$ infusion.

The tissue concentration of ^{3}H-E$_1$ was nearly equal to the plasma concentration or slightly elevated after the ^{3}H-E$_1$ infusion. However after ^{3}H-E$_2$ infusion, the radioactive tissue concentration of E$_1$ is about 13 times higher in endometrium and five times higher in myometrium compared to the ^{3}H-E$_1$ level in plasma.

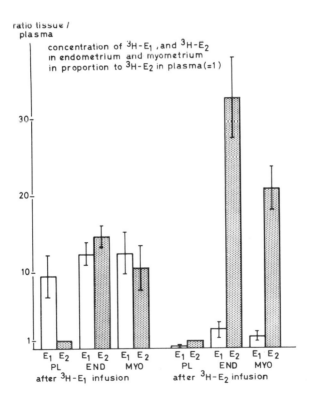

Fig. 2. Concentrations of ^{3}H-oestrone and ^{3}H-oestradiol in the subcellular fractions of endometrium and miometrium in proportion to ^{3}H-E$_2$ in plasma.

Table I shows the concentrations of ^{3}H-E$_1$ and ^{3}H-E$_2$ in the subcellular fractions of endometrium and myometrium. All concentrations are expressed in proportion to the activity of unconjugated ^{3}H-E$_2$ in plasma. These concentrations are also given for three patients with endometrial carcinoma. In addition, in most cases the total ^{3}H activity in plasma and the ^{3}H-E$_1$ concentration in plasma are given in a similar way. Estradiol is highly concentrated in the nuclear fraction and to a lesser degree in the receptorbound fraction of the cytosol in normal postmenopausal endometrium and myometrium. In the patients with endometrial cancer no consistent pattern of ^{3}H-E$_1$ and ^{3}H-E$_2$ concentrations is seen. In one patient (WM) an extremely high tissue/plasma gradient of ^{3}H-E$_1$ and ^{3}H-E$_2$ was found. The histological diagnosis of the tumour in this case was well-differentiated adeno-acanthoma. Well-differentiated adeno-carcinoma of the endometrium was diagnosed in the other cancer patients. The endometria of women without carcinoma were classified by the pathologist as atrophic endometria.

DISCUSSION

The use of the labelled oestrogen infusion technique gives information on the oestrogen uptake and on oestrogen interconversions by target tissues. At the concentrations we used in this study no change in the blood levels of endogenous oestradiol and oestrone was produced. Therefore, the handling of the radioactive oestrogens *in vivo* by endometrium, myometrium and endometrial carcinoma represents physiological conditions, in which the labelled oestrogens will reflect the endogenous situation in the tissues. Oestradiol appears to be the most important oestrogen in endometrium and myometrium of postmenopausal women without carcinoma. This finding confirms the conclusion of our preliminary report (Thijssen *et al.*, 1978). In a recent publication of King *et al.* (1980), E$_2$ is described as the major endometrial oestrogen after treatment of postmenopausal women with pharmacological doses of oestrogens. Both findings are consistent with the excellent *in vitro* work of Tseng and Gurpide (1973) showing the uptake of E$_2$ and E$_1$ by slices of human endometrium.

Figure 1 and Table I clearly demonstrate that the E$_2$/E$_1$ ratio in plasma is no reflection of their ratio in endometrium, myometrium and endometrial carcinoma. Considering the use of subphysiological doses of ^{3}H-E$_1$ or ^{3}H-E$_2$ in our study one should expect an identical tissue/plasma gradient for ^{3}H-E$_1$ and ^{3}H-E$_2$ after either labelled E$_1$ or E$_2$ infusion. However, both ^{3}H-E$_2$ and ^{3}H-E$_1$ tissue/plasma gradient were found higher after ^{3}H-E$_2$ infusion. Arguments can be derived from this discrepancy that: (a) E$_2$ and not E$_1$ is responsible for the tissue concentration of oestrogens in target cells; (b) the intracellular increase of E$_1$ is produced by interconversion from E$_2$ in the cell; (c) although a steady state in plasma concentrations of ^{3}H-E$_1$ and ^{3}H-E$_2$ is reached in 10 h during ^{3}H-E$_1$ infusion, no equilibrium in their tissue concentrations is established in this period. Probably the tissues have not been exposed long enough to plasma ^{3}H-E$_2$ which first has to be derived from ^{3}H-E$_1$ by interconversion.

These findings leave no important place for E$_1$ at the cellular level in postmenopausal endometrium and myometrium, as especially in the nuclear fraction

Table I. Ratios of the subcellular concentrations of ^3H-E_1 and ^3H-E_2 in endometrium and myometrium (DPM/g) to the plasma concentration (DPM/ml) of ^3H-E_2 (= 1) after infusion of a subphysiological dose of ^3H-E_2 or ^3H-E_1. Abreviations used: C = cytosol; f = free; b = receptorbound; N = nucleus.

Patient	Endometrium ^3H-E_1			Endometrium ^3H-E_2			Myometrium ^3H-E_1			Myometrium ^3H-E_2			Plasma Total ^3H	Plasma ^3H-E_1
	Cf	Cb	N	Cf	Cb	N	Cf	Cb	N	Cf	Cb	N		
After ^3H-E_2 infusion														
RA	1.4	0.8	1.5	3.6	8.4	27.7	1.5	0.2	0.6	0.6	4.8	20.9	8.8	0.5
BR	1.4	0.8	1.2	1.6	12.4	21.6	1.0	0.0	0.2	0.6	4.4	11.0	9.8	0.3
SH	0.0	0.3	0.1	1.6	9.0	11.7	0.2	0.2	0.5	1.1	5.9	12.1	4.3	0.2
M	*0.9*	*0.6*	*0.9*	*2.3*	*9.9*	*20.3*	*0.9*	*0.1*	*0.4*	*0.8*	*5.0*	*14.7*	*7.6*	*0.3*
SEM	*0.5*	*0.2*	*0.4*	*0.7*	*1.3*	*4.7*	*0.4*	*0.1*	*0.1*	*0.2*	*2.9*	*3.1*	*1.7*	*0.1*
After ^3H-E_1 infusion														
DU	17.3	3.3	26.7	2.6	7.7	22.8	2.3	3.5	10.7	1.8	0.8	6.9	n.d.	18.0
FR	2.8	15.5	1.8	0.9	3.0	6.7	3.7	2.5	6.5	1.8	4.7	4.1	n.d.	12.4
KR	2.8	1.4	1.3	4.3	0.2	4.1	1.3	0.4	4.2	1.4	1.3	1.0	n.d.	10.4
HE	2.3	2.6	2.7	0.7	0.5	8.5	2.4	0.4	1.4	0.7	0.3	1.7	11.0	2.5
GR	4.2	4.5	4.4	0.5	1.5	11.7	2.8	6.0	3.8	0.0	1.8	18.7	18.6	4.3
M	*5.9*	*5.5*	*7.4*	*1.8*	*2.6*	*10.8*	*2.5*	*2.6*	*5.3*	*1.1*	*1.8*	*6.5*	*14.8*	*9.5*
SEM	*2.9*	*2.6*	*4.9*	*0.8*	*1.4*	*3.3*	*0.4*	*1.0*	*1.6*	*0.3*	*0.8*	*3.2*	*3.8*	*4.3*
After ^3H-E_1 infusion in endometrial carcinoma														
WM	59.5	15.8	594	238	26.0	288							332	39.0
BA	1.2	6.2	7.4	0.5	1.0	4.4							71.6	13.2
SC	33.2	8.1	14.0	47.2	14.7	47.9							100	11.0
M	*21.3*	*10.0*	*205*	*95.2*	*13.9*	*113*							*168*	*21.0*
SEM	*19.2*	*2.9*	*195*	*72.9*	*7.3*	*88.6*							*82.8*	*4.0*

E_2 is the major oestrogen. The wide variation in intracellular concentrations of $^3H\text{-}E_1$ and $^3H\text{-}E_2$ in the endometrial carcinomata does not permit conclusions on their significance.

Work is in progress to extend these data, including $^3H\text{-}E_2$ infusions in patients with endometrial cancer. The following conclusions can be made.

(a) E_2 is the most important tissue oestrogen.

(b) The E_1/E_2 ratio in plasma of postmenopausal women does not reflect this ratio in endometrium and myometrium.

(c) The uptake of E_2 by the tissue is mainly responsible for the tissue/plasma gradient.

(d) Intracellular E_1 in target tissues is partly derived of interconversion from E_2 in the cell.

(e) A wide variation in intracellular concentrations of E_1 and E_2 is found in individual endometrial carcinoma tissues.

REFERENCES

King, R. J. B., Dyer, G., Collins, W. P. and Whitehead, M. I. (1980). *Journal of Steroid Biochemistry* **13**, 377.

Poortman, J. Thijssen, J. H. H. and Schwarz, F. (1973). *Journal of Clinical Endocrinology and Metabolism* **37**, 101.

Thijssen, J. H. H., Wiegerinck, M. A. H. M., Mulder, G. and Poortman, J. (1978). *Frontiers of Hormone Research* **5**, 220.

Tseng, L. and Gurpide, E. (1973). *Endocrinology* **93**, 245.

THE *IN VITRO* CONVERSION OF ANDROSTENEDIONE TO OESTRONE BY ADIPOSE TISSUE FROM NORMAL WOMEN AND WOMEN WITH ENDOMETRIAL CANCER

E. J. Folkerd, M. J. Reed and V. H. T. James

Department of Chemical Pathology, St. Mary's Hospital Medical School, London UK

INTRODUCTION

The contribution to oestrone production from the extragonadal conversion of androstenedione *in vivo* has been shown to increase with age (Hemsell *et al.,* 1974) but it is not increased in women with endometrial cancer when compared with normal women of similar age and weight (MacDonald *et al.,* 1978).

Extragonadal aromatization has been demonstrated *in vitro* in various tissues such as adipose tissue (Schindler *et al.,* 1972; Nimrod and Ryan, 1975; Perel and Killinger, 1979), cultured human fibroblasts (Schweikert *et al.,* 1976) and liver (Smuk and Schwers, 1977; Frost *et al.,* 1980). Conditions associated with increased peripheral conversion of androstenedione to oestrone, such as ageing (Hemsell *et al.,* 1974) and obesity (Edman and MacDonald, 1978; MacDonald *et al.,* 1978), are also associated with endometrial cancer. It is not clear whether the increased conversion is dependent upon the plasma production rate of androstenedione or the efficiency of aromatization.

The present study was carried out to determine whether the *in vitro* conversion of androstenedione to oestrone by adipose tissue was related to the age of the subject, and also to examine the efficiency of aromatization in subjects with endometrial cancer, or endometrial hyperplasia, a condition that often precedes endometrial cancer.

Serono Symposium No. 39, "The Menopause: Clinical, Endocrinological and Pathophysiological Aspects", edited by P. Fioretti, L. Martini, G. B. Melis and S. S. C. Yen, 1982. Academic Press, London and New York.

MATERIALS AND METHODS

Chemicals

[7α-³H] Androstenedione (15Ci/mol) and [4-¹⁴C] oestrone (55mCi/mmol), Radiochemical Centre Amersham, were purified by paper chromatography before use. Light petroleum (100° to 120° fraction): to toluene: methanol: water (10:40: 40:10) was used as a solvent system. All cofactors were obtained from Sigma Chemical Company.

Tissue Preparation

Subcutaneous adipose tissue was obtained from the abdominal wall of subjects undergoing gynaecological surgery. The tissue was rinsed in 0.1M phosphate buffer pH 7.4, and fibrous tissue removed by dissection. The tissue was suspended in 0.1M phosphate buffer pH 7.4 containing $MgCl_2$ (5mM) and nicotinamide (10mM) at a concentration of 1g/ml and homogenized using a glass homogenizer. An aliquot of the soluble fraction obtained after centrifugation of the homogenate was taken for protein estimation by the method of Lowry et al. (1951) and the remained was used for incubation.

Incubation of Adipose Tissue

The procedure used for tissue incubation was based on that described by Nimrod and Ryan (1975). Cofactors were added to the aqueous phase of the tissue homogenate to give the following concentrations: glucose 6 phosphate (10mM), NAD (2mM), NADP (2mM), ATP (mM) and glucose 6 phosphate dehydrogenase (2 units/ml). The incubation mixture also contained [7α-³H] androstenedione (1–2μCi) and tracer amounts (0.01–0.04μCi) of [4-¹⁴C] oestrone to allow correction for losses during purification.

Tissue preparations were incubated in air for 3 h at 37 °C with continuous shaking. Control samples omitting the tissue or with boiled tissue were included in each study. At the end of the incubation methanol was added to give a 50% aqueous solution.

Extraction

The incubation mixture was extracted with ether (3 × 1 vol) and the combined extracts taken to dryness under nitrogen. The oestrone was isolated as described by Frost et al. (1980). The method involved a preliminary separation of oestrogens from androgens by phenolic partition (Brown, 1955) followed by column chromatography on Sephadex LH-20 with toluene: methanol (85:15ᵛ/v) as solvent and three successive thin layer chromatography steps: (1) dichloromethane: ethyl acetate (8:2ᵛ/v); (2) cyclohexane: ethyl acetate (1:1ᵛ/v) and (3) toluene: ethyl acetate (6:4ᵛ/v). The ³H/¹⁴C ratio of the final product was determined and this ratio was used to calculate the amount of product formed according to the formula:

$$\text{Product (pmole)} = \frac{^3\text{H}/^{14}\text{C Product (cpm/cpm)} \times {}^{14}\text{C oestrone added (cpm)}}{\text{Specific Activity Androstenedione (cpm/pmole)}}$$

adapted from Tseng and Gurpide (1974).

The pmoles of product formed were related to the mg tissue protein and the final results expressed as pg oestrone/mg tissue protein/3h.

Table I. The conversion of androstenedione to oestrone by adipose tissue from normal women.

Subject	Age (years)	Weight (Kg)	Height (cm)	Conversion (pg oestrone/mg tissue protein/3h)
JS	24	60.33	170	7.65
MR	25	60.33	167	5.88
MK	28	52.62	160	7.68
MKE	28	63.50	162	1.88
KS	32	50.80	157	0.70
BS	32	63.50	160	2.56
DG	36	54.43	170	1.06
CS	36	73.03	162	2.43
DF	37	60.33	160	1.35
KG	38	58.97	163	0.51
SW	40	60.78	160	20.76
MD	41	58.06	155	1.17
GR	41	66.68	172	17.30
AW	42	58.06	162	12.60
EO	43	53.98	152	17.50
SM	43	50.80	157	44.00
SS	43	59.40	152	2.30
FS	44	79.38	157	34.58
AM	45	50.80	162	39.15
PM	47	57.61	160	16.03
RS	47	78.02	157	2.25
JM	49	50.80	152	7.90
NS	50	69.85	160	38.97
RW	61	69.85	155	10.60
KJ	68	69.85	167	4.72

RESULTS

Aromatization of Androstenedione by Normal Adipose Tissue

The data obtained using normal adipose tissue are presented in Table I. The efficiency of aromatization appeared to increase with age at least up until the time of the menopause (Fig. 1). The postmenopausal subjects that have been studied have had conversion rates below 11 pg oestrone/mg tissue protein/3h, indicating that the efficiency of aromatization may decline in later years.

The degree of obesity of the overweight normal subjects studied was obtained by subtraction of the subjects normal weight from their actual weight. Normal weights were calculated using the formula of Lorenz:

$$\text{Normal weight (kg)} = \text{Height (cm)} - 100 - \frac{\text{Height} - 150}{4}$$

taken from Vermeulen and Verdonck (1978).

The regression line for the correlation of the conversion of androstenedione to oestrone and age was calculated by the method of least squares and is shown in Fig. 2. The correlation coefficient of the two variables was 0.22 and was not statistically significant at the 5% level of significance.

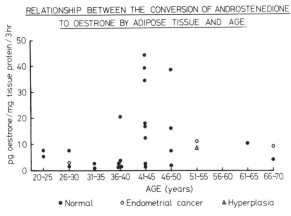

Fig. 1. The conversion of androstenedione to oestrone in adipose tissue obtained from normal women aged between 20 and 70 and women with endometrial cancer or endometrial hyperplasia. The mean conversion (3.17 pg oestrone/mg tissue protein/3h) for the 10 normal premenopausal (20–39 years) women was significantly lower ($P < 0.005$) than the mean (19.50 pg oestrone/mg tissue protein/3h) for the 13 normal perimenopausal women (40–50 years).

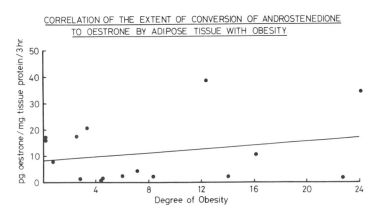

Fig. 2. The correlation between the extent of conversion of androstenedione to oestrone in adipose tissue and degree of obesity in 16 normal women. The correlation coefficient for these two variables was 0.22 and was not significant at the 5% level of significance.

**Aromatization of Androstenedione by
Adipose Tissue from Subjects with
Endometrial Cancer**

The three subjects studied so far with endometrial cancer and the one subject with endometrial hyperplasia did not show an elevated conversion of androstenedione to oestrone in subcutaneous adipose tissue compared with normal women of similar age and weight. The results are shown in Table II.

In contrast to the results obtained using subcutaneous tissue, a very high conversion of androstenedione to oestrone (104pg oestrone/mg tissue protein/3h) was found in a sample of omental adipose tissue obtained from the intraperitoneal cavity of the woman (MR) aged 51 with endometrial cancer.

DISCUSSION

The results of the present study, in agreement with the findings of Schindler *et al.* (1972), Nimrod and Ryan (1975) and Perel and Killinger (1979), show that adipose tissue is capable of aromatizing androstenedione *in vitro*, and is therefore a possible site for the peripheral formation of oestrogens.

Table II. The conversion of androstenedione to oestrone in adipose tissue from women with endometrial cancer or hyperplasia.

Subject	Age (years)	Weight (Kg)	Conversion (pg oestrone/mg tissue protein/3h)	History
AP	27	–	2.54	Adenocarcinoma PCO
MR	51	68.9	11.71	Well differentiated papillary adenocarcinoma
JH	71	70.0	9.55	Well differentiated adenocarcinoma
HH	55	63.5	8.90	Moderate cystic glandular hyperplasia

MacDonald *et al.* (1978) found that the conversion of androstenedione to oestrone *in vivo* was related to body weight. It could be suggested, therefore, that obesity might account for the high conversion values found for the 40–50 year age group (mean 19.50pg oestrone/mg tissue protein/3h) compared with the 20–39 year age group (mean 3.17pg oestrone/mg tissue protein/3h). However, it was found that adipose tissue from obese subjects was not significantly more efficient at aromatization *in vitro* than that from subjects of normal weight indicating that the increased conversion observed *in vivo* is a result of an increase in the mass of adipose tissue rather than a change in aromatase activity. In addition, some women in the 40–50 year age group had high conversion values *in vitro* even though they were up to 12kg under their expected weight and, therefore, a factor other than obesity must be sought to account for the relationship between age and aromatization.

There is a possible explanation for the high conversion value observed in two of the women in the 40–50 year age group. Both women were receiving norethisterone therapy, a synthetic progestagen which may, like progesterone, inhibit 5α-reductase activity (Frederiksen and Wilson, 1971). The resulting increase in available androstenedione and decrease in the intracellular concentration of 5α-reduced aromatase inhibitors (Siiteri and Thompson, 1975) could account for the high conversion observed.

The three subjects studied with endometrial cancer and the patient with endometrial hyperplasia did not show an increased conversion of androstenedione to oestrone compared with normal women of similar age and weight. A sample of omental adipose tissue obtained from the intraperitoneal cavity of the patient (MR) aged 51 with endometrial cancer did, however, show a very high conversion rate (104pg oestrone/mg tissue protein/3h) indicating that aromatization may be elevated in adipose tissue in subjects with endometrial cancer but not uniformly throughout the body.

The role, if any, of altered peripheral production of oestrogen in the development of endometrial cancer remains uncertain. The factors which mediate androgen-oestrogen conversion are not understood and the interpretation of the results of *in vivo* isotopic studies are clearly complicated by the problem that adipose tissue from different sites within the same subject differs considerably in its ability to affect aromatization. Furthermore, the degree of exposure of individual target tissue to oestrone does not necessarily indicate the extent to which oestrone is converted to oestradiol in these tissues, which may be more important in relation to normal or abnormal hormonal effects. Finally, the role of other hormones, e.g. progesterone, in mediating further metabolic transformations is also likely to be important.

ACKNOWLEDGEMENTS

This work was supported by a grant from the Campaign for Cancer Research. We gratefully acknowledge the assistance of staff at the Samaritan Hospital in supplying the samples of adipose tissue used in this investigation.

REFERENCES

Brown, J. B. (1955). *Biochemical Journal* **60**, 185.
Edman, C. D. and MacDonald, P. C. (1978). *American Journal of Obstetrics and Gynecology* **130**, 456.
Frederiksen, D. W. and Wilson, J. D. (1971). *Journal of Biological Chemistry* **246**, 2584.
Frost, P. G., Reed, M. J. and James, V. H. T. (1980). *Journal of Steroid Biochemistry* (in press).
Hemsell, D. L., Grodin, J. M., Brenner, P. F., Siiteri, P. K. and MacDonald, P. C. (1974). *Journal of Clinical Endocrinology and Metabolism* **38**, 476.

Lowry, O. M., Rosebrough, N. J., Farr, A. L. and Randall, R. L. (1951). *Journal of Biological Chemistry* **193**, 265.

MacDonald, P. C., Edman, C. D., Hemsell, D. L., Porter, J. C. and Siiteri, P. K. (1978). *American Journal of Obstetrics and Gynecology* **130**, 448.

Nimrod, A. and Ryan, K. (1975). *Journal of Clinical Endocrinology and Metabolism* **40**, 367.

Perel, E. and Killinger, D. W. (1979). *Journal of Steroid Biochemistry* **10**, 623.

Schindler, A. E., Ebert, A. and Friedrich, E. (1972). *Journal of Clinical Endocrinology and Metabolism* **35**, 627.

Schweikert, H. U., Milewich, L. and Wilson, J. D. (1976). *Journal of Clinical Endocrinology and Metabolism* **43**, 785.

Siiteri, P. K. and Thompson, E. A. (1975). *Journal of Steroid Biochemistry* **6**, 317.

Smuk, M. and Schwers, J. (1977). *Journal of Clinical Endocrinology and Metabolism* **45**, 1009.

Tseng, L. and Gurpide, E. (1974). *Endocrinology* **94**, 419.

Vermeulen, A. and Verdonck, L. (1978). *Clinical Endocrinology* **9**, 59.

OESTRADIOL PRODUCTION AND FACTORS THAT INFLUENCE THE INTERCONVERSION OF OESTRONE AND OESTRADIOL IN POSTMENOPAUSAL WOMEN WITH ENDOMETRIAL HYPERPLASIA, ENDOMETRIAL CANCER OR CIRRHOSIS

M. J. Reed, C. T. Noel, E. A. Johns, D. L. Jones and V. H. T. James

Department of Chemical Pathology, St Mary's Hospital Medical School, London, UK

INTRODUCTION

The concept that oestrogens are in some way involved in the development of endometrial cancer has stimulated many investigations into steroid production and metabolism in women with this disorder (James and Reed, 1980). After the menopause, when endometrial cancer most frequently occurs, oestrone is the main plasma oestrogen and it is now established that this oestrone is formed by aromatization of androstenedione in peripheral tissues (Siiteri and MacDonald, 1973).

Initial studies, carried out in obese postmenopausal women with endometrial cancer, suggested that oestrone production was elevated and a role for oestrone in the development of endometrial cancer postulated (Siiteri *et al.*, 1974). Subsequent studies, however, showed that when allowance was made for excess weight, there was no increase in oestrone production (MacDonald *et al.*, 1978; Reed *et al.*, 1979a).

Recent evidence has suggested that oestradiol rather than oestrone is the active oestrogen at the cellular level (Thijssen *et al.*, 1978; Morse *et al.*, 1979) and thus the role of oestrone may be as a prehormone for oestradiol formation. There is, however, little information about the production rates of oestradiol in normal

Serono Symposium No. 39, "The Menopause: Clinical, Endocrinological and Pathophysiological Aspects", edited by P. Fioretti, L. Martini, G. B. Melis and S. S. C. Yen, 1982. Academic Press, London and New York.

postmenopausal women and no reports, as far as we are aware, of oestradiol production rates in postmenopausal women with endometrial cancer or endometrial hyperplasia.

In the present study, the production rates of oestradiol have been measured in four postmenopausal women with endometrial cancer and two with endometrial hyperplasia, a possible predisposing condition for endometrial cancer. Production of oestradiol in two postmenopausal women with cirrhosis was also measured as there is some controversy about the risk for the development of endometrial cancer in this group of women (Speert, 1949; Brewer and Foley, 1953). As little is known about the factors that influence the interconversion of oestrone and oestradiol, this aspect of oestrogen metabolism was investigated in relation to body weight, age and plasma concentrations of progesterone and dehydroepiandrosterone sulphate (DHA-S).

Plasma hormone levels, the production rates of oestradiol and the interconversion of oestrone and oestradiol were measured by standard procedures previously described (Reed *et al.*, 1979b; Jones *et al.*, 1980).

RESULTS

The values obtained for the production rates of oestradiol, together with the number of years that have elapsed for each subject since the menopause, are shown in Fig. 1. Where a number of years have elapsed since the menopause,

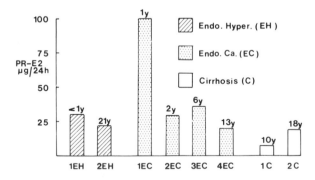

Fig. 1. Production rates of oestradiol (PR-E$_2$) in postmenopausal women with endometrial hyperplasia (EH), endometrial cancer (EC) or cirrhosis (C). The number of years elapsed since the menopause is shown for each subject.

production of oestradiol was 7.4–22.2 μg/24 h. Higher production rates of oestradiol were found in some subjects studied for up to six years after the menopause. For one subject, where only one year had elapsed since the menopause, production of oestradiol was greatly increased, in spite of plasma levels of FSH, LH and progesterone in the postmenopausal range.

Similar values for the conversion of oestrone to oestradiol were found for all subjects (range 3.0–8.1%) and for the conversion of oestradiol to oestrone in

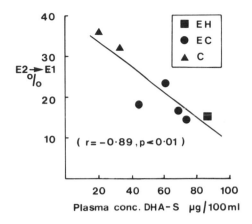

Fig. 2. Correlation between the conversion of oestradiol to oestrone ($[\rho]_{BB}^{E2E1}$) and plasma levels of dehydroepiandrosterone sulphate* (DHA-S) for women with endometrial hyperplasia (EH), endometrial cancer (EC) or cirrhosis (C). (*39.4 μg/100 ml = 1 μmol/1 litre).

women with endometrial cancer or hyperplasia (range 14.7–23.8%). However, values for the conversion of oestradiol to oestrone were significantly higher (31.9 and 35.7%) in the subjects studied with cirrhosis.

No significant correlations were found between the conversion of oestrone to oestradiol ($[\rho]_{BB}^{E1E2}$) and body weight, age or plasma levels of progesterone or DHA-S. Similarly, there was no correlation between the conversion of oestradiol to oestrone ($[\rho]_{BB}^{E2E1}$) and age or plasma concentrations of progesterone. A correlation was found between $[\rho]_{BB}^{E2E1}$ and body weight ($r = -0.58$), although it was not significant for the small number of subjects so far studied. As shown in Fig. 2 there was a statistically significant negative correlation between $[\rho]_{BB}^{E2E1}$ and plasma concentrations of DHA-S ($r = -0.89, P < 0.01$).

DISCUSSION

The continued production of oestradiol by postmenopausal women is confirmed by the results of the present investigation. Where a number of years have elapsed since the menopause, oestradiol production was similar to the 11–25 μg/24 h reported for normal postmenopausal women by Pratt and Longcope (1978). Increased production of oestradiol was found in some subjects for up to 6 years after the menopause and was considerably elevated in one woman who had endometrial cancer. The continued, and in some subjects, elevated production of oestradiol throughout the climacteric, presumably reflecting continued ovarian production, at a time when progesterone production is minimal, may be related to the development of endometrial cancer.

Values for the conversion of oestrone to oestradiol, apart from one subject with endometrial cancer and for the conversion of oestradiol to oestrone for subjects with endometrial cancer or hyperplasia, were similar to those for normal postmenopausal women (Longcope, 1978). Transfer constants for the conversion of oestradiol to oestrone by the two women with cirrhosis were elevated. Increased conversion of oestradiol to oestrone has also been reported in cirrhotic men (Olivo et al., 1975).

As there is some evidence of adrenocortical hyperfunction in women with endometrial cancer (Sommers and Meissner, 1957; Calström et al., 1979), the significant negative correlation found between the values for the conversion of oestradiol to oestrone and plasma levels of DHA-S prompted us to postulate a possible role for DHA-S, or a metabolite of DHA-S, in the regulation of oestradiol metabolism.

Our hypothesis, summarized in Fig. 3, postulates that elevated levels of DHA-S, leading to elevated tissue levels of DHA-S or possibly 5α-androstene-3β,17β-diol (A'diol), influences the metabolism of oestradiol in a way that may be related to the development of endometrial cancer. Reduced conversion of oestradiol to oestrone could result in increased exposure of target tissues to oestradiol, the active cellular oestrogen.

Although further work is required to substantiate or refute this hypothesis it

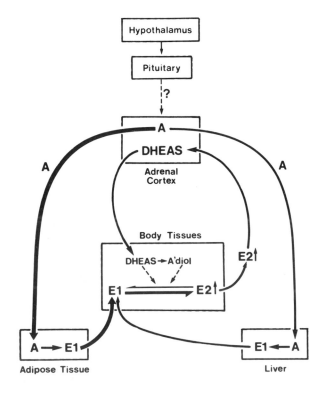

Fig. 3. Summary of an hypothesis postulating that dehydroepiandrosterone sulphate (DHEA-S) or its metabolite 5α-androstene-3β, 17β-diol (A'diol) influences the metabolism of oestradiol (E₂) to oestrone (E₁).

can provide an explanation for a number of factors known to alter the risk for the development of endometrial cancer. In normal postmenopausal women a significant correlation ($r = 0.71, P < 0.02$) was found between plasma levels of DHA-S and body weight. In obese women, generally considered to be at greater risk for developing endometrial cancer, increased plasma levels of DHA-S would be associated with reduced conversion of oestradiol to oestrone and thus increased exposure to oestradiol. Increased secretion of DHA-S has also been shown to occur in hypertension (Shao *et al.*, 1970), also considered by some to be associated with an enhanced risk for the development of endometrial cancer.

Conversely, reduced production of DHA-S and the associated increase in the conversion of oestradiol to oestrone, as found for the two cirrhotic women in the present study, could, by reducing tissue exposure to oestradiol, result in a lower risk for endometrial cancer. These data therefore support the original observation of Brewer and Foley (1953) that women with cirrhosis do not have an increased risk of developing endometrial cancer.

Finally, as it has been shown in postmenopausal women that oestrogens can stimulate DHA-S production (Abraham and Maroulis, 1975), it is possible that an initial stimulation of the adrenal cortex, at some time during the menopausal transition, is perpetuated by the increased plasma levels of oestradiol which could arise from reduced conversion of oestradiol to oestrone.

ACKNOWLEDGEMENT

This work was supported by a grant from the Cancer Research Campaign.

REFERENCES

Abraham, G. E. and Maroulis, G. B. (1975). *Obstetrics and Gynaecology* **45**, 271.
Brewer, J. I. and Foley, T. J. (1953). *Obstetrics and Gynaecology* **1**, 67.
Calström, K., Damber, M.-G., Furuhjelm, M., Joelsson, I. Lunell, N.-O. and Schoultz, B. (1979). *Acta Obstetrica Gynaecologica Scandinavia* **58**, 179.
James, V. H. T. and Reed, M. J. (1980). *In* "Progress in Cancer Research and Therapy" (S. Iacobelli, R. J. B. King, H. R. Lindner and M. E. Lippman, Eds), 13. Raven Press, New York (in press).
Jones, D. L., Jacobs, H. S. and James, V. H. T. (1980). *In* "Progress in Cancer Research and Therapy" (A. R. Genazzani, J. H. H. Thijssen and P. K. Siiteri, Eds), 15. Raven Press, New York (in press).
Longcope, E. (1978). *In* "Endocrinology of the Ovary" (R. Scholler, Ed.), pp. 23–33. Editions Sepe, Paris.
MacDonald, P. C., Edman, C. D., Hemsell, D. L., Porter, J. C. and Siiteri, P. K. (1978). *American Journal of Obstetrics and Gynecology* **130**, 448.
Morse, A. R., Hutton, J. D., Jacobs, H. S., Murray, M. A. F. and James, V. H. T. (1979). *British Journal of Obstetrics and Gynaecology* **86**, 981.
Olivo, J., Gordon, G. G., Rafii, F. and Southren, A. L. (1975). *Steroids* **26**, 47.
Preatt, J. H. and Longcope, C. (1978). *Journal of Clinical Endocrinology and Metabolism* **46**, 44.
Reed, M. J., Hutton, J. D., Baxendale, P. M., James, V. H. T., Jacobs, H. S. and Fisher, R. P. (1979a). *Journal of Steroid Biochemistry* **11**, 905.

Reed, M. J., Hutton, J. D., Beard, R. W., Jacobs, H. S. and James, V. H. T. (1979b). *Clinical Endocrinology* **11**, 141.

Shao, A., Nowaczynski, W., Kuchel, O. and Genest, J. (1970). *Canadian Journal of Biochemistry* **48**, 1308.

Siiteri, P. K. and MacDonald, P. C. (1973). *In* "Handbook of Physiology, Section 7, Endocrinology" (G. B. Astwood and R. O. Greep, Eds.). American Physiological Society, Washington.

Siiteri, P. K., Schwarz, B. E. and MacDonald, P. C. (1974). *Gynecologic Oncology* **2**, 228.

Sommers, C. S. and Meissner, W. A. (1957). *Cancer* **10**, 516.

Speert, H. (1949). *Cancer* **2**, 597.

Thijssen, J. H. H., Wiegerink, M. A. H. M. and Poortman, J. (1978). *Journal of Steroid Biochemistry* **9**, 893 (Abs. 392).

PLASMA STEROIDS IN NORMAL AND PATHOLOGICAL MENOPAUSE

J. Hustin[1], J. Duvivier[2] and R. Lambotte[1]

*Departments of Gynaecology and Obstetrics[1] and Clinical Biochemistry[2],
University of Liège, Belgium*

INTRODUCTION

The postmenopausal ovarian function is normally limited to the production of some C19 androgenic steroids (Vermeulen, 1976). In an early work, we demonstrated that a number of elderly patients displayed clinical evidence of sustained hormonal production even several years after the menopause (Gregoire and Hustin, 1969). Some of these patients were eventually suffering from endometrial carcinoma.

Endocrinological studies dealing with the urinary excretion of steroids were then conducted. It appeared that many patients had elevated urinary levels of oestrogens, especially oestriol, which were suppressible by dexamethasone (Hustin, 1973). Today, there is still controversy as regards the carcinogenetic action of exogenous oestrogens. Moreover, we were impressed by a frequent histological picture in menopausal hyperplastic endometria, which was quite reminiscent of oestro-androgenic influence (Hustin *et al.*, 1974). Therefore, we suggested that many patients with menopausal pathology, including endometrial cancer, might have a persistent hormonal secretion, predominantly androgenic. The present study was undertaken in order to confirm that hypothesis. It deals with different series of postmenopausal patients, with and without endometrial cancer. Six different steroids have been assayed in their serum. Results have been submitted to statistical evaluation.

Serono Symposium No. 39, "The Menopause: Clinical, Endocrinological and Pathophysiological Aspects", edited by P. Fioretti, L. Martini, G. B. Melis and S. S. C. Yen, 1982. Academic Press, London and New York.

MATERIALS AND METHODS

Fifty-one patients were investigated. All had been undergoing the menopause for at least 3 years. They were divided into three groups: ten normal women, without evidence of disease, as controls (T); twelve patients, with uterine bleeding but without evidence of cancer, were included in the "hyperhormonal" (H) series; finally 29 patients, with histologically proven endometrial cancer, constituted the cancer group (C). There were 15 patients without any previous treatment and 14 who were already under progestin treatment (medroxyprogesterone acetate 1 gm i.m. per week).

Twenty ml of blood was drawn from each patient in a fasting state, and was allowed to clot. Serum was then collected and frozen at $-20\,°C$. All samples were assayed simultaneously.

Oestrone (E_1), Oestradiol (E_2), Oestriol (E_3), δ-4-androstenedione (A), testosterone (T), progesterone (Pg) and 17-α-Hydroxyprogesterone (170 HPg) were evaluated on each serum sample according to classic radioimmunoassay techniques (Abraham, 1974) with, however, the chromatographic modifications already described by one of us (Duvivier and Germeau, 1976).

RESULTS

Detailed results are reported in Table I. For each group mean values, and standard error of mean are given. Comparison of various means according to Student's t-test disclosed that the hyperhormonal (H) group had higher E_2 levels than controls ($t = 3.12$, d.f.:22; $P < 0.01$); mean E_1 and E_2 values of cancer patients were also elevated but no significant difference could be drawn with group C when all cancer patients were considered. However, if untreated patients alone were considered, the sum of E_1 and E_2 was significantly higher in this group ($t = 2.85$, d.f. = 22; $P < 0.01$).

There was no significant difference in serum oestrogen between group H and C. Cancer patients under medroxyprogesterone treatment had E_1 and E_2 values intermediate between untreated cancers and control patients, but no statistical difference could be drawn.

E_3 was at very low values (below 0.1 pmole/ml) in all three groups. If E_1 or E_2 levels or their sum were plotted against age no correlation appeared whatsoever. However the influence of being overweight was significant. In a limited series it appeared that E_2 levels exceeded 0.22 nmoles/litre in only one out of eight normal weight patients, while in seven overweight patients, E_1 and/or E_2 were found markedly elevated in five instances.

C19 androgens (A and T) were significantly higher in the plasma of patients belonging to the hyperhormonal (H) group ($P < 0.01$ as compared with the T group, and $P < 0.01$ as compared with the whole C group). Untreated cancer patients also had moderately high A and T levels, while medroxyprogesterone treated ones did not differ from controls. There was however no significant difference between the cancer subgroups except when plasma A and T were summed up: untreated cancer patients were then significantly different from the treated ones ($P < 0.05$; Fig. 1).

Table I. Plasma steroids[a].

Groups	E_1	E_2	E_3	A	T	Pg	17OHPg
T	0.08 ± 0.01	0.06 ± 0.01	0.1 ± 0.05	2.73 ± 0.44	1.07 ± 0.14	0.4 ± 0.01	2.5 ± 0.5
H	0.21 ± 0.07	0.16 ± 0.04	0.06 ± 0.01	3.12 ± 0.5	2.26 ± 0.4	—	—
C (Whole series)	0.16 ± 0.03	0.17 ± 0.04	0.07 ± 0.01	3.95 ± 0.69	1.12 ± 0.15	1.7 ± 0.4	4.5 ± 0.6
C Untreated	0.19 ± 0.04	0.19 ± 0.05	0.07 ± 0.01	5.07 ± 0.57	1.45 ± 0.2	2.2 ± 0.6	4.7 ± 0.7
C Progestin treated	0.13 ± 0.02	0.17 ± 0.04	0.07 ± 0.01	2.76 ± 0.47	0.90 ± 0.1	1.2 ± 0.3	4.2 ± 0.5

[a]Mean ± SE, nmoles/litre.

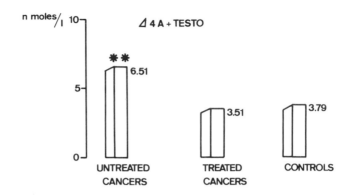

Fig. 1. Sum of plasma androgens Δ4A = δ-4-androstenedione; testo = testosterone. Progestin treated patients do not differ from controls while untreated patients have significantly higher values. (****P* < 0.01).

Plasma Pg and 17 OH Pg were constantly low in all series. However, cancer patients had a mean 17 OH Pg slightly higher than other groups ≅4 nmoles/litre) but this elevation was not significant, owing to the wide scatter of individual values. It must be noted that medroxyprogesterone treatment did not influence plasma values of C21 steroids and emphasized that this drug did not interfere with the assays used in the present study.

Lastly, we tried to draw correlations between different assays within each clinical group. It appeared that, in all three groups, a real correlation could be drawn between plasma A and T ($r = 0.83$ for all groups; Fig. 2). E_1 and A were similarly correlated ($r = 0.56$; Fig. 3). No correlation was found between E_1 and E_2 except perhaps in the treated cancers subgroup, but the usually very low values did not allow precise statistical analysis. There was no correlation between Pg and 17 OH Pg levels in the H and C groups. However, correlation was present in the T group and progestin treated cancer patients; both curves were indeed very similar (Fig. 4).

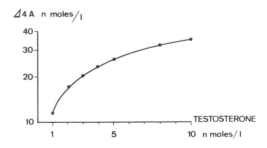

Fig. 2. Correlation between plasma δ-4 androstenedione (Δ4A) and testosterone; (all groups pooled).

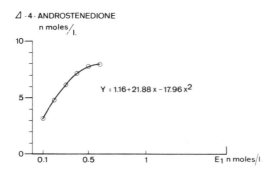

Fig. 3. Correlation between plasma E_1 and A; ($r = 0.56$; all groups pooled).

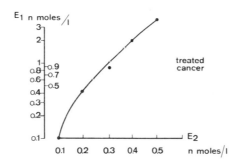

Fig. 4. Progestin treated cancers. Possible correlation between plasma E_1 and E_2 ($r - 0.39$).

DISCUSSION

We demonstrate in this study that patients with pathological menopause, associated or not with endometrial cancer, have often high serum androgen levels (A and T). This finding is in agreement with the earlier work of Calanog *et al.* (1977), but, quite recently, Schenker *et al.* (1979) did not measure high levels of T in endometrial cancer patients. In our study, T alone did not appear to be very discriminating between the different series. Cancerous patients under progestin treatment have androgen levels not unlike those of controls.

This overall decrease is significant and is rather similar to that observed in postmenopausal women placed under corticosteroids therapy (Marshall *et al.*, 1978). It is known that medroxyprogesterone acetate possesses corticosteroid like properties (Anderson, 1972). The drug reduction of plasma androgen could be explained by this effect. It also appears that there is a modest increase of serum oestrogens, especially E_2, in the pathological groups. However it must be noted that the overall increase is obviously correlated to the importance of being over-weight (Edman *et al.*, 1978) which is preferentially found in pathological states. Conversely oestriol was at very low levels. Serum oestrogens did not, in our studies, correlate with age, a finding at variance with the recent work of Badawy *et al.*

(1979). These authors suggest that the gradual decrease in oestrogens could be linked to a similar decrease in plasma A, which was well documented for oophorectomized women by Crilly *et al.* (1979).

We have demonstrated in our series that there was a correlation between serum A and oestrone. This could appear logical since it is known that in postmenopause, E_1 is preferentially derived from plasma A through an extraglandular aromatization (Edman *et al.*, 1978). However, neither partition according to group nor to age influenced this correlation.

The correlation which exists between their respective plasma levels shows that androstenedione is also linked with testosterone in the steroid metabolism. Vermeulen (1976) has already suggested a common origin (ovarian) of both steroids. Tseng and Gurpide (1975) have demonstrated that uterine levels of 17-β-steroid dehydrogenase were considerably increased by the administration of progestins. Now, in our series of progestin treated patients, oestrogen levels are low, and this may be due to the already mentioned decrease in androgens. Nevertheless, in this subgroup only, there seems to be a correlation between plasma E_1 and E_2. One can postulate that it could reflect the stimulation of target cell 17-β-dehydrogenase.

Lastly, we have demonstrated a correlation between the low levels of Pg and 17 OH Pg in two groups, namely controls and progestin treated patients. In the last subgroup, most endometrial samples possessed 17-α-steroid dehydrogenase (Hustin and Kremers, 1975). It may be that the relation between both steroids is partly due to this enzymatic activity.

In conclusion, we demonstrate in this study that plasma levels of steroids may reflect the capabilities of the organism to maintain an endocrine activity after the menopause. In pathological groups the normal hormonal ratio is often shifted towards an androgenic preponderance. Now, in paraneoplastic endometria or in cases of postmenopausal hyperplasia, there are frequent histological changes suggestive of androgenic influence (unpublished observations). We think that there might be a link between endometrial pathology and this imbalance in the oestrogen-androgen ratio. Medroxyprogesterone might thus act immediately at the cellular level by inducing its potent progestational effect. The drug could also reduce the endocrine imbalance, i.e. the androgen preponderance, and thus suppress the improper stimulus which might cause abnormal endometrial growth.

REFERENCES

Abraham, G. E. (1974). *In* "Radioimmunoassay and related procedures in Medicine", Vol II, 3–28. International Atomic Energy Agency, Vienna.

Anderson, D. G. (1972). *American Journal of Obstetrics and Gynecology* **113**, 195–208.

Badawy, S. Z. A., Elliott, L. J., Elbadawi, A. and Marshall, L. D. (1979). *British Journal of Obstetrics and Gynaecology* **86**, 56–63.

Calanog, A., Sall, S., Gordon, G. G. and Southren, A. L. (1977). *American Journal of Obstetrics and Gynecology* **129**, 553–556.

Crilly, R. G., Marshall, D. H. and Nordin, B. E. C. (1979). *Clinical Endocrinology* **10**, 199–201.

Duvivier, J. and Germeau, P. (1976). *Journal of Chromatography* **129**, 471–472.

Edman, C. D., Aiman, E. J., Porter, J. C. and MacDonald, P. C. (1978). *American Journal of Obstetrics and Gynecology* **130**, 439–447.

Gregoire, L. and Justin, J. (1969). *In* "Le Cancer et les glandes endocrines" (H. P. Klotz, Ed.), p. 301. L'Expansion, Paris.

Hustin, J. (1973). "Etude du contexte endocrinien du cancer endométrial". Thesis, University of Liège.

Hustin, J. and Kremers, P. (1975). *The Journal of Clinical Endocrinology and Metabolism* **41**, 419–421.

Hustin, J., Cession, G. and Duvivier, J. (1974). *Annales d'Anatomie Pathologique* **19**, 117–126.

Marshall, D. H., Crilly, R. and Nordin, B. E. C. (1978). *Clinical Endocrinology* **9**, 407–412.

Schenker, J. G., Weinstein, D. and Okon, E. (1979). *Cancer* **44**, 1809–1812.

Tseng, L. and Gurpide, E. (1975). *Endocrinology* **97**, 825–833.

Vermeulen, A. (1976). *The Journal of Clinical Endocrinology and Metabolism* **42**, 247–253.

ENDOCRINE CORRELATIONS IN POSTMENOPAUSAL ENDOMETRIAL CANCER

D. Marchesoni, B. Mozzanega, M. Gangemi and G. B. Nardelli

Obstetric and Gynaecological Department, University of Padua, Padua, Italy

INTRODUCTION

Recent studies have shown that significative increases of oestradiol and prolactin plasma levels may be found in women with endometrial cancer, whereas testosterone plasma levels appear to be normal (Benjamin and Deutsch, 1976; Gurpide, 1978; Marchesoni, 1980).

As is well known, the plasma oestradiol levels positively influence prolactin secretion through a sensitization mechanism (Archer, 1977). Moreover, oestradiol can originate from testosterone through processes of peripheral aromatization (Speroff *et al.*, 1978). Thus it is conceivable to compare the correlation coefficients between prolactin and oestradiol and oestradiol and testosterone, relative to postmenopausal age, in patients without endometrial pathology and in patients with endometrial cancer.

SUBJECTS, METHODS AND RESULTS

In our series, 20 patients were free from any endometrial pathology, 20 were affected with a histologically proven endometrial cancer. Correlation coefficients are expressed by regression lines.

In the first group the menopausal duration, expressed in months, is 86.65 ±

Serono Symposium No. 39, "The Menopause: Clinical, Endocrinological and Pathophysiological Aspects", edited by P. Fioretti, L. Martini, G. B. Melis and S. S. C. Yen, 1982. Academic Press, London and New York.

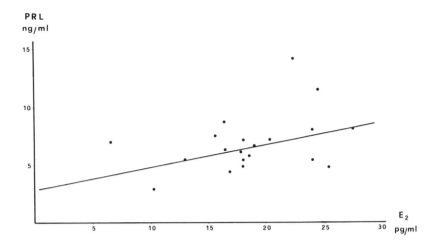

Fig. 1. Correlation between prolactin and oestradiol in control patients.

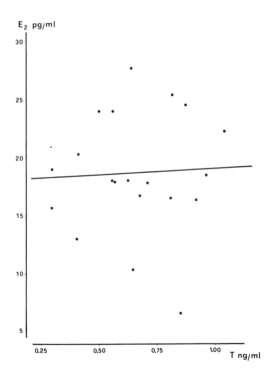

Fig. 2. Correlation between oestradiol and testosterone in control patients.

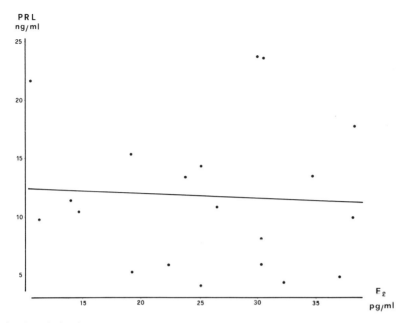

Fig. 3. Correlation between prolactin and oestradiol in cancer patients.

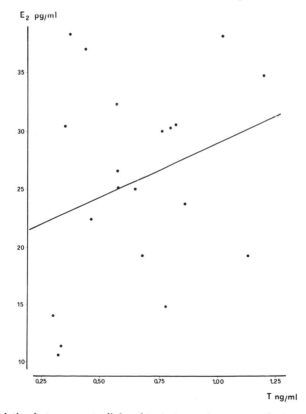

Fig. 4. Correlation between oestradiol and testosterone in cancer patients.

17.78 with a percentage variation coefficient of 91.74; the mean plasma levels are 6.48 ± 2.52 ng/ml for prolactin, 18.61 ± 5.16 pg/ml for oestradiol and 0.66 ± 0.21 ng/ml for testosterone. In the second group the menopausal duration, expressed in months, is 142.48 ± 30.28 with a percentage variation coefficient of 60.71; the mean plasma levels are 11.75 ± 4.87 ng/ml for prolactin, 25.72 ± 5.48 pg/ml for oestradiol and 0.65 ± 0.26 ng/ml for testosterone.

In the first group (Figs 1 and 2) the correlation between prolactin and oestradiol is expressed by $y = 0.193 \cdot x + 2.89$ with $r = 0.439$ ($P < 0.05$); the correlation between oestradiol and testosterone is expressed by $y = 1.236 \cdot x + 17.794$ with $r = 0.0516$ ($P = NS$). In the second group (Figs 3 and 4) the correlation between prolactin and oestradiol is expressed by $y = -0.041 \cdot x + 12.802$ with $r = 0.058$ ($P = NS$); the correlation between oestradiol and testosterone is expressed by $y = 9.265 \cdot x + 19.698$ with $r = 0.283$ ($P = NS$).

CONCLUSIONS

The above mentioned data show the absence of any significant correlation between oestradiol and testosterone, both in the controls and in affected patients; a significant correlation is found in the control patients between prolactin and oestradiol, whereas the same correlation has not been found in affected patients.

We therefore think we can conclude that the high prolactin plasma levels in endometrial cancer don't seem to give adequate justification for the high oestradiol plasma levels.

REFERENCES

Archer, D. F. (1977). *Fertility and Sterility* 28, 125.
Benjamin, F. and Deutsch, S. (1976). *American Journal of Obstetrics and Gynecology* 126, 638.
Gurpide, E. (1978). *Cancer* 38, 503.
Marchesoni, D. (1980). *European Journal of Gynecological Oncology* 1, 32.
Speroff, L., Glass, R. H. and Kase, N. G. (1978). *In* "Clinical Gynecological Endocrinology and Infertility". Williams and Wilkins Co., Baltimore.

PLASMA ANDROSTENEDIONE CONCENTRATIONS IN PRE— AND POSTMENOPAUSAL WOMEN AND IN ENDOMETRIAL PATHOLOGY

D. Mango, P. Scirpa, F. Battaglia, L. Casarella and P. Fiorillo

Department of Obstetrics and Gynecology, Catholic University, Largo Gemelli, Rome, Italy

INTRODUCTION

During the reproductive period the extraglandular aromatization of ovarian and adrenal androstenedione to oestrone contributes 10-50% of the blood's oestrogen production, which mainly originates from the ovary (MacDonald *et al.*, 1976). Since the ovarian function is sensibly reduced, the peripheral conversion of adrenal androstenedione after menopause to oestrone becomes the almost exclusive source of blood oestrogens (Siiteri and MacDonald, 1973; Grodin *et al.*, 1976). Although plasma androstenedione is also reduced in this period (Longcope, 1974), the extent of its conversion increases with aging (Hemsell *et al.*, 1974), obesity (Edman *et al.*, 1978; MacDonald *et al.*, 1978), hepatic disease (Edman *et al.*, 1975; Gordon *et al.*, 1975) and hyperthyroidism (Southern *et al.*, 1974).

A higher androstenedione production has been found in cases of polycystic ovarian disease (Siiteri and MacDonald, 1973), hypertecosis (Aiman *et al.*, 1978) and ovarian tumours (Aiman *et al.*, 1975; MacDonald *et al.*, 1976; Aiman *et al.*, 1977). All these conditions have been implicated in inducing increased risk for endometrial cancer (Siiteri, 1978). However, as far as the role of androstenedione conversion to oestrone in the development of endometrial cancer is concerned, the "estrone hypothesis" of Siiteri *et al.* (1974), conflicting results have been reported

Serono Symposium No. 39, "The Menopause: Clinical, Endocrinological and Pathophysiological Aspects", edited by P. Fioretti, L. Martini, G. B. Melis and S. S. C. Yen, 1982. Academic Press, London and New York.

(Hausknecht and Gusberg, 1973; Rizkallah *et al.*, 1975; Calanog *et al.*, 1977; MacDonald *et al.*, 1978; Nisker *et al.*, 1978; Reed *et al.*, 1979).

In this study we have determined the androstenedione plasma levels by a new, sensitive and specific radioimmunoassay method, during the reproductive and menopausal periods in a large number of healthy women or women affected by dysfunctional, pre-neoplastic and neoplastic endometrial pathology. Preliminary data about ovarian pathology are also presented.

MATERIALS AND METHODS

Fifty normal women during the reproductive period (18-35 years), 25 in the premenopausal period (40-48 years) and 50 in the postmenopausal period (50-70 years) were examined.

Eighty-eight patients with pre- and postmenopausal uterine bleeding were hospitalized and the diagnosis was verified by fractional curettage. Those patients who were found to have only atrophic or proliferative or irregularly mature endometrium, were ranked as being affected by dysfunctional bleeding in premenopause (21 cases, group A) and in postmenopause (21 cases, group B). Twenty-three patients in the pre- and postmenopausal periods presented glandular hyperplasia of endometrium, of simple, cystic or adenomatous kind, and therefore were considered in the same group (group C). Finally, 22 patients in the postmenopausal period presented endometrial adenocarcinoma (group D). Ten patients affected by adenocarcinoma of the ovary (all stages) and six affected by non-endocrine benign ovarian tumours (two cases of ovarian cysts, two cases of polycistic ovary, two cases of dermoid cysts) have been preliminary examined. Some of the outpatients and a few hospitalized ones were receiving antihypertensive agents, and/or digitalis and oral hypoglycaemic medications; none had received oestrogen treatment for at least 4 weeks before examination. Several of the examined women were obese.

Plasma androstenedione determinations were performed by a sensitive, specific and accurate radioimmunoassay, without chromatography (Montemurro *et al.*, 1980). The antiserum has been raised in New Zealand rabbits, inoculated with 11α-hydroxy-androst-4-ene-3,17-dione-hemisuccinate bovine serum albumin and showed high affinity to the former steroid (K_d = 7.6 × 10^{-11} M). The method consists of an initial n-hexane extraction of plasma, spiked with a tracer amount of tritiated androstenedione (for the calculation of recovery) and followed by a conventional radioimmunoassay of the plasma extract.

Table I.   Plasma androstenedione concentrations in normal women.

Age (years)	No. of cases	Androstenedione ng/ml (mean ± SD)
18–35	50	0.93 ± 0.32
40–48	25	0.88 ± 0.30
50–70	50	0.52 ± 0.17

RESULTS

As it may be seen in Table I, plasma androstenedione concentrations resulted 0.93 ± 0.32 ng/ml (mean ± SD) during reproductive age and 0.88 ± 0.30 ng/ml during the 5th decade of life (Premenopausal women), while significantly lower values were obtained during the postmenopausal period (0.52 ± 0.17 ng/ml; $P < 0.001$).

Table II shows that plasma androstenedione concentrations in subjects with dysfunctional uterine bleeding in premenopause (group A) and in postmenopause (group B) are similar to those obtained in healthy women of the same age. On the other hand, significantly higher values were obtained in subjects affected by endometrial hyperplasia (group C, $P < 0.02$). Androstenedione concentrations in patients with endometrial cancer in postmenopause (group D) do not differ from those obtained in normal women. Androstenedione levels in patients with ovarian adenocarcinoma and benign ovarian pathology resulted 1.56 ± 0.61 ng/ml and 2.03 ± 1.03 ng/ml, respectively (Table III).

Table II. Plasma androstenedione concentrations in endometrial pathology.

	No. of cases	Androstenedione ng/ml (mean ± SD)
(A) Dysfunctional uterine bleeding in premenopause	21	0.93 ± 0.38
(B) Dysfunctional uterine bleeding in postmenopause	21	0.54 ± 0.24
(C) Endometrial hyperplasia	23	1.20 ± 0.51
(D) Endometrial adenocarcinoma	22	0.55 ± 0.27

Table III. Plasma androstenedione concentrations in ovarian pathology (preliminary data).

	No. of cases	Androstenedione ng/ml (mean ± SD)
Ovarian adenocarcinoma	10	1.56 ± 0.61
Benign ovarian tumours	6	2.03 ± 1.03

DISCUSSION

It is well established that androstenedione is a prehormone for extraglandular oestrogen formation. This mechanism, although active throughout the reproductive years, represents the almost exclusive source of blood oestrogens in puberty and after the menopause. Although many physiological and pathological conditions (i.e. age and obesity) may increase the conversion rate of androstenedione to oestrone, it has been found that plasma androstenedione concentration is the main determinant of plasma oestrone (Marshall *et al.*, 1978). During the reproductive and premenopausal years, when both the ovaries and the adrenal glands contribute to the androstenedione production, plasma androstenedione concentrations resulted 0.93 ± 0.32 ng/ml and 0.88 ± 0.30 ng/ml respectively. These values are not significantly different from those obtained in the cases of dysfunctional uterine bleeding in premenopause. During the postmenopausal period the plasma androstenedione concentrations significantly fall to mean values of 0.52 ± 0.17 ng/ml, and, although our data do not consider the relative contributions of adrenal glands and the ovary, this is probably due to the reduced ovarian production. The fact that androstenedione values are lower than those obtained by other authors (Longcope, 1974; Judd *et al.*, 1974; Greenblatt *et al.*, 1976) seems to be ascribed to the higher specificity of our antiserum. Like our observations in the premenopause, the concentrations of androstenedione in the postmenopause, in cases of dysfunctional uterine bleedings, do not differ from the values observed in normal women of the same age.

Regarding the controversial role of androstenedione conversion to oestrone in the development of endometrial cancer, our results indicate significantly higher values in cases of endometrial hyperplasia than in normal women, while androstenedione values are within the normal range in the presence of endometrial cancer in the postmenopause. These results are in agreement with those of Reed *et al.* (1979), who found normal androstenedione concentrations in four women affected by endometrial cancer. Conversely Calanog *et al.* (1977) obtained significantly higher values in 14 patients affected by the same disease. On the other hand, Reed *et al.* (1979) did not find an increased conversion of androstenedione to oestrone in presence of endometrial cancer.

The high androstenedione plasma levels obtained by us in nonendocrine ovarian tumours may be explained in terms of steroid secretion by the hyperplastic stromal cells of the ovary, according to MacDonald *et al.* (1976) and Aiman *et al.* (1977).

On the basis of these results it seems that the "oestrone hypothesis" (Siiteri *et al.*, 1974) cannot be confirmed in the presence of endometrial adenocarcinoma. However, the high androstenedione values in patients with endometrial hyperplasia and ovarian disease (both high risk conditions for the development of endometrial cancer) suggest that this hormonal alteration may be only present before the development of endometrial neoplasia.

ACKNOWLEDGEMENTS

This work was partly supported by a grant from the Ministero della Pubblica Istruzione, Italy.

REFERENCES

Aiman, E. J., Edman, C. D., Siiteri, P. K. and MacDonald, P. C. (1975). *Gynecology Investigation* **6**, 21.
Aiman, E. J., Nalick, R. H., Jacobs, A., Porter, J. C., Edman, C. D., Vellios, F. and MacDonald, P. C. (1977). *Obstetrics and Gynecology* **49**, 695.

Aiman, E. J., Edman, C. D., Worley, R. J. and MacDonald, P. C. (1978).
Obstetrics and Gynecology **51**, 1.

Calanog, A., Sall, S., Gordon, G. G. and Southern, A. L. (1977). *American Journal of Obstetrics and Gynecology* **129**, 553.

Edman, C. D., MacDonald, P. C. and Combes, B. (1975). *Gastroenterology* **69**, 819,

Edman, C. D., Aiman, E. J., Porter, J. C. and MacDonald, P. C. (1978). *American Journal of Obstetrics and Gynecology* **130**, 439.

Gordon, G. G., Olivo, J., Rafii, F. and Southren, A. L. (1975). *Journal of Clinical Endocrinology and Metabolism* **40**, 1018.

Greenblatt, R. B., Colle, M. L. and Mahesh, V. B. (1976). *Obstetrics and Gynecology* **47**, 383.

Grodin, J. M., Siiteri, P. K. and MacDonald, P. C. (1976). *Journal of Clinical Endocrinology and Metabolism* **36**, 207.

Hausknecht, R. U. and Gusberg, S. B. (1973). *American Journal of Obstetrics and Gynecology* **116**, 981.

Hemsell, D. L., Grodin, J. M., Brenner, P. F., Siiteri, P. K. and MacDonald, P. C. (1974). *Journal of Clinical Endocrinology and Metabolism* **38**, 476.

Judd, H. L., Judd, G. E., Lucas, W. E. and Yen, S. S. C. (1974). *Journal of Clinical Endocrinology and Metabolism* **39**, 1020.

Longcope, C. (1974). *In* "The Menopausal Syndrome" (R. B. Greenblatt, V. B. Mahesh and P. G. MacDonough, Eds), 6–11. Medcom Press, New York.

MacDonald, P. C., Rombaut, R. P. and Siiteri, P. K. (1967). *Journal of Clinical Endocrinology and Metabolism* **27**, 1103.

MacDonald, P. C., Grodin, J. M., Edman, C. D., Vellios, F. and Siiteri, P. K. (1976). *Obstetrics and Gynecology* **47**, 644.

MacDonald, P. C., Edman, C. D., Hemsell, D. L., Porter, J. C. and Siiteri, P. K. (1978). *American Journal of Obstetrics and Gynecology* **130**, 448.

Marshall, D. H., Crilly, R. and Nordin, B. E. C. (1978). *Clinical Endocrinology* **9**, 407.

Montemurro, A., Johnson, M. W., Barile, G. and Youssefnejadian, E. (1980). *Journal of Steroid Biochemistry* (in press).

Nisker, J. A., Ramzy, I. and Collins, J. A. (1978). *American Journal of Obstetrics and Gynecology* **130**, 546.

Reed, M. J., Hutton, J. D., Baxendale, P. M., James, V. H. T., Jacobs, H. S. and Fisher, R. T. (1979). *Journal of Steroid Biochemistry* **11**, 905.

Rizkallah, T. H., Tovell, H. M. M. and Kelly, W. G. (1975). *Journal of Clinical Endocrinology and Metabolism* **40**, 1045.

Siiteri, P. K. (1978). *Cancer Research* **38**, 4360.

Siiteri, P. K. and MacDonald, P. C. (1973). *In* "Handbook of Physiology, Section 7, Endocrinology" (G. B. Astwood and R. O. Greep, Eds). American Physiological Society, Washington.

Siiteri, P. K., Schwarz, P. E. and MacDonald, P. C. (1974). *Gynecologic Oncology* **2**, 228.

Southren, A. L., Olivo, J., Gordon, G. G., Vittek, J., Brener, J. and Rafii, F. (1974). *Journal of Clinical Endocrinology and Metabolism* **38**, 207.

SECTION VI
CLINICAL PATHOLOGY OF THE POSTMENOPAUSE

PRECOCIOUS OVARIAN FAILURE

P. T. Tho and P. G. McDonough

Department of Obstetrics and Gynecology, Medical College of Georgia, Augusta, Georgia, USA

INTRODUCTION

Menopause is physiologic and refers to the cessation of ovarian activity related to aging. Precocious menopause includes all pathologic conditions causing ovarian failure prior to the normal timing of physiologic ovarian exhaustion. The conditions or causes predisposing to premature gonadal failure may be present during fetal life, at birth, in childhood or develop during early reproduction life. The common diagnostic denominator is the elevation of pituitary gonadotropins as a result of a decrease in estrogen production and loss of the negative feedback mechanism. The precise etiology of premature ovarian failure in many instances is obscure. Ovarian failure is usually a consistent sequela of sex chromosome privations, but other known and presumed causes are not necessarily consistent etiologic agents. Irrespective of the cause, ovarian failure is not necessarily an all or none phenomenon. Follicular depletion may be incomplete and a few residual follicles under the effect of elevated gonadotropins may produce periodic bursts of estrogenic activity and even fertility. A comprehension of causes and pathologic mechanisms producing premature ovarian failure is facilitated by a thorough knowledge of both ovarian morphogenesis and the ontogeny of the human hypothalamic pituitary ovarian axis.

Serono Symposium No. 39, "The Menopause: Clinical, Endocrinological and Pathophysiological Aspects", edited by P. Fioretti, L. Martini, G. B. Melis and S. S. C. Yen, 1982. Academic Press, London and New York.

OVARIAN MORPHOGENESIS AND ONTOGENY OF THE FOLLICULAR
APPARATUS

The cytogenetic sex of an embryo is determined at conception but the ovary does not become morphologically distinct until the 6th to 8th week of intrauterine life. At approximately 4 weeks of embryonic development, the genital ridge develops, consisting structurally of an external layer of coelomic epithelium covering an internal core of mesenchyme. At 5 weeks, the indifferent gonadal anlage is formed with incorporation of the primitive germ cells into the genital ridge. The primitive germ cells have an extragenital origin. They migrate from the entoderm of the yolk sac and the hindgut into the gonadal primordia by amoeboid movement. Their migration has been traced, using alkaline phosphatase as a marker. Their journey is complete by the 5th week and no germ cells are found in the extragenital sites after 8 weeks. Mitotic multiplication of the initial germ cell endowment continues in the ridge until the original number is increased to approximately 100 000.

Histologic differentiation of the gonad begins promptly after the arrival of the primitive germ cells. The indifferent gonad is transformed into a testis or an ovary, depending upon the genetic constitution of the germ cells in the gonadal primordium. Differentiation occurs earlier in the testicular line at 4–6 weeks and later in the ovarian line at 6–8 weeks. Testicular formation is controlled by the masculinizing determinant localized on the short arm of the Y chromosome. The primordial germ cells with intact XY sex chromosomal complement congregate in the medullary area and are arranged in cords, the precursors of the seminiferous tubules. The primordial germ cells, having XX genotype and also rare XY genotype devoid of genetically active short arm Y material congregate essentially in the cortical area to form the primitive ovarian anlage. The primordial germ cells, now termed oogonia, continue to multiply rapidly by mitosis. Active mitotic proliferation ceases by the 20th week, giving a finite fetal oogonial endowment reaching 6–7 million by this time. The oogonia become primary oocytes when they enter the first meiotic division, indicating the first stage of ovarian exocrine maturation.

After the cessation of mitotic division, the oogonium enters an interphase in which DNA synthesis occurs in preparation for the first meiotic division. This phase is called preleptotene and is followed by the leptotene stage in which the chromosomes become thicker and more identifiable. In the next stage, or zygotene, the germ cell chromosomes begin to pair, forming 23 homologous bivalents. These chromosomes, arranged in bivalents or pairs, condense and undergo spiralization. During this process, synapsis or crossing over occurs, mediated by the chromatids which are formed by the longitudinal splitting of each of the paired chromosomes. The chromatids break and rejoin during spiralization with exchange of paternal and maternal DNA material, resulting in gene reassortment. Following this pachytene stage, the chromosomes become more diffuse and the oocyte enters a prolonged arrested quiescent state known as dictyotene. The dormant dictyotene stage is terminated only if the primary oocyte is to be ovulated or undergo precocious maturation leading to atresia. Most of the primary oocytes are in this arrested prophase (dictyotene) by 28 weeks of fetal life.

The initial stages of this meiotic process begin in oogonia that are not surrounded by follicular cells. However, early in meiotic prophase, the oocytes are quickly enveloped by a single layer of flattened granulosa cells. This oocyte-single layer granulosa complex constitutes the primordial follicule. Later in development, the granulosa cells surround the oocytes completely, forming the primary follicles. Oocyte survival depends in some way upon the integrity of this complete follicular ring. This enveloping, or mantling process, which takes place from the 16th fetal week until shortly after birth, seems to require the presence in the oocyte of two intact active X chromosomes (Franchi and Baker, 1973). Anatomical and presumably biochemical inactivation of one of the X chromosomes occurs in all female somatic cells by the 50th day (Migeon and Kennedy, 1975). In the human oocyte, both X chromosomes are presumed active as evidenced by full expression of both G_6PD alleles on electrophoretic patterns (Gartler *et al.*, 1973). Gartler *et al.* (1975) suggested that the primordial germ cells and oogonia are X inactivated and that reactivation of the second X chromosome occurs as the germ cells enter into meiosis. It is possible, however, that human germ cells are never subject to X chromosome inactivation. In the 45,X female, the oocytes go through their growth with half of the normal X chromosome activity. This marked deficiency of X linked products might affect meiotic control mechanisms and accelerate the primary oocyte through the complete meiotic cycle prematurely, leading to excessive follicular atresia and depletion. Jirásek (1976) suggests that X chromosome privation in germ cells is associated with an incomplete follicular mantle, resulting in degeneration of the oocyte shortly after formation of the primary follicles. Whether a deficiency of X chromosome activity thwarts mantle formation leading to accelerated uncontrolled meiosis is enigmatic.

Follicular growth begins at 20 weeks of fetal life when the primary oocyte starts to enlarge and the granulosa cells multiply. After 24 weeks, the multiplication of granulosa cells results in the formation of multi-layered primary follicles and a few antral follicles. These antral follicles are encapsulated by epitheloid theca interna cells which presumably are capable of some steroidogenesis. The follicle population can be categorized morphologically into two pools of non-proliferating and proliferating follicles (Schwartz *et al.*, 1974). The latter are characterized by an increase in the numbers of granulosa cells surrounding the oocyte. Once a follicle enters the proliferating pool, it must proceed onto maturation and ovulation or it degenerates by atresia. The oocyte and follicle population therefore declines throughout the ovary life span. Follicular growth and atresia constitute a continuous basic biological phenomenon that starts at 6 months of fetal life, continues during childhood and into the reproductive years. It manages to continue uninterrupted in spite of pregnancy, lactation and other acyclic events (Peters *et al.*, 1975). Information obtained from hypophysectomized animals indicates that exogenous FSH and LH can induce follicular maturation. Pituitary gonadotropins seem to be responsible in some way for the proliferative events leading to follicular maturation and atresia.

ONTOGENY OF THE HYPOTHALAMUS PITUITARY GONADAL CIRCUIT AND DIAGNOSIS OF OVARIAN FAILURE

The follicle is the functional subunit of the ovary under hypothalamic pituitary control. Follicular depletion resulting in estradiol reduction and gonadotropin elevation is the basic anatomical and biochemical event of primary ovarian failure.

Follicular maturation and atresia are continuous uninterrupted processes from fetal ovarian organogenesis to the time of menopausal exhaustion. Nevertheless, age related differences and pathologic aberrations in hypothalamic pituitary control mechanism may alter the different stages of maturation of the follicle.

Since maternal concentrations of FSH and LH are low, amniotic fluid gonadotropins are most likely of fetal origin. In both sexes, FSH and LH appear in fetal serum and amniotic fluid at about 11-12 weeks, increase to peak levels between 14-20 weeks, then decline promptly to low values that persist until term. The low third trimester values are presumably due to fetal pituitary inhibition by placental estrogens. This observation seems to suggest that the negative feedback mechanism matures and becomes operative after midgestation. Gonadotropin levels are much higher in the female than in the male fetus and the difference seems to indicate that maturation of the negative feedback mechanism by steroids occurs earlier in males than in females or that feedback of androgens is established before that of estrogens. The rapid fall of serum gonadotropins in both male and female fetuses after midgestation coincides with the marked rise in fetal estrogen levels of placental origin. This suggests that the low set point for negative feedback in the prepubertal child is not fully developed until late in infancy or early childhood. Neonatal withdrawal of placental estrogens elicits a brisk increase in pituitary gonadotropin secretion. This increase begins at the end of the first week of life and continues until about 3 months of age. There is a decline to a nadir around 3 to 4 years of age, reflecting pituitary suppression by ovarian steroids (Winter *et al*. 1971). Nevertheless, the ovary in childhood is sensitive to pituitary hormones and considerable numbers of oocytes in the proliferative follicles attempt to mature precociously. In the absence of full hypothalamic control, this maturation cannot culminate in ovulation and such follicles are destined to degenerate. The period from 4 to 8 years is characterized by low levels of gonadotropins and estradiol. The pituitary response to Gonadotropin Releasing Hormone (GnRH) during this time of low baseline gonadotropin is characterized principally by a greater FSH than LH release. After the age of 8, with the approach of puberty there is a progressive higher set point for negative feedback. Accompanying this decrease in the sensitivity of hypothalamic receptors to sex steroids is an increased secretion of gonadotropins and consequent stimulation of sex steroid output. This change in sensitivity appears to correlate with general somatic and central nervous system maturation, resulting in increased secretion of GnRH. This decreased sensitivity is a major determinant of the increased gonadotropin secretion at puberty. The germ cell population at puberty has been reduced to 300 000 from which only 300 will finally ovulate over the subsequent 35-40 years of adult life. For every successful ovulatory cycle, approximately 1000 follicles will become atretic. The adolescent hypothalamic pituitary ovarian unit finally matures to the point that the follicle stimulated by FSH secretes sufficient estradiol to trigger a midcycle ovulatory surge of LH and FSH followed by a luteal rise in serum progesterone level. This development of positive feedback is the last step in hypothalamic pituitary ovarian maturation. Estradiol plays a key role in the maturation of the pubertal axis and maintenance of the recycling mechanism. It maintains follicular sensitivity to FSH by inducing FSH receptors, enhances follicle response to LH by working synergistically with FSH to induce LH receptors and triggers ovulation through its positive feedback effect on the LH surge (McNatty, 1978).

At approximately 40 years of age, the ovary has a few thousand residual follicles which are less and less sensitive to FSH stimulation and have decreased ability to synthesise estradiol. Estradiol levels fall and with removal of this feedback inhibition gonadotropin levels become elevated. During the early premenopausal years, monotropic exacerbated late luteal increments of FSH levels constitute the earliest biochemical change portending ovarian failure (Sherman and Korenman, 1975). At this time estradiol is in the low normal range and no significant change has been observed in serum LH and progesterone values. The progression from this sporadic monotropic increase of FSH to a persistent elevation of both gonadotropins and low estradiol has been observed. Physiologic ovarian failure occurs at the mean age of 50. It is preceded by approximately 10 years of gradual endocrine changes related to follicular depletion. Premature ovarian failure can occur at any age before 35 years. Diagnosis of ovarian failure beyond 11-12 years of age is based principally upon castrate levels of pituitary gonadotropins. Diagnosis in childhood and infancy requires some knowledge of the similarities and differences between normal and agonadal children. In agonadal infants and children, the overall biphasic pattern of gonadotropin secretion is qualitatively similar to that observed in normal females, although the levels of FSH and LH are increased above the age specific normal range. Conte *et al.* (1980) observed this biphasic pattern in both basal and GnRH stimulated gonadotropin levels. Although the increase is significant under 5 years of age and striking after age of 11 years, in some agonadal girls between 5 and 11 years of age, both basal and readily releasable gonadotropins are comparable to values in normal prepubertal children (Conte *et al.*, 1980). The biochemical and functional diagnosis of ovarian failure is not always evident in some agonadal prepubertal children in this age group on the basis of both basal gonadotropin concentrations and response to GnRH. The marked decrease in circulating gonadotropins and gonadotropin reserve to values within and only slightly greater than the range for age matched normal children, in the absence of functional gonads, suggests a central nervous system inhibitory mechanism which is independent of negative gonadal feedback mechanism and which restrains gonadotropin synthesis and secretion and inhibits puberty between early childhood and adolescence in normal females.

The ranges of ovarian function seen in individuals who have or develop ovarian failure are best comprehended when one appreciates the numerous factors contributing to normal ovarian development and function. These factors, discussed under ovarian morphogenesis are summarized here as:

(1) Absence of genetically active Y material and the presence of two intact and genetically active X chromosomes in the germ cell line.
(2) Germ cell migration to the ridge.
(3) Mitotic activity in the ridge.
(4) Development of granulosa cell mantle.
(5) Normal transformation of the oogonium into a primary oocyte with controlled arrest of development at the dictyotene stage.
(6) Physiologic response of primary follicle to fetal FSH.

Pathology interfering with these normal mechanisms may produce ovarian failure. Knowledge of the normal hypothalamic pituitary ovarian axis at different ages assists in the diagnostic evaluation of individuals suspect for ovarian failure.

Intrauterine diagnosis of ovarian failure is suggested in the presence of a sex chromosome anomaly incidently identified during amniotic fluid karyotyping for a genetic reason. However, endocrine confirmation of ovarian failure during fetal life is impossible, since the normal fetal ovary is functionally quiescent and the negative feedback in the fetus is operated by the fetal estrogens of placental origin. After puberty, the biochemical diagnosis is essentially obvious with basal gonadotropin determinations. Basal gonadotropins and complementary GnRH stimulated gonadotropins mostly provide for separating the normal prepubertal child from a prepubertal agonadal child. These studies may not however substantiate definitive evidence of ovarian failure in the child between 5 and 11 years of age because of overlapping gonadotropin levels during this period of life.

ETIOLOGY OF PREMATURE OVARIAN FAILURE

Since the X chromosome privation is consistently associated with primary ovarian failure, two broad cytogenetic categories of this entity can be recognized. Patients with absent or deleted X chromosome material form a group of individuals with Chromosomally Incompetent Ovarian Failure (CIOF). Patients having normal intact sex chromosome constitution comprise a group of Chromosomally Competent Ovarian Failure (CCOF) individuals.

CIOF Group

Two consistent clinical correlates in the CIOF subjects are short stature and failure of gonadal development. Although shortness represents a constant clinical stigmata of CIOF, other important somatic anomalies comprise cardiovascular renal malformations, essentially coarctation of the aorta and horseshoe kidney. Two intact active X chromosomes in the germ cells are necessary for normal somatic development and follicular formation. Genotype phenotype correlations seem to suggest that the gonadal determinants are located near the centromere on both the long and short arm of the X chromosome. Statural determinants are probably located on the short arm of the X chromosome, but exceptions to this generalization have been reported. Examination of embryonic, fetal and neonatal ovaries with 45,X or X chromosome mosaicism indicate normal germ cells up until 4 months of fetal life and mostly poor follicular formation and rapid germ cell atresia thereafter (Conen and Glass, 1963; Carr *et al.*, 1968; Kohn *et al.*, 1977). The granulosa layer surrounding the 45,X primary oocytes appears to be incomplete. Atretic utilization of these defective primary oocytes seems to be markedly accelerated. One might speculate that dose related X deficiency limits follicular growth and the meiotic control mechanisms are lost with rapid abnormal progression through all the stages of meiosis (Burgoyne and Biggers, 1976). Structural abnormalities of the Y chromosome such as 46,X,i(Yq) or deletion of the Y chromosome short arm have been reported in individuals with female phenotype, short stature and gonadal dysgenesis (Böök *et al.*, 1973). This can be well correlated with the hypothesis that ovarian morphogenesis requires both absence of the genetically active Y chromosome material and presence of two intact genetically active X chromosomes.

Among 82 patients seen in our institution with primary ovarian failure, 52, or 63%, presented with sex chromosome anomalies (Fig. 1). The most common geno-type in this CIOF group is X chromosome mosaicism (27/52, or 51%). The classical 45,X constitutes only 32% (18/52) of the chromosomally incompetent group. The most frequent chromosome mosaicism is 45,X/46,XY. The increased incidence of identical twinning in sibships involving 45,X/46,XY form seems to suggest a post segmentation divisional error following an attempt for 46,XY identical twinning. The abnormal morphology of the paternal Y chromosome, if demonstrated, might have a causal relationship with this cytogenetic anomaly. There appears to be no consistent correlation between the relative representation of 45,X and 46,XY cell lines to modify toward streak or testicular formation. More patients in this group of 45,X/46,XY individuals have bilateral streak gonads than sexual ambiguity with one streak on one side and one testis on the other side. Since there is a high incidence of neoplastic formation associated with the Y component, gonadal extirpation is mandatory in both masculinized and non-masculinized 45,X/46,XY subjects. This is also applicable to 46,XY geno-types presenting with privation of the Y chromosome short arm material. Among our nine patients with 45,X/46,XY, 3 had gonadoblastomas.

The principal single cell line chromosomal anomalies in CIOF patients are 45,X and 46,X,i(Xq). The classical 45,X aberration should alert some precaution since an XY cell line might be missed if generous cell counts are not carried out and supplemented with H- Y antigen studies to detect a 46,XY cell line.

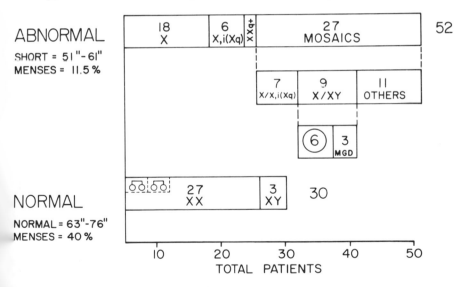

Fig. 1. Patients beyond 12 years with primary ovarian failure (N = 82)—sex chromosomes constitutions.

(From McDonough, P. G., Byrd, J. R., Tho, P. T. and Mahesh, V. B: Phenotypic and cyto-genetic findings in 82 patients with ovarian failure—changing trends. *Fertility and Sterility* 28, 638; 1977. Reproduced with the permission of the publisher, The American Fertility Society).

The genotype with long arm X isochromosome 46,X,i(Xq) should require periodic evaluation of the thyroid, since thyroid autoimmune disorders are frequently associated with this X chromosome constitution. One case of Hashimoto thyroiditis and one case of thyroid carcinoma out of six patients with long arm X isochromosome were present in our series. A practical point concerning this genotype is that it is not infrequent to mistake a long arm isochromosome X with a normal X chromosome if some banding technique is not used. Combined short stature and ovarian failure should call for suspicion of miskaryotyping if the report is normal 46, XX. All our patients with CIOF are short with a height of less than 63 inches. Cardiovascular renal anomalies were identified in 12 of the 52, or 23%, of the CIOF patients. Among our 52 patients with CIOF, 11.5% experienced a short menstrual life. We do not have any CIOF patients becoming pregnant. There have been increasing reports of fertility in patients with CIOF under estrogen replacement therapy. The most likely explanation is that estrogen enhances the response of follicles to FSH and causes an increased receptor content for FSH and LH (Richards *et al.*, 1976).

CCOF Group

Unlike the CIOF patients, the individuals with intact sex chromosomes and ovarian failure (CCOF) present with normal female phenotype, normal stature with heights greater than 63 inches. They have either 46,XX or 46,XY sex chromosome constitutions and represent 30 out of 82 patients (36%) with primary ovarian failure. The intact chromosomes guarantee normal stature. Ovarian failure with deficient estrogen production delays epiphyseal closure leading to increased final height. These patients escape the diagnosis of ovarian failure at younger ages. They usally present at chronologic age of puberty for evaluation of sexual infantilism and amenorrhea. Forty percent of the CCOF females in our series have a brief menstrual history. None of the CCOF patients in our series has reported a history of pregnancy. Determination of FSH levels is the clue in diagnosing ovarian failure in this group. Most of these individuals have streak gonads except for the patients with Savage Syndrome, in which the follicular apparatus is well preserved (Jones and DeMoraes-Ruehsen, 1969). Diagnostic laparoscopy and ovarian biopsy are necessary for gonadal visualization and histologic distinction between follicular depletion and follicular dormancy type of ovarian failure. The etiologies of CCOF are diverse and mostly ill defined (Table I).

XY Forms of CCOF

XY Gonadal Dysgenesis of Swyer's Syndrome

This form is infrequent, but constitutes an important group, since its diagnosis requires gonadal extirpation for the patient and a search for other affected female siblings in the family (McDonough *et al.*, 1977a). Testicular regression occurring before the production of mullerian inhibiting factor is the most likely pathologic mechanism. These patients have normal female external genitalia, mullerian systems, bilateral streak gonads, elevated gonadotropin concentrations and H-Y antigen studies may be positive (Dorus *et al.*, 1977) or negative (Ghosh *et al.*,

Table 1. Etiologies of 46,XX forms of chromosomally competent ovarian failure (CCOF).

(1) Autosomal recessive
(2) Environmental factors

 (a) Virus
 (b) Radiation therapy
 (c) Cytotoxic drugs

(3) Autosomal abnormalities
(4) Autoimmune disease
(5) Infectious process – Infiltrative disease
(6) Myotonia dystrophica
(7) Ataxia telangiectasia
(8) 17α Hydroxylase deficiency
(9) Resistant ovary syndrome

1980). Although sexual infantilism and primary amenorrhea are the usual features of this entity, occasionally XY gonadal dysgenesis patients were described with fairly well developed breast tissue. Neoplasia of the streak gonads, usually a gonadoblastoma or, rarely, a dysgerminoma frequently occurs in patients with 46,XY gonadal dysgenesis (Schellas, 1974; Amarose *et al.*, 1977). All patients diagnosed as having 46, XY gonadal dysgenesis should have their ridges removed. Gonadoblastoma was present at laparotomy in two of the three XY gonadal dysgenesis patients in our series. All three patients were sexually infantile and amenorrheic. No renal anomalies were present in our series of three 46,XY gonadal dysgenesis patients. Horseshoe kidney was recently reported in association with this entity (Swanson and Chapler, 1978). Familial aggregation has been documented by reports of affected sibs, concordant monozygotic twins and affected individuals in a sibship with transmission through unaffected females (Espinear *et al.*, 1970). Vertical transmission and absence of parental consanguinity clearly suggests the possible role of an X linked gene. With the advent of H- Y antigen, two forms of XY gonadal dysgenesis can be identified. In the 46,XY gonadal dysgenesis individual with negative H- Y antigen typing, failure of testicular development is due to a mutational suppression of the testis determining gene, located on the Y short arm by a regulatory gene of the X chromosome. In the 46,XY gonadal dysgenesis individuals with positive H- Y antigen typing, gonadal maldevelopment is due to a functional absence of H- Y antigen due to deficiency of specific gonadal receptors for H- Y antigen (Wachtel, 1979).

XY Agonadism or Empty Pelvis Syndrome

First described by Overzier and Linden, this entity comprises complete absence of the gonads and wolfian and mullerian systems. The individuals in this category present usually at puberty for evaluation of sexual infantilism and primary amenorrhea. They have normal female external genitalia with absence of the vagina. No gonadal structures, mullerian or wolfian derivatives are found at laparotomy. They resemble the XY gonadal dysgenesis patients by their phenotype and genotype, but they lack internal genitalia and vagina (Dewhurst *et al.*, 1963; Penney and Betz, 1977). In these individuals perhaps the fetal testis was functional for a sufficient time to induce mullerian duct inhibition, but not long enough to maintain wolfian duct development.

XX Forms of CCOF

Most of these patients have streak gonads as the only anatomic abnormal finding and the prevailing consensus as to etiology is recessive inheritance. The genetic theory is probably an oversimplification of the problem and etiologic factors in this group are likely diverse (Table I).

Single Gene Etiology, Autosomal Recessive

Most of these individuals are phenotypic females with streak gonads resulting in an eunochoid habitus, primary amenorrhea, lack of secondary sexual development. Their gonadal streaks are identical to that seen in CIOF patients. As in the patients with X chromosome anomalies, they have a wide spectrum of residual follicular population and a significant percentage of the 46,XX gonadal dysgenesis patients have estrogenic function with fairly good breast development and a menstrual history, varying from one menses to several years of monthly periods, but mostly oligohypomenorrhea. Among our series of 27 patients with 46,XX CCOF, 12 have normal female secondary sex characteristics and experience an abbreviated menstrual history. None of them has presented a normal long-term menstrual life, nor has become pregnant (McDonough *et al.*, 1977a). Gonadal visualization by laparoscopy or laparotomy was performed in 24 of the 27 CCOF patients and the gonadal morphology was consistently rudimentary streak gonads. The only exceptions were two patients in whom normal ovarian contour was preserved, but the ovaries were reduced in size (approximately 2 cm x 1 cm) and bilateral ovarian biopsy in both instances revealed only fibrous stroma with absence of follicular apparatus. It is difficult to predict any correlation between gonadal morphology and ovarian endocrine activity. Familial aggregration, parental consanguinity and association with neuroauditory abnormalities in affected siblings seem to support the hypothesis of autosomal recessive inheritance (Nazareth *et al.*, 1977). In our series of 27 patients with 46,XX constitution genotype, are two sets of sisters: one pair concordant for ovarian failure have SS and SA genotype for sickle cell hemoglobin (McDonough and Byrd, 1970).

Environmental Etiology

Competent 46,XX ovarian failure may occasionally occur as a result of a pre- or postnatal environmental insult interfering with germ cell endowment. Extrinsic factors can prevent migration, disturb early mitotic activity in the genital ridge, disrupt meiotic pairing of chromosomes or disrupt the follicular apparatus of the fully developed ovary. Viruses, radiation and cytotoxic drugs have been known as etiologic factors that can cause ovarian failure.

Virus

Morrison *et al.* (1975) have reported three cases of premature ovarian failure due to mumps oophoritis which was acquired *in utero* at term, at puberty and later in reproductive life, respectively with positive mump skin test and elevated antibody titer at the time of evaluation for ovarian failure. The myxovirus might have destroyed directly the follicles in a fully developed ovary in these particular cases. We have in our series of CCOF patients a monozygotic twin discordant for ovarian failure with her otherwise identical twin sister. Both twins had rubella at the age of 2 years with much higher fever in the affected twin than her normal twin. The monozygotic twin situation and the clinical history of viral illness suggest that environmental insult is most likely the etiology for rapid follicular atresia and consequently ovarian failure (McDonough *et al.*, 1977b).

Radiation

Ovarian failure has been recently reported following inadvertent ovarian irradiation in patients with Hodgkin's disease. In a retrospective study of 22 patients with Hodgkin's disease, Thomas *et al.* (1976) found that doses of irradiation to the ovaries above 500 rads was associated with endocrine ovarian failure. Such doses consistently occurred with the inverted Y exposure in which 3500 rads were delivered to the paraaortic, iliac and inguinal nodes. The ovaries were transposed to a midline position (bilateral midline oophoropexy) where they were shielded from the direct beam of radiation in an attempt to preserve their function. Only one of the 12 patients so treated and whose ovaries were estimated to have received 650 and 700 rads on either side, became pregnant 6 years after therapy, but no gonadotropin values are available for this particular case. All the other 11 subjects had FSH levels in the castrate range (Thomas *et al.*, 1976). Baker *et al.* (1972) used the same midline oophoropexy – ovarian shielding technique on eight young females ages 16 to 33 with Hodgkin's disease. The patients received, after staging surgery and oophoropexy, 3800 rads to the paraaortic, pelvic and inguinal nodes over 58 days and only 450–500 rads were estimated to be received by the ovaries. Four of the eight so treated patients resumed menstruation and one became pregnant 6 years after irradiation. No endocrine monitoring was performed in this series (Baker *et al.*, 1972). Himelstein-Braw and Faber (1977) studied the histology of the ovaries in 12 children who died between the ages of 5 months and 6 years and who had received besides surgery for abdominal tumors, either no additional therapy, chemotherapy alone, abdominal radiation alone, or combined abdominal irradiation and chemotherapy. Actively growing ovaries were found only among children who received no chemotherapy or only a short course. Quiescent ovaries were observed in all children who received chemotherapy over more than 2 months. In addition to inhibition of follicular growth, a marked reduction in the number of nongrowing follicles was observed in patients who received abdominal radiation either alone or combined with chemotherapy. Chemotherapy composed of Vincristine and cyclophosphamide was given continuously until death, which occurred between 1 week to 14 months after treatment. The abdominal radiation dose used in this series was 2500 rads, full course fractionated over a 30 day period (Himelstein-Brawl and

Faber, 1977). Shalet *et al.*, (1976) reported low estradiol and elevated FSH in all 18 patients who received during childhood (at age 1–13 years) abdominal radiation (2000–3000 rads over 25–44 days) for abdominal tumors. Seven of these females received in addition, Actinomycin D, Vincristine, Cyclophosphamide in single or combined regimen and there was no difference between the endocrine profile in these patients and the rest of the group who received radiation therapy alone (Shalet *et al.*, 1976). One of our patients received 1200 rads through posterior low back ports at 2 years of age and presented at the age of 13 with ovarian failure. The above observations indicate that while short-term chemotherapy has no effect on follicular growth, prolonged chemotherapy and abdominal radiation both inhibit follicular growth and destroy the small, nonproliferating follicles.

Cytotoxic Drugs

Cytotoxic agents used in malignant as well as in non-malignant conditions have been reported to induce reversible and permanent ovarian failure. Busulphan or Myleran used by a female patient known as having chronic granulocytic leukemia from 6 weeks to 36 weeks gestation induced multiple fetal malformations and severe gonadal hypoplasia. This patient received throughout her previous pregnancy radiation therapy to the spleen and chemotherapy with 6-mercaptopurine and delivered a normal child (Diamond *et al.*, 1960). This seems to implicate Busulphan as the agent responsible for the multiple malformations and ovarian hypodevelopment in the fetus.

Cyclophosphamide is another alkylating agent reported as having deleterious effects upon the ovary. No oocytes were found in the ovaries of a 46,XX 4 year old girl who died after 29 months of cyclophosphamide for juvenile rheumatoid arthritis (Miller *et al.*, 1971). In another series of 22 women receiving cyclophosphamide over 12 to 39 months for progressive glomerulonephritis or rheumatoid arthritis, 17 became amenorrheic with decreased estrogen and elevation of urinary gonadotropins. Of six of these patients who had ovarian biopsies, two had oocytes present and none showed follicle maturation. Only one of these patients with biochemical ovarian failure resumed normal ovarian function 10 months after stopping treatment (Warne *et al.*, 1973). Kumar *et al.* (1972) reported his series of eight patients receiving cyclophosphamide for nephrotic syndrome over no more than 9 months. Six of them developed amenorrhea which recovered on cessation of therapy (Kumar *et al.*, 1972). Examination of the ovaries of leukemic children who died after courses of chemotherapy of variable length suggested that the disease does not disturb follicular growth, but that treatment with cytotoxic agents for more than 2 months causes inhibition of follicular growth. Prolonged treatment over 1–2 years with alkylating agents such as cyclophosphamide destroys the small follicles through direct effect on the granulosa cells (Himelstein-Braw *et al.*, 1978). Other cytotoxic agents have induced premature ovarian failure, as shown by the use of single agent or combined regimen given cyclically to premenopausal breast cancer patients. After 6 months of chemotherapy, there was a significant fall of plasma E_1 and E_2 concentration and increase in FSH and LH to the castrate range (Rose and Davis, 1977). From these studies, there appears to be no disease related ovarian susceptibility, but rather a progressive loss of ovarian function related to treatment duration.

Ovarian Failure Associated with Autosomal Anomalies

Although gonadal dysgenesis has been clearly associated with sex chromosome rearrangement and accepted to be related to an autosomal recessive gene in case of normal genotype, it has recently been reported in association with autosomal aberrations, mostly Trisomy 18 (Russell and Altschuler, 1975), Trisomy 13 (Kennedy *et al.*, 1977), chromosome of group D (Lázló *et al.*, 1976; Cohen *et al.*, 1967; Shapiro *et al.*, 1978). In all the six Trisomy 18 and the four Trisomy 13 fetuses and infants of Kennedy's series and in all the 13 Trisomy 18 female infants and children of Russell's series, varying degrees of histologic gonadal mal-development were described, such as fewer multilayer follicles, reduced numbers of primordial follicles, pyknotic follicle cells, nests of pregranulosa cells, presence of mesothelial clefts and abnormal masses of stroma cells. There is a preponderance in the literature of D group chromosome aberrations associated with 46,XX gonadal dysgenesis. Lázló *et al.* (1976) reported that 5–26% of 200 metaphase cells in all the six patients of his series with ovarian hypoplasia and intact sex chromosomes, contained a D ring most likely belonging to autosome 15 on fluorescent and Giemsa bandings. The autosomal aberrations might cause difficulty in meiotic pairing, as in X chromosome aneuploidy, resulting in premature fol-licular growth and accelerated follicular atresia. The incompatibility with life beyond early childhood in Trisomies 13 and 18 hinders any further investigation of ovarian development associated with these autosomal abnormalities. Although autosomal defects might occur in individuals with 46,XX gonadal dysgenesis as a coincidental event, the associated gonadal histologic features and the frequency of certain autosomal anomalies seen in association with ovarian hypoplasia seem to lend support to the hypothesis that in addition to the sex chromosome, autosomal gene effects are involved in controlling ovarian development.

Immunologic Etiology

Immunologic studies in patients with ovarian failure have defined a small group of patients with high circulating antiovarian antibody titers. By immunofluorescence methods, the circulating antibodies from the patients with idiopathic Addison's disease and premature ovarian failure were demonstrated to react with normal human theca interna of the ovary, interstitial cells of the testis, adrenal cortex and placental trophoblast (Irvine *et al.*, 1968). This suggests that antigens are shared between steroid producing tissues and that the antigens are probably related to enzymes involved in various pathways of steroid biosynthesis. In one of the six patients with coexistent adrenal and premature ovarian failure of Irvine's series, histologic features of a possible autoimmune etiology were described. While there was no evidence of any immunologic attack against the patient's own primordial follicles, the follicular epithelium of larger follicles showed immunofluorescence staining with her own serum and also the lymphocytic and plasma cell infiltra-tion which would lead to follicular destruction. Coulam and Ryan (1979) by radioiodinating protein extracted from normal premenopausal ovarian tissue, observed a definite increase in binding of antibodies in the sera of patients with premature menopause as compared to control sera. Association of clinical failure of the ovary, adrenal cortex, thyroid, parathyroid with organ specific autoantibodies seems to suggest that primary ovarian failure may be part of a poly-endocrine autoimmune disorder. However, while autoantibodies to cytoplasmic components of the ovary have been found in patients with premature ovarian failure and other immune disorders, the ovarian antigens and the autoimmune mechanism responsible for the destruction of the ovarian tissue remain to be elucidated.

Infectious Process - Infiltrative Diseases

Destruction of the ovarian parenchyma and its constituents is more commonly seen in chronic than in acute oophoritis.

(1) Tuberculosis — the ovary is much less involved than the tube. Rarely granulomatous infiltration or extensive caseation destroys the ovarian tissue sufficiently to cause ovarian failure (Ylinen, 1961).

(2) Sarcoidosis, actinomycosis and schistosomiasis involve the ovaries to a much lesser extent than the endometrium, cervix, fallopian tubes, and rarely the granulomatous process destroys the entire ovarian parenchyma.

(3) Infiltrative diseases, such as β thalassemia and mucopolysaccharidosis, rarely cause extensive infiltration of the ovary to cause ovarian failure.

Myotonia Dystrophica in Association with Ovarian Failure

In this disorder, myotonia and muscular atrophy are accompanied by testicular atrophy in the male and premature ovarian failure in the female (Harper and Dyken, 1972). The occurrence of myotonia dystrophica and premature ovarian failure in chromosomally intact individuals suggests that the gene controlling gonadal development may be closely linked to the gene producing myotonia dystrophica. The gene causing myotonia dystrophica is an autosomal dominant gene, transmitted from affected individuals to 50% of their offspring. A satisfactory study of the incidence of gonadal failure within a myotonia dystrophica pedigree is however not available.

Ataxia Telangiectasia in Association with Ovarian Failure

This syndrome of oculocutaneous telangiectasia and cerebellar ataxia has been suggested to be due to a demyelinating process and to have an autoimmune basis. The affected individuals may succumb by midadolescence to sinopulmonary infection or lymphoreticular malignancy. Ovarian dysgenesis and even dysgerminoma have been described at autopsy. It has been speculated that mesenchymal involvement in ataxia telangiectasia could be associated with abnormal germ cell migration in early intrauterine life, since the germ cells are intimately in contact with mesenchyme during their travel from their extra-gonadal origin into the genital ridge (Miller and Chatten, 1967). The frequency of this association, especially the occurrence of ovarian neoplasia in these patients should urge the clinician to consider appropriate cytogenetic and endocrine studies and possible gonadal visualization in search for gonadal abnormalities in these patients.

17 Hydroxylase Deficiency

Impaired 17 alpha hydroxylation of progesterone and pregnenolene causes estrogen and androgen deficiency and excessive production of mineralocorticoid precursors of aldosterone. These patients present with symptoms of sexual immaturity, primary amenorrhea and hypertension accompanied by high serum gonadotropins and undetectable serum androgens and estrogens (Goldsmith *et al.*, 1967). This disorder provides a unique model for demonstrating the importance of intraovarian estrogen production for optimal follicular development. Large cysts, primordial and early primary follicles were described in ovarian biopsies from these women (Mallin, 1969).

Resistant Ovary Syndrome

It has been postulated as resulting from deficient FSH hormone receptor on the follicular cell membrane. Ovarian biopsies from these women show only primordial follicles with no progression to follicular maturation. These patients usually present with primary amenorrhea, hypoestrogenism, hypergonado- tropism, but normal secondary sex characteristics and may respond to ovulation induction with excessive doses of exogenous gonadotropins. A successful pregnancy was recently reported in a patient with resistant ovary syndrome sub- sequent to estrogen replacement therapy (Shangold *et al*, 1977).

APPROACH TO DIAGNOSIS

Six diagnostic steps will aid in an appropriate evaluation of premature ovarian failure, essentially in an adolescent patient:

(1) Serum gonadotropin determination by RIA. Elevated gonadotropins, especially FSH, constitute the most sensitive diagnostic test of primary ovarian failure. A level of FSH above 50 mIU/ml mostly signifies markedly decreased, or absent follicles. This test is indicated in all adolescents with short stature, sexual infantilism, hypoestrogenic vaginal smear associated with primary or secondary amenorrhea. It should also be included in the recycling failure workup in patients complaining of infertility, since anovulation and refractoriness to ovulation induc- tion therapy are not unusually preliminary signs of permanent ovarian failure. This diagnosis should be established as soon as possible, so that these young females can cease their futile search for fertility. Since the diagnosis of ovarian failure is a serious one for the patient and since the gonadotropins fluctuate considerably, it should be made only after at least two serum gonadotropin deter- minations and the gonadotropin assay should be repeated in 6 months to see whether the pituitary gonadotropins are consistently elevated. In a prepubertal or adolescent child who is potentially subject to have ovarian failure because of X chromosome privation or because of a history of abdominal radiation or chemo- therapy, a normal or low level of gonadotropins does not rule out the diagnosis of ovarian failure, even in the presence of some sexual development. Periodic gonadotropin determinations will allow to establish the diagnosis by the time of

further hypothalamic pituitary maturation. Administration of GnRH by inducing exaggerated responses after the age of 12, would clarify the ambiguous serum values.

(2) Cytogenetic studies. Chromosome analysis with G-banding and C-banding is essential in the diagnosis of specific structural anomalies of the X chromosome or of a mosaic genotype with or without a Y component. Buccal smear provides for visualization of the genetically inactive late replicating X chromosome and the genetically inactive fluorescent portion of the Y chromosome. Although it cannot replace the karyotyping, it serves as a helpful double check to eliminate any possibility of laboratory mislabelling. One patient in our series was referred for evaluation of growth retardation, sexual delay with a 46,XX karyotype. Repeat karyotyping in our laboratory and in another cytogenetic laboratory elaborated the diagnosis of 45,X/46,XY.

Both chromosome studies and buccal smear cannot however, identify the genetically active nonfluorescent portion of the Y chromosome, which codes for testicular structures.

(3) H-Y antigen studies. These studies in the near future would be of a great help in uncovering an undetectable XY cell line in some 45,X ovarian failure patients or identifying a chromosome fragment or a ring chromosome which still constitutes a problem with the current cytogenetic techniques.

(4) Identification of associated anomalies:

(a) An IVP and a careful evaluation of the cardiovascular system are crucial steps as soon as the diagnosis of chromosomally incompetent ovarian failure is established, since a coartation of the aorta or a renal anomaly may pose a serious threat to the life expectancy of these patients.

(b) Thyroid evaluation, including antithyroid antibodies should be performed on all patients with ovarian failure. Autoimmune thyroiditis not only is frequently seen in association with a long arm isochromosome X, but also with a 46,XX ovarian failure of immunologic etiology.

(c) Patients with a Y component or positive H-Y antigen studies should have prophylactic gonadal extirpation because of high potential of neoplastic formation. Gonadoblastoma, which is the most frequent tumor associated with dysgenetic gonads tends to undergo degeneration and rarely metastasizes unless the germ cell element predominates in which case they behave biologically as a dysgerminoma. The possibility of adrenal hypofunction associated with gonadal dysgenesis should always be kept in mind, especially when the patient is subject to surgery or any stress situation, so that adrenal insufficiency can be early recognized and appropriately treated.

(d) Routine 2 h postprandial blood glucose level determination is appropriate in patients with gonadal dysgenesis who are at increased risk for diabetes mellitus.

(5) Gonadal visualization. The easy availability of serum gonadotropin radioimmunoassay has rendered endoscopic visualization and ovarian biopsy unnecessary. Laparoscopic inspection and histologic examination may fail to distinguish ovarian failure from an unstimulated ovary and the presence of a few scattered primordial follicles is an unusual finding in ovarian failure. Furthermore, gonadal visualization has no place in patients known to have a Y chromosome. Laparotomy and gonadal extirpation should be performed at any age as soon as the diagnosis i

made because of a 25% incidence of neoplasia associated with gonadal dysgenesis and the presence of a Y component in the genotype. The real controversy for diagnostic laparoscopy and ovarian biopsy in ovarian failure revolves around a few distinctive cases with high levels of gonadotropins who exhibit numerous primordial follicles, suggestive of an FSH receptor defect and an ovary resistant to gonadotropins. Another indication for diagnostic laparoscopy in patients with ovarian failure is the presence of masculinization which hints a possibility of ridge tumor (McDonough *et al.*, 1967).

(6) Bone age determination. An AP film of the hand for skeletal age and AP film of the pelvis for iliac epiphysis visualization and documentation of estradiol secretion are helpful in the adolescent group for assessment of ovarian activity and post-therapeutic monitoring.

COUNSELLING AND THERAPY

In the adolescent girl with ovarian failure, counselling aims to give her a prospective idea of her future height, sexual development and reproductive performance. Usually when a proper reassurance and a candid explanation are given, the situation is readily accepted and future life planned accordingly. In the young female seeking fertility, laparoscopic or laparotomy ovarian biopsy would aid the physician to identify the rare patient with resistant ovary syndrome who may benefit from a high dose of exogenous gonadotropins for ovulation induction (Johnson and Peterson, 1979). The young infertile female is mostly frustrated in knowing of her slim chance for reproductive performance. They usually accept the situation and cease their future efforts for fertility. They should also be informed of the rare possibility of becoming pregnant while on replacement therapy.

All patients with premature ovarian failure ultimately need hormonal replacement therapy with periodic evaluation of blood sugar, triglycerides and of the endometrium. In patients with a Y chromosome, prophylatic extirpation of the gonads is mandatory at any age as soon as the diagnosis is established, because of the high malignant potential of these dysgenetic gonads. Hormonal replacement can be initiated with ethinyl estradiol, 20 micrograms and Provera, 10 mg. a day for the last 7 days of the monthly ethinyl estradiol course, until breast development is complete. This sequential regimen is advisable to the infertile patient with ovarian failure who may conceive on such estrogen replacement regimen. Low dose combined therapy would be used for those patients who do not desire pregnancy.

CONCLUSION

Comprehending ovarian failure in phenotypic females with privations of sex chromosomes is better now than one decade ago. Continued inquiry into X inactivation in somatic and germ cells, coupled with dose related growth effects of X chromosomes should provide further insight into genetic factors affecting ovarian development.

Ovarian failure in chromosomally intact subjects will be a source of continued mystery and requires clearer separation of genetic and environment factors. New methods to identify ovarian receptor defects and more specific ovarian antibodies for a clear delineation of immunologic ovarian failure offer promise. It should be a challenging field of endeavor in the future for the geneticist, endocrinologist and immunologist.

In both chromosomally incompetent and competent individuals, recent radioimmunoassay techniques have provided interesting information in the ontogeny of steroid-gonadotropin dynamics, especially in the hypothalamic pituitary ovarian feedback mechanism before full maturation in adult life. Improved techniques in identification and quantitation of H- Y antigen should further clarify the genetic aspect of gonadal differentiation and development and aid in better preventing neoplastic formation in these patients bearing dysgenetic gonads.

REFERENCES

Amarose, A. P., Kyriazis, A. A., Dorus, E. and Azizi, F. (1977). *American Journal of Obstetrics and Gynecology* **127**, 824.

Baker, J. W., Morgan, R. L., Peckham, M. J. and Smithers, D. W. (1972). *Lancet* **1**, 1307.

Böök, J. A., Eilon, B., Halbrecht, I., Komlos, L. and Shabtay, F. (1973). *Clinical Genetics* **4**, 410.

Burgoyne, P. A. and Biggers, J. D. (1976). *Developmental Biology* **51**, 109.

Carr, D. H., Haggar, R. A. and Hart, A. G. (1968). *American Journal of Clinical Pathology* **19**, 521.

Cohen, M. M., Capraro, V. J. and Takagi, N. (1967). *American Journal of Human Genetics* **30**, 313.

Conen, P. E. and Glass, I. H. (1963). *Journal of Clinical Endocrinology and Metabolism* **23**, 1.

Conte, F. A., Grumbach, M. M., Kaplan, S. L. and Reiter, E. O. (1980). *Journal of Clinical Endocrinology and Metabolism* **50**, 163.

Coulam, C. B. and Ryan, R. J. (1979). *American Journal of Obstetrics and Gynecology* **133**, 639.

Dewhurst, C. J., Paine, C. G. and Blank, C. E. (1963). *Journal of Obstetrics and Gynecology of the British Commonwealth* **70**, 675.

Diamond, I., Anderson, M. I. and McCreadie, S. R. (1960). *Pediatrics* **25**, 85.

Dorus, E., Amarose, A. P., Koo, G. and Wachtel, S. (1977). *American Journal of Obstetrics and Gynecology* **127**, 829.

Espinear, E. A., Veal, A. M. O., Sands, V. E. and Fitzgerald, P. H. (1970). *The New England Journal of Medicine* **283**, 6.

Franchi, L. L. and Baker, T. G. (1973). *In* "Human Reproduction, Conception and Contraception" (E. S. E. Hafez and T. N. Evans, Eds) 53–83. Harper and Row, Hagerstown.

Gartler, S. M., Liskay, R. M. and Gant, N. (1973). *Experimental Cell Research* **82**, 464.

Gartler, S. M., Andina, R. and Gant, N. (1975). *Experimental Cell Research* **91**, 454.

Ghosh, S. N., Shah, P. N. and Gharpure, H. M. (1980). *Nature* **276**, 180.

Goldsmith, O., Solomon, D. H. and Horton, R. (1967). *The New England Journal of Medicine* **277**, 673.

Harper, P. S. and Dyken, P. R. (1972). *Lancet* **2**, 53.

Himelstein-Braw, R. and Faber, M. (1977). *British Journal of Cancer* **36**, 269.

Himelstein-Braw, R., Peters, H. and Faber, M. (1978). *British Journal of Cancer* **38**, 82.

Irvine, W. J., Chem, M. M. W. and Scarth, L. (1968). *Lancet* **2**, 883.

Jirásek, J. E. (1976). *In* "Disorders of Sexual Differentiation" (J. L. Simpson, Ed.), 75–92. Academic Press, New York.

Johnson, R. and Peterson, E. P. (1979). *Fertility and Sterility* **31**, 35.

Jones, G. S. and De Moraes-Ruehsen, M. (1969). *American Journal of Obstetrics and Gynecology* **104**, 597.

Kennedy, J. R., Freeman, M. G. and Bernirschke, K. (1977). *Obstetrics and Gynecology* **50**, 13.

Kohn, G., Cohen, M. M., Beyth, Y. and Ornoy, A. (1977). *Journal of Medical Genetics* **14**, 120.

Kumar, R., Biggart, J. D., McEvoy, J. and McGeown, M. G. (1972). *Lancet* **12**, 12.

László, J., Gaál, M. and Bösze, P. (1976). *Clinical Genetics* **9**, 61.

Mallin, S. R. (1969). *Annals of Internal Medicine* **70**, 69.

McDonough, P. G. and Byrd, J. R. (1970). *International Journal of Gynecology and Obstetrics* **8** (2), 193.

McDonough, P. G., Greenblatt, R. B., Byrd, J. R. and Hastings, E. V. (1967). *Obstetrics and Gynecology* **29**, 54.

McDonough, P. G., Byrd, J. R., Tho, P. T. and Mahesh, V. B. (1977a). *Fertility and Sterility* **28**, 638.

McDonough, P. G., Tho, P. T. and Byrd, J. R. (1977b). *Fertility and Sterility* **28**, 251.

McNatty, K. P. (1978). *Clinics in Endocrinology and Metabolism* **7**, 577.

Migeon, B. R. and Kennedy, J. B. (1975). *American Journal of Human Genetics* **27**, 233.

Miller, M. E. and Chatten, J. (1967). *Acta Paediatrica Scandinavia* **56**, 559.

Miller, J. J., Williams, G. F. and Leissring, J. C. (1971). *The American Journal of Medicine* **50**, 530.

Morrison, J. C., Givens, J. R., Wiser, W. L. and Fish, S. A. (1975). *Fertility and Sterility* **28**, 251.

Nazareth, H. R. S., Farah, L. M. S., Cunha, A. J. B. *et al.* (1977). *Human Genetics* **37**, 117.

Penney, L. L. and Betz, G. (1977). *American Journal of Obstetrics and Gynecology* **127**, 299.

Peters, H., Byskov, A. G., Himelstein-Braw, R. and Faber, M. (1975). *Journal of Reproduction Fertility* **45**, 559.

Richards, J. S., Ireland, J. J., Rao, M. C., Bernath, G., Midgley, A. R. and Reichert, L. E. (1976). *Endocrinology* **99**, 1562.

Rose, D. P. and Davis, T. E. (1977). *Lancet* **1**, 1174.

Russell, P. and Altschuler, G. (1975). *Pathology* **7**, 149.

Schellas, H. F. (1974). *Obstetrics and Gynecology* **44**, 298.

Schwartz, N. B., Anderson, C. H., Neguin, L. G. and Ely, C. A. (1974). *In* "The Control of the Onset of Puberty" (M. M. Grumbach, G. D. Grave and F. E. Mayer, Eds), 367–385. John Wiley and Sons, New York.

Shalet, S. M., Beardwell, C. G., Jones, P. H. M., Pearson, D. and Orrell, D. H. (1976). *British Journal of Cancer* **33**, 655.

Shangold, M. M., Turksoy, R. N., Bashford, R. A. and Hammond, C. B. (1977). *Fertility and Sterility* **28**, 1179.

Shapiro, L. R., Graves, Z. R., Warburton, D. and Huss, H. A. (1978). *Birth Defects* **14**, 167.

Sherman, B. M. and Korenman, S. G. (1975). *Journal of Clinical Investigation* **55**, 699.

Swanson, J. A. and Chapler, F. K. (1978). *Obstetrics and Gynecology* **51**, 237.

Thomas, P. R. M., Winstanley, D., Peckham, M. J., Austin, D. E., Murray, M. A. F. and Jacobs, H. S. (1976). *British Journal of Cancer* **33**, 226.

Wachtel, S. S. (1979). *Obstetrics and Gynecology* **54**, 671.

Warne, G. L., Fairley, K. F., Hobbs, J. B. and Martin, F. I. R. (1973). *New England Journal of Medicine* **289**, 1159.

Winter, J. S. D., Faiman, C. and Reyes, F. I. (1971). *In* "Morphogenesis and Malformation of the Genital System" (R. J. Blandau and D. Bergsma, Eds). Vol. XIII, 41–58.

Ylinen, O. (1961). *Acta Obstetrica Gynecologica Scandinavia* **40** (Suppl 2) 1, 214.

EVALUATION OF FUNCTIONAL OVARIAN CAPACITY IN CASES WITH PREMATURE MENOPAUSE

H. Meden-Vrtovec and B. Vrtovec

*Department of Gynaecology and Obstetrics, University of Ljubljana,
Slajmerjeva Ljubljana, Yugoslavia*

INTRODUCTION

When occurring in young women, disappearance of menstrual bleeding with high plasma gonadotropins characterizes the clinical laboratory picture named "premature menopause". Nevertheless we cannot take these clinical laboratory data as proof of functional ovarian follicle loss, because they are also present in cases of resistant ovarian syndrome and Netter's ovarioplegic amenorrhoea. The aim of this study is to identify different aetiological groups on the basis of their responsiveness to exogenous gonadotropin administration.

MATERIALS AND METHODS

This study was performed on 12 women, aged 24–37, with clinical vasomotor signs of *climax precox* (palpitations, night sweats, hot flushes). All subjects had positive sex-chromatin and karyotype 46 XX. Treatment with progesterone (50 mg/day for 3 days) failed to induce menses. Oestrogen treatment (5 mg/day of oestradiol-dypropionate for 5 days) induced uterine bleeding, thus excluding uterine factors of secondary amenorrhoea.

Blood samples were taken three times over a 3 month period for FSH, LH

Serono Symposium No. 39, "The Menopause: Clinical, Endocrinological and Pathophysiological Aspects", edited by P. Fioretti, L. Martini, G. B. Melis and S. S. C. Yen, 1982. Academic Press, London and New York.

and prolactin evaluation. Samples of 24 h urine were collected for determination of pregnandiol, oestriol, 17-OH and 17-KETO steroids.

Gonadotropins [15 doses of Pergonal (Serono) and 15.000 i.v. hCG (Pregnyl-Organon)] were administered to the subjects over a 13 day period.

RESULTS

Repeated gonadotropin evaluation revealed hypergonadotropic values (FSH > 50 mIU/ml, LH > 50 mIU/ml) in all cases; prolactin concentrations were within the normal range (5–25 ng/ml). The 24 h urine 17-OH and 17-KETO steroids showed normal values, while pregnandiol and oestriol were low in all cases (Table I).

Table I. Clinical and laboratory data of 12 cases with hypergonadotropic amenorrhoea

Patient	Age	Menarche	Years of spontaneous cycles	Prolactin (ng/ml)	24 h urine			
					pgn (mg)	E_2 (μg)	17-KS (mg)	17-OH (mg)
B.M.	31	15	1	5.5	1.1	98	11.3	13.1
P.N.	31	14	10	6.5	0.8	42	6.5	7.1
P.T.	28	13	11	6.4	1.1	48	13.1	9.9
S.G.	28	11	16	10.2	1.0	62	5.8	10.8
G.A.	23	14	7	10.1	1.0	52	9.6	8.3
R.C.	25	15	9	7.8	1.4	43	11.1	10.9
P.N.	24	13	7	6.8	1.0	50	7.2	8.2
P.M.	31	13	17	11.6	1.1	83	8.1	11.2
O.R.	37	14	22	12.9	1.6	61	8.4	15.1
M.M.	28	13	12	13.4	1.0	24	10.0	4.4
M.S.	24	15	6	6.2	0.8	34	11.2	8.3
K.C.	31	11	8	7.1	0.9	56	11.3	10.9

pgn = pregnandiol (normal values: proliferative phase 0.8–1.5 mg/24 h urine; secretory phase 2.1–2.4 mg/24 h urine). E_2 = oestriol (normal values: 10–80 μg/24 h urine). 17-KS = 17-KETO steroids. 17-OH = 17-hydroxy steroids.

Gonadotropin administration had no effects on cervical mucus and failed to induce menstrual bleeding in 10 out of 12 subjects.

On the contrary, patient R.C. showed marked cervical reaction and menstrual bleeding following gonadotropin treatment; spontaneous menses occurred in this subject three cycles later. Patients P. T. also showed marked cervical reaction and menstrual bleeding following gonadotropin administration. Spontaneous menstruation did not occur, but menstrual bleeding was induced by repeated gonadotropin treatment. Laparoscopic ovarian biopsy revealed the presence of ovarian follicles in all 12 subjects.

DISCUSSION

Hypergonadotropic secondary amenorrhoea is generally considered as resulting from the loss of functional ovarian follicles (Goldenberg *et al.*, 1973). Usually premature menopause is really the clinical sign of primary ovarian failure, but we must keep in mind the existence of gonadotropin resistant ovary syndrome. This syndrome is characterized by clinical vasomotor signs of premature menopause, amenorrhoea and high gonadotropin levels, with presence of ovarian follicles (Koninckz and Bronsens, 1977; Wright and Jacobs, 1979). The same clinical picture was also described by Netter (1957), but the author showed that ovarian failure could depend on the stress and he called this syndrome "ovarioplegic amenorrhoea" of hypothalamic origin.

Our data showed that gonadotropin treatment induced menstrual bleeding only in two out of 12 subjects with clinical laboratory evidence of "premature menopause" and bioptic finding of primordial follicles in the ovary. These results led us to postulate the existence of resistance for endogenous gonadotropins in the two subjects responsive to exogenous gonadotropin administration. On the contrary, the unresponsive group of subjects could represent the evidence of ovarioplegic amenorrhoea. Contrasting results have been reported with regard to the effects of gonadotropin treatment in this last syndrome. Jones and Moraes-Ruehsen (1969) described positive effects of high dose gonadotropin administration, with induction of ovulation, while Starup *et al.* (1971) did not obtain the same results.

In our opinion gonadotropin test could permit aetiological identification of two different syndromes within the uniform group characterized by clinical evidence of premature menopause, hypergonadotropic amenorrhoea and present ovarian follicles.

REFERENCES

Dewhurst, C. J., de Koos, E. B. and Ferreira, H. P. (1975). *British Journal of Obstetrics and Gynaecology* **82**, 341.

Goldenberg, R. L., Grodin, J. M. and Rodbard, D. (1973). *American Journal of Obstetrics and Gynecology* **116**, 1003.

Jones, G. S. and Moraes-Ruehsen, M. (1969). *American Journal of Obstetrics and Gynecology* **104**, 597.

Kononckx, P. R. and Bronsens, I. A. (1977). *Fertility and Sterility* **28**, 926.

Linquette, M. and Dupont-Lecompte, J. (1973). *In* "Précis d'endocrinologie" (V. M. Linquette, Ed.), 745. Masson and Cie, Paris.

Netter, A. (1957). *Les Annales d'Endocrinologie* **18**, 1014.

Starup, J., Sele, V. and Henriksen, B. (1971). *Acta Endocrinologica (Kbh)* **66**, 248.

Wright, C. S. and Jacobs, H. S. (1979). *British Journal of Obstetrics and Gynaecology* **86**, 389.

CORONARY HEART DISEASE IN WOMEN: A CLINICAL ANGIOGRAPHIC AND HORMONAL STUDY

G. Gasperetti, R. De Caterina, I. Simonetti, S. Innocenti[1], A. M. Paoletti[1], G. B. Melis[1] and A. Maseri

CNR Clinical Physiology Institute, Department of Obstetrics and Gynaecology[1], University of Pisa, Pisa, Italy

NEW CONCEPTS ON ISCHAEMIC HEART DISEASE

Traditionally, diagnosis, therapy and prevention of coronary artery disease have been centred on coronary atherosclerosis. However in spite of an overwhelming statistical association between coronary atherosclerosis and the clinical manifestations of coronary heart disease, there is growing evidence that this association is not a direct one. This conclusion is based on several observations:

(1)   The prevalence of coronary atherosclerosis in the general population, evidenced by autopsy studies, is nearly 10 times higher than the number of symptomatic patients (Enos *et al.*, 1953; Baroldi, 1978).
(2)   The severity of symptoms correlates poorly with the severity of coronary atherosclerosis (Friesinger and Smith, 1972).
(3)   About 10% of patients with angina pectoris or myocardial infarction have normal coronary arteries or exhibit no critical stenosis of their coronary tree (Gorlin, 1978).
(4)   The severity of coronary atherosclerosis is similar in patients with "stable" and "unstable" angina (Fuster *et al.*, 1975; Neill *et al.*, 1977).
(5)   About 10% of patients with electrocardiographically proven "unstable" angina had to be excluded from randomized surgical trials because their coronary lesions were not severe enough (Bertolasi *et al.*, 1974; Conti, 1976; Conti: personal communication).

Serono Symposium No. 39, "The Menopause: Clinical, Endocrinological and Pathophysiological Aspects", edited by P. Fioretti, L. Martini, G. B. Melis and S. S. C. Yen, 1982. Academic Press, London and New York.

The classic definition of "angina pectoris" as given by Friedberg (1966), and also recorded in the Glossary of the National Heart and Lung and Blood Institute's Task Force Report on Atherosclerosis (1971, 1977) has conditioned our thinking with the extrapolated notion that the only important variable in the development of acute transient myocardial ischaemia is coronary atherosclerotic stenosis resulting in a limited blood supply that is unable to meet excessive increases in myocardial demand. The stimulus to challenge this traditional concept has come from studies of "variant" angina (Prinzmetal *et al.*, 1959), which have now expanded to other forms of angina at rest. "Variant" angina has been shown to be caused not by increased myocardial demand but by coronary vasospasm (Maseri *et al.*, 1975, 1976). This is now considered a proven hypothesis (Meller *et al.*, 1976). On the basis of observations performed on a large number of patients, we have come to the conclusion that "variant" angina is frequent when appropriately sought (Maseri *et al.*, 1977). Moreover "variant" angina is not a discrete syndrome but, rather, represents one extreme of a continuous spectrum of acute myocardial ischaemia caused by coronary vasospasm. Indeed, our observations suggest that coronary vasospasm may result in varying degrees of ischaemia with variable electrocardiographic changes with or without typical chest pain (Maseri *et al.*, 1977; 1978b). Coronary vasospasm may also cause sudden coronary death (Maseri *et al.*, 1978b) and may evolve into myocardial infarction (Maseri *et al.*, 1978a).

These views seem to be gaining acceptance (Hillis and Braunwald, 1978). Thus, coronary vasospasm, superimposed on a variable degree of coronary atherosclerosis, appears to be an important modulating factor in the genesis of acute myocardial ischaemia with or without typical pain, which may result in "unstable" angina pectoris, myocardial infarction, and/or sudden cardiac death. Other modulating factors responsible for the occurrence of acute transient myocardial ischaemia have been proposed, and one may anticipate that as research continues in this area, they will be objectively identified, as was the case of coronary spasm.

ISCHAEMIC HEART DISEASE IN FEMALES

Mortality from ischaemic heart diseases (IHD) increases progressively with age both in males and females; however, the incidence is considerably lower in women particularly in the premenopausal age in the white population (Figs 1-4). It is not clear whether the relatively higher incidence of death from IHD in young coloured females is related to an earlier menopausal development in this group. No brisk increase in the incidence of death from IHD can be observed in white nor in coloured females after the menopausal age, rather some form of protection may be suspected relative to males in all age groups leading to approximately a decade delay in the incidence of fatal IHD (Figs 1-4).

Furman (1968) suggested that differences in the incidence of myocardial infarction between males and females of menopausal age could be due to a greater number of male subjects being vulnerable to early fatal coronary artery disease before the 5th decade of life.

However, little is actually known about the relative prevalence of non-fatal IHD in the female population. The frequent finding of normal coronary arterio-

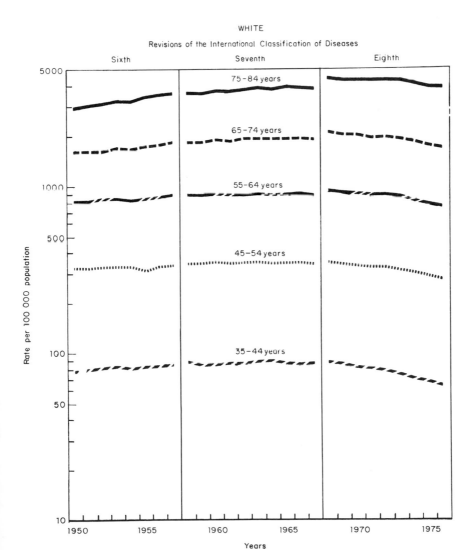

Fig. 1. Death rates for ischaemic heart disease per 100 000 population, by age for the white male population: USA, 1950-76-con. From: Chartbook for the Conference on the Decline in Coronary Heart Disease Mortality. National Center for Health Statistics, USA, 1980.

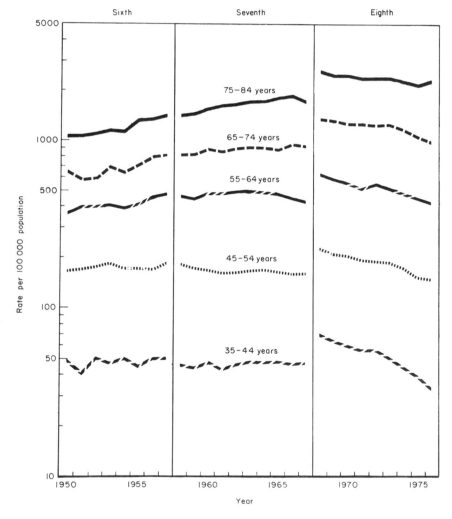

ALL OTHER

Revisions of the International Classification of Diseases

Fig. 2. Death rates for ischaemic heart disease per 100 000 population, by age for the non-white male population: USA, 1950–76–con. From: Chartbook for the Conference on the Decline in Coronary Heart Disease Mortality. National Center for Health Statistics, USA, 1980.

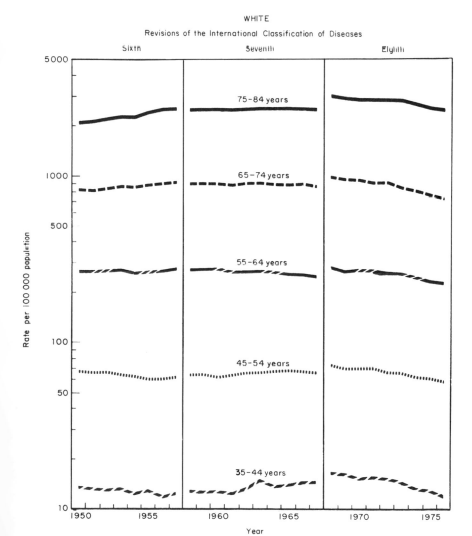

Fig. 3. Death rates for ischaemic heart disease per 100 000 population by age for the white female population: USA, 1950–76–con. From: Chartbook for the Conference on the Decline in Coronary Heart Disease Mortality. National Center for Health Statistics, USA, 1980.

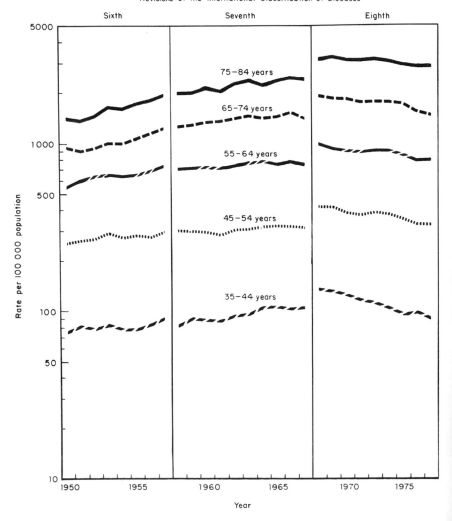

ALL OTHER

Revisions of the International Classification of Diseases

Fig. 4. Death rates for ischaemic heart disease per 100 000 population by age for the non-white female population: USA, 1950–76–con. From: Chartbook for the Conference on the Decline in Coronary Heart Disease Mortality. National Center for Health Statistics, USA, 1980.

grams in women with angina pectoris (Likoff *et al.*, 1967; Neill *et al.*, 1968; Eliot and Bratt, 1969; Ciraulo, 1975) and myocardial infarction (Glancy *et al.*, 1971; Cheng *et al.*, 1972; Ciraulo, 1975) suggests a major role of functional factors such as coronary spasm as a cause of myocardial ischaemia, in the absence of significant coronary atherosclerosis.

Therefore we decided to undertake a study about: (1) the frequence of documented acute myocardial ischaemic episodes in the patient population admitted to our institute; (2) the gynaecological and hormonal profile in the pre- and postmenopausal women with documented myocardial ischaemic episodes relative to a control population in order to try and identify factors predisposing the development of clinical manifestation of IHD.

METHODS

We revised the discharge diagnosis of all patients referred to our Institute from January 1st 1978 to December 31st 1979. During these 2 years a total of 624 patients with known or suspected heart disease were admitted; an objective diagnosis of myocardial ischaemic episodes was established when the following criteria were met: (1) documented infarction by unequivocal symptoms, ECG signs, enzymes; (2) documented typical ECG ischaemic S-T/T changes during typical pain (spontaneous or induced by provocative tests).

The percentage of males and females admitted, and the relative incidence of documented myocardial ischaemic episodes is listed in Table I. Out of the 111

Table I. Sex distribution and incidence of IHD in the patient population.

	Patients admitted	Patients with documented ischaemic episodes
Males	513 (82.2% of the total)	399 (77.7%)
Females	111 (17.8% of the total)	67 (60.3%)
Total	624	456 (74.7%)

females admitted, 67 had objectively proven myocardial ischaemic episodes. Among these we extensively studied a subpopulation of 34 patients who were submitted to coronary arteriography. Exercise stress testing was performed in all these last subjects and ergonovine test in 20 of them (Table II).

In this group of 34 patients and in the other 29 chosen with the same criteria (objectively documented episodes of myocardial ischaemia and coronary arteriographic study) among females admitted in past years, information on the gynaecological profile was obtained by a self-administered questionnaire [the first (Table III) for the group of premenopausal women and the second (Table IV) for the group of climacteric subjects]. In 25 of these 63 patients we also performed hormonal studies. These included assays of different proteic and steroid hormones in blood samples collected between 9 and 10 a.m. Those samples were withdrawn

Table II.   Female population with documented IHD.

		Total	Pre-M	Post-M
	No. of patients	34	17	17
Finding at	Normal CA	20	11	9
coronary	One-vessel disease	4	2	2
arteriography	Two-vessel disease	8	3	5
	Three-vessel disease	2	1	1
Exercise stress	No. of patients	34	17	17
testing	Positive	21	9	12
Ergonovine	No. of patients	20	9	11
maleate test	Positive	5	3	2

once from postmenopausal subjects and twice (10 days before and 10 days after spontaneous menses) from normally menstruating women. Circulating levels of gonadotropins (LH, FSH), prolactin (PRL), oestradiol (E_2), progesterone (P), oestrone (E_1), dehydroepiandrosterone (DHA) and its sulphate (DHA-S), androstenedione (A), testosterone (T) and dihydrotestosterone (DHT) were measured by specific radioimmunoassay (RIA) methods. While proteic hormones were directly assayed in the plasma using previously described RIA methods (Fioretti *et al.*, 1978; Melis *et al.*, 1977), E_2 and P were measured after plasma extraction with diethylether (Fioretti *et al.*, 1974).

The other steroid hormones were assayed by RIA after purification by means of a celite chromatography as previously described (Facchinetti and Genazzani, 1978).

RESULTS

Prevalence

Female admissions for IHD were only 17.8% of the total. Episodes of myocardial ischaemia could be documented in 60.3% of females vs 78% of males. Angina pectoris was present in 82% of females vs 68.7% of males. A myocardial infarction was present in 38.8% of females vs 67.4% of males with documented ischaemic episodes.

Coronary Arteriography

In our female patients with documented episodes of myocardial ischaemia the incidence of coronary atherosclerotic involvement is shown in Table II. In particular, the incidence of a finding of normal coronary arteries in this female population (58.8%) was considerably higher than the corresponding male control (9.8%).

Table III. Questionnaire for the study of the menstrual cycle in premenopausal women

---

NAME   SURNAME   AGE

FAMILY HISTORY

Mother's menstrual cycle: cycle
                          flow
                          length of period

PATIENT HISTORY

Menarche: age
           flow
           length of period

Successive menstruation: cycle
                          flow
                          length of period

Spotting before or after menstruation   YES   NO

Haemorrhaging between periods   YES   NO

Have you taken hormones?   Name of drug used

Have you used the pill?   Name of pill used

How long between first sexual intercourse and first conception?

Number of pregnancies

Number of deliveries

Number of miscarriages and the month of pregnancy in which they occured

MENSTRUAL SYMPTOMS

Nausea, fluid retention, weight increase, breast tenderness, headache, muscular cramps, giddiness, chloasma, vaginal discharge, depression, decreased libido, acne, hirsutism, hair loss, oily skin or scalp, appetite increase, abdomen tenderness, premenstrual syndrome (breast tenderness + giddiness + depression).

In what phase of the cycle are the symptoms prevalent?

Just before menstruation—in the middle of the cycle—after menstruation

---

Electrocardiographic Stress Testing

Maximal exercise stress testing, performed by cycloergometer, was positive (1 mm or more rectilinear or downsloping S-T segment depression) in 21 out of 34 (61.7%). Ergonovine maleate test was positive in five out of 20 women (25%) Table II).

Table IV. Questionnaire for the study of the menstrual cycle in climacteric women

NAME	SURNAME	SOCIAL CONDITION

FAMILY HISTORY

Mother's menstrual cycle: cycle
                             flow
                             length of period

PATIENT HISTORY

Menarche: age
                flow
                length of period

Successive menstruation: cycle
                              flow
                              length of period

Spotting before or after menstruation	YES	NO
Haemorrhaging between periods	YES	NO

Have you taken hormones?   Name of drug used

Have you used the pill?   Name of pill used

How long between first sexual intercourse and first conception?

Number of pregnancies

Number of deliveries

Number of miscarriages and the month of pregnancy in which they occurred

Last menstruation: date
                        flow
                        length of period

MENSTRUAL SYMPTOMS

Breast tenderness, headache, chloasma, spotting before and after menstruation, haemorrhaging between periods, abdomen tenderness.

CLIMACTERIC SYMPTOMS

Hot flushes, sweating, heart palpitations, allergic manifestations (asthma), irritability, character modifications, headache, depression, pain in the joints, weight increase, obesity, diabetes, high blood pressure

Findings in Pre- and Postmenopausal Women

When the female population with documented ischaemic episodes and coronary angiographic findings was subdivided into two subsets, pre- and postmenopausal, no significative difference in the incidence of coronary atherosclerotic involvement and in the response to stress testing was found (Table II).

Response to the Questionnaire

Twenty-nine premenopausal patients with IHD were examined by means of the above mentioned questionnaire (Table III). The statistical analysis of results considering the incidence of mastodynia, headache, weight increase and nausea in the group under study in comparison to 30 control subjects examined with the same questionnaire, showed a significantly ($P < 0.01$) higher incidence of those symptoms in subjects with IHD. A similar difference was evident relative to the incidence of the same symptoms in normal populations of the same age group (Table V).

Since the incidence of premenstrual syndrome is considered to be linked to an increased activity of oestrogens (Janowsky *et al.*, 1973), the patients with IHD seem to show a greater incidence of hyperoestrogenism in comparison with the control population. In postmenopausal women (Table VI) a great incidence of hot

Table V. Incidence of premenstrual symptoms in patients with ischaemic heart disease.

No. of patients: 29		Mean age: 44.6 (range 27–55 years)
Symptoms	% Frequency	% Normal frequency
Mastodynia	72.41	10
Headache	44.82	15–20
Weight increase	34.48	4–8
Nausea	34.48	2–4

Table VI. Incidence of climacteric symptoms in patients with ischaemic heart disease

No. of patients: 34		Mean age: 55.35 (range 42–67 years)
Symptoms	% Frequency in IHD patients	% Normal frequency
Hot flushes	73.52	
Sweating	55.88	75% of climacteric women have no
Irritability	47.05	symptoms (W. D. Odell, 1979)
Depression	44.11	

flushes, sweating, irritability and depression was observed. When the percentage of those symptoms, which are commonly considered signs of deficient oestrogenic activity, was taken into account, it was significantly greater ($P < 0.01$) than that reported in a group of control subjects examined with the same questionnaire.

Hormonal Profile

In the group of premenopausal women the levels of most of the assayed hormones were within the normal range for the follicular phase of the menstrual cycle (Fig. 5). Only a slight, but not statistically significant, decrease in some steroids (particularly E_1, DHA, and DHA-S levels) was observed in comparison with control subjects of the same age group. However important differences were observed in the group of patients with IHD when the levels of E_2 and P were measured in the second part of the cycle (Fig. 6). A higher incidence of anovulatory cycle and, consequently, a relative hyperoestrogenism, was observed relative to the control subjects of the same age group. No significant differences were observed between postmenopausal IHD patients and control subjects of the same age group (Fig. 7).

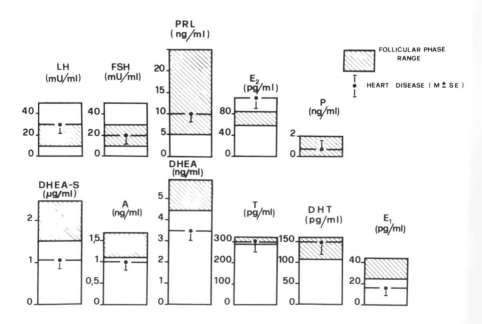

Fig. 5. Basal levels of different hormones in premenopausal patients with IHD during the follicular phase of the menstrual cycle.

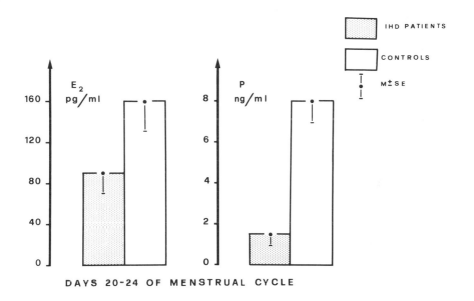

Fig. 6 Basal levels of 17-β-oestradiol (E_2) and progesterone (P) during luteal phase of the menstrual cycle in patients with IHD: a higher incidence of anovulatory cycle and, as a consequence, a relative hyperoestrogenism may be observed.

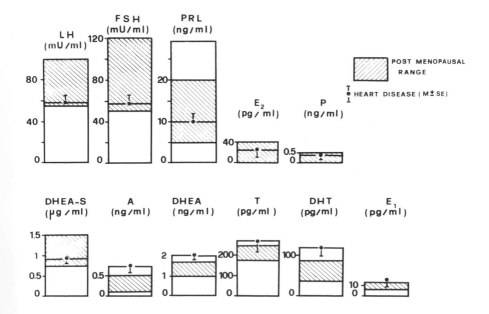

Fig. 7. Basal levels of different hormones in postmenopausal patients with IHD.

DISCUSSION AND CONCLUSIONS

Our findings are consistent with the existence of a lower incidence of IHD in females both in the pre- and in postmenopausal age groups relative to males; furthermore they show that in the presence of objectively documented myocardial ischaemic episodes, the incidence of coronary atherosclerosis is significantly lower in females than in males, with a greater than 50% (64.7% pre- and 52.9% postmenopausal) incidence of angiographically normal coronary arteries vs 9.8% for males.

These observations substantiate the hypothesis of a major role of functional factors such as coronary vasospasm, which could be proven angiographically during an anginal episode in two patients in this series.

The preliminary results on the hormonal profile of these patients seem to suggest that relative or absolute hyperoestrogenism may be observed in premenopausal women. Both the questionnaire and endocrine studies suggest that these patients were affected by luteal defect, anovulatory cycle and by the majority of premenstrual symptoms which characterize hyperoestrogenism (Janowsky et al., 1973).

On the other hand, in the postmenopausal group a higher incidence of the climacteric symptoms was observed while the same incidence of premenstrual symptoms as observed in premenopausal group (see above) could be deduced by history through analysis of the self-administered questionnaire.

It may be pointed out that a higher incidence of climacteric symptoms may be observed in patients who were suffering from hyperoestrogenism during the fertile life, as commonly observed in the clinical experience. On the other hand, when patients with gonadal disgenesis are considered, climacteric symptoms may be achieved only after some cycles of oestrogenic treatment have been performed. These observations suggest that the high incidence of climacteric symptoms in our patients may be related to the existence of a previous hyperoestrogenic state which was present in premenopausal life. Whether the hyperoestrogenism could represent a factor increasing the susceptibility of the coronary arteries to vasoconstrictive stimuli requires independent evidence.

In turn, local coronary hypersensitivity was postulated as a provisional working hypothesis in the genesis of coronary spasm which may result from a variable combination of local hypersensitivity and of a series of varied vasoconstrictive stimuli (Maseri et al., 1980). The possibility that a relative or absolute hyperoestrogenism could favour the susceptibility of coronary vessels to spasm, is supported by the observations that coronary arteries have receptors for oestrogens (S. S. C. Yen, personal communication); therefore contraceptive steroids may increase the risk for myocardial infarction not only with their effect on coagulation and platelet aggregation, but probably also with a direct effect on the coronary vessels. Similar studies may contribute to develop a rational therapeutic approach to IHD.

ACKNOWLEDGEMENTS

This work was partially supported by CNR (Rome, Italy) through the "Biology of Reproduction" project and grant No. 79.01891.04.

REFERENCES

Arteriosclerosis. A report by the National Heart and Lung Institute Task Force on Arteriosclerosis, Vol. 1, p. 36. US Department of Health, Education and Welfare, Public Health Service National Institutes of Health, DHEW Publication No. (NIH) 72-137, June 1971.

Arteriosclerosis. The Report of the 1977 Working Group to Review the 1971 Report by the National Heart and Lung Institute Task Force on Arteriosclerosis, p. 36. US Department of Health, Education and Welfare, Public Health Service, National Institutes of Health, DHEW Publication No. (NIH) 78-1526, December 1977.

Baroldi, G. (1978). *American Heart Journal* **96**, 139-143.

Bertolasi, C. A. Trongè, J. E., Carreño, C. A. *et al.* (1974). *American Journal Cardiology* **33**, 201-208

Cheng, T. O., Bashour, T., Singh, B. K. and Kelser, G. A. (1972). *American Journal Cardiology* **30**, 680.

Ciraulo, D. A. (1975). *American Journal Cardiology* **35**, 923.

Conti, C. R. (1976). *American Journal Cardiology* **37**, 896-902.

Eliot, R. S. and Bratt, G. (1969). *American Journal Cardiology* **23**, 633.

Enos, W. F., Holmes, R. H. and Beyer, J. C. (1953). *JAMA* **152**, 1090-1093.

Facchinetti, F. and Genazzani, A. R. (1978). *Journal Nuclear Medicine Allied Sciences* **22**, 419.

Fioretti, P., Genazzani, A. R., Facchinetti, F., Nasi, A., Melis, G. B. and Paoletti, A. M. (1974). Atti LVI^ Congresso Nazionale Società Italiana Ostetricia e Ginecologia, 637-716.

Fioretti, P., Melis, G. B., Paoletti, A. M., Parodo, G., Caminiti, F., Corsini, G. U. and Martini, L. (1978). *Journal of Clinical Endocrinology and Metabolism* **47**, 1336-1340.

Friedberg, C. K. (1966). *In* "Disease of Heart", W. B. Saunders, Philadelphia.

Friesinger, G. C. and Smith, R. F. (1972). *Circulation* **46**, 1173-1184.

Furman, R. H. (1968). *Annales New York Academy of Sciences* **149**, 822.

Fuster, V., Frye, R. L., Connolly, D. C., Danielson, M. A., Elveback, L. R. and Kurland, L. T. (1975). *British Heart Journal* **37**, 1250-1255.

Glancy, D. L., Marcus, M. L. and Epstein, S. E. (1971). *Circulation* **44**, 495.

Gorlin, R. (1978). *In* "Primary and Secondary Angina Pectoris" (A. Maseri, G. A. Klassen, M. Lesch, Eds), 71-79. Grune & Stratton, New York.

Hillis, L. D. and Braunwald, E. (1978). *New England Journal Medicine* **299**, 695-702.

Janowsky, D. S., Berens, S. C. and David, J. M. (1973). *Psychosomatic Medicine* **35**, 143-153.

Likoff, W., Segal, B. L. and Kasparian, H. R. (1967). *New England Journal Medicine* **276**, 1063.

Maseri, A., Mimmo, R., Chierchia, S., Marchesi, C., Pesola, A. and L'Abbate, A. (1975). *Chest* **68**, 625-633.

Maseri, A., Parodi, O., Severi, S. and Pesola, A. (1976). *Circulation* **56**, 280-288.

Maseri, A., L'Abbate, A., Pesola, A., Ballestra, A. M., Marzilli, M., Severi, S., Maltinti, G., De Nes, M., Parodi, O. and Biagini, A. (1977). *Lancet* **1**, 713-717.

Maseri, A., L'Abbate, A., Baroldi, G., Chierchia, S., Marzilli, M., Ballestra, A. M., Severi, S., Parodi, O., Biagini, A., Distante, A. and Pesola, A. (1978a). *New England Journal Medicine* **299**, 1271-1277.

Maseri, A., Severi, S., De Nes, M., L'Abbate, A., Chierchia, S., Marzilli, M., Ballestra, A. M., Parodi, O. and Biagini, A. (1978b). *American Journal Cardiology* **42**, 1019-1035.

Maseri, A., Chierchia, S. and L'Abbate, A. (1980). *Circulation* (Dec.) (in press).

Melis, G. B., Mameli, M., Cardia, S., Genazzani, A. R., Milia, A., Nasi, A., Paoletti, A. M., Puddu, R. and Fioretti, P. (1977). *Acta Europea Fertilitatis* **8**, 283–296.

Meller, J., Pichard, A. and Dack, S. (1976). *American Journal Cardiology* **37**, 938–940.

Neill, W. A., Kassebaum, D. C. and Judkins, M. P. (1968). *New England Journal Medicine* **279**, 789.

Neill, W. A., Ritzmann, L. W. and Selden, R. (1977). *American Heart Journal* **94**, 439–444.

Odell, W. D. (1979). *In* "Endocrinology" Vol. III, (L. J. Degroot, Ed.), p. 1489. Grune and Stratton, New York.

Prinzmetal, M., Kennamer, R., Merliss, R., Wada, T. and Bor, N. (1959). *American Journal Medicine* **27**, 375–388.

CARDIOVASCULAR APPARATUS AT CLIMACTERIC
(MULTIDISCIPLINARY STUDY ON 138 CASES)

F. Bottiglioni, A. S. Villecco[1], D. De Aloysio and E. Pisi[1]

*Institute of Obstetric and Gynaecological Pathology and
1st Institute of Special Medical Pathology and Clinical Methodology[1],
University of Bologna, Bologna, Italy*

INTRODUCTION

The relationships between cardiovascular pathology and climacteric as well as the pathogenetic processes involved, are still not fully understood (Oliver and Boyd, 1959; Novak and Wilmhas, 1960; Manchester *et al.*, 1971; Leone, 1975; Kannel *et al.*, 1976; Elkeles, 1977; Oliver, 1977; Jullian *et al.*, 1977; Zuspan, 1979).

Is there a cardiovascular disease which is favoured by and dependent on menopause? Our long-term research is aimed at clarifying this problem. Therefore the data here presented are only a starting-point and a guide-line.

METHODS

One hundred and thirty-eight recent postmenopausal women (0–5 years from cessation of menstruation) were taken as a sample. Out of them, 52 were oophorectomized and 86 had undergone a natural menopause. These women were attending the Menopause Clinic of the University of Bologna, and were used for epidemiological and statistical research*.

* Our data are preliminary, because the number of cases in the sample is not yet sufficient for use in statistical tests (χ Square, Cramer's V., contingency coefficient, symmetric lambda, asymmetric lambda).

Serono Symposium No. 39, "The Menopause: Clinical, Endocrinological and Pathophysiological Aspects", edited by P. Fioretti, L. Martini, G. B. Melis and S. S. C. Yen, 1982. Academic Press, London and New York.

Table I. Characterizing factors homogeneously distributed.

(A) Clinical–anamnestic data

Average height (cm)	160 ± 6
Age at menarche (years)	13 ± 2
0	21%
1	32%
> 1	47%
Familiar anamnesis of cardiovascular disease	
father	21%
mother	32%
Smoking (more than five cigarettes/day)	31%
Previous hormone treatment (during last 5 years and for at least 6 consecutive months)	47%

(B) Laboratory data — Percentages of normal values

HORMONES :	
17 β-oestradiol (less than 50 pg/ml)	100
LH (more than 30 mUI/ml)	84
FSH (more than 30 mUI/ml)	87
ACTH	89
TSH	64
STH	93
HPRL	98
T_3	79
T_4	95
Aldosterone	81
LIPIDS :	
Phospholipids	53
Esterified cholesterol	100
NEFA	89
Triglycerides	91
Kilomicrons	99
α-lipoproteins	89
β-lipoproteins	81
RO-lipoproteins	79
β/pre-β ratio	81
ENZYMES :	
Alkaline phosphatase	98
SGOT	96
SGPT	98
γGT	93

(C) Laboratory data   Percentage of normal values

ELECTROLYTES :

Plasmatic
- Ca — 100
- P — 95
- Na — 100
- K — 93

Urinary
- Ca — 95
- P — 87

CLOTTING FACTORS :

Platelets (> 150.000 per ml)	93
Normotest	86
Euglobulin lysis time	57
Antithrombine III	98
PAT (up to 3)	91

HAEMATOLOGIC DATA

Leucocytes	89
Erythrocytes	95
IIb	90
Ht	59
MCV	94
MCH	79
MCHC	85

OTHER DATA:

Vanylmandelic acid	98
Total proteinaemia	100
Fractionated proteinaemia :	
Albumine	92
α_1-globuline	100
α_2-globuline	97
β-globuline	84
γ-globuline	72
A/G ratio	81
Plasma creatinine	100
Urinary creatinine	84
Uricaemia	100

Table II. Characterizing factors heterogeneously distributed

(A) Clinical-anamnestic data		Natural menopause	Oophorectomy
Average age (years)		52 ± 3	46 ± 7
Average age at menopause (years)		49 ± 3	41 ± 7
profession	housewife	52.3%	42.3%
	inferior rank	7.0%	17.3%
	freelance	9.3%	11.5%
	employee	27.9%	26.9%
	superior rank	1.2%	0%
	retired	2.3%	1.9%
level of education	low	43%	53.8%
	medium	27.6%	25%
	high	20.9%	19.2%
	university	9.3%	1.9%
Miscarriages	yes	27.9%	48.1%
	no	72.1%	51.9%
Average weight (kg)		66 ± 11	62 ± 9
Ponderal index	normal	52.0%	59.1%
	less than 10 kg above normal value	21.3%	27.3%
	more than 10 kg above normal value	26.7%	13.6%
Diet	more than 3000 cal	65.2%	78.9%
	less than 3000 cal	34.8%	21.1%

(B) Endocrine profile		Natural menopause	Oophorectomy
Cortisol	<	5.2%	6.1%
	normal	75.3%	85.7%
	>	19.5%	8.2%
Testosterone	normal	90.2%	96.1%
	>	9.8%	3.9%
Insulin	<	32.9%	43.1%
	normal	59.5%	41.2%
	>	7.6%	15.7%

(C) Laboratory data		Natural Menopause	Oophorectomy
Sideraemia	<	6.8%	15.9%
	normal	93.2%	84.1%
Azotaemia	normal	96.4%	90.2%
	>	3.6%	9.8%
Glycaemia	normal	93.8%	100%
	>	6.5%	0%

Coleste-rolaemia	{ normal	53.2%	73.5%
	{ >	46.8%	26.5%
Total lipids	{ normal	84.6%	95.9%
	{ >	15.4%	4.1%
Urinary Na	<	27.6%	12.5%
	normal	65.8%	81.3%
	>	6.6%	6.3%
Urinary K	<	17.6%	6.3%
	normal	82.4%	93.8%
Pre β lipo-proteins	normal	83.3%	92.9%
	>	16.7%	7.1%
β + pre β/RO+ α ratio	{ < 3.0	72.7%	53.8%
	{ > 3.0	27.3%	46.2%

Table III. Climacteric disturbances connected with cardiovascular apparatus

	Whole sample (%)	Natural menopause (%)	Oophorectomy (%)
Palpitation	23.1	19.8	28.8
Precordialiga	26.8	32.9	17.6
Perspiration	74.6	77.9	69.2
Flushing	78.9	79.1	78.8
Vertigo	30.4	34.9	23.1
Asthenia	47.1	47.1	48.1
Headaches	31.8	29.1	36.5
Anxiety	57.9	61.6	51.9
Insomnia	50.0	46.5	55.8

Description of Sample

The sample is characterized by clinical-anamnestic and biohumoral factors, of which some are homogeneously (Table I) and others heterogeneously distributed (Table II) in the two groups (oophorectomy and natural menopause).

As for the distribution of heterogeneous factors, the statistical analysis shows that the women with natural menopause are generally older, overweight and economically more prosperous (clinical-anamnestic factors) and are characterized by a greater frequency of hypercortisolemia, hypertestosteronemia, glyco- and lipo-metabolic alterations and hypokaliemia (bio humoral factors).

As far as climacteric disturbances of the cardio-vascular apparatus are concerned, it was discovered from the heterogeneous distribution that natural postmenopausal women are more prone to precordialgia and vertigo; oophorectomized women are more prone to palpitation (Table III).

CARDIOVASCULAR PARAMETERS

We have studied certain cardiovascular alterations such as arterial hypertension (mainly systo-diastolic, border line: 150/95 mmHg) and certain electrocardiographic alterations (ischaemic and nonischaemic patterns as well as disturbances of rhythm). These alterations, in fact, have a paramount influence on the standards of cardiovascular morbidity and mortality.

Table IV. Systo-diastolic arterial pressure in recent (naturally and oophorectomized) postmenopausal women

Systo-diastolic arterial pressure	Whole sample (100%)	Natural menopause (62.1%)	Oophorectomy (37.9%)
Normal	77.3%	81.5%	72.0%
Increased	22.7%	19.5%	28.0%

Table V. ECG patterns in recent (naturally and oophorectomized) postmenopausal women

Electrocardiographic diagnosis	Whole sample (100%)	Natural menopause (50.9%)	Oophorectomy (39.1%)
Normal	52.6%	51.9%	53.8%
Ischaemic patterns	6.0%	6.2%	5.8%
Non-ischaemic patterns	27.1%	32.1%	19.2%
Disturbances in rhythm	14.3%	9.9%	21.2%

Hypertension

This considion, present in 22.7% of the sample, is more frequent in oophorectomized women (28%) than in natural postmenopausal women (19.5%) (Table IV). The rate of incidence is similar to that referred to in the literature (Pubbl. 1000, 11(13); Washington D. C., Ministero P. I., 1966), where a group made up of both men and women of the same age as our group is taken as an example.

The fact that hypertension occurs more frequently in recent oophorectomized women seems to be in contrast with the fact that they are younger.

Electrocardiographic Alterations

Ischaemic patterns are present in 6% of the sample, and there are no notable differences between natural postmenopausal (6.2%) and oophorectomized women (5.8%) (Table V). Non-ischaemic patterns (i.e. secondary repolarization alterations) are present in 27.1% of the sample, and are more frequent in natural postmenopausal women (32.1%) than in the oophorectomized ones (19.2%). Disturbances of rhythm, present in 14.3% of cases, are more frequent in oophorectomized women (21.2%) than in natural postmenopausal women (9.9%).

RELATIONSHIPS BETWEEN HYPERTENSION AND ELECTROCARDIO-GRAPHIC PATTERNS

We analysed electrocardiographic patterns in relation to arterial pressure and vice versa in natural postmenopausal women (Table VI) and in oophorectomized women (Table VII). Our data show:

(1) In the group of natural postmenopausal women:
(a) a higher incidence of ischaemic (13.3% v 4.6%) and non-ischaemic patterns (53.3% v 27.7%) in women suffering from hypertension in relation to those with normal blood pressure;
(b) a lower incidence of disturbances of rhythm in women suffering from hypertension in relation to those with normal blood pressure (6.7% v 10.8%);
(c) a higher incidence of hypertension in patients with ischaemic (40.0%) and non-ischaemic patterns (30.8%);
(d) 3.7% of cases of women with ischaemic patterns and 22.5% of cases with non-ischaemic patterns, both not associated with hypertension.
(2) In the group of oophorectomized women.
(a) an increased frequency of ischaemic (14.3% v 2.8%) and non-ischaemic patterns (28.6% v 16.7%) and disturbances in rhythm (28.6% v 16.7%) in women suffering from hypertension in relation to those with normal blood pressure;
(b) a higher frequency of hypertension (66.7% v 33.3%) in patients with ischaemic patterns and a lower frequency of hypertension in women with non-ischaemic patterns (40.0% v 60.0%);
(c) 2.0% of cases with ischaemic patterns and 12.0% of cases with non-ischaemic patterns, both not associated with hypertension.

According to the above results, it may be said that women in natural post-menopause (obviously older) are more subject to ischaemic heart diseases electro-cardiographically documented; myocardial ischaemia seems to have no relation to the menopause but rather to old age, and disturbances in rhythm are more frequent in oophorectomized women and seem to have some bearing with the event of menopause.

CLIMACTERIC DISTURBANCES CONNECTED WITH CARDIO-VASCULAR APPARATUS

These disturbances were correlated with hypertension (Table VIII) and electro-cardiographic patterns (Table IX); the analysis of these correlations shows that

Table VI. Relationships between the electrocardiographic pattern and arterial pressure in natural menopause.

| | ECG diagnosis in natural menopause | | | | |
	Normal	ECG ischaemic patterns	ECG non-ischaemic patterns	Disturbances in rhythm	Total ROW
Systo-diastolic arterial pressure — normal	37[a] 56.9%[b] 90.2%[c] 46.2%[d]	3 4.6% 60.0% 3.7%	18 27.7% 69.2% 22.5%	7 10.8% 87.5% 8.8%	65 81.3%
increased	4 26.7% 9.8% 5.0%	2 13.3% 40.0% 2.5%	8 53.3% 30.8% 10.0%	1 6.7% 12.5% 1.2%	15 18.8%
Column total	41 51.3%	5 6.3%	26 32.5%	8 10.0%	80 100.0%

[a] count; [b] row %; [c] col %; [d] tot %.

Table VII. Relationships between the electrocardiographic pattern and arterial pressure in oophorectomy.

	ECG diagnosis in oophorectomy				
	Normal	ECG ischaemic patterns	ECG non-ischaemic patterns	Disturbances in rhythm	Total ROW
Systo-diastolic arterial pressure — Normal	23[a] 63.9%[b] 85.2%[c] 46.0%[d]	1 2.8% 33.3% 2.0%	6 16.7% 60.0% 12.0%	6 16.7% 60.0% 12.0%	36 72.0%
Increased	4 28.6% 14.8% 8.0%	2 14.3% 66.7% 4.0%	4 28.6% 40.0% 8.0%	4 28.6% 40.0% 8.0%	14 28.0%
Column total	27 54.0%	3 6.0%	10 20.0%	10 20.0%	50 100.0%

[a] count; [b] row %; [c] col %; [d] tot %.

Table VIII. Climacteric disturbances connected with cardiovascular apparatus in recent postmenopause in relation to hypertension

	Hypertension	
	Yes (%)	No (%)
Palpitation	23.3	22.5
Precordialgia	30.3	28.0
Perspiration	63.3	77.5
Flushing	73.3	81.4
Vertigo	35.7	25.7
Asthenia	43.3	46.5
Headaches	30.0	32.4
Anxiety	53.3	57.8
Insomnia	33.3	53.9

Table IX. Climacteric disturbances connected with cardiovascular apparatus in recent postmenopause in relation to the electrocardiographic pattern

	ECG diagnosis			
	Normal (%)	ECG ischaemic patterns (%)	ECG non-ischaemic patterns (%)	Disturbances in rhythm (%)
Palpitation	25.7	25.0	22.2	10.5
Precordialgia	18.6	37.5	47.2	22.2
Perspiration	72.9	75.0	75.0	78.9
Flushing	80.0	62.5	80.6	84.2
Vertigo	30.9	28.6	27.8	31.6
Asthenia	49.3	37.5	50.0	36.8
Headaches	32.9	37.5	25.0	42.1
Anxiety	61.4	50.0	52.8	57.9
Insomnia	57.1	50.0	36.1	57.9

there is a greater incidence of vertigo (35.7% v 25.7%) and a lesser incidence of insomnia (33.3% v 53.9%) in women suffering from hypertension; in patients presenting electrocardiographic alterations there is a lower frequency of palpitations in women with disturbances in rhythm (10.5%); a greater incidence of precordialgia in women with ischaemic (37.5%) and non-ischaemic (47.2%) patterns; a lower frequency of flushing in women with ischaemic patterns (62.5%) and of insomnia in those with non-ischaemic patterns (36.1%).

FACTORS INFLUENCING HYPERTENSION AND ELECTRO-CARDIOGRAPHIC ALTERATIONS

The incidence of hypertension was higher in women who had gained weight, in those with familial anamnesis of cardiovascular diseases, in those with diabetes mellitus (both latent and manifest), in those with hypercholesterolemia, in those with increased T_3-T_4 values, in those with increased blood urea nitrogen and in those with hypokaliemia (Table X).

The incidence of ischaemic alterations was greater in women who had gained weight, in those with dysfunction of the thyroid, in those with hypercoagulation, in those with hypercortisolemia and in those who had undergone substitutive hormone treatment in the past (Table XI).

Table X. Frequency of hypertension in relation to clinical-anamnestic and biohumoral factors.

Increased in women with:	Unvaried in women with:
(1) Ponderal index (+)	(1) Smoking (more than 5 cigarettes per day)
(2) Familial anamnesis of cardiovascular diseases (+)	
	(2) Previous hormone treatment
(3) Glycemia (+)	(3) Cortisol (+) and (−)
(4) Normo-test (+)	(4) Aldosterone (+) and (−)
(5) PAT (more than 3)	(5) TSH (+) and (−)
(6) Cholesterolemia (+)	(6) Testosterone (+)
(7) T_3 and T_4 (+)	(7) STH (+)
(8) Azotemia (+)	(8) Plasmatic K (+)
(9) Plasmatic K (−)	(9) Hb and Ht (−)
	(10) Gamma GT (+)
	(11) Antithrombin III (−)
	(12) Platelets (−)
	(13) Euglobulin lysis time (+) and (−)

CONCLUSIONS

The data of our sample show that a whole group of clinical and biohumoral factors, which are connected in part with menopause and in part with the natural life of a woman, may concur in determining some cardiovascular diseases during postmenopausal years.

The latter seem to be of more importance than the former, but it is at present impossible to establish how much they are influenced by gonadal failure. However if such an influence exists it should act on metabolic, endocrine and haemoco-agulative disorders.

Table XI. Frequency of electrocardiographic ischaemic alterations in relation to clinical-anamnestic and biohumoral factors.

Increased in women with:	Unvaried in women with:
(1) Ponderal index (+)	(1) Smoking (more than 5 cigarettes per day)
(2) Previous hormone treatment	
(3) T_3 (+) and (−)	(2) Familial anamnesis of cardiovascular diseases
(4) T_4 (+)	(3) TSH (−)
(5) Anti-thrombine III (−)	(4) Cortisol (+)
(6) PAT (greater than 3)	(5) Aldosterone (+)
(7) Euglobulin lysis time (+)	(6) STH (+)
	(7) Testosterone (+)
	(8) Cholesterol (+)
	(9) NEFA (+)
	(10) Triglycerides (+)
	(11) Plasmatic K (+)
	(12) Hb and Ht (−)
	(13) Glycemia (+)
	(14) Azotemia (+)
	(15) Platelets (−)
	(16) Normo-test (+) and (−)
	(17) Euglobulin lysis time (−)

REFERENCES

Elkeles, A. (1977). *British Medical Journal* 1, 1215–16.

Gordon, T., Kannel, W. B., Hjortland, M. C. and McNamara, P. M. (1978). *Annales Internal Medicine* 89 (2), 157–161.

Kannel, W. B., Hjortland, M. C. and McNamara, P. M. (1976). *Annales Internal Medicine* 85 (4), 447–52.

Jullian, G., Gichtenaere, J. C. and Gerard, R. (1977). *Nouvelle Press Medicale* 6 (13), 1125–28.

Leone, U. (1975). *Minerva Ginecologica* 27 (10), 812–15.

Manchester, J. H., Herman, M. V. and Gorlin, R. (1971). *American Journal of Cardiology* 28, 33.

Novak, E. R. and Wilmhas, P. J. (1960). *American Journal Obstetrics and Gynecology* 80, 863.

Oliver, M. F. (1977). *British Medical Journal* 1 (6073), 1414.

Oliver, M. F. and Boyd, G. S. (1959). *Lancet* 2, 690.

Suamborg, G. *et al.* (1977). *Clinica Chimica Acta* 79 (2), 229–307.

Zuspan, F. P. (1979). *Annales Internal Medicine* 90 (3), 439–440.

CORONARY HEART DISEASE AND ITS RISK FACTORS IN POSTMENOPAUSAL AGE

G. Morra[1], P. Cavallo-Perin[2], R. Sorbo[1], E. Pisu[2], G. Pagano[2] and G. Lenti[1]

*Cattedra di Clinica Medica A[1], Cattedra di Semeiotica Medica[2]
Department of Internal Medicine, University of Turin, Turin, Italy,*

INTRODUCTION

Cardiovascular disease and in particular coronary heart disease (CHD) has been the most important cause of death in Italy in the last 2 decades (Compendio Statistico Italiano, 1978).

Several long-term prospective studies (Kannel *et al.*, 1971; Wilhelmsen *et al.*, 1973; Reid *et al.*, 1976) have confirmed the role of hypercholesterolemia and hypertension as independent factors predicting the increased likelihood of CHD. Other variables such as plasma triglycerides (Kannel *et al.*, 1971), body weight (Reid *et al.*, 1976), blood glucose (Fuller *et al.*, 1975) and uric acid (Stamler *et al.*, 1972) may be related to the prevalence of CHD. CHD prevalence seems to be higher in men than in women of similar age (Elmfeldt *et al.*, 1975) and some differences before and after menopause exist (Kannel *et al.*, 1975).

Since the characteristics of the correlation between CHD and risk factors in the two sexes are not yet well defined, particularly in the Italian population, the objects of the present study are to study the prevalence of CHD in a group of women in postmenopausal age and in a control group of men with similar age; to compare the pattern of some variables in the two sexes; and to evaluate the risk factor frequence and its relation to CHD in these sex groups.

Serono Symposium No. 39, "The Menopause: Clinical, Endocrinological and Pathophysiological Aspects", edited by P. Fioretti, L. Martini, G. B. Melis and S. S. C. Yen, 1982. Academic Press, London and New York.

G. Morra et al.

SUBJECTS AND METHODS

A group of 2703 postmenopausal women, aged 58.8 ± 10.1 years were selected from a random population sample of three country towns near Turin and examined in a Public Medical Centre for 5 years (1973-1977). A group of 1421 males, aged 59.3 ± 9.9 years, were selected from the same population sample and examined in the Centre during the same period. The participation rate in the study was 92% in females and 89% in males.

A general health questionnaire was compiled to obtain information about family history of diabetes and vasculopathy, history of diabetes, hypertension and smoking habits; height (m), weight (Kg) and radial blood pressure (systolic and diastolic) were measured. A resting ECG was recorded and evaluated by Minnesota Code (Rose and Blackburn, 1968). A venous blood sample for determination of blood glucose, total cholesterol, triglycerides and uric acid was drawn in the morning after fasting and biochemical estimations were carried out by enzymatic methods.

CHD affected patients were identified; these included subjects with previously recognized myocardial infarction and subjects ECG positive for ischaemia evaluated by Minnesota Code. The hypertensive group was defined as including subjects with positive anamnesis for hypertension and subjects with systolic blood pressure of 170 mmHg and more and/or diastolic of 100 mmHg or more, in two different determinations after a rest of 30 min in recumbent position (Rose, 1976). The obsese group was defined as including subjects with BMI (body mass index = weight/height^2) of 28 or more, according to the range variation recorded in other studies (Goldbourt and Medalie, 1979). The diabetic group was defined as including subjects with positive personal anamnesis for diabetes mellitus and subjects whose fasting blood glucose was 120 mg/dl or more in two different determinations. The following upper limit values were considered to permit the recognition of the risk factors for CHD: hypertriglyceridemia of 200 mg/dl or more (Schettler and Nüssel, 1975); hypercholesterolemia of 260 mg/dl or more (Schettler and Nüssel, 1975); hyperuricemia of 7 mg/dl or more in males and 5.7 mg/dl or more in females (Thefeld *et al.*, 1973).

The differences between females and males of the mean values of the variables measured, of risk factor frequencies and of the prevalence of CHD were evaluated by χ^2 and *t*-test; multiple regression analysis was performed using SPSS.

RESULTS

The prevalence of CHD was significantly higher in women than in men (Fig. 1). The mean values of the variables studied were all significanlty higher in CHD females than in normals; in males, only blood pressure, age and cholesterol showed higher values in CHD patients than in normals.

Figure 2 gives the frequence of CHD when each risk factor is present or absent respectively in females and males. Hypertension seems to be important in conditioning the presence of CHD in the two sexes. Hypercholesterolemia, obesity, diabetes and family history of vasculopathy seem to be important only in females, while smoking and being over 60 years of age seem to be relevant only in males.

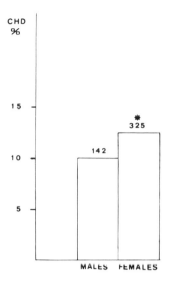

Fig. 1. Percentage prevalence of CHD in males and females. The difference between the % frequency of CHD in males and females was evaluated by χ^2 test. $*P < 0.05$. Males 1.421; females 2.703; age matched.

Figure 3 gives the risk factor frequency in females and males of the CHD patients group. While the frequency of hypercholesterolemia in females is higher than in males, the frequency of smoking and hyperuricemia is higher in males ($P < 0.001$). Besides, the risk related to age, obesity, diabetes and hypertriglyceridemia is distributed in the two sexes without any significant difference.

DISCUSSION

The higher CHD prevalence in postmenopausal women than in males contradicts the results of other community studies in which the prevalence of CHD is about 3-6 times higher in men than in women in the age group 45 to 54 years (Elmfeldt *et al.*, 1975; Wilhelmsen *et al.*, 1977).

The different implication of the risk factors in conditioning the prevalence of CHD in the two sexes (Fig. 2), not confirmed by others (Kannel and Castelli, 1972), could in part explain the discrepancy described above. In particular, among smokers, the frequency of CHD is higher both in males and females, but in this last group the difference does not reach statistical significance owing to the negligible number of smokers in females (Fig. 3). So, if smoking does have some influence on a higher prevalence of CHD in females as well, the number of CHD associated risk factors is greater in females than in males (Fig. 2). Furthermore, the mean values of all variables are significantly higher in CHD females and not in males, and many such variables are significantly and positively related to one another. These results suggest a heavier coronary risk profile in women than in men.

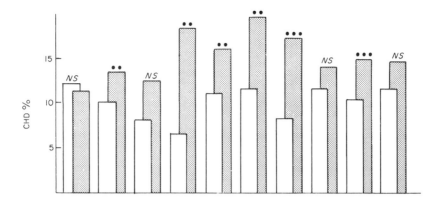

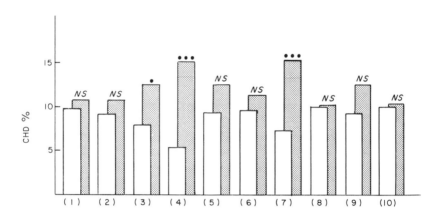

Fig. 2. Percentage frequency of CHD in presence (filled columns) and in absence (white columns) of each risk factor. Risk factors are, from left to right, in order: family history of diabetes (1), family history of vasculopathy (2), smoking (3), ageing > 60 (4), obesity (5), diabetes (6), hypertension (7), hyperuricemia (8), hypercholesterolemia (9), hypertriglyceridemia (10). The differences between the % frequencies of CHD in presence and in absence of each risk factor were evaluated by x^2 test. The top graph shows the results for females (N = 2703) and the bottom graph for males (N = 1421). $\bullet P < 0.05$; $\bullet\bullet P < 0.01$; $\bullet\bullet\bullet P < 0.001$.

Nevertheless, in the CHD group, the higher frequency of hypercholesterolemia in females and the higher frequency of smoking and hyperuricemia in males cannot solely explain why the females suffered CHD more than males.

Since in the postmenopausal period the protective effect of the female hormone pattern disappears, the prevalence of CHD may be related to the presence of traditional risk factors such as family history of vasculopathy, ageing, obesity, hypertension (similar distribution in both sexes). Since CHD prevalence is higher in

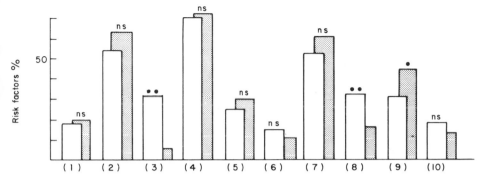

Fig. 3. Percentage frequency of risk factors in CHD males (white columns) and CHD females (filled columns). Risk factors are, from left to right, in order: family history of diabetes (1), family history of vasculopathy (2), smoking (3), ageing > 60 (4), obesity (5), diabetes (6), hypertension (7), hyperuricemia (8), hypercholesterolemia (9), hypertriglyceridemia (10). The differences between the % frequency of every risk factor in males and females were evaluated by χ^2 test. $\bullet P < 0.01$; $\bullet\bullet P < 0.001$.

females, there are probably as yet unidentified factors which are important for CHD in this sex. Such factors may be connected with the lipid metabolism of the vessel wall, the coagulation system, or even with the sensitivity of the myocardium to hypoxia or its tendency to react with catecholamine release. In an experimental study (Wolinsky, 1973), a different reactivity of the vessel wall in male and female animals was reported. Similar sex differences with respect to the sensitivity of the myocardium in humans are not known at present, but are worthy of investigation.

REFERENCES

Chapman, J. M. and Massey, F. J. (1964). *Journal of Chronic Diseases* 17, 933.
Compendio Statistico Italiano. Ed. by Istituto Centrale di Statistica (1978), p. 59.
Elmfeldt, D., Wilhelmsen, L., Tibblin, G., Vedin, J. A., Wilhelmsson, C. and
   Bengtsson, C. (1975). *Journal of Chronic Diseases* 28, 173.
Fuller, J. H., McCartney, P. and Colwell, L. M. (1975). (abstract) *Diabetologia*
   11, 343.
Goldbourt, V. and Medalie, J. H. (1979). *American Journal of Epidemiology*
   109, 296.
Kannel, W. B. and Castelli, W. P. (1972). *Medical Times* (New York) 100, 173.
Kannel, W. B., Castelli, W. P., Gordon, T. and McNamara, P. M. (1971). *Annals
   of Internal Medicine* 74, 1.
Kannel, W. B., Hjortland, M. and McNamara, P. (1975). *Abstract of Conference
   on CVD Epidemiology*, Tampa, Florida, 10–11 March.
Reid, D. D., Hamilton, P. J. S., McCatney, P., Rose, G., Jarret, R. J. and Keen, H.
   (1976). *Lancet* 2, 979.
Rose, G. (1976). *Postgraduate Medical Journal* 52, 452.
Rose, G. A. and Blackburn, H. (1968). *In* "Cardiovascular Survey Methods".
   World Health Organization. Monograph Series, 56, 149.

Schettler, G. and Nüssel, E. (1975). *Arbeitmedizine Sozialmedizine Präventivmedizine* **10**, 25.

Stamler, J., Berkson, D. M. and Lindberg, A. (1972). *In* "The Pathogenesis of Atherosclerosis" (R. W. Wissler and J. C. Geer, Eds), p. 41. Williams and Wilkins, Baltimore.

Thefeld, W., Hoffmeister, H., Bush, E. W., Koller, P. U. and Vollman, J. (1973). *Deutsche Medizine Wochenschrift* **98**, 380.

Wilhelmsen, L., Weden, H. and Tibblin, G. (1973). *Circulation* **48**, 950.

Wilhelmsen, L., Bengtsson, C., Elmfeldt, D., Vedin, A., Wilhelmsson, C., Tibblin, G., Lindquist, O. and Wedel, H. (1977). *British Heart Journal* **39**, 1179.

Wolinsky, H. (1973). *Circulation Research* **33**, 183.

CARDIOVASCULAR RESPONSES DURING MENOPAUSAL FLUSHES

J. Ginsburg and J. R. Swinhoe

Academic Department of Medicine, Royal Free Hospital Medical School, Pond Street, London, UK

INTRODUCTION

Hot flushes are probably the commonest accompaniment of the menopause and occur in over 80% of women (Mulley and Mitchell, 1976). Although the characteristic sensation of increased heat together with reddening of the skin in the blush areas of the face and neck during the flush were attributed to altered autonomic activity as long ago as 1889 (Glaevecke, 1889), neither the mechanism responsible for this phenomenon nor the precise nature of the accompanying circulatory changes are known.

Current therapy for the flush is empirical. In order that rational therapy may be developed, we require knowledge of the underlying mechanisms involved. We have therefore undertaken a study of the peripheral circulatory changes occurring during hot flushes and present the initial data herewith.

PATIENTS AND METHODS

The patients studies were those presenting at our Endocrine outpatients with complaints of frequent severe hot flushes and who had not previously been treated with oestrogen or other medication. Fifty-six women aged between 47 and 54 years were initially incorporated in the study. However, hot flushes did not occur

Serono Symposium No. 39, "The Menopause: Clinical, Endocrinological and Pathophysiological Aspects", edited by P. Fioretti, L. Martini, G. B. Melis and S. S. C. Yen, 1982. Academic Press, London and New York.

spontaneously in the laboratory and could not be provoked in 38 of these women. The results presented here are therefore based on data derived from 18 of these women, 12 of whom flushed spontaneously during the recording session and six in whom a hot flush was provoked by stressful mental arithmetic.

Limb blood flow was measured by venous occlusion plethysmography using water filled plethysmographs as in our previous studies of the peripheral circulation (Ginsburg and Duff, 1958; Ginsburg and Cobbold, 1960; Beaconsfield *et al.*, 1972). Hand and forearm flow were measured in all 18 subjects and calf flow in four of the women.

Experiments were conducted in standardized laboratory conditions with a constant ambient and plethysmograph temperature. Subjects lay down and rested for 15 min on arrival in the laboratories after which pulse and blood pressure were measured and the plethysmographs placed in position. Recordings of limb blood flow were then made for 20 min. If a flush did not occur spontaneously during this period, stressful mental arithmetic (Fenel *et al.*, 1959) was applied for 2 min. This provoked a hot flush in six women.

Limb blood flow was measured at 30 s intervals throughout, except during a hot flush or when stressful mental arithmetic was applied, in which case recordings were made more frequently, at 10 or 15 s intervals. Blood pressure was measured by auscultation with a standard sphygmomanometer. Pulse rate was calculated from the plethysmographic tracing every 30 s during resting phases and every 15 s during a hot flush.

At the end of each recording session the volume of the limb within the plethysmograph was measured by water displacement and limb blood flow calculated and expressed in ml/100 ml tissue/min.

With the onset of a flush, women frequently became restless. It was therefore not possible to obtain continuous recordings every 15 s throughout the flush in all 18 patients. However, six women remained still and relaxed throughout and in these frequent uninterrupted recordings were possible. Analysis of the detailed pattern of change, as shown in Fig. 1, is based on data derived from studies in the six women who remained still, whereas the overall mean changes in flow, as illustrated in Fig. 2, refer to measurements in the larger group of 18 which included the six in whom continuous recordings were made.

RESULTS

The pattern of change in peripheral blood flow during the flush is constant in both direction and time. The earliest indication of a hot flush is a rapid rise in hand flow to reach a peak some $2\frac{1}{2}$ min after the onset of symptoms. Hand flow then falls rapidly and symmetrically to settle at around control values.

In the six women studied in detail, hand flow increased from a mean resting value of 8.7 ml blood/100 ml tissues/min, to a peak of 29.4 ml (Fig. 1). Hand flow then fell and reached resting values after a further $2\frac{1}{2}$ min. There was a highly significant mean percentage increase ($P < 0.001$) in hand flow, overall, of 250% (Fig. 2).

Forearm flow increased *pari passu* with the rise in hand flow but to a lesser extent. There was no sharp peak in forearm flow. The mean change in the group

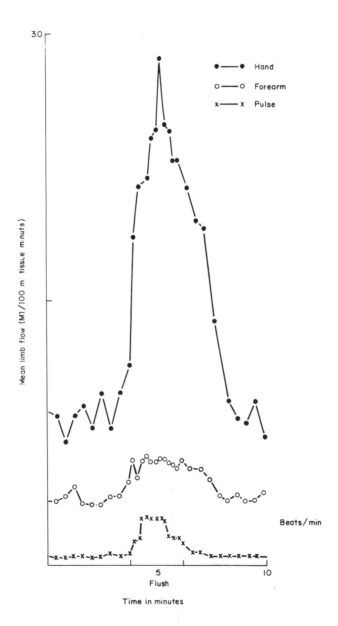

Fig. 1. Mean hand (crosses) and forearm (open circles) flow and pulse rate (closed circles) in six women during a menopausal flush (see methods).

of six was from 3.9 ml initially, in the control period, to 5.9 ml concomitantly with the peak in hand flow (Fig. 1). There was a highly significant ($P < 0.001$) overall increase in mean forearm flow of 50% (Fig. 2).

In the four women in whom calf flow was measured, the pattern of response resembled that of forearm rather than hand flow, there being no sharp peak and a mean rise in flow of 100%. However this increase is not significant.

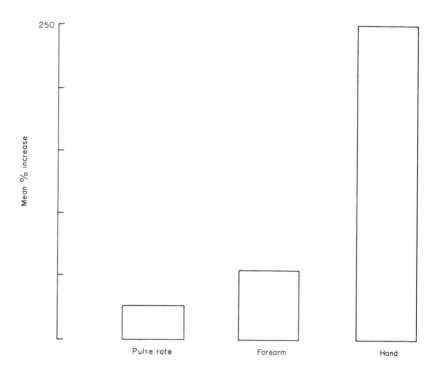

Fig. 2. Mean % change in pulse rate, forearm and hand flow in 18 women during a menopausal flush.

An increase in pulse rate was also observed during the flush, the maximum rise in the six women being eight beats/min $2\frac{1}{2}$ min after the start of the flush (Fig. 1). There was a significant ($P < 0.01$) increase in mean pulse rate in the group of 18 patients of 25% (Fig. 2). However pulse rate fell earlier than hand or forearm flow and control pulse levels were regained at a time when both forearm and hand flow were still elevated. There was no significant alteration in blood pressure either during or after the flush.

DISCUSSION

A major problem in studying the mechanism of the hot flush has been the difficulty of eliciting responses in standardized laboratory conditions. The involuntary movements which may occur during the hot flush have vitiated previous attempts to obtain continuous electrocardiographic and pulse rate recordings. The flush, moreover, is a very variable phenomenon and whilst it may be evoked by stress, stress itself provokes circulatory changes (Fenel *et al.*, 1959).

It is therefore of considerable importance that we were able to obtain accurate and continuous measurements of limb flow during the hot flush. In these circumstances a clearly defined unequivocal pattern of circulatory response is apparent. Our study has shown that a dramatic increase in hand flow occurs rapidly and consistently to reach a peak within $2\frac{1}{2}$ min of the onset of symptoms. There is a simultaneous but less marked increase in forearm and calf flow but with no apparent sharp peak. Changes in pulse rate parallel those in forearm and calf flow initially but fall to reach control rates slightly earlier.

Circulatory responses in the hand essentially reflect alterations in skin flow. The results of our study would therefore suggest there is considerable rise in skin flow during the hot flush. The extent to which the increase in forearm flow reflects changes in blood vessels of the skin as opposed to those of skeletal muscle cannot however be determined from the present data alone. This requires separate determination of flow at different levels of the forearm, for example by strain gauge plethysmography (Clarke *et al.*, 1958), and investigations to determine this are currently in progress. Although calf flow also rose during the flush the increase was not significant. This finding would not support the simultaneous occurrence of vascular change in skeletal muscle during the flush. The fact that minimal changes were recorded in blood pressure would also suggest that changes in muscle flow are overall slight, unless a major distribution of regional blood flow had occurred to maintain blood pressure at the same time.

Although stress may on occasion provoke hot flushes and indeed it was used for this purpose in the present study, the pattern of circulatory change during stress differs from that observed during the hot flush. During stressful mental arithmetic, there is a variable change of flow, with a fall in hand flow in some women (Fenel *et al.*, 1959). Forearm flow increased consistently but the rise during stress was always less than that observed during the hot flush (Fig. 3).

What is the stimulus to the marked increase in hand and hence in skin flow that we have demonstrated? Blood flow through the distal parts of the extremities is governed by variations in vasoconstrictor tone and these regions are specialized for temperature control. Disturbance of the peripheral mechanisms for thermoregulatory control may therefore occur during the flush, as evidenced clinically by the sensation of heat frequently experienced and the distribution of skin reddening. We have no current information as to the factors responsible for any such disturbance of thermoregulatory control but the parallelism between menopausal flushes and the flushing observed after alcohol in subjects taking chlorpropamide (Leslie *et al.*, 1979) and the claim that endorphins may be involved in this particular response (Leslie *et al.*, 1979) have led to the suggestion that endorphins might be a central mediator determining the onset of the menopausal hot flush (Lightman

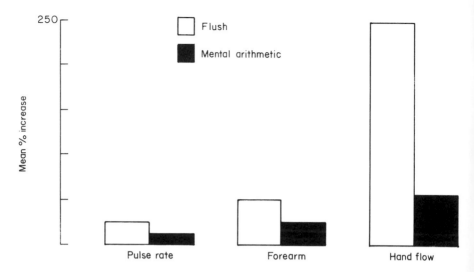

Fig. 3. Mean % change in pulse rate forearm and hand flow in 18 women during a meno-pausal flush (open histograms) and during stressful mental arithmetic (solid histograms) (see methods).

and Jacobs, 1979). It is therefore of interest that in recent studies naloxone, an antagonist of endorphin, was found to reduce the frequency and intensity of hot flushes (Lightman and Jacobs, 1979).

Not all women flush, Some never do and the most intense responses seem to occur with rapid change as after surgical removal of the ovaries or abrupt discontinuation of therapy. This would further suggest that other factors are involved, possibly an alteration of vascular reactivity in the menopause, an aspect which we are presently investigating.

There are many potential hazards of oestrogen therapy, which is in any event contra-indicated or unacceptable to many women. It is therefore important that more information is obtained on precisely what happens in the hot flush and how it is triggered. In the light of these and other results, it should be possible to develop alternative forms of therapy for the many women with severe disabling menopausal hot flushing.

REFERENCES

Beaconsfield, P., Ginsburg, J. and Rainsburg, R. (1972). *New England Journal of Medicine* **287**, 209.

Clarke, R. S. J., Ginsburg, J. and Hellon, R. F. (1958). *Journal Physiology* **140**, 318.

Fenel, V., Hejl, Z., Jirka, J., Madlafousek, J. and Brod, J. (1959). *Journal Clinical Science* **18**, 491.

Ginsburg, J. and Cobbold, A. F. (1960). *In* "Adrenergic Mechanisms" (Vane *et al.*, Eds), 173–189. Churchill, London.

Ginsburg, J. and Duff, R. S. (1958). *Circulation Research* **6**, 751.
Glaevecke, W. (1889). *Archives Gynakologie* **35**, 1.
Leslie, R. D. G., Pyke, D. A. and Stubbs, W. A. (1979). *Lancet* **I**, 341.
Lightman, S. L. and Jacobs, H. S. (1979). *Lancet* **II**, 1071.
Mulley, G. and Mitchell, J. A. A. (1976). *Lancet* **1**, 1397.

CLIMACTERIC ALTERATIONS OF LOW URINARY TRACT

S. Bettocchi and F. P. Selvaggi

I^ Clinica Ostetrica e Ginecologica, e Insegnamento di nefrologia di interesse chirurgico, Università di Bari, Bari, Italy

INTRODUCTION

The common embryological origin and the close anatomical relations between the lower urinary tract and the genitalia give a logical explanation for the high frequency of bladder and urethral complaints in postmenopausal females. It is not our intention to remind everyone of the multiplicity of hormonal changes in the physiological development of a woman and the considerable effect they have on the lower urinary tract. Here we shall describe the most common phenomena and complaints that patients in the climacteric age refer to us almost every day.

These phenomena and complaints can be strictly linked either to anatomical changes or to functional changes or both. From a urological point of view stress incontinence is the typical complaint of these women and is related to the anatomical changes of the pelvic floor and the organs of the pelvis. Moreover incontinence can be complicated by infections, chronic urinary retention and by modifications and complaints related to endocrine problems. However, in this paper we will consider only problems due to endocrine disturbances of the climacteric age because they are less known although probably more common.

These pathologies can be divided into two groups: the first and most frequent one is the group which includes the so-called "syndromes" presented by patients with a wide variety of symptoms but with very poor or no objective signs; the second one includes lesions that can be very clearly documented.

In the first group we can include the poorly defined "urethral syndrome" of

Serono Symposium No. 39, "The Menopause: Clinical, Endocrinological and Pathophysiological Aspects", edited by P. Fioretti, L. Martini, G. B. Melis and S. S. C. Yen, 1982. Academic Press, London and New York.

the English authors; in the second we can put lesions such as the urethral caruncle, the senile urethritis, the spontaneous thrombosis of the urethral vein and the mucosal urethral prolapse.

Typically the patient with "urethral syndrome" complains of dysuria, frequency, urgency, suprapubic pressure, low back pain or pelvic pain, general discomfort and occasional dyspaurenia. The urological evaluation is usually normal and so are all the diagnostic urological aids, such as i.v. pyelography, cystoscopy, urethral calibration, cystourethrography, urodynamic tests and perineal electromyography. Usually it is not possible to document a urinary tract infection, except in very rare instances.

Senile atrophy has been considered as the causal factor as well as psychic problems, allergies, and urethral obstructions. Few facts are certain, like the high incidence of hysterectomy and pelvic surgery in these patients, and also of endometriosis. Recently Bruce *et al.* (1973) have recovered through the use of culture swabs, micro-organisms such as *Streptococcus faecalis* and *Enterobacter*, significantly more frequently in patients with this syndrome than in a control group of asyntomatic women. These micro-organisms are not usually recovered through a routine "clean catch" culture nor by suprapubic aspiration, but they harbour in the vagina, vestibule and urethra and, according to Stamey *et al.* (1971) and Elkins and Cox (1974), they can be the cause of the syndrome.

If this "urethral syndrome" still appears unclear, poorly differentiated from other diseases and not generally accepted, the natural involution of the vesical trigone and urethra is something completely different. This involution is strictly correlated with those of the female genital organs and it is dependent on the common hormonal dependence. In fact, many years ago it was demonstrated that there are areas of epithelium, present at the level of the trigone, similar to those of the vagina. In normal circumstances these areas contain cells with high glycogen content and go through the same menstrual changes as the vaginal epithelium. Biopsy of patients with trigonitis has shown areas of metaplasia, similar to those of the vaginal epithelium, which are particularly sensitive to androgens and oestrogens. The clinical picture of the "senile or hypoestrogenic cystopathy" appears to be well recognised so far since it is characterized by typical cystoscopic findings such as trigonal hyperemia, squamous metaplasia of the trigone and pseudopolyps of the bladder neck. Such findings, though not always present, constantly correspond to very impressive symptoms. In fact the patients give a history of frequent or occasional nicturia, urgency to urinate, incontinence, burning related or not to the micturition, and pain in the external genitalia, hypogastrium and perineal area. Such a picture can be further confused by the presence of a urinary tract infection. As is known, in postmenopausal women these infections are very common because of atrophy of trigone and urethra, hypoestrogenism and anatomical changes of the bladder base, with chronic urinary tension. On the other hand a correct urological evaluation is essential for a diagnostic approach of those lesions of the lower urinary tract strictly correlated with the endocrine disturbances. Here we can only give a short description of the most frequent pathologies.

Urethral Caruncle

This is the common type of lesion of the female urethra in climacteric age. Clinical examination shows a small tumour well circumscribed, pedunculated or sessile, embedded within the mucosa of the distal urethra, typically on the edge of the inferior lip of the meatus. Patients complain of intermittent urination; spotting following friction from pads and use of toilet paper. The caruncle may be confused with a variety of similar lesions of the distal urethra such as polyps, hemangiomas, and varicose veins and, in particular, with the redundant or prolapsed urethral mucosa. They can be distinguished by their morphologic characteristics, which indicate their vascular origins. The differential diagnosis in the precocious stages of urethral carcinoma can be very difficult so that a biopsy will often be necessary.

Senile Urethritis

It is probably the least known lesion of the climacteric age and almost always confused with the "urethral syndrome". Clinical examination should reveal a urethral orifice, often reddened and hypersensitive, in contrast to the diagnosis and the pallor of the vaginal epithelium. The posterior lip of the meatus presents some eversion of the mucosa, mostly due to the shortening of the urethral vaginal wall. Endoscopy usually demonstrates a reddened and granular urethral mucosa with urethral stenosis in some instances. Differential diagnosis with urethral caruncle can be difficult and urinary-cytology, which always shows atrophic changes, can be useful.

Thrombosis of the Urethral Vein

Spontaneous thrombosis of the vein which occupies the flow of the distal urethra can occur. The patient suffers from a sudden local pain and, shortly there-after, a mass appears at the level of the urethral meatus. This mass is usually purple and protudes from the posterior lip of the orifice, and it is quite tender. It can be differentiated from the caruncle by the sudden onset and the gradual resolution without treatment in most instances. Evacuation of the clot is seldom recommended.

Mucosal Urethral Prolapse

It is not a very common pathology in the climacteric age but it can be seen more often in young girls under 18 years of age. However in the postmenopausal women it can be caused by several factors such as stress, coughing and Valsalva-like manoeuvres which act on an athrophic urethra. It appears as a red soft lump which protrudes from the urethral meatus around the entire circumference and, if not promptly reduced, may become gangrenous. Typically it causes an irritating sense of heaviness and mass in the genitalia, painful urination and easy bleeding due to possible ulceration. The differential diagnosis includes polyps, condyloma, cysts, periurethral abscess and granuloma. Vaginal examination and biopsy are sometimes necessary for an accurate diagnosis.

Urethral Diverticulum

It is not common principally because the gynaecologist does not look for it. It occurs more frequently in the 4th decade and appears to be more common in

Negroes than in Caucasians with a ratio of six:one (Andersen, 1967). It is not always possible to appreciate a soft mass in the middle part of one of the lateral walls of the urethra, but compression on the anterior vaginal wall against the pubis should push out the content of the little pocket as a purulent discharge from the urethral meatus. The aetiology is still controversial but it is conceivable that urethral diverticula could result from repeated infections of the paraurethral glands during postmenopauseal years. These infections lead to subsequent inflammation, obstruction, and finally cystic enlargement of these glands with formation of the small submucosal pockets. Symptoms range from minimal local discomfort to repeated urinary tract infection; in many patients the classic "three D's" of diverticulum can be seen: dribbling, dyspareunia and dysuria (Jacob, 1978). In some instances a stone can be formed within the sack of diverticulum and the patient presents a hard palpable mass on the anterior vaginal wall. The differential diagnosis has to be done with urethral cysts, vaginal tumours, and infection of the Skene's glands.

Clinical Study

Throughout the last 8 years clinical and urodynamic studies were performed among a group of about one thousand women for urological diseases related to gynaecological problems. Out of them, a homogenous group of 85 patients has been well classified so far. The subjects were 40-70 years old; a third had surgical menopause (Table I). Serum LH and FSH levels were evaluated to be sure that all patients were in postmenopause. Urodynamic tests were performed in all cases: subjects showing even small signs of an irritable bladder were not included in the study group.

Table I. Patients with climacteric low urinary tract troubles.

Age	No.	of	cases	Surgical menopause
40–45	4	=	4.7%	3
46–50	14	=	16.5%	8
51–55	26	=	30.6%	12
56–60	16	=	18.8%	1
61–65	14	=	16.5%	3
66–70	11	=	12.9%	1
	85		100%	28 (32.9%)

Table II. Appearance of urinary symptoms and onset of menopause.

Years after menopause	Physiologic menopause	Surgical menopause
1	26.3	53.5
1–5	35	2.5
6–10	10.5	14.2
10	28	7.1

RESULTS

The urinary symptoms appeared at different time intervals after the menopause (Table II). Fifty per cent of the surgical menopause patients experienced symptoms a few months after surgery, while in the others complaints appeared over a 10 year period. In 45% of the patients the main complaint was "stress incontinence" (Table III). A urinary tract infection was present in only few cases, about 5%, but 23.2% had dysuric problems (burning, frequency, etc.) with clear urine; 26% had mostly urgency; and in 14 cases more than one symptom was present. Table IV shows the percentage of urinary symptoms which occurred in the patients as obtained from an accurate anamnesis. They were various, sometimes alone or often associated with one another. Table V summarizes the non-urinary troubles directly related to the climacteric age in women. In particular, 91% of women suffered from psychological discomforts such as anxiety and depression which could be correlated in some way to dysparcunia and loss of libido observed in about 35% of subjects. The clinical examination in most women showed an average of 85% of findings indicating dystrophic external genitalia and 77% of cystocele and/or urethrocele (Table VI). Bacteriological findings of the vagina and urina are summarized in Table VII. Whereas the vaginal culture gave no reasons for speculation (apart from a moderate increase in the frequency of candida), about 21% of patients showed urinary tract infections (with a significant bacterial concentration

Table III. First complaint of urinary symptoms.

Dysuric problems (with clear urine)	23 (23.2%)
Urgency	26 (26.3%)
Urinary tract infections	5 (5.1%)
Incontinence	45 (45.1%)

In 14 cases more than one symptom was present

Table IV. Urinary symptoms in postmenopausal women.

Symptom	%
Stress incontinence	67
Nicturia	62.3
Urgency	47
Frequency	42.3
Hipogastric pain	32.9
Back pain	28.2
Previous UTI	28.2
Intermittent flow	20
Straining	18.8
Hematuria	15.2
Enuresis	3.5
Acute urinary retention	3.5

Table V. Non-urinary troubles of postmenopausal subjects.

Symptom	%	Symptom	%
Hypertension	21.1	Breast discomfort	18.8
Hot flushes	56.4	Hair loss	40
Headache	32.9	Osteoarticular pain	76.4
Insomnia	31.7	Vulvovaginal burning	25.8
Tachycardia	32.9	Dyspareunia	36.4
Anxiety–depression	91.7	Decrease of libido	35.2

Table VI. Clinical examination.

	%
Dystrophic genitalia	85.8
Urethro-cystocele	77.6
Rectocele	37.6
Urethal caruncle	27
Urethral pain	17.6
Uterine fibromatosis	14

and germs not always related to *E. Coli*) which could justify the above symptoms in this group. Cystoscopic findings (Table VIII) were completely normal in 16% of patients. The comparison between cytological findings in the vagina and those in the lower urinary tract (Table IX) showed that in 50% of the patients hypotrophic alterations were present, whereas in spite of very impressive symptoms, in 25% no alteration was found.

CONCLUSIONS

The diagnostic approach to lower urinary tract complaints, related to the climacteric age, deserves close attention by the gynaecologist. Women with very impressive symptoms have been submitted to anti-bacterial treatment for many years in spite of negative bacteriological findings. In our opinion a few and very simple tests, possibly provided by a multidisciplinary service, could permit correct diagnosis, rational therapy and successful results in the approach to urological diseases of postmenopausal women.

Table VII. Bacteriological findings.

Vagina	%	Urine	%
Positive:	54.1	Positive:	21.1
Non-specific flora	54.3	*E. Coli*	38.8
Candida	36.9	*Proteus*	22.2
Trichomonas Vaginalis	8.7	*Klebsiella*	22.2
		Staphylococcus A.	15.5
		Mixed flora	11.1

Table VIII. Cystoscopic Findings.

	%
Normal	16.4
Superficial ulceration	9.4
Cystitis ⎧ Pseudo-polypomatosis	17.6
⎩ Cystic	35.2
Squamous metaplasia	16.4
Trigonitis	40

Table IX. Cytological Findings.

	Vaginal (%)	Urinary (%)
Normal	23.5	25.8
Hypotrophic	52.9	50.5
Atrophic	21.1	21.1
Marks oestrogenic activity	2.3	2.3

REFERENCES

Andersen, M. J. F. (1967). *Journal of Urology* **98**, 96.

Bruce, A. W., Chadwick, P. and Hassan, A. (1973). *Canadian Medical Association Journal* **108**, 973.

Elkins, I. B. and Cox, C. E. (1974). *Journal of Urology* **111**, 88.

Jacob, E. (1978). *In* "Gynecological and Obstetric Urology", p. 325. Saunders, Philadelphia.

Stamey, T. A., Timothy, M. and Millar, M. (1971). *Californian Medical Journal* **115**, 1.

DEPRESSIVE STATES DURING THE MENOPAUSE: A PRELIMINARY STUDY OF ENDOCRINOLOGICAL, SOCIOENVIRONMENTAL AND PERSONALITY FACTORS

P. Castrogiovanni[3], I. Brunori De Luca[2], G. Teti[2], I. Corradi[1], G. Moggi[2], R. Zecca[2], S. Murru[2], D. Silvestri[4] and P. Fioretti[2]

Istituto di Clinica Psichiatrica[1], Clinica Ostetrico-Ginecologica[2], Cattedra di Psicologia[3], Laboratorio di Endocrinologia del CNR[4] dell'Università di Pisa, Pisa, Italy

INTRODUCTION

The menopause may be said to begin and develop on a primarily biological plane, since it may be identified with the end of the reproductive cycle, which is inaugurated by the menarche. The clinical and symptomatological troubles which most disturb women, however, are found on an almost exclusively psychological or psychopathological level. Even in the absence of precise epidemiological data, the menopause Syndrome is known to affect a high proportion of women for many years, and it often induces them to consult a gynaecologist.

Only to a very small extent this Syndrome consists of neurovegetative phenomena, such as hot flushes and perspiration, which are the only symptoms (besides atrophic vaginitis), recognized to be certainly due to hormonal changes (Aylward, 1976; Utian and Serr, 1976).

Besides these symptoms, there are much more worrying and debilitating subjective ones (Van Keep and Prill, 1975), whose depressive basis may sometimes be easily recognized and sometimes more indirectly identified. Depressive mood, anxiety, irritability, insomnia, loss of interest and various kinds of somatization, which may mask the depressive nature of the clinical picture, are very often found, though to widely varying degrees (Brown, 1976).

Serono Symposium No. 39, "The Menopause: Clinical, Endocrinological and Pathophysiological Aspects", edited by P. Fioretti, L. Martini, G. B. Melis and S. S. C. Yen, 1982. Academic Press, London and New York.

Despite the severity of such psychic phenomena, surprisingly few investigations based on precise experimental data have been carried out to discover the essential pathogenetic factors responsible for the onset and persistence of depressive states during the menopause (Hertz *et al.,* 1971; Schneider *et al.,* 1977). Most references to this subject spring from generic statements about the role played by hormonal changes, inferred from not unequivocal results of hormonal therapy. In fact, it is well known that such therapy does not give satisfactory results in all trials, and that a clearly antidepressive activity is only found with very high doses (Kerr, 1976), probably as a result of interference with MAOs (Klaiber *et al.,* 1979). In the literature there is complete agreement in admitting that the conclusions drawn from the studies by the authors who have investigated this topic are conflicting (Ballinger, 1976; Campbell, 1976).

METHODS

There is a clear need for experiments whose aim is to determine whether anxious-drepressive states appearing in concomitance with the menopause (including pre- and postmenopausal periods) are related to changes in hormonal levels, or to other kinds of factors, such as socio-environmental or personality factors. Standard methodologies which express psychosocial and psychopathological data in quantitative form allow correlation with biological data. Especially during the early stages of an approach to the problem, the use of questionnaires and self-rating scales seems to meet those needs, as they accurately reflect a woman's subjectivity and give it a quantitative form which allows statistical elaboration. The SAD (Self-Rating Scale for Repression, Cassano and Castrogiovanni, 1977), is made up of 31 items, and gives a total score and factor scores; the former expresses the global evaluation of the syndrome and the latter the importance of some specific sectors, each of which is grouped under a general heading: "Depression", "Anxiety", "Insecurity", "Somatic Symptoms", "Changes during the Day", and "Withdrawal from Life". The 16 PF (16 Personality Factors of Cattel), is one of the best known questionnaires used in studying personality, which is defined in terms of 16 bi-polar traits ("Secure"/ "Insecure", "Emotive"/"Mature", and so on). The QSA (Socio-Environmental Questionnaire) (Cassano and Castrogiovanni, 1977) allows the personal data on the patient and her family to be recorded and explores the influences affecting the patient and her attitude to her environment from birth to full maturity (attitude of her family, degree of its permissiveness, sexual education, stability of the original family unit, schooling, identification with her social and cultural environments, sexual life, acceptance of her family and her occupation).

The present study, which was based on these instruments, also included an evaluation of plasma levels of the pituitary and ovarian hormones which are mainly affected by the menopause: LH, FSH, prolactin, testosterone, progesterone, and oestrogens [oestrone (E_1), oestradiol (E_2), and oestriol (E_3)].

Blood was collected by venipuncture in heparinized tubes, centrifuged and then the plasma stored. Seven days later the collection was repeated and, for each subject, the plasma samples were pooled and stored at $-20\,^{\circ}C$ until assay.

LH, FSH and prolactin levels were determined by a double antibody radioimmunoassay*. The limits of sensibility in these assays were lmIU/ml for LH and FSH, and 0.5 ng/ml for prolactin. Oestrone, oestradiol, oestriol, progesterone and testosterone levels were measured by radioimmunoassay procedures after ether extraction. These assays had a sensitivity of 8, 5 and 4 pg/ml, and 0.075 and 0.6 ng/ml respectively. For each hormone, all samples were run in triplicate and the values reported are the means of the results obtained. Besides this, the vaginal cyto-hormonal test was carried out, and the degrees of vaginal maturation was calculated according to the technique of Wachtel (1975).

SAMPLE

This methodology was used with women randomly chosen among those who came as out-patients for a gynaecological examination on account of signs of menopause (amenorrhoea) at a fairly early stage, without any concomitant organic pathology or a history of noteworthy psychopathological disturbances. The mean age was 49 years, and the age of 82% of the patients fell within the 45-55 year range (Fig. 1).

Half of the chosen women had amenorrhoea uninterruptedly for at least 6 months, while the other half had their last menstruation less than 6 months previously; all of the latter had experienced periods of amenorrhoea or menstrual

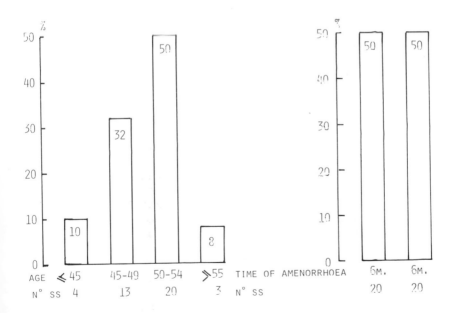

Fig. 1. Distribution of 40 women during perimenopause according to age and time of amenorrhoea.

*All specific antisera were kindly supplied by A. Cappellini from Biodata S.p.A. (Italy).

irregularity (Fig. 1). It is, in fact, well known that depressive states often appear for the first time at the earliest stages of the menopause, or may actually appear before it, acting as a warning signal.

The heterogenicity of the sample, which was ensured by choosing women at different stages of the menopausal process, had the advantage of facilitating the identification of the eventual correlations between the psychopathological picture and hormonal levels. The mean hormonal levels in the sample (Table I)

Table I. Mean values and standard deviation of hormonal rates in 40 women of perimenopausal age.

	Mean values	SD	Normal levels during menopause
LH (mIU/ml)	54.72	31.63	50 – 100
FSH (mIU/ml)	57.17	33.95	50 – 100
P (ng/ml)	0.427	0.835	0.075 – 0.30
T (ng/ml)	0.937	0.640	0.2 – 0.8
E_1 (pg/ml)	33.95	16.28	23 – 42
E_2 (pg/ml)	33.65	28.97	10 – 34
E_3 (pg/ml)	17.72	17.28	4 – 12
PRL (ng/ml)	13.37	6.87	5 – 25

confirmed the foregoing. Hormonal values, in fact, were mostly within the normal range for the menopause. The exceptions were progesterone, testosterone, and E_3, whose levels slightly exceeded the upper limits of the range, so providing evidence of the persistence of the "peripheral" endocrine function in some women, even if at levels far below those found at a fertile age.

The socio-environmental data show that the sample was representative of the population of a provincial town. Most of the women were married and had children; 40% had been educated up to primary level, 20% up to junior secondary school, 20% up to senior secondary school, and 15% had a university degree. Their mean economic position was within the middle range; 50% were housewives and 28% were teachers.

On the psychological plane, as evaluated by the mean QSA scores, the samples showed a good level of acceptance of their occupational environment and this was correlated with a good level of acceptance of their school environment. They also showed a fairly good degree of integration within family life, whereas their degree of socialization was rather poor, and their sexual life was inhibited.

RESULTS

The distribution of the subjects' total SAD scores, which express the severity of their anxious-depressive states, approximates to a Gaussian curve (Fig. 2). For 21 (53%) of the 40 women examined, the *total* SAD score was above 50. This value has been identified in previous analysis as dividing clinically significant levels of depression from those which may be considered normal. An examination of the scores of the *single SRSD items* makes it clear that only few women (22%)

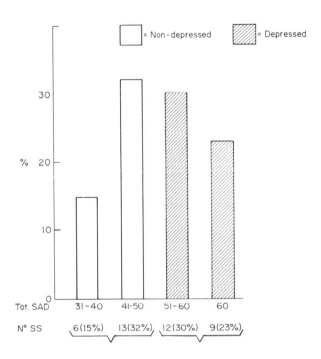

Fig. 2. Distribution of 40 women during perimenopause according to the SAD total score. □ = non-depressed; ■ = depressed.

deny the presence of a depressed state of mind, or of nervous tension with disphoria (20%); one of the most frequent symptoms was asthenia, which was reported in 88% of all cases, even if only "sometimes" in 45%; palpitations were often reported too (70%), but they were mostly not very severe (62% of the women had them "sometimes"). In the sample examined, probably partly as a result of the patients' original cultural background and social class, sexual activity was reported to be at a very low level; only 30% declared it to be unchanged, while 27% declared a total loss of sexual desire. The menopause is not accompanied by a feeling of uselessness of life, or only to a moderate degree; 92% of these women did not experience this feeling. Lastly, 70% of women referred the menopause disturbances to be globally insignificant (25%) or slight (45%).

To provide an answer to the specific queries which can be made about the factors most closely linked with depressive symptomatology, the total SAD scores were examined in relation to the hormonal, socio-environmental and personality data, partly by means of parametric tests (degree of correlation), and partly by means of non-parametric ones (χ^2 test).

In addition, using univariate tests (analysis of variance), the hormonal, socio-environmental and personality data for the women who were "depressed" (with a total SAD score above 50) were compared with those for the women who were "not depressed" (with a total SAD score below 50).

The degree of correlation between the severity of depressive symptomatology, as assessed by total SAD scores, and plasma levels of LH, FSH, progesterone, testosterone, oestrogens and prolactin was decidely low, and in any case far from being statistically significant (Table II). Similarly, there were no significant correlations between hormonal levels and the various symptomatological factors explored by SAD ("Depression", "Anxiety", "Insecurity", "Somatic Symptoms", "Changes during the Day" and "Withdrawal from Life"), except that between progesterone and "Withdrawal from Life", which is difficult to interpret (Table II).

Table II. Degree of correlation between *sad scores* and *hormonal* levels in 40 women of peri-menopausal age.

	LH	FSH	P	T	E_1	E_2	E_3	PRL
SAD total score	0.05	−0.06	0.16	−0.06	0.07	0.02	0.00	0.14
F Depression	0.05	−0.14	0.20	−0.04	0.04	0.00	−0.01	0.16
A Anxiety	−0.02	−0.01	0.03	0.00	0.14	0.08	0.00	0.07
C Sensitivity	0.04	−0.14	0.15	0.03	−0.04	−0.05	0.03	0.01
T Somatic symptoms	0.10	0.13	0.28	−0.19	−0.04	−0.02	−0.01	0.05
O Diurnal variations	0.11	0.12	−0.08	−0.22	−0.03	−0.11	0.03	0.26
R Suicide	0.01	−0.13	0.34[a]	0.00	0.00	0.06	0.02	0.07
S								

[a] $P < 0.05$.

Table III. Mean values and variance analysis of hormonal levels in 21 depressed and 19 non-depressed women of perimenopausal age.

	Mean values		F ratio	P
	Depressed (SRDS total > 50)	Non-depressed (SRDS total < 50)		
LH	56.23	53.05	0.09	NS
FSH	55.28	59.26	0.13	NS
P	0.41	0.44	0.01	NS
T	0.78	1.10	2.42	NS
E_1	35.09	32.68	0.20	NS
E_2	32.04	35.42	0.12	NS
E_3	17.33	18.15	0.02	NS
PRL	14.38	12.26	0.92	NS

The mean hormonal patterns for "depressed" and "non-depressed" patients almost coincide. The differences between these two sub-groups are not significant for any of the hormones considered (Table III).

Also the distribution of the results of the cytohormonal test for these two sub-groups (Fig. 3) show no significant differences. Most of the "depressed"

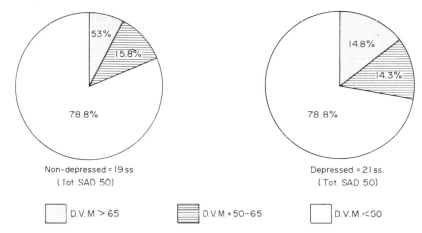

Fig. 3. Distribution of 40 women depressed and non-depressed during perimenopause according to the cyto-hormonal test (degree of vaginal maturation = DVM) (χ^2 = NS).

women (71.4%) and of those who are "not depressed" (71.8%), had values of vaginal maturation below 50 ("hypoestrinic" values).

Similarly, comparison between the 12 women who considered the degree of their disturbances to be "moderate" or "considerable" and the other 28 who considered them to be "insignificant" or "slight" did not reveal significant differences between their hormonal levels. Nevertheless, discriminant analysis identifies a function which, even if at levels below significance, seems to be a characteristic of these women who report the most severe disturbances. These women have lower plasma levels of LH, FSH, progesterone, testosterone and prolactin than the others, but a higher level of oestrogens.

The anxious-depressive state appears to be independent of the main personal data, too. The "depressed" patients do not differ from the others as regards age, duration of amenorrhoea, marital status, having or not having had children, order of birth in the family, educational level, kind of occupation or economic position (Table IV).

PERSONALITY TRAITS

The severity of the anxious-depressive symptomatology seems to be significantly correlated with the "Depression/Elation", "Dependance/Self-Sufficiency", and "Relaxation/Tension" factors in the 16 PF scale (Table V). Thus the severity of psychic disturbances seems to be the greatest in women who can be defined as having a tendency to be "taciturn, reserved, introverted, with a languid, depressed

Table IV. Distribution of depressed and non-depressed women during perimenopause.

	Depressed	Non-Depressed	Total	χ^2 test
Age:				
45	3	3	6	
46–50	9	9	18	NS
50	9	7	16	
Last menstruation				
< 6 months	10	10	20	
> 6 months	11	9	20	NS
Marital status:				
Single	2	1	3	
Married	19	17	36	NS
Widow	0	1	1	
Children:				
Yes	18	16	34	
No	3	2	5	NS
Order of birth:				
Only child	3	1	4	
Firstborn	3	3	6	
Not first or last	10	9	19	NS
Lastborn	5	6	11	
Education:				
Junior school	15	11	26	
High school	6	8	14	NS
Occupation:				
Housewife	11	9	20	
Teacher	6	5	11	NS
Economic position:				
Good	7	6	13	
Fairly good	7	7	14	
Middling	4	3	7	NS
Poor	0	1	1	

mood, slow-thinking, reticent, pessimistic, worried, bad-tempered, and melancholy" ("Depression"); "those who prefer to work and take decisions together with others, who need social approval and admiration, who are conventional and easily influenced, and lacking in determination" ("Dependence"); "tense, excitable, restless, impatient, irritable, overworked but incapable of staying idle" ("Tension").

These same three factors reveal significant differences between the 16 PF scores for "depressed" and "non-depressed" patients; discriminant analysis allows the identification of a function which distinguishes between the two groups, especially in terms of "Dependence", "Tension" and "Depression", in a decreasing order (all three values are above 0.40).

Table V. Analysis of correlations between *total SRDS scores* and *16 PF factors* in 40 women during perimenopause.

Factors		R	
A – Cold	Warm	NS	"Taciturn, reserved, intro-
B – Dull	Lively	NS	vered; languid and depressed
C – Immature	Mature	NS	mood, slow thinking reticent,
E – Passive	Aggressive	NS	pessimistic, worried, bad-
F – Depressed	Elated	-0.31 ($P < 0.05$)	tempered, melancholy".
G – Inconstant	Constant	NS	
H – Timid	Bold	NS	"Prefers to work and take
I – Insensitive	Sensitive	NS	decisions together with
L – Trusting	Suspicious	NS	others, needs social approval
M – Conformist	Anti-conformist	NS	and admiration; easily
N – Simple	Sophisticated	NS	influenced and conventional,
O – Self-confident	Insecure	NS	lacking in determination".
O1 – Conservative	Innovative	NS	
O2 – Dependent	Independent	-0.34 ($P < 0.05$)	
O3 – Easy-going	Self-controlled	NS	"Tense, excitable, restless,
O4 – Relaxed	Tense	-0.39 ($P < 0.01$)	impatient, unstable, over-
			worked, but incapable of
			remaining idle".

It is not easy to determine which of these characteristics are present before the psychopathological disturbances begin, and so constitute a stable feature of the pre-morbid personality, and which are an expression or a symptom of the anxious-depressive state.

Some of the above mentioned features (e.g.: depressive mood, slow thinking, tendency towards isolation, pessimism, tendency to be worried, tension and restlessness) recall the typical features of the depressive picture, and may be considered an expression of that picture; whereas other kinds of behaviour (e.g. need for social approval and admiration, tendency to be easily influenced, conventionality, psychoasthenic traits, hyperactivity even when tired, and reservedness), resemble the classical characteristics of the pre-depressive personality (both in the sense of the *"Typus melancholicus"* of Tallenback, and in that of the compulsive-obsessive personality).

Therefore it seems possible to hypothesize that the second group of traits are specific elements, capable of favouring the onset of depression during the menopause, analogously with what happens to depressive states whose onset is related to other events in various periods of the patient's life.

The severity of anxious-depressive symptoms in these patients is negatively correlated with all the psycho-social features explored by the QSA. This confirms the significance of the connections between depressive experience and environment (Cassano *et al.,* 1977). Statistically significant correlations are immediately recognizable with some scales (attitude of the parents to the birth of the subject, permissiveness, cultural level, acceptance of own occupation). These correlations, together with the analytical comparison between women who are "depressed" and those who are not, which reveals significant differences in favour of the latter as regards attitude to own birth and to childhood before school age, cultural level and integration within the family, allow the conclusion that the women who have a depressive picture during their menopause report a childhood characterized by a detached attitude in their parents, a lack of affection, and a strict upbringing. In their maturity these women are less learned and less closely integrated with their families and/or working environments.

CONCLUSIONS

The frequency and severity of subjective symptomatology during the menopause, which is characterized by depressed mood, anxiety, irritability and somatization, are not correlated to the plasma levels of the hormonal secretions most strongly affected by the end of the reproductive cycle. Different levels of gonadotrophins (LH,FSH), oestrogens (oestrone, oestradiol, oestriol), progesterone, testoterone and prolactin do not correspond to the presence or absence of anxious-depressive states or their severity. Thus it is not the type or severity of endocrinological changes that determines psychic disturbances. The menopause itself as a biological event, in the sense of an upheaval in hormonal balance, together with external factors typical of the menopause (the irregularity and discontinuance flow, changes in physical appearance etc.), stands out as an element common to all women at this stage in life and, therefore, as a necessary but not sufficient condition for an explanation of the onset of psychological states which only affect a certain, even if considerable, proportion of the female population. Other characteristics of the endocrinological process may be involved, such as the speed at which this change takes place, but not the merely quantitative aspects, such as hormonal plasma levels.

Personality and socio-environmental factors seem to allow sharper differentiation between the women suffering from anxious-depressive disturbances and the others. The onset of a psychopathological picture is, in fact, related to the presence of personality factors of pre-depressive type (dependance, conventionality, anxiety and devotion to duty) together with a difficult childhood and a low degree of acceptance of the environment during adulthood. The anxious-depressive syndromes of the menopause may thus be defined as the result of the concurrence of a number of factors; personality and socio-environmental factors, interacting with endocrinological changes, have a key role in triggering off the subjective symptomatology. This multifactorial aetiology accounts for apparently contradictory results reported in the literature, where therapeutic successes have been attributed both to the administration of oestrogens, and to psychopharmacological treatments and psychotherapy.

The methodology used in this study, which is based on self-assessment, has confirmed the role of psychosocial factors in the genesis of the menopause syndrome, but can do no more than explore the most superficial levels of the patient's experience. Confirmation of these results, together with a more precise definition of casual links, may emerge from further research which must be carried out on the plane of individual investigation on deeper psychological processes and specific biographical and existential connections.

In this way it will be possible to clarify whether the onset of the menopause affects a particular personality situation, which interacts with the socio-environmental contest, so that it is no more than an aspecific triggering factor, or whether it is a specific causal agent which assumes a particular form by individual problems and by a given cultural formation.

REFERENCES

Aylward, M. (1976). *In* "The Management of Menopause and Post-Menopausal Years". (S. Campbell, Ed.). MTP, Lancaster, England.

Ballinger, C. B. (1976). *In* "The Management of the Menopause and Post-Menopausal Years". (S. Campbell, Ed.). MTP, Lancaster, England.

Brown, M. C. (1976). *In* "The Management of Menopause and Post-Menopausal Years". (S. Campbell, Ed.). MTP, Lancaster, England.

Campbell, S. (1976). *In* "The Management of the Menopause and Post-Menopausal Years". (S. Campbell, Ed.). MTP, Lancaster, England.

Cassano, G. B. and Castrogiovanni, P. (1977). S.A.D. — Scala di Autovalutazione per las Depressione. *International Committee for Prevention and Treatment of Depression*

Cassano, G. B., Castrogiovanni, P., Ghiozzi, M. and Principe, S. (1977). *In* Atti XXXIII Congresso S.I.P., Napoli, 29 Ottobre-1 Novembre 1977, CLUED, Verona.

Hertz, D. G., Steiner, J. E., Zuckermann, H. and Pizanti, S. (1971). *Psychotherapy and Psychosomatics* **19**, 47.

Kerr, M. D. (1976). *In* "The Management of Menopause and Post-Menopausal Years" (S. Campbell, Ed.). MTP, Lancaster, England.

Klaiber, E. L., Browerman, D. M., Vogel, C. and Kobayashi, Y. (1979). *Archives of General Psychiatry* **36**, 550.

Schneider, M. A., Brotherton, P. L. and Hailes, J. (1977). *Medical Journal of Australia.* **30**, 162.

Utian, W. H. and Serr, D. (1976). *In* "Consensus on Menopause Research" (P. A. Van Keep, R. B. Greesboht and M. Albeaux-Fernet, Eds). MTP, Lancaster, England.

Van Keep, P. A. and Prill, H. J. V. (1975). *In* "Estrogens in the Post-Menopause. Frontiers of Hormone Research". (P. A. Van Keep and C. Lauritzen, Eds). Karger, Basel, Switzerland.

Wachtel, E. G. (1975). *In* "Estrogens in Post-Menopause. Frontiers of Hormone Research". (P. A. Van Keep and C. Lauritzen, Eds). Karger, Basel, Switzerland.

SECTION VII
THE AGED COUPLE: SEXUAL BEHAVIOUR AND SOCIAL PROBLEMS

ROLE OF BRAIN DOPAMINE IN THE REGULATION OF MALE SEXUAL BEHAVIOUR

P. Falaschi, G. Fraiese, A. Rocco, P. Pompei and G. L. Gessa[1]

*Istituto di Clinica Medica Generale V, Università di Roma, Rome,
Italy and Istituto di Farmacologia Medica, Università di Cagliari,
Cagliari, Italy*[1]

INTRODUCTION

The stimulatory role of brain dopamine (DA) on male sexual behaviour is well established. Apomorphine, a potent DA agonist, and L-Dopa, a DA precursor, increase the copulatory behaviour in rats. Haloperidol, a DA blocker, is able to prevent this effect and also to suppress the spontaneous copulatory behaviour in male rats (Tagliamonte *et al.*, 1974).

Data which seem to confirm the stimulatory action of the brain dopaminergic system on sexual behaviour have also been reported in man. L-Dopa treatment is capable of increasing sexual activity in parkinsonian patients (Hyyppa *et al.*, 1970; O'Brien *et al.*, 1971). Improvement in libido and sexual performance has been observed during bromocriptine therapy in acromegalic patients (Wass *et al.*, 1977). Bromocriptine is a potent DA agonist compound. It is interesting to notice that the sexual improvement, in acromegalic subjects, is independent of basal prolactin (PRL) levels which can be normal. This stimulatory effect on sexual behaviour occurs either in patients complaining of impotence before treatment or in patients who had supposed themselves to be sexually normal. Furthermore the effect of the DA agonist, bromocriptine, on the sexual behaviour of acromegalic patients is so rapid and potent that its stimulatory action sometimes precedes GH normaliza-

Serono Symposium No. 39, "The Menopause: Clinical, Endocrinological and Pathophysiological Aspects", edited by P. Fioretti, L. Martini, G. B. Melis and S. S. C. Yen, 1982. Academic Press, London and New York.

tion. Besser and his colleagues (unpublished observation) noticed that piribedil, another DA agonist compound, given by infusion, caused, in normal volunteers, erection after a few minutes. This immediate effect was probably due to the stimulation of central and, perhaps, of peripheral dopaminergic mechanisms of erection. In fact, DA receptors and DA containing neurons have also been found outside the CNS, in the pelvis, in the vas deferens and in the penis (Thorner, 1975) (Fig. 1). Thus DA could also play a role in the peripheral mechanisms of erection.

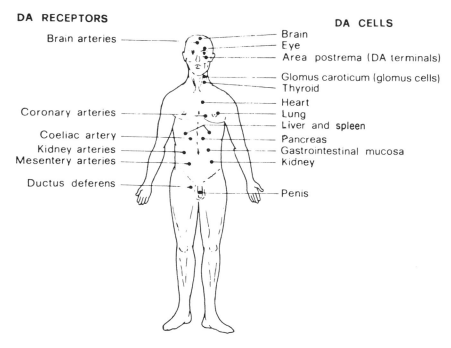

Fig. 1. Sites of DA receptors and DA containing cells (from Ungerstedt, 1978, modified).

IMPOTENCE IN HYPERPROLACTINAEMIA

In man hyperprolactinaemia causes impotence, loss of libido, gynecomastia and/or galactorrhoea, seminal volume reduction, sometimes oligo- or azoospermia. PRL secretion is under a tonic inhibition by hypothalamic DA. Many *in vivo* and *in vitro* tests show that DA is able to inhibit PRL release at pituitary level (Mac Leod and Lehmeyer, 1974; Yeo *et al.*, 1979). Bromocriptine and other DA agonist compounds which directly stimulate DA receptors reduce PRL secretion at the pituitary level. Excellent results have been obtained with bromocriptine treatment in impotent patients with PRL secreting pituitary adenomas (Thorner *et al.*, 1977). During bromocriptine PRL is reduced while libido and potency improve; when therapy is stopped sexual abnormalities come back together with elevated PRL levels.

It is not clear which is the pathogenesis of impotence during hyperprolactinaemia. At the moment only hypotheses can be advanced. First, hyperprolactinaemia could directly inhibit the mechanisms which modulate sexual behaviour. Secondly, a disturbance of cerebral dopaminergic activity could induce both hyperprolactinaemia and impotence. Finally, hyperprolactinaemia could interfere with the dopaminergic control of sexual behaviour.

The good results obtained during bromocriptine therapy could be due to the normalization of PRL levels but also to the direct action of the compound on dopaminergic mechanisms modulating sexual behaviour. Recent experiments in rats did not show any inhibitory effect of hyperprolactinaemia on sexual behaviour. These experiments were performed either inducing hyperprolactinaemia with pituitary implants under kidney's capsule (Scapagnini *et al.*, 1980), or administering domperidone, a potent DA blocker which does not cross the blood brain barrier and does not interfere with DA activity inside the CNS (Benassi-Benelli *et al.*, 1980). In these experimental conditions no inhibitory effect on male rat sexual behaviour was observed, but sometimes a stimulatory action was reported.

In order to have a quantitative evaluation of sexual behaviour disturbances and to establish the variations during pharmacological treatment we use a vis and libido rating scale (VLRS) which consists of 11 items on the topics listed in Table I. The questions on topics 1 to 8 are expressed in terms of degrees of

Table I. Vis and Libido Rating Scale of sexual behaviour disturbances (from Davies *et al.*, 1976, modified).

11 items on the following parameters	
1	Interest in sex
2	Success in ejaculation
3	Premature ejaculation
4	Frequency of intercourse
5	Intercourse latency
6	Spontaneous erections
7	Frequency of masturbation
8	Duration of erection
9	Quality of erection
10	Depression
11	Anxiety

severity (ranging from -2 to $+2$), while questions on topics 9 to 11 are expressed in the form of graded analogue scales. The total score is the algebraic addition of the scores of each question. The total score in normal males ranges from 10 to 16.

As far as hyperprolactinaemic effects on sexual behaviour are concerned we studied a group of male volunteers during the administration of Metoclopramide (M), a DA receptor block, one of the most potent PRL secretagogues (Falaschi *et al.*, 1978). During the experiment (M 10 mg t.d.s. for 6 weeks), four subjects showed loss of libido and three lack of spontaneous erections. Plasma testosterone (T) levels did not show any significant variations, as well basal levels of FSH and LH and their response to GnRH (100 mcg i.v.). It was concluded, therefore, that M-induced hyperprolactinaemia caused the libido and potency disturbances. It is possible however that this DA receptor blocking drug might directly affect central or peripheral dopaminergic mechanisms which control sexual behaviour.

In order to understand better the relationships between DA blockers, PRL and sexual behaviour we studied a group of psychotic patients during chronic neuro-leptic treatment (Table II).

Table II. Hormonal and VLRS evaluations in psychotic patients during chronic neuroleptic treatment in comparison with normal controls.

	PRL[a]	LH[a]	T[a]	VLRS[a]
Fluphenazine	7.9	9.0	430	+5
decanoate (N = 7)	(4.1–13.7)	(4.8–12.0)	(303–585)	(− 1:+6)
Haloperidol	7.6	7.2	395	+4
(N = 9)	(3.8–12.5)	(4.2–10.1)	(351–560)	(− 3:+7)
Combination of	14.6	5.7	405	+3
drugs (N = 32)	(9.0–30.5)	(3.9– 9.8)	(277–610)	(− 3:+5)
Controls (N = 10)	6.7	7.6	470	+3
	(4.3–10.6)	(5.5–10.9)	(330–680)	(+ 10:+16)
[a]mean (range)	PRL: ng/ml − LH: mIU/ml − T: ng%			

On the basis of treatment administered, patients were divided into three groups (Table II). The first group took fluphenazine decanoate, which is a depot DA blocker (25 mg i.m. monthly), the second group took haloperidol, a potent DA receptor blocker (3 mg x *os* daily) and, finally, the third group took a combination of neuroleptic drugs, such as penfluridol (20 mg x *os* weekly), chlorpromazine (100 mg x *os* daily) and thioridazine (50 mg x *os* daily). In all groups plasma LH and T levels were normal. Morning basal PRL levels did not show in the first two groups significant modifications in comparison with a group of normal subjects of matched age, as already reported in the literature (Beumont *et al.*, 1974). The group combination of the drugs showed a slight PRL elevation. All the subjects had a decrease in sexual activity as shown by the VLRS score. Preliminary results obtained during neuroleptic washout (placebo or benzodiazepines) indicate a tendency in recovering sexual function (libido and spontaneous erections). It is tentative therefore to advance the hypothesis that neuroleptics, as DA blockers, could act on cerebral system controlling sexual behaviour independently from the PRL modifications induced by drugs.

The data previously reported on bromocriptine treatment of hyperprolactinaemic impotence and the evidences both in animal and man of the stimulatory role of the DA system on sexual behaviour led us and other investigators to perform a similar trial on normoprolactinaemic impotence but, unfortunately, no significant variations were observed between bromocriptine and placebo treatment. Thus it is possible that other neurotransmitters such as serotonin, enkephalins, ACTH like peptides could play a role in the so-called normoprolactinaemic psychogenic impotence.

BRAIN DOPAMINE AND PREMATURE EJACULATION

In rats DA agonist compounds are able to induce premature ejaculation (Table III) characterized by a decrease both in the number of intromissions preceding ejaculation (intromission frequency) and in the interval between the first intromission to the first ejaculation (ejaculation latency) (Gessa *et al.*, 1980). This effect of DA agonist is prevented by centrally acting DA receptor blockers such as (—) sulpiride and M but not by domperidone which was reported not to cross the blood brain barrier (Table III).

Table III. Apomorphine (APO), N-n-propyl-Norapomorphine (NPA) and L-Dopa induce premature ejaculation in rats. This effect is prevented by centrally acting DA receptor blockers. Values are means ± SE from at least 10 animals. L-Dopa, APO and NPA are given 30 min prior to mating test with receptive females (Paglietti *et al.*, 1978). Antagonists are given 30 min before APO (from Gessa *et al.*, 1980).

Treatment	Dose/kg	Ejaculation latency	Intromission frequency
		Seconds	*Number*
Saline	—	565.6 ± 113	13.1 ± 1.4
APO	25 μg	288.5 ± 56^{a}	4.3 ± 1.1^{a}
NPA	6 μg	293.8 ± 62^{a}	4.8 ± 0.8^{a}
L-Dopa + Ro4–4602	100 + 50 μg	388.5 ± 88^{a}	7.2 ± 1.2^{a}
Metoclopramide + APO	0.1 μg + 25 μg	487.5 ± 102	11.5 ± 1.6
(—) Sulpiride + APO	5 mg + 25 μg	583.6 ± 120	14.1 ± 1.8
Domperidone + APO	3 mg + 25 μg	295.6 ± 56^{a}	4.9 ± 1.3^{a}

^{a} $P < 0.01$ in respect to saline treated.

These results show that brain DA plays a key role on ejaculation and also suggest that an excessive brain dopaminergic activity could be responsible for premature ejaculation in man. On the basis of the above reported animal data we performed a double blind cross-over trial with M and placebo in a group of patients with premature ejaculation as isolated symptom. The modifications of premature ejaculation were evalulated using a premature ejaculation scale which consists of 4 degrees of severity (Table IV).

Ten patients (aged 24–45) with premature ejaculation took 10 mg of M or

Table IV. Premature ejaculation scale.

1 Ejaculation ante portas
2 Ejaculation immediately after penetration
3 Ejaculation within 1 min of penetration
4 Ejaculation after 1 min of penetration

Table V. Hormonal (mean ± SE) and VLRS (mean ± SE) evaluations in basal conditions (mean of two different evaluations), during placebo and metoclopramide treatment in 10 men complaining of premature ejaculation.

	BAS	Placebo			Metoclopramide		
		30	60	90	30	60	90
PRL (ng/ml)	8.3 ± 0.7	5.3 ± 0.4	6.0 ± 0.4	9.8 ± 0.5	$38.9 ± 2.3^c$	$14.7 ± 1.4^b$	9.0 ± 0.4
T (ng%)	653 ± 33	582 ± 27	670 ± 41	626 ± 35	719 ± 38	610 ± 22	538 ± 25
FSH (mIU/ml)	4.5 ± 1.7	6.7 ± 2.1	5.8 ± 0.9	5.9 ± 1.1	4.6 ± 1.3	5.3 ± 1.0	5.0 ± 1.1
LH (mIU/ml)	7.5 ± 2.0	7.0 ± 2.0	8.1 ± 1.7	6.4 ± 1.3	8.0 ± 2.2	6.6 ± 1.5	6.8 ± 1.6
VLRS	1.8 ± 0.2	2.2 ± 0.2	1.9 ± 0.2	1.5 ± 0.1	2.5 ± 0.3	$2.7 ± 0.2^a$	$2.9 ± 0.2^b$

^{a} $P < 0.02$; ^{b} $P < 0.01$; ^{c} $P < 0.001$.

placebo tablets at 8.00 and 20.00 h for two periods of 3 months treatment with 1 month interval. In basal conditions (two evaluations on different days) and at monthly intervals during treatment, plasma levels of T, FSH, LH and PRL were determined together with the premature ejaculation scale. During placebo and M administration plasma T, FSH and LH levels did not show any modifications. Plasma PRL levels, which were elevated after 30 and 60 days from the beginning of therapy, came back to the normal range after 90 days (Table V), as previously reported during neuroleptics (Beumont *et al.*, 1974).

As for the premature ejaculation scale, the total score during M is significatively higher after 60 ($P < 0.02$) and 90 days ($P < 0.01$) in comparison with the basal scale (Table V). These results therefore, confirm the hypothesis that a dopaminergic hyperactivity can be involved in the genesis of premature ejaculation.

AGEING AND SEXUAL BEHAVIOUR

Various animal and human studies have recently focused the importance of a lack of central dopaminergic activity in the pathogenesis of ageing and dementia. In particular DA synthesis (Samorajski, 1975), uptake (Jonec and Finch, 1975) and content (Carlsson and Winblad, 1976) seem to be reduced in the senescent mammalian brain.

The integrity of central dopaminergic transmission has a key role in the control of emotions, motility and hormone secretion, functions which are altered during ageing. As for the decreased sexual activity in the aged man, many pathogenetic explanations have been claimed. Several authors demonstrated a reduced testicular androgen production in the aged animal (Meites *et al.*, 1982) and man (Serio, 1982).

Our working hypothesis on sexuality in the aged man is that a reduced DA function in the CNS could be responsible for the decreased sexual activity. Many studies however are necessary to confirm this stimulating hypothesis.

ACKNOWLEDGEMENT

We thank Miss Tiziana Buongiorno for her skillful technical assistance.

REFERENCES

Benassi-Benelli, A., Ferrari, F. and Pellegrini-Quarantotti, B. (1980). *Archives Internationales de Pharmacodynamic et de Therapie*, in press.
Beumont, P. J. V., Corker, C. S., Friesen, H. G., Kolakowska, T., Mandlebrote, B. M., Marshall, J., Murray, M. A. F. and Wiles, D. H. (1974). *British Journal Psychiatry* **124**, 420.
Carlsson, A. and Winblad, B. (1976). *Journal of Neural Transmission* **38**, 271.
Casacchia, M., Meco, G., Carchedi, F., Di Ceglie, M., Falaschi, P., Rocco, A., Pompei, P. and Frajese, G. (1979). *In* "Neuroendocrine correlates in neurology and psychiatry" (E. E. Muller and A. Agnoli, Eds). Developments in neurology, Vol. 2. pp. 211 Elsevier/North-Holland Biomedical Press, Amsterdam.

Davies, T. F., Mountjoy, C. Q., Gomez-Pan, A., Watson, M. J., Hanker, J. P. and Besser, G. M. (1976). *Clinical Endocrinology* 5, 601.

Falaschi, P., Frajese, G., Sciarra, F., Rocco, A. and Conti, C. (1978). *Clinical Endocrinology* 8, 427.

Gessa, G. L., Benassi-Benelli, A., Falaschi, P. and Ferrari, F. (1980). *In* "Endocrinology 1980". Proceedings of Sixth Int. Congress of Endocrinology (Australian Academy of Science, Ed.) p. 619.

Hyyppa, M., Rinne, U. R. and Sonninen, V. (1970). *Acta Neurologica Scandinavia.* Suppl. 43, 223.

Jonec, V. and Finch, C. W. (1975). *Brain Research* 91, 197.

Mac Leod, R. M. and Lehmeyer, J. E. (1974). *Endocrinology* 94, 1077.

Meites, J., Henry Huang, H. H. and Steger, R. W. (1980). In the present volume.

O'Brien, C. P., Digiacomo, J. N., Fahn, S. and Schwarz, G. A. (1971). *Archives General Psychiatry* 24, 61.

Paglietti, E., Pellegrini-Quarantotti, B., Mereu, G. P. and Gessa, G. L. (1978). *Physiological Behaviour* 20, 559.

Samorajski, T. (1975). *In* "Aging" (H. Brady, D. Hartman and J. M. Ordy, Eds), vol. 1. Raven Press, New York.

Scapagnini, U., Rizza, V., Drago, F., Canonico, P. L., Pellegrini-Quarantotti, B., Ragusa, N., Clementi, G., Prato, A., Marchetti, B. and Gessa, G. L. (1980). *In* "Central and peripheral regulation of prolactin function" (R. M. Mac Leod and U. Scapagnini, Eds), pp. 293. Raven Press, New York.

Serio, M. (1982). In the present volume, p. 457.

Tagliamonte, A., Fratta, W., Del Fiacco, M. and Gessa, G. L. (1974). *Pharmacology Biochemistry and Behavior* 2, 257.

Thorner, M. O. (1975). *The Lancet,* i, 662.

Thorner, M. O., Edwards, C. R. W., Hanker, J. P., Abraham, G. and Besser, G. M. (1977). *In* "The testis in normal and infertile man" (P. Troen and H. R. Nankin, Eds). pp. 351. Raven Press, New York.

Wass, J. A. H., Thorner, M. O., Morris, D. V., Rees, L. H., Stuart-Mason, A., Jones, A. E. and Besser, G. M. (1977). *British Medical Journal* 1, 875.

Yeo, T., Thorner, M. O., Jones, A., Lowry, P. J. and Besser, G. M. (1979). *Clinical Endocrinology* 10, 123.

ANDROGENS AND SEXUAL BEHAVIOUR

G. Magrini

*Clinical Biochemistry Division, Medicine Department, CHUV,
Lausanne, Switzerland*

INTRODUCTION

It has been demonstrated in many mammalian species that androgens are
necessary for male sexual behaviour. In rats, for instance, testosterone was shown
to restore normal sexual behaviour in asexual castrates within 1 or 2 weeks.
Androgens are also generally believed to be necessary for normal sexual
responsiveness in the human male and female. However, the evidence is limited
and sometimes conflicting (Magrini, 1979; Magrini and Felber, 1980).

Sexual steroids appear to be so related to somatic maturation at puberty, to
the modification during menopause or to the somatic consequences of castration
that it has long been assumed that decline of sexual behaviour and erotism with
age is sex-hormone-dependent. The gonadal steroids appear to have mood
elevating, psychotonic effects. Recent studies suggest that the metabolism of CNS
hormones is modulated by endogenous and exogenous gonadal steroids: therefore, many postmenopausal symptoms may be gonadal hormone-dependent.

Correlations between sexual behaviour and level of circulating sex steroids,
both androgen and oestrogen of either andrenocortical or gonadal origin,
are however not evident. Although it is established that the level of circulating sex
steroids diminishes with age, a clear sex difference appears in the sharp, menopausal diminution of the female and the slowly progressive diminution of the
male. Some women do not decrease but rather maintain or increase their sex life
postmenopausally. Some men with the diagnosis of "andropause" become
sexually apathetic long before their androgen levels can be implicated.

Serono Symposium No. 39, "The Menopause: Clinical, Endocrinological and Pathophysiological Aspects", edited by P. Fioretti, L. Martini, G. B. Melis and S. S. C. Yen, 1982. Academic
Press, London and New York.

In all vertebrate species so far studied, castration sooner or later results in disappearance of mating behaviour. At present, we can at least conclude, from animal experiments, clinical experience and substitution therapy that testosterone is very important also in humans, for the maintenance of the secondary male sex characteristics and for normal sexual functions, libido and potency.

TESTOSTERONE PATTERNS

In blood, testosterone is bound to sex-hormone-binding globulin and only the small free fraction is available to receptors and thus biologically active. In order to exert its effects testosterone needs to be converted into 5α-dihydrotestosterone (5α-DHT) in some target tissues; in others it works directly and in hypothalamic areas aromatization to oestrogens may be required. Testosterone is not secreted continually from the testes but rather in short secretory spikes, which usually occur during the day; they are preceded by LH peaks. The mean plasma testosterone levels have diurnal variation with high concentrations in the morning and lower values in the evening.

When one is investigating correlations between sexual behaviour and plasma androgens, it can be misleading to draw conclusions from single plasma testosterone determinations, because of the short-term and diurnal variations in plasma testosterone occuring in normal men. Multiple samples rather than single determinations are necessary in such studies. Three samples per hour may provide a better basis. So far, hardly any studies on behavioural aspects fulfil these requirements. On the other hand, it has been shown that plasma testosterone may be significantly and drastically reduced by physical exercise and stress over hours or days. On the contrary, it has been reported that short term exhausting exercise can produce a 30% increase in plasma testosterone, measured at the end of a 30 min period. It can be observed therefore that exercise produces alterations in plasma testosterone levels depending on the type of exercise. Moreover, prolonged psychological stress alone may also suppress plasma testosterone concentrations (Kreuz et al., 1972). In studying correlations between sexual activity and plasma androgen levels, these findings should then be kept in mind.

Testosterone levels in plasma vary through life from the foetal period to senescence. One observes a typical profile with a first peak at about 12 weeks of gestation, a second peak shortly after birth and a sharp increase to adult levels during puberty. Whereas the sexual differentiation and masculinization of the genitalia and consequential problems of gender identity are related to the foetal peak, the peak after birth may be especially important for programming hypothalamo-pituitary centres which participate in gonadal feedback control.

Plasma testosterone levels are quite stable from the termination of puberty to about 50–55 years of age, and thereafter decrease slowly. On the other hand, it is interesting to point out that even with relatively low circulating levels of androgens, sexual activity can be initiated (i.e. before puberty) or maintained, as observed in many hypogonadal subjects.

Extensive studies have been carried out on seasonal variations in reproductive functions of various mammalian species. The rhesus monkey also shows a clear circannual pattern of conception rates, which persists under controlled laboratory conditions when exogenous stimuli such as photoperiods, considered strong signals for seasonality, are excluded. Because man is continually exposed to artificial light through the year, circannual cyclic phenomena are much less obvious than in animals. However, some circannual rhythmicity of reproduction is still to be found in humans. Thus, some authors, in different countries, have shown that the highest conception rates may be found in summer and the lowest in winter. It is not known if this seasonality is mainly due to the contribution of men or women. A correlation between plasma testosterone levels and sexual activity in men depending on the season has been however observed. Plasma testosterone concentrations of five men in Paris showed seasonal variations with the lowest concentrations in spring and peak values in September; the frequency of sexual activity followed the pattern of plasma testosterone concentrations (Reimberg *et al.*, 1978).

ANDROGENS, LIBIDO AND SEXUAL FUNCTION

Androgens, which originate chiefly from the adrenal gland, seem to be primarily responsible for female libido, even though the mechanism is poorly understood. Androgens from the testes, especially testosterone, affect male libido. Oestrogen administration to normal women does not seem to increase libido, however, removal of the ovaries will decrease it and oestrogen replacement may reverse this castration effect. Very early it has been shown that there are enhancing effects of exogenous androgens on the sexual interest and response of some women. Removal of the women's source of endogenous androgens, that is by ovariectomy and adrenalectomy, has been said to result in almost complete loss of sexual interest which does not follow ovariectomy alone (Wexenberg and Finkbeiner, 1960). Moreover clinical studies suggest that exogenous androgen may stimulate female libido, however, it is not clear whether androgen action is directly on the brain or is also due to other mechanisms. It was observed that prepubertal females with congenital adrenal hyperplasia may have early and exaggerated sexual desire, whereas andrenalectomy and hypophysectomy produce practically total loss of female libido, which can be restored by testosterone. Some workers have also suggested that female libido may vary through the menstrual cycle and may be correlated with some hormonal levels. Until now however there have been no scientifically controlled studies of relevance.

Experiments with rhesus monkeys have shown that attractiveness of the female rhesus to the male is dependent on oestrogens, whereas her proceptively, i.e., behaviour by her that invites sexual activity, seem to be dependent on androgens (Baum *et al.*, 1977).

Studies in women

Carney *et al.*, (1978) evaluated the effects of combining androgen therapy with counselling in sexually unresponsive women. In the study, involving 32 couples, the authors compared the effect of testosterone undecanoate (10 mg daily sublingually) with those of diazepam (10 mg daily), both therapies combined with their normal method of counselling. The authors reported significant effects on a number of variables associated with sex, all in favour of testosterone, both at the end of the treatment and 6 months later.

However, in a second study (Bancroft, 1980) on 14 women who attributed their loss of the sexual responses to oral contraceptives, using a therapy with oral androstenedione (which is peripherally converted also in testosterone—20 mg daily for 2 months), compared with placebo in a double blind cross-over design, the authors could not find any significant differences between androstenedione and placebo. Only one woman showed a convincing behavioural response to androstenedione. The authors suggest that these negative findings might depend on either: (a) androgens are not important for the problem in these women; (b) androgens are useful only if combined with counselling; or (c) the dose of androstenedione was too low.

Studies in Men

Even though there is widespread use of androgen in the treatment of hypogonadal men, its efficacy in restoring sexual behaviour to hypogonadal subjects has not been established in appropriately controlled behavioural studies. For this reason, Davidson (1980) injected six adult males, aged 32-65, two out of these affected by gonadal failure and four by secondary hypoganadism, with testosterone enanthate or vehicle once every 4 weeks i.m., in a double blind experiment. Two doses of testosterone (100 and 400 mg) were administered for approximately 5 months. Frequencies of erections, including nocturnal erections and coitus, showed significant dose-related responses to androgen treatment and closely followed the variations in the circulating testosterone level.

A similar double blind placebo controlled study was also recently performed by Bancroft (1978) on 12 hypogonadal men during the original replacement therapy, during a period of no treatment and while the patients were receiving placebo or oral testosterone undecanoate (80 mg twice daily) for a period of 8 weeks each.

Many behavioural and sexual parameters were recorded. Bancroft (1978) observed that all the seven patients that have completed the trial showed convincing sexual responses during the new androgen, having failed to show any response during placebo. These studies seem convincing as regards the specificity and rapidity of the powerful effects of testosterone in the adult males, at least when blood levels change from hypogonadal to physiologic and supra-physiologic levels.

We have seen above that androgens seem necessary for normal sexual functions and thus it might have been supposed that endocrine alterations may be present even in men with "psychogenic" impotence in whom organic lesions and hypogonadism cannot be found. In many studies on psychogenic impotence, no significant differences in plasma testosterone levels could be detected from normal men. However, Leydig cell function test by HCG stimulation revealed an impaired endocrine capacity of the testes in psychogenic impotent patients (Nieschlag et al., 1971). Since such an impaired capacity may be found in other primary non-endocrine diseases, this impairment might be a consequence of impotence rather than a cause, as pointed out by Nieschlag et al., (1971). Recent data from Pirke et al., (1979) which are in agreement with previous observations of Ansari (1975), Comhaire and Vermeulen (1975) and other authors, indicate that androgen deficiency does not contribute to the development of psychogenic erectile impotence. On the other hand, lowered plasma levels of testosterone were reported by other authors. It is possible that either the reduced sexual activity of the patients or the stressful circumstances originating from the patients' fears of reduced sexual "performance" could explain the decrease in testosterone levels observed in many patients.

On the other hand, the effects of testosterone undecanoate and placebo on sexual potency of 29 impotent men aged 45–75 were studied in a double blind experiment (Benkert *et al.*, 1979). These patients had a reduced or non-existent capacity to have an erection during intercourse and no clinical signs of endocrinological pathology.

Pharmacotherapy with testosterone was not found to be more effective than placebo in restoring sexual potency to those sexually impotent patients who did not have lowered androgen plasma levels, confirming previous observation indicating that androgen therapy alone seems useless, in absence of androgen deficiency, except for a placebo effect.

Extraepatic tissues seem to be the major sources of circulating 5α-Dihydrotesterone, the biologically active androgenic metabolite, that predominantly originates from testosterone. On the other hand, we know that androgens, as well as oestradiol (which may originate from conversion of testosterone in peripheral tissues, included the brain), are not only taken up by gonadal or adrenal target tissues but are also accumulated in sensitive brain cells, located in areas of the CNS considered implicated in sexual responses and behaviour. It appears therefore of interest to observe whether significant changes in this peripheral metabolism take place, in studying sexual behaviour.

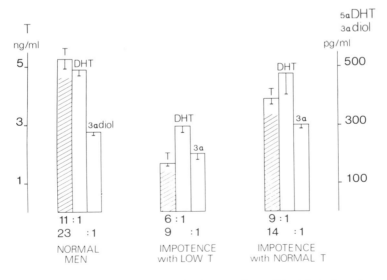

Fig. 1. Mean plasma androgen levels and ratios in normal men (N = 18), in "psychogenic" impotence with lowered testosterone levels (N = 15) and with normal testosterone levels (N = 15).

452   G. Magrini

A recent endocrine investigation performed in our Division on over more than 100
impotent patients, indicates that psychogenic impotence, in the majority of cases
is not associated with significantly decreased basal testosterone levels, in agreement with the observations of Comhaire and Vermeulen (1975) and of Pirke *et al.*,
(1979). On the contrary, (Fig. 1) we observed in many impotent men that the
conversion of testosterone into its active metabolites 5α-DHT and 5α, 3α-andro-
stanediol (3α-diol), as reflected by the ratio of plasma levels, appeared significantly increased compared to normal range.

Therefore, we studied this androgenic metabolism in two groups of 75 psychogenic impotent men, each group presenting either normal or decreased plasma
testosterone levels, in order to verify if a decrease in basal testosterone is accompanied by a corresponding decrease in its 5α metabolites. As shown in Fig. 1, in
each group the 1st column represents the mean plasma testosterone levels, the 2nd
and the 3rd columns represent the mean levels of 5α-DHT and 3α-diol respectively.
In the group with low testosterone, the levels of 5α-DHT and 3α-diol were not
corresponding lowered, therefore the ratios between testosterone and its metabolites also decreased to 6 : 1 and 9 : 1 respectively, suggesting an increased 5α conversion of testosterone, or anyway, an increased formation of 5α metabolites. In
the patients where testosterone levels were not significantly decreased, the plasma
ratios between androgens remained in the normal ranges.

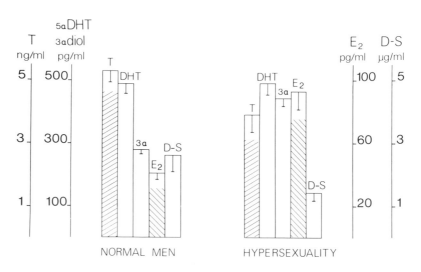

Fig. 2. Mean plasma sexual steroid levels in normal men (N = 18) and in "hypersexuality"
(N = 3).

It would appear to be interesting to know, on the other hand, if androgen
levels may be increased in so-called "hypersexuality". Hypersexuality may
perhaps be defined, according to Friedman, as a change in the sexual activity of an
individual, which is in excess of what either partner had come to expect from the
other. Hypersexual behaviour is probably not correlated with an excess of endo-

genous sex steroids, but scientific reports on hormonal data are lacking. In this preliminary investigation, (Magrini *et al.*, 1980) we measured the plasma levels of sex steroids in three patients apparently showing hypersexual behaviour. As shown in Fig. 2, testosterone as well as 5α-DHT levels were close to normal controls (1st and 2nd columns), but the levels of the metabolite 3α-diol and even more, those of the oestrogen 17β-oestradiol (E_2) were clearly increased. Therefore the hormonal balance did not apparently seem to be in favour of a hyperandrogenism, as the adrenal dehydroepiandrosterone sulphate (D-S) also appeared normal or even lowered.

ANDROGENS AND PROLACTIN

On the other hand, androgen levels seem to be influenced by prolactin (PRL): PRL seems able to interfere with testicular and adrenal steroidogenesis, as well as with the uptake and/or the metabolism of androgen in target organs.

In man, hyperprolactinaemia is often associated with impotence and impaired libido. Whatever the mechanism, it is now clear that an important and reversible pertubation implicated in impaired sexual response has been identified. Partial or complete impotence, associated with impaired libido, were reported by Franks *et al.*, (1978), in 26 of the 29 hyperprolactinemic patients studied. When the excessive PRL secretion was effectively suppressed, plasma testosterone levels increased significantly and sexual potency returned to normal. However, Buvat *et al.*, (1977), confirming reports of other authors, found normal PRL levels in more than 90% of the 103 impotent patients studied: thus, hyperprolactinemia does not seem to provide an explanation of most cases of idiopatic impotence with normal testosterone levels. On the opposite side, although the meaning of hypoprolactinemia or of lowered PRL levels is still not well defined, it seems to us that this aspect of PRL secretion may be important, considering that physiological circulating levels of PRL were shown by Bartke (1971) to be necessary for normal steroidogenesis.

We found normal or even low PRL levels (Fig. 3) in most of the impotent patients studied recently, in agreement with recent preliminary reports of Deutsch and Sherman (1978) and of Buvat *et al.* (1977); these authors found lowered PRL levels, compared to their normal ranges, in a consistent proportion of patients with secondary impotence. The mean PRL levels in the group of psychogenic impotents, (Fig. 3, 2nd column) as well as in seven depressive patients (the 3rd column), although still in the range considered as normal, were significantly lowered ($P < 0.02$) compared to the mean of normal controls. Mean testosterone levels were lowered as well, in the same groups, but oestradiol on the contrary remained normal. Also the mean levels of the 5α-metabolites of testosterone were still in the normal range. Jacobi *et al.* (1979) showed that treatment with bromocriptine, lowering PRL levels induced a significant increase in 5α-reductase activity and 5α-DHT formation in patients with advanced prostatic carcinoma. This observation may fit with these data in impotent patients with low PRL levels, which suggest an increased 5α metabolism, and with our previous reports (Magrini *et al.*, 1979) in normal men, indicating on the contrary a decrease in 5α reductase and aromatase activity during drug-induced hyperprolactinemia.

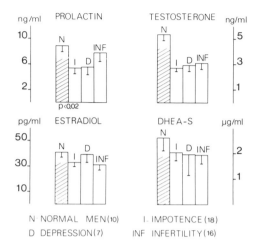

Fig. 3. Mean plasma prolactin and sexual steroid levels in normal men, in "psychogenic impotence", in depressive patients and in infertile men.

CONCLUSIONS

These studies support the role and the necessity of androgens for male sexual function and responsiveness. In the female, it is more than probable that androgens are necessary, however, further work is needed to establish this. At present we can at least observe that the relationship between androgens and sexuality in the human female is complex and probably even more so than in the male. Moreover, there are certainly considerable variations between individuals, and although androgens seem to play a role in human sexuality, sexual responses are modulated by such a great number of influences that any hormonal contribution tends to be masked by the primal role of psychological and psychosocial determinants: we know that many aspects of sexual behaviour may be inhibited, with advancing age, by the myth that sex is for the young. However, the biological parameter of androgen levels may limit and condition the other determinants.

REFERENCES

Ansari, J. M. (1975) *British Journal Psychiatry* **127**, 337.
Bancroft, J. (1978). *In* "Biological determinants of sexual behaviour", p.209. Wiley, New York.
Bancroft, J. (1980). *In* "Medical Sexology", p.210. PSG Publishing Co., Massachussetts.
Bartke, A. J. (171). *Journal of Endocrinology* **49**, 317.
Baum, M. J., Everitt, B. J., Herbert, J. and Keverne, E. B. (1977). *Archives Sexual Behaviour* **6**, 173.
Benkert, O., Witt, W., Adam, W. and Leitz, A. (1979). *Archives Sexual Behaviour* **8**(6), 471.

Buvat, J., Fossati, P. *et al.* (1977). *Problèmes Actuels Endocrinologie Nutrition* **21**, 165.

Comhaire, F. and Vermeulen, A. (1975). *Journal of Clinical Endocrinology* **40**, 824.

Carney, A., Bancroft, J. and Mathews, A. (1978). *British Journal of Psychiatry* **133**, 339.

Davidson, J. M. (1980). *In* "Medical Sexology", p.198. PSG Publishing Co., Massachussetts.

Deutsch, S. and Sherman, L. (1978). *61th Annual Meeting of Endocrine Society*, p. 350.

Franks, S., Jacobs, H. S., Martin, N. and Nabarro, J. D. (1978). *Clinical Endocrinology (Oxf.)* **8**, 277.

Kreuz, L. E., Rose, R. M. and Jennings, R. (1972). *Archives General Psychiatry* **26**, 279.

Jacobi, G. H., Altwein, J. E. and Hohenfellner, R. (1979). *Klinik Wochenschroe* **57**, 49.

Magrini, G. (1979). *Médical Hygienes* **37**, 1781.

Magrini, G. and Felber, J. P. (1980). *Médical Hygienes* **38**, 1304.

Magrini, G., Iselin, H., Ebiner, J. R. and Felber, J. P. (1979). *Archives of Andrology* **2**, 141.

Magrini, G., Büber, V. and Felber, J. P. (1980). *5th Annual Meeting of the American Society of Andrology Chicago − Journal of Andrology* **1**, 2.

Nieschlag, E., Rohr, M. and Wombacher, H. (1971). *Klinik Wochenschroe* **49**, 91.

Pirke, K. M., Kockott, G., Aldenhoff, J., Besinger, V. and Feil, W. (1979). *Archives Sexual Behaviour* **8**(1), 41.

Reinberg, A., Lagoguey, M., Cesselin, F., Tonitou, Y., Legrand, J. C., Delassale, A., Antreassian, J. and Lagoguey, A. (1978). *Acta Endocrinologica (Kbh)* **88**, 417.

Wexenberg, S. E. and Finkbeiner, J. A. (1960). *Psychosomathic Medicine* **22**, 435.

ENDOCRINE CHANGES OF TESTICULAR ACTIVITY
IN AGEING

M. Serio, G. Forti, G. Fiorelli and M. Mannelli

Endocrinology Unit, University of Florence, Florence, Italy

It is generally accepted that in the aging male the testicular endocrine function declines. Nevertheless the decline of androgen testicular secretion in aging is accompanied by variations in extraglandular metabolism of steroids which could modify the androgenic impregnation independent of glandular function.

ANDROGENS

The human testis secretes testosterone (T) and other androgens such as androstenedione (Δ), dehydroepiandrosterone (DHEA), 5α-androsten-3β, 17β-diol (A-diol), dihydrotestosterone (DHT) (Serio *et al.*, 1979) and 5α-androstan-3α, 17β-diol (3α-diol) (Moneti *et al.*, 1980). Unfortunately while circulating T originates almost exclusively from testicular secretion, the other androgens also originate from adrenal secretion and/or peripheral conversion from steroid precursors (Serio *et al.*, 1979). Therefore only the circulating T can be considered a true index of testicular secretion. However we must consider, that the circulating levels of T can be modified by variations in the metabolic clearance rate (MCR) and in testosterone binding globulin (TBG). In fact during senescence there is an increased TBG capacity (Vermeulen *et al.*, 1972) and a reduction in hepatic blood flow (Ruol and Curri, 1975). As a consequence of these phenomena the MCR of this steroid is reduced in aging. This finding can explain why in some old men plasma T is in the normal adult range, although a marked decrease of blood production rate (BPR) is present (Rubens *et al.*, 1974; Baker *et al.*, 1976).

Serono Symposium No. 39, "The Menopause: Clinical, Endocrinological and Pathophysiological Aspects", edited by P. Fioretti, L. Martini, G. B. Melis and S. S. C. Yen, 1982. Academic Press, London and New York.

In relation to the above mentioned problems the measurement of androgens in the spermatic venous blood can be considered a more precise index of testicular secretion. We did so in a large number of subjects during anaesthesia for surgical intervention for hernia repair (Giusti *et al.*, 1975; Serio *et al.*, 1977; Serio *et al.*, 1979). We found a significant decrease of Δ_4 and Δ_5 androgens in spermatic venous blood with increasing age (Serio *et al.*, 1979). Also DHT levels were found to be significantly reduced (Giusti *et al.*, 1975).

The decrease in androgen secretion by the human testis has been considered essentially due to a primary testicular origin as indicated by the moderate but statistically significant increase in LH (Stearns *et al.*, 1974) and by a reduced response to HCG stimulation in old subjects (Rubens *et al.*, 1974).

The cause of this primitive testicular deficiency may be a reduction of the Leydig cell number and/or a reduction in the blood supply (Serio *et al.*, 1979). More recently an impairment of the mechanism of action of LH at the testicular level has been also hypothesized (Harman *et al.*, 1979).

OESTROGENS

While androgen secretion is reduced in advancing age, several authors have found a pronounced increase in circulating 17β-oestradiol (E_2) and in the E_2/T ratio (Pirke and Doerr, 1973; Kley *et al.*, 1973; Baker and Hudson, 1974; Rubens *et al.*, 1974).

The increase in plasma E_2 concentration with age is probably due to a decrease in MCR and an unchanged BPR of this steroid (Baker *et al.*, 1976). Although testicular (Serio *et al.*, 1979) and adrenal secretions (Vermeulen and Verdonk, 1976) of aromatizable androgens show a pronounced decrease with age, the unchanged BPR of E_2 may be due to an increase in its direct testicular secretion, which accounts for about 25–40% (Longcope *et al.*, 1968), or to an increase in the peripheral aromatization of androgens. The latter hypothesis is strongly favoured by the finding of an increase in the transfer constant of androstenedione (Mac Donald *et al.*, 1967) and of T to E_2 (Baker *et al.*, 1976) with age.

Going back to the former hypothesis we measured E_2 in spermatic venous blood and we did not find any significant increase in senescence (Mannelli *et al.*, 1979). However in the same subjects we demonstrated that both Δ and T were decreased with age (Mannelli *et al.*, 1979). Therefore the absence of a decrease in E_2 should be explained by an increased aromatization at the testicular level similar to that observed in the other aromatizing tissues.

CONCLUSION

The decreased secretion of testicular androgens seems to be the main phenomenon in male senescence, but the increase of aromatizing activity at the peripheral level increases E_2 circulating concentrations and the E_2/T ratio. As a consequence there is an increase in TBG capacity and a reduction in the free T fraction available for the tissues.

ACKNOWLEDGEMENTS

This paper was supported by a grant (No. 76.0034.85) from the Reproductive Biology Programme of the National Research Council.

REFERENCES

Baker, H. W. G. and Hudson, B. (1974). *Clinics in Endocrinology and Metabolism* 3, 507-532.

Baker, H. G. W., Burger, H. G., de Kretser, D. M., Hudson, B., O'Connor, S., Wang, C., Mirovics, A., Court, J., Dunlop, M. and Rennie, G. C. (1976). *Clinical Endocrinology* 5, 349-35.

Giusti, G., Gonnelli, P., Borrelli, D., Fiorelli, G., Forti, G., Pazzagli, M. and Serio, M. (1975). *Experimental Gerontology* 10, 241-245.

Harman, S. M., Martin, C. E. and Tsitouras, P. D. (1979). Proceedings of the Conference on the Endocrine Aspects of Aging, Bethesda, Maryland, October 18-20 (in press).

Kley, H. K., Nieschlag, E., Bidlingmaier, F. and Kruskemper, H. L. (1973). *Hormone Metabolic Research* 6, 213-218.

Longcope, C., Layne, D. S. and Tait, J. F. (1968). *Journal of Clinical Investigation* 47, 93-106.

Mac Donald, P. C., Rombant, R. P. and Siiteri, P. K. (1967). *Journal Clinical Endocrinology and Metabolism* 27, 1103-1111.

Mannelli, M., Borrelli, D., Gonnelli, P., Fiorelli, G., Forti, G. and Serio, M. (1979). *International Journal Andrology* 2, 131-135.

Moneti, G., Pazzagli, M., Fiorelli, G. and Serio, M. (1980). *Journal Steroid Biochemistry* (in press).

Pirke, K. M. and Doerr, P. (1973). *Acta Endocrinologica* 74, 792-798.

Rubens, R., Dhont, M. and Vermeulen, A. (1974). *Journal Clinical Endocrinology and Metabolism* 39, 40-45.

Ruol, A. and Curri, G. (1975). *In* "Gerontologia e geriatria" (F. M. Antonini and C. Fumagalli, Eds), Vol. 2, 195-224. Wassermann, Milan.

Serio, M., Cattaneo, S., Borrelli, D., Gonnelli, P., Pazzagli, M., Forti, G., Fiorelli, G., Giannotti, P. and Giusti, G. (1977). *In* "Androgens and Antiandrogens" (L. Martini and M. Motta, Eds), pp. 67-75. Raven Press, New York.

Serio, M., Gonnelli, P., Borrelli, D., Pampaloni, A., Fiorelli, G., Calabresi, E., Forti, G., Pazzagli, M., Mannelli, M., Baroni, A., Giannotti, P. and Giusti, G. (1979). *Journal Steroid. Biochemistry* 11, 893-897.

Stearns, E. L., Mac Donnell, J. A., Kaufman, B. J., Padua, R., Lucman, T. S., Winter, J. S. D. and Faiman, C. (1974). *American Journal Medicine* 57, 761-766.

Vermeulen, A. and Verdonk, L. (1976). *Journal Steroid Biochemistry* 7, 1-10.

Vermeulen, A., Rubens, R. and Verdonk, L. (1972). *Journal Clinical Endocrinology and Metabolism* 34, 730-735.

EFFECT OF HUMAN SEMINAL PLASMA ON GONADOTROPIN POST-CASTRATION RISE IN ADULT MALE RATS

M. De Murtas, A. Nasi, F. Caminiti and F. Menchini Fabris[1]

Department of Obstetrics and Gynaecology, School of Medicine, University of Cagliari, Cagliari, Italy; and Andrologic Centre, First Medical Clinic, School of Medicine, University of Pisa, Pisa, Italy[1]

INTRODUCTION

Recent studies have clarified that the testes may secrete a polypeptide which inhibits specifically FSH secretion (Chari, 1977). Inhibin-like activity has been detected in rete testis fluid (Setchell, 1974), testicular tissues (Keogh *et al.*, 1976), spermatozoa (Lugaro *et al.*, 1974) and seminal plasma (Franchimont *et al.*, 1976). Some experimental data suggest that inhibin could be elaborated by Sertoli cells (Steinberger and Steinberger, 1976) and/or by germinal epithelium (Franchimont, 1972). The synthesis of inhibin by these structures may contribute to clarifying the pathway of plasma gonadotropins in cases of oligospermia and azoospermia (De Kretser *et al.*, 1978). Conflicting results have been reported about the presence of inhibin in the ejaculate (Chari *et al.*, 1978) and about the effects of human seminal plasma on gonadotropin secretion (Franchimont, 1972). In this work the effect of human seminal plasma, collected by normal and oligospermic hypergonadotropic subjects, on serum levels of FSH and LH in castrated male rats, has been examined.

Serono Symposium No. 39, "The Menopause: Clinical, Endocrinological and Pathophysiological Aspects", edited by P. Fioretti, L. Martini, G. B. Melis and S. S. C. Yen, 1982. Academic Press, London and New York.

MATERIALS AND METHODS

Human seminal plasma was taken by the subjects who requested a spermatogram to our laboratory. As normal seminal plasma was assumed the plasma recovered from the ejaculates whose seminal values were: number $\geq 40.10^6$/ml; motility $\geq 50\%$; abnormal morphology $< 10\%$. The seminal plasma of the subjects with a spermatogram lower than -10000/ml was collected separately. Ejaculates were centrifuged (4000 r.p.m. for 15 min) for removing spermatozoa and the surnatant was kept at $-20\,^\circ$C until use. Blood samples were collected from the antecubital vein, and plasma levels of FSH and LH were assayed by radioimmunoassay (Biodata, Milan, Italy). For the experiment subjects with a normal spermatogram and normal levels of FSH (5-20 mUI/ml) and LH (5-20 mUI/ml) or subjects with a spermatogram lower than -10000/ml and FSH plasma values higher than 20 mUI/ml were selected. Sixteen adult male Sprague-Dawley rats, weighing 300-400 g, were used: twelve rats were submitted to surgical castration and then maintained for 3 weeks in a light and temperature controlled room.

The first group of four castrated rats received normal seminal plasma intraperitoneally at dose of 0.5 ml every 8 h for 48 h and were killed 4 h after the last injection; the second group of four castrated rats were treated with oligospermic seminal plasma with the same schedule. The third group of castrated rats and the group of intact rats were treated by saline. All the rats were killed by decapitation and blood samples were collected by exsanguination. Serum levels of FSH and LH were evaluated by radioimmunoassay (NIAMD system). Statistical analysis was performed by the t paired test.

RESULTS

FSH and LH serum levels in adult male intact rats were in the normal range; as expected, surgical castration induced a marked increase of both gonadotropins (Table I). Normal seminal plasma administration induced a significant ($P < 0.05$) decrease in FSH serum levels while no effect was observed on LH levels. Oligospermic seminal plasma was ineffective in modifying FSH post-castration rise while it induced a significant decrease in serum LH ($P < 0.05$).

Table I. Serum levels of FSH and LH in 3 week castrated male rats after i.p. administration of human normal (NSP) and oligospermic (OSP) seminal plasma. NSP induces a significant decrease in FSH post-castration rise and is ineffective on LH; on the contrary OSP determines a significant inhibition of LH without affecting FSH. The values are reported as mean $\pm$ S.E.

	Intact (4)	Castrated (4)	Castrated + NSP (4)	Castrated + OSP (4)
FSH ng/ml	211.7 ± 12.5	816.2 ± 64.8	$398.0^a \pm 73.5$	720.6 ± 65.8
LH ng/ml	31.1 ± 4.1	320.4 ± 109.3	280.6 ± 87.2	$159.1^a \pm 18.6$

$^aP < 0.05.$

DISCUSSION

It is well known that FSH secretion and spermatogenesis are strictly correlated (Swerdloff *et al.*, 1971); this observation is also supported by considering that severe damage of seminiferous tubules, such as Sertoli-cell-only syndrome, total tubular hyalinosis etc., is characterized by an increase in FSH plasma levels (de Kretser *et al.*, 1978). This abnormal FSH pattern has been partially clarified by the isolation of a specific FSH inhibiting factor, inhibin, from the seminal plasma (Franchimont *et al.*, 1976). The secretion rate and the exact way through which inhibin reaches the blood from the testes still remain unclear (Chari *et al.*, 1978). The different inhibitory effect of normal and oligospermic seminal on FSH levels observed by Franchimont (1972), has raised the question of the biological significance of inhibin. Steinberger (1980) hypothesized that an overproduction of inhibin, by suppressing FSH, could explain the pathogenesis of oligospermia with low FSH plasma levels. On the other hand, it is not unlikely that the increase in FSH plasma levels observed in oligospermia with severe damage of the seminiferous tubules, could result from a decreased synthesis of inhibin. The present data have shown that human seminal plasma of normal and oligospermic subjects determines the different effect on FSH and LH serum levels. The inhibitory effect of oligospermic seminal plasma on FSH post-castration rise is slight and not statistically significant while the inhibition on LH secretion is more marked ($P < 0.05$); on the contrary normal seminal plasma induces a significant decrease ($P < 0.05$) in FSH whereas it is ineffective on LH. The LH decrease observed after oligospermic seminal plasma treatment could be due to the negative feedback effect exerted by the high concentrations of DHT (Nieschlag *et al.*, 1978). The slight decrease in FSH levels could be due either to lowered inhibin synthesis or to delayed and/or absent FSH response to steroid effect (Negro-Vilar and DePaolo, 1980). The inhibitory effect of normal seminal plasma on FSH post-castration rise could be explained by the presence in the ejaculate of inhibin, which is not reabsorbed in the head of the epididymis, as hypothesized by Setchell and Sirinathsinghji (1972) and by Chari *et al.* (1978). Further studies are needed in order to clarify the importance of inhibin in oligospermia and in the pituitary testicular function.

REFERENCES

Chari, S. (1977). *Endokrinologie Band.* **70**(1), 99.
Chari, S., Duraiswami, S. and Franchimont, P. (1978). *Acta endocrinologica* **87**, 434.
de Kretser, D. M., Rich, K., Kerr, J. B. and Lee, V. W. K. (1978). *In* "Recent progress in Andrology" (A. Fabbrini and E. Steinberger, Eds), p. 31. Academic Press, New York and London.
Franchimont, P. (1972). *Journal of Royal College of Physiology London* **6**, 283.
Franchimont, P., Chari, S. and Demoulin, A. (1976). *Journal of Reproductive Fertility* **44**, 335.
Keogh, E. J., Lee, V. W. K., Rennie, G. C., Burger, H. G., Hudson, B. and de Kretser, D. M. (1976). *Endocrinology* **98**, 997.
Lugaro, G., Casellato, M. M., Mazzola, G., Fachini, G. and Carrea, G. (1974). *Neuroendocrinology* **15**, 62.

Negro-Vilar, A. and De Paolo, L. (1980). *In* "International symposium on oligospermia", June 30–July 2, L'Aquila (Italy). Abstract 67.

Nieschlag, E., Wickings, E. J. and Mauss, J. (1978). *In* "Recent progress in Andrology" (A. Fabbrini and E. Steinberger, Eds), p. 101. Academic Press, New York and London

Steinberger, A. (1980). *In* "International symposium on oligospermia", June30–July 2, L'Aquila (Italy). Abstract 26.

Steinberger, A. and Steinberger, E. (1976). *Endocrinology* **99**, 918.

Setchell, B. P. (1974). *Journal of Reproductive Fertility* **37**, 165.

Setchell, B. P. and Sirinathsinghji, D. J. (1972). *Journal of Endocrinology* **53**, 434.

Swerdloff, R. S., Walsch, P. C., Jacobs, H. S. and Odell, W. D. (1971). *Endocrinology* **88**, 120.

FEMALE SEXUALITY AFTER SIXTY YEARS OF AGE

W. Pasini

*Unit of Psychosomatic Gynaecology and Sexology, Medical School,
University of Genève, Geneva, Switzerland*

INTRODUCTION

Before Kinsey, sexuality in the aged woman was totally ignored; at best, it was evoked in a negative way. Then Kinsey appeared and in spite of the small number of patients over 60 he included in his study it appeared that the sexuality of woman did not disappear at that age but decreased progressively. According to McCary (1973), only the conjugal coitus diminishes in an important way, and Kinsey's report (1953) indicates that 84% of the women of this age have still a certain form of sexual activity. It seems that this fact is more influenced by social factors than biological causes.

Pfeiffer *et al.* (1973) point out that the decline of sexuality in the woman has an epidemiological cause: the average age of the women in the United States is from 7–8 years higher than that of the men. It is known to be the same in France. In this situation, the decrease of sexual interest in the elderly women would not have a physiological basis, but a psychological function of protection: having no longer the opportunity to satisfy her libido, the woman would inhibit it.

PAIN AND CLAIM FOR HELP

The physiological changes which affect the genital organs of the woman in old age can lead to dyspareunia. Contrarily to vaginismus, the superficial or deep dyspareunia has always at least an organic component, which means that the

Serono Symposium No. 39, "The Menopause: Clinical, Endocrinological and Pathophysiological Aspects", edited by P. Fioretti, L. Martini, G. B. Melis and S. S. C. Yen, 1982. Academic Press, London and New York.

anamnesis and the gynaecological examination have never to be neglected. But pain and dyspareunia are also often the expression of a hysterical syndrome of conversion: the complaint becomes an appeal for help, an infantile manner to avoid sexuality which is no more easy to express; it could even be a form of aggressivity toward the partner.

Certain women who complain of coital dyspareunia seem to wish to say to their partner: "Not only do you no longer give me any pleasure, but you hurt me; this means that you can't call yourself a man".

There are also claims for help where, beneath dyspareunia and pain, we discover a trouble of sexual identity hidden until then by the realization of the reproductive function. When the latter vanishes and loses its function off screen, the underlying trouble comes out during the menopause or later. These women are a heavy load for the male gynaecologists and generalists: they discharge their hostility toward men in general on the therapist. In addition to the quest for help, there is in these repeated consultations for dyspareunia and pelvic pain an agressive attempt to bring about the failure of the therapist in order to prove his incompetence.

SYNDROMES OF PATIENTS OPERATED MANY TIMES

Certain women turn this aggressivity against themselves, provoke the irritability of the physician who will be voluntarily or involuntarily induced to resort to surgery. This means Cottes, hysterectomies, appendix and vesicles. We are so well acquainted with these women with their dozens of scars. Even if we will not overpsychiatrize, the syndrome of Münchhausen remains a reality.

It is necessary then to make an investigation of the "psychosomatic type" in case of pain in the aged woman, and to analyze the "utilization" adopted in other areas of the body. Dyspareunia can effectively be associated with perineal pains, with cystitis, where it is useful to investigate whether it is somatic or not. We have also to find out the pruritis of perineal pains which can permit to discover an infection, diabetes but also indicate a sexual ambivalence.

Sometimes a dyspareunia is associated with pelvic algias, the investigation of which, with its psychological approach, is much more justified if the apparition of the pains is spread out and remote.

SEXUALITY AND IMAGERY OF THE BODY

From an intrapsychical point of view, sexual behaviour is linked to the way the woman perceives her erotism, her body and her person. Erotism finds its origin in fantasy and in this fantastic life that is not altered by age. The only difficulty of the aged woman in this respect is to share her fantasy because of an excess of shyness often present at that age. But it can also happen that age brings confidence in oneself and that, sure of her sexual identity, the aged woman ventures to express herself in the couple without applying to the doctor.

But sexuality is also experienced in the body and in fantasy; the body changes with age, losing its attributes, the aesthetic function, the erotico-relational function, and sometimes its efficiency.

Sexuality in old age depends a great deal on the way the woman integrates the image of her changing body. In situations where body had anaesthetic function, a value by its surface and its relational value, sexuality receives a serious repercussion, because there is progressively a lack of aphrodisiac represented by the look and the desire of the other partner. It is the drama of hysterical or infantile women, as well of those who age badly. On the contrary, the women who see their body as something to be enjoyed besides the erotic pleasure, and who feel at ease with themselves, integrate much more easily the modifications due to their age, and sexuality is for them not affected.

AND WHAT ABOUT RELATIONSHIP?

As far as sexology is concerned, the changes of the aged woman can be more easily corrected, by means of oestrogens, than the sexual decline of the partner. How many men, when they perceive the first sexual failure, refuse to look into themselves and prefer to ask for a check-up. In looking for an exterior solution, they also seek new experiences, most of the time with younger partners; this situation creates for their wives the double inconvenience of less sexual intercourse (creating vaginal atrophy as well as narcissistic injury).

DYSPAREUNIA AND CULTURE

Does there exist a biological basis for the fact that the sexuality of the man is experienced as a pleasure, and that of the woman as a sign of pain, for the woman goes through painful experiences such as the menarche, and defloration, and the delivery? It would be excessive to give to these biological facts a cultural reinforcement which would perpetuate the old tendency which considers that the man has the monopoly of the pleasure and the woman that of pain, her only pleasure being to have children. It is therefore necessary to avoid the opinion that sexuality in old age is observed only in the exclusive sense of pain. This pain can have a iatrogenic causality, because pain is perhaps the only symptom by which women can express their suffering and their appeal.

I am convinced that, in cases of vomiting during pregnancy, dyspareunias and pelvic algias, these troubles will disappear, as soon as the physician takes time to listen to the patient, in the symbolic sense of her suffering, and will be touched by the sexual demands and not speak of suffering but of pleasure. At that time, the symptom having no more value, we shall perhaps see a diminution of the above mentioned disturbances. In order to reach this aim, it needs a double modification: modification of the woman who has to define her identity through the positive dimension of her sexuality and a medico-social modification to overpass the double taboo of old age and sexuality which does not refuse a new identity to the woman.

REFERENCES

Abraham, G. and Pasini, W. (1975). *In* "Introduction à la sexologie médicale", Chap. 21. Payot, Paris.

Kinsey, A. (1953). "Sexual behaviour in the human female". Saunders, Philadelphia.

McCary, J. L. (1973). "Human sexuality". D. Van Nostrand Co., New-York.

Pasini, W. (1979). L'anamnèse sexologique en gynécologie, *Contr. Fert. Sex.*, Paris Vol. 7, No. 1, 1979, pp. 51–56.

Pfeiffer, E., Gleen, C. and Davis, B. A. (1973). Determinants of sexual behavior in middle and old age. *Journal of the American Geriatric Society* **22**, 481.

THE MALE CLIMACTERIC SYNDROME

G. F. Menchini Fabris, B. Bianchi and C. Basile Fasolo

*Postgraduate School of Andrology, 1st Medical Clinical, Pise University,
Pisa, Italy*

INTRODUCTION

Endocrinological Findings

Many authors (Coppage and Cooner, 1965; Kent and Acone, 1965; Frick, 1969; Vermeulen *et al.*, 1972), using different methods (double isotope derivative, competitive binding assay, gas-chromatography, RIA) found that plasma testosterone levels do not decrease significantly during aging or at least until 70 years of age. A slow decline then follows, but it is not unusual to find 90 year old men who have testosterone levels within the normal range (Vermeulen, 1977). Blood testosterone is bound to several proteins, SHBG (sex hormone binding globuline), CBG (cortisol binding globuline) and serum albumine.

During aging, the affinity of SHBG towards testosterone rises (Vermeulen *et al.*, 1972), reducing the free fraction of testosterone with a significant decrease of free dihydrotestosterone (DHT) (Doerr and Pirke, 1973). The increase of binding capacity of SHBG causes a decrease of testosterone free fraction (AFTC, apparently free testosterone concentration), which is believed to be the metabolic active fraction. There is, also, a progressive increase of those β-reduced metabolites of testosterone which are biologically inactive, and at the same time, a decrease of biologically active α-reduced metabolites (Tamm and Voigt, 1971; Vermeulen *et al.*, 1972). This could be linked to a lessened enzymatic activity specific for androgens (Wilson, 1971) or to reduced androgen receptors in target organs (Shain, 1973). As for other adrenal androgens, dehydroepiandrosterone (DEA)

Serono Symposium No. 39, "The Menopause: Clinical, Endocrinological and Pathophysiological Aspects", edited by P. Fioretti, L. Martini, G. B. Melis and S. S. C. Yen, 1982. Academic Press, London and New York.

and its sulphate (DEA-S) decrease without changes in other adrenal hormones (Vermeulen, 1977). Doerr and Pirke (1973) and Rubens *et al.* (1974) found a progressive rise of total and free oestradiol.

Vermeulen (1977) reports a small, but significant, rise of values of oestrone and oestradiol, and a more significant increase of oestradiol/testosterone ratio. Basal plasma levels of gonadotropins (FSH and LH) rise slightly (Nieschlag *et al.*, 1973; Rubens *et al.*, 1974; Steins *et al.*, 1975; Vermeulen, 1977). The pituitary response to stimulation with LH-RH is maintained (Longcope, 1973; Nieschlag *et al.*, 1973; Rubens *et al.*, 1974; Vermeulen, 1977). The testicular response to standardized stimulation with HCG (5000 U.I./D for 3 days) decreases (Nieschlag *et al.*, 1973), confirmed by Vermeulen (1977).

HISTOLOGIC ASPECTS OF MALE GENITAL TRACT

Testes

During the aging process, testis shows a slow progressive hypotrophy, never arriving at complete atrophy. We can observe a progressive thickening and sclerosis of basal membrane (Engle, 1942; Honore, 1978), a progressive sclerosis and disorganization of tubules, with degeneration of spermatids and spermatocytes (Sniffen, 1950; Honore, 1978).

Sometimes, Leydig cells appear hyperplastic (Honore, 1978), sometimes flat and less frequent. Sertoli cells are for the most part preserved, but they tend to grow thin. Also focal mononuclear orchitis, capsular smooth muscle hyperplasia and dilatation of rete testis have been observed (Honore, 1978).

Prostate

According to Mostofi and Price (1973), physiologic atrophy in the prostate may involve the epithelium, the acini or the stroma. In atrophy of the prostate, epithelial cells are cuboidal; the cytoplasm is granular and reticulated, cell boundaries are distinct and there is no scalloping towards the lumen.

The somewhat hyperchromatic nucleus fills at least half the cell. Later, the cells become flatter and the cytoplasm more homogeneous and acidophilic. There is associated atrophy of the acini and the stroma. Acinar atrophy usually involves an entire lobule, within which the acini are smaller, collapsed and closely packed; some contain a granular acidophilic material. In its early stages, stromal atrophy consists of proliferation of fibroblasts around the acini, followed by hyalinization of the collagen.

Seminal Vesicles

The data so far published are incomplete.

SEXUAL AND BEHAVIOURAL ASPECTS

According to Masters and Johnson (1970), the most important factor in maintaining sexual efficiency in the aging male, is the continuation of normal sexual rapport. The same authors (1966), in a study carried out on 39 males, aged 51-89, found some changes in the sexual response of the older male in respect to those observed in the younger male. The changes are as follows: necessity of a longer stimulation time to obtain erection; once erection is achieved, it persists for a longer time (increase of *plateau* period), caused by an increased capacity to control ejaculation, sometimes, there is the presence of phenomon of "inverse refractory period" — the man achieves and loses the erection without ejaculation. Then, the refractory period follows, as if the man had ejaculated. In other words, what normally appears after the resolution period, now appears in the phase of excitement; decrease of potency of the ejaculatory stream. Often, there is only one expulsion period with a trickling of seminal fluid.

Therefore, there is a decrease in the sensation of the inevitability of ejaculation, caused by reduction of the expulsive contractions and a subsequent decrease of psychosexual satisfaction, the penis becomes flaccid more rapidly and a longer refractory period follows.

The same authors attribute importance to decreased sexual tension levels and to reduced responsiveness during intercourse. The causes may be the following: monotony in the sexual relationship: often, the wife forgets the need to keep the sexual relationship alive and frustrates the husband; economical preoccupations of the husband: the necessity to achieve a social status, which will provide security for the future; physical and mental exhaustion; excess of food and drink; physical and mental illness and fear of failure.

Later, the same authors, in addition to their previous findings, say that the aging male achieves orgasm with increased pleasure. Moreover, they considered the decreased need to ejaculate as advantageous for the male, in that it allows him to rapidly achieve a subsequent erection. Many sexual complaints could be attributed to unpreparedness and misinformation of the couple towards changes in sexual function, during aging.

Case studies carried out on 628 middle-aged males (Martin, 1977) and more than 900 other middle-aged men (Fabris and Davis, 1978) found decreased sexual activity because of aging. Henker (1977), from 486 patients, selected 50 middle-aged men and found cardiovascular symptoms in 41 patients, sexual inadequacy in 50 (in 30 impotence, in 12 reduced libido) emotional problems (anxiety, depression, excessive smoking, sleep disturbances) in all 50 patients, and concluded that "It appears evident that the male climacteric is an indefinite syndrome composed of several constellations of physical, sexual and emotional symptoms brought about by a complex interaction of hormonal, psychological, situational and physical factors".

METHODS

For this study, 62 middle-aged men showed apparent or evident psychic disturbances, sexual impairment and physical complaints, resembling the male climacteric. The patients were between the ages of 50 and 73 years, average age 56 years. They were free of any evident organic disease or diseases of the genital apparatus. All patients were examined physically. The examination included an andrologic inspection and personal interview regarding their sexual activity and these data were collected by means of an andrologic standardized form. The patient was asked to suspend any sexual activity for a 24 h period from the sampling time. Blood samples were drawn between 9 and 10 a.m. Plasma levels of FSH, LH, prolaction and testosterone were determined by radioimmunoassay.

RESULTS

Thirteen patients showed hot flushes, 22 vasomotor symptoms, 11 sweating, 32 appeared psychologically troubled (depression, anxiety, irritability, sleep disturbances). Fifty-eight patients complained of sexual impairment, particularly secondary impotence (according to Nijs, 1974) (45), incapacity to ejaculate (5), premature ejaculation (5) and reduced libido (3). Four patients did not demonstrate sexual symptoms. Physical examination showed reduced body hair in 12 patients, from which 11 presented hypotrophic testes (Prader's method).

Ten patients showed signs of prostatitis (acute or chronic), but without any precise subjective symptoms; in four, benign prostatic hypertrophy was found. Gonadotropins (FSH and LH) and prolactin were found in the normal range. Average values for FSH were 2.35 ng/ml (0.70-9.00), for LH 2.66 ng/ml (0.50-8.00) and for prolactin 11.27 ng/ml (3.6-28.5). Testosterone was found at the lower limit of the normal range, with an average value of 3.90 ng/ml (1.2-5.9).

DISCUSSION

Our data are in agreement with those of the literature. The frequency of sexual inadequacy is comparable to the findings of Masters and Johnson (1970). Studying 56 middle-aged men (50-79 years), they found primitive impotence in one patient, secondary impotence in 28, premature ejaculation in 19 and no sexual symptoms in eight patients.

Also the hormonal values are in agreement with those of other authors (Vermeulen et al., 1972; Nieschlag et al., 1973). Further study will have to be carried out to know the roles of prolactin and the organo-receptors for androgens. A higher frequency was found for symptoms like sweating, hot flushes and psychological disturbances (Kies, 1974), but their aetiopathogenesis is still unknown. We suggest a psychosomatic origin or an emphasized kenestopathy already present before middle age. Cohen (1977) and Masters and Johnson (1970) asked as a basis for their research: "Does andropause exist?" At present, we are in agreement with Kaplan (1974): "We cannot consider andropause as a loss of reproductive capacity. Instead, the idea is valid for a few psychosexual reactions in a declining sexuality, and therefore we prefer to use "male climacteric syndrome". However, further and in depth studies must be conducted towards a better understanding of the changes presented by the aging male.

REFERENCES

Cohen, J. (1977). "Les sterilités et hipofertilités masculines". Masson, Paris, New York, Barcelone, Milan.
Coppage, W. S. and Cooner, A. E. (1965). New England Journal of Medicine 273, 902-907

Doerr, P. and Pirke, K. M. (1973). *Acta Endocrinologica* Suppl. **177**, 123.

Engle, E. J. (1942). *In* "Problems of ageing" (E. Cowdry, Ed.). The Williams and Wilkins Co, Baltimore.

Fabris, G. and Davis, R. (1978). "Il mito del sesso. Rapporto sul comportamento sessuale degli italiani". A. Mondadori, Milan.

Frick, J. (1969). *Urologic International* **24**, 481–501.

Henker, F. O. (1977). *Psychosomatics.* Vol. **18**, 5, 23–27.

Honore, L. H. (1978). *Gerontology* 24/1, 58–65.

Kaplan, H. S. (1974). "The new sex therapy". Brunnel Mazel, New York.

Kent, J. R. and Acone, A. B. (1965). 2nd Symp. *Steroid Hormones*, Ghent Excerpta Medica Foundation 31–35.

Kies, N. (1974). *Medizininische Weltie* **25**, 228.

Kley, H. K., Nieschlag, E., Bidlingmaier, F. and Kruskemper, H. L. (1971). *Hormone Metabolic Research* **6**, 213.

Longcope, C. (1973). *Steroids* **21**, 461–471.

Martin, C. E. (1977). *In* "Sessuologia" (J. Money and H. Masaph, Eds), Vol. 2, 1034–1049. Borla, Roma.

Masters, W. H. and Johnson, V. E. (1966). "Human sexual response". Little, Brown and Co., Boston.

Masters, W. H. and Johnson, V. E. (1970). "Human sexual inadequacy". Little, Brown and Co., Boston.

Mostofi, F. K. and Price, F. B. (1973). *In* "Tumors of the male genital system". Armed Forces Institute of Pathology.

Nieschlag, E. (1978). *In* "Female and male climacteric. Current Opinion 1978" (P. A. Van Keep, D. M. Serr and R. B. Greenblatt, Eds), 2nd International Congress on the Menopause, Jerusalem, June 1978.

Nieschlag, E., Kley, K. H., Wiegelmann, W., Solbach, H. and Gandkrüskemper, H. L. (1973). *Deutsche Medizinische Woschenschrift (Stuttgart)* **98**, 1281–1284.

Nijs, P. (1974). *Medikon* **3**, 29–36.

Rubens, R., Dhont, M. and Vermeulen, A. (1974). *Journal of Clinical Endocrinology* **39**, 40–45.

Schmidt, II. (1968). *Symp. Dtsch. Ges. Endokrinol.* **17**, 165–174. Springer-Verlag, Berlin.

Shain, S. A. (1973). *In* "Symposium on the Normal and Abnormal of Growth of the Prostate" (M. Goland, Ed.), 712–730. Charles C. Thomas, Springfield, Illinois.

Sniffen, R. C. (1950). *Archives of Pathology* **50**, 259.

Steins, P., Hornung, D., Lindenmayer, D. and Theile, L. (1975). *21 Symp. Dtsch. Ges. Endokrinol Acta Endocrinol.* Suppl. 193–68.

Tamm, J. and Voigt, K. D. (1971). *Schweizenische Medizinische Wochenschrift (Basel)* **101**, 1078–1083.

Vermeulen, A. (1977). *In* "The testis in normal and infertile men" (E. Nonkin, Ed.). Raven Press, New York.

Vermeulen, A., Rubens, R. and Verdonck, L. (1972). *Journal of Clinical Endocrinology* **33**, 730–735.

Wilson, J. D. (1971). *In* "17 Symp. Dtsch. Ges. Endokrinol". Springer-Verlag, Berlin.

THE SEXUALITY OF THE ELDERLY MAN: BEYOND SEX

I. Simeone

*Centre de Gériatrie, Départment de Médicine et de Psychiatrie,
Université de Genève, Geneva, Switzerland*

INTRODUCTION

The sexuality of man confronts us with problems of sexuality in its broadest significance, more symbolic and basically, in its truest aspect which extends beyond the simple, functional genital activity. The sexual behaviour of the elderly man is much less bound with physiological or endocrinological changes than with the numerous social and psychological factors of which he is both object and subject. Briefly, the physiological changes are:

(1) The time needed for erection is longer compared to the young, but once it occurs the duration is longer, much longer than in the young.

(2) The quantity of seminal fluid in ejaculation is reduced and the jet is less strong. Ejaculation may not occur.

(3) The pleasure derived from orgasm is no longer as violent as in the past.

(4) The subjective need for ejaculation is less strong and this lessening permits continuation of sexual activity until an advanced old age.

(5) The number of sexual rapports diminish in frequency with aging.

(6) The phase of resolution which follows ejaculation will be much more rapid.

(7) The period which follows ejaculation can call a refractory phase during which stimulation has no further effect and which can prolong itself for hours or even a day or two.

Serono Symposium No. 39, "The Menopause: Clinical, Endocrinological and Pathophysiological Aspects", edited by P. Fioretti, L. Martini, G. B. Melis and S. S. C. Yen, 1982. Academic Press, London and New York.

It is naturally necessary to recall the important drop in the quantity of testosterone which, in absolutely no way precludes the possibility having rapports as satisfactory as in the past. Thus, the elderly man can continue to have a happy sexual life until a very late age if he has a partner, if he has the desire, if he is in good health and if he has always enjoyed a regular sex life.

IMPOTENCE IN ELDERLY MEN

But if one "ages sexually as one has lived", why do we see so many cases of impotence (Finkle, 1973)? At this point we must discuss the numerous social and psychological factors past and present, blending with one another, in order to compose the polymorphous portrait of the elderly man today. For example, it must not be forgotten that he stems from a moral and religious ideology totally different from that of today. Equally, it must not be forgotten that aging does not present the same characteristics for everyone: it is a highly variable process. Gerontology tells us that age is not bound only with the chronological passage of time but that it is closely bound to the individual biological and psychosocial characteristics of each person. At 70 years of age one may be decrepit or still quite young, one may have left long ago all sexual manifestations or be more active than during his youth or compared to other younger subjects. But to return to impotence and one of its possible explanations one should recall with Simone de Beauvoir (1970) that "it is in his penis that a man identifies all his life and where he feels endangered".

On the one hand one has the impression that the elderly man is "castrated" by his social *milieu*, by the education he has received, by family pressure. On the other hand he gives us the impression that he "autocastrates" himself for numerous other reasons. We can enumerate many possibilities which in the last analysis are the real "traps" into which the elderly man permits himself to be caught, and we know that failure today will make him fear the worst tomorrow. In this way the vicious circles repeat themselves easily. One example of a "trap" is the myth of "performance" and quantitative accomplishment rather than qualitative. When there is less frequency the elderly man immediately fears the worst. Then there is the idea that sexual rapport must necessarily be accompanied by an orgasm, so if once it is not, the fear immediately brings forth the spectre of impotence. The fear of losing the male agressive role codified by his culture, of seeing his own "virile superiority" disappear will accelerate the process of avoiding any sexual opportunity, the origin of eventual frustration. As though this wasn't enough one has the impression that the elderly man conforms with too much resignation to the social norms of today which expect that old age be asexual, at all costs. Thus, the elderly many complying with abandoning all sexual activities, with having been able to liberate himself from the temptation of the flesh, can feel proud to have, in this way, escaped a feeling of ridicule, and is convinced that he is more respectable and esteemed in his family and social circle, as though the loss of passion were the most important means of achieving wisdom. But, on the other hand, this behaviour may be an easy way out in the face of exterior pressures. The refuge in anonymity may be a convenient way to cease the struggle and to resign himself.

Impotence is thus the symptom of a narcissistic appraisal of negative life, the image of one's self, of one's own body regarded from now on with disgust and uneasiness.

SEXUALITY AND AGING

But we can also ask another question. What is the positive dimension of sexuality which is acquired with aging? Gone is the one-dimensional urgency which characterized younger sexual behaviour. Other methods of relationship appear with one's self and others—more intense and more affective. For example—the discovery of an old affective symbiosis (with the mother) who forms the first sexual behaviour of the child, the search for a pleasure which may be more intense and more subtle perhaps because it is the last. The fantasy life may become richer and make better the acceptance of reality, the truer identity, because the superfluous has disappeared but the essential has become even more evident. A certain part of sexuality is finally 'sublimated" with aging for a better search "of things unrelated to time and place", the arts, music, nature, etc. (Werwoerdt, 1976). One can affirm that "in aging man must learn to die" (Abraham, 1971) and that the proximity of death need not prevent him from living. It should even stimulate the desire to live more intensely in a more authentic search for himself. But often the contrary happens; that he is submerged in aging, for him synonymous with death and the anguish which is present becomes amplified by social devaluation and affective solitude.

Before this choice, fundamental and obligatory, which consists of accepting his age and struggling against what is lost by replacing it with other, better qualities, if he does not emerge victorious and stronger, he will express neurotic illusory reflections, regrets for what he has not been and he may finally, in the end, take refuge in depression or hypochondria. The first sign of this defeat or this renunciation may be autocastration from which stems the thought that the pathological aging of man, born under the sign of impotence, may finally become the renunciation of life in face of the fear of death.

REFERENCES

Abraham, G. (1971). *Médecine et Hygiène,* **29**, 2031–3032.
De Beauvoir, S. (1970). *In* "La Viellesse", Vol. 1, 336–381. Gallimard, Paris.
Finkle, A. L. (1973). *Journal of Geriatric Psychiatry* **6**, 70–79.
Werwoerdt, A. (1976). *In* "Clinical geropsychiatry", 255–265. Williams and Wilkins, Baltimore.

THE CLIMACTERIC PROBLEMS AMONG A HOMOGENOUS GROUP OF WORKING WOMEN IN GENOA: PLAN FOR A MENOPAUSE CENTRE

R. Cirillo and S. Garzarelli, (Gruppo Menopausa 150 ore FLM)

Divisione Ostetrico-Ginecologica, Ospedali Civili di Sampierdarena, Corso O. Scassi, Genoa, Italy

INTRODUCTION

The idea for this study came from a group of working women who got together to confront and study collectively the problems related to the climacteric and who came to us for medical advice. It seemed to us a good opportunity to extend the theme to a larger group of women (a homogenous group of women factory workers) in order to draw from it a plan of diagnostic-therapeutic treatment adequate to women's real needs. For such purposes, a 43 item questionnaire was divided and distributed to 200 women selected according to age and then further subdivided into groups according to Jaszmann's (1973) classification. The particularity of the work lies in the fact that questions were posed by women to other women thereby eliminating the conditioning of the doctor-patient relationship. The questions confront the climacteric as an interrelated physical-social phenomenon, an integral part of the experience lived by each woman.

PSYCHOLOGICAL AND PHYSICAL SYMPTOMS

The more common symptoms, as shown in Table I, are bone pain, weight gain, irritability, sight loss and anxiety. Hot flushes, sweating, headache and insomnia,

Serono Symposium No. 39, "The Menopause: Clinical, Endocrinological and Pathophysiological Aspects", edited by P. Fioretti, L. Martini, G. B. Melis and S. S. C. Yen, 1982. Academic Press, London and New York.

Table I.   Age-related changes of psychological and physical findings. (The symptoms are listed according to their frequency).

All groups together	Group A	Group B	Group C_1-C_2	Group C_3-C_5	Group[b] C_6-C_9
(A) Bone pain	B	E	G^a	A	A
(B) Weight increase	T	A	C	B	Z
(C) Anxiety	A	C	D	G^a	B
(D) Irritability	C	F	E	I^a	E
(E) Sight loss	Q	L	A	E	O
(F) Paresthesia	H^a	H^a	I^a	F	C
(G) Hot flushes[a]	F	D	B	D	T
(H) Poor memory[a]	L	B	N	L	L
(I) Sweating[a]	D	M	T	T	G^a
(L) Palpitation	V	I^a	H^a	C	F
(M) Cries easily	U^a	N	M	Q	Q
(N) Depressive mood	E	G^a	L	R	H^a
(O) Sleepiness	N	P	F	Z	M
(P) Melancholy	G^a	T	R	S^a	I^a
(Q) Cystitis	I^a	S^a	V	O	D
(R) Vertigo	M	O	S^a	M	P
(S) Insomnia[a]	P	R	O	H^a	R
(T) Headache		U^a	P	U^a	V
(U) Atrophic vaginitis[a]		V		P	U^a
(V) Breast symptoms		Q		N	S^a
(Z) Decrease in height					N

[a] Symptoms responsive to oestrogen therapy; [b] Jaszmann' classification: Group A: premenopausal women with regular menstrual cycle; Group B: women with irregular menstrual cycle; Group C_1-C_2: women in the first 2 years of menopause; Group C_3-C_5: women, 3-5 years after menopause; Group C_6-C_9: women, 6-9 years after menopause.

usually more responsive to oestrogen therapy, are less frequent in our study than in the International Health Foundation survey (van Keep, 1970).

The frequency of the symptoms varies according to the age of the patients and they tend to occur together in the older women; this is in agreement with Jaszmann's (1973) results.

The psychological changes are already present in a great number of premenopausal patients (Group A); with age, their behaviour undergoes a modification from an active to a passive one. The vasogenic symptoms are more frequent in the first 2 years of menopause (Group C_1-C_2) and they disappear with age. Muscular pain, sight loss and weight gain are the more frequent findings in all groups and they increase with age. The data suggest that hormonal therapy is helpful only in a limited number of cases and for a short period of time (Group C_1-C_2). The symptoms with a higher incidence do not respond to pharmacological treatment, but are alleviated by a balanced diet, exercise, physiotherapy and rehabilitation of ocular muscles. The emotional problems are best relieved with the improvement of the family and social environment and with a better acceptance and understanding of the menopause itself.

Table II. Age related changes in sexual and social behaviour (responses in %).

Questions :		Group A	Group B	Group C_1–C_2	Group C_3–C_5	Group[a] C_6–C_9
(1) Women who have read about the menopause		17%	27%	//	//	//
(2) Women who feel the need to discuss the menopause with other women		27%	52%	20%	44%	//
(3) Women who have changed their self-image		38%	47%	40%	44%	//
(4) Women who feel underloved		11%	14%	40%	33%	//
(5) Women with altered libido	increased	6%	11%	//	//	66%
	no change	68%	45%	80%	88%	66%
	decreased	26%	44%	20%	22%	34%
(6) Women who contemplate changing partners		22%	38%	//	//	//
(7) Women who want to go on working		22%	23%	20%	22%	//
(8) Women who want to retire		5%	//	20%	22%	//
(9) Women who have menopause-related difficulties in working performance		//	20%	60%	44%	//

[a] Jaszmann's Classification.

AGE RELATED CHANGES IN SEXUAL AND SOCIAL BEHAVIOUR IN MENOPAUSAL WORKING WOMEN

Table II illustrates the need of premenopausal women to understand the physiology of menopause and to share their knowledge with other women.

Data about sexual activity and social attitudes are best derived from the women in Group B. Despite the decline in libido, many of those women contemplate changing their partner. This is an indication that the decline in sexual activity is not related to the changes of the menopause but rather to an evolution of the sexual relationship itself. Postmenopausal women are less cooperative in discussing their sexual problems.

Data suggest that non-professional or even menial jobs are a means of self assurance to many women so that few of them wish for retirement despite a decline in working performance due to menopause-related symptoms.

DEVELOPMENT OF THE WORKING GROUP ON THE MENOPAUSE

We are working women from 40 to 55 years of age, members of this group on the menopause. We tried to find an answer to our problems by reading and discussing together many books on the subject. It was even difficult to analyze our feelings about the menopause: it is frightening because it is a step towards death or is it a disease to be studied by physicians? We found through our readings that the menopause is usually treated as a medical problem and we discussed the hormonal treatment with the physicians of a local hospital. We found that it was difficult to analyze individually all the aspects of the problems and that it was important to discuss them between us.

RESULTS OF OUR MEETING

It is difficult to evaluate the physiological components apart from the emotional, psychological, sexual and social problems of the premenopausal women.

The experience of this working group indicates that there is some analogy between adolescence and menopause; but while young women derive self-assurance from achieved sexual maturity, older women are faced with the decline of old age, loneliness and despair. Excessive reliance upon hormonal replacement therapy must be avoided because this may prevent the achievement of a new self confidence by the woman. An active and rich life can by itself prevent some of the menopausal symptoms such as hot flushes.

Schedule for a "Menopause Centre" in Genoa

For further development of this activity, we plan to create within the established medical facilities a centre for the prevention, therapy and counselling of menopause-related problems. The laboratory facilities for hormonal, histological and chemical tests will be provided by the Hospital. The centre will also offer treatment of the articular and ocular affections of menopausal patients. Special care will be devoted to improve the social opportunities of the women in their 50's and the general attitude of the society towards the moneopause and old age.

REFERENCES

Jaszmann, L. J. B. (1973). *In* "Epidemiology of Climacteric and Post Climacteric Complaints" (P. A. van Keep and C. Lauritzen, Eds), 22–34. S. Karger, Basel.
Van Keep, P. A. (1970). International Health Foundation, Geneva.

SECTION VIII

THERAPEUTIC APPROACHES TO CLIMACTERIC DISTURBANCES: BENEFITS AND RISKS

THERAPEUTIC STRATEGIES: OESTROGEN SUPPLEMENTATION

N. Siddle, S. Campbell and M. Whitehead

Department of Obstetrics and Gynaecology, King's College Hospital Medical School, Denmark Hill, London, UK

INTRODUCTION

This chapter discusses the management of patients with low oestrogen produc tion due to gonadal failure. Although the causative mechanisms are varied and include gonadal dysgenesis, premature ovarian failure of any aetiology and mid-life follicular exhaustion, there is a common denominator in that the short- and long-term sequelae of oestrogen deprivation can be partially or completely controlled by exogenous oestrogen therapy. The treatment of other causes of low oestrogen production, such as hyperprolactinaemia and anorexia nervosa, in which ovarian function is disturbed but potentially normal is different in that the aim is to restore normal ovarian steroidogenesis. Oestrogen treatment, therefore, is not indicated and these conditions will not be considered further.

Defining the best strategy of hormone treatment involves answering a number of questions:

Why treat ovarian failure?
Which patients should be treated?
What are the hazards of treatment and how can they be minimized?
What regimes should be prescribed?
What is the pharmacology of the drugs available?
How long should treatment last?

Serono Symposium No. 39, "The Menopause: Clinical, Endocrinological and Pathophysio-logical Aspects", edited by P. Fioretti, L. Martini, G. B. Melis and S. S. C. Yen, 1982. Academic Press, London and New York.

Although the answers to the above questions determine general prescribing policies the management of each patient results from an individual benefit/risk analysis. As the decision to commence therapy is essentially made by the patient she must be fully informed of all beneficial and potentially adverse effects.

It is impossible to reproduce the pattern of ovarian steroidogenesis during the menstrual cycle with exogenous hormone therapy. Thus, although modern treatment aims to approximate the physiological in the belief that this will minimize the adverse effects, exogenous therapy is pharmacological. For this reason the term "hormone replacement therapy" is inappropriate and is best modified to "hormone treatment".

THE DIAGNOSIS OF OVARIAN FAILURE

Oestrogen treatment will be of no benefit if endogenous production is adequate and therefore the latter must first be evaluated.

There is rarely any doubt about the diagnosis of ovarian failure in the patient who is in her fifties and who has ceased to menstruate. The presence of amenorrhoea, vasomotor instability, urogenital atrophy and reduction in well-being allow the diagnosis to be made clinically. Gonadal dysgenesis will be diagnosed following investigation for primary infertility/amenorrhoea and the other constitutional features, which may aid diagnosis, will depend upon the precise nature of the underlying abnormality. Excluding these two categories, there will remain a group of patients who have symptoms of oestrogen deficiency which may or may not be due to ovarian failure. Unfortunately, low plasma oestrogen levels are not a reliable guide to diagnosis. Weight-loss related amenorrhoea, hypopituitarism and hyperprolactinaemia may all result in a low oestrogen state despite the presence of intact ovaries and normal steroidogenesis will be resumed when the primary condition has been treated.

Patients with ovarian failure, however, always have a secondary rise in gonadotropin levels and this is much more reliable in distinguishing gonadal failure from other causes of hypo-oestrogenism. There is an overlap between the postmenopausal and mid-cycle ranges of LH so that FSH levels are a better discriminant. An FSH level in plasma greater than 50 IU/l is pathognomonic of ovarian failure and will usually be associated with low plasma oestradiol levels and an inverted oestradiol–oestrone ratio (Chakravarti *et al.*, 1976). Sporadic ovarian activity is occasionally seen up to 4 years after the menopause (Vermeulen and Verdonck, 1979), and therefore a single gonadotropin measurement may be misleading. Gonadotropin concentrations will be suppressed in patients who have recently received exogenous oestrogens.

Gonadotropin levels may be unreliable when used for the diagnosis of idiopathic premature ovarian failure. Approximately 20% of women who develop "premature" ovarian failure, with all the above features, resume ovulation and may conceive within 5 years (O'Herlihy *et al.*, 1980). Thus it is unwise to assume a totally hopeless prognosis for fertility on the basis of raised gonadotropins alone. Ovarian biopsy to look for the presence of primordial follicle may be justified in this group but carries the risk of tubal damage.

WHY TREAT OVARIAN FAILURE?

The principal reason for treating patients with ovarian failure is to relieve the symptoms of oestrogen deficiency. Patients with gonadal dysgenesis are treated to allow normal sexual development and function even though they remain infertile. Until recently there was no evidence to support a suggestion that hormone treatment could prevent against heart disease in middle-aged women and insufficient evidence to justify the universal prescription of oestrogens to prevent against osteoporosis. These situations are currently under review. There is now a report (Ross, 1981) of a reduction in mortality in ischaemic heart disease in patients receiving natural oestrogens but confirmation of these observations is required before any dramatic change in prescribing policy can be recommended. More especially, women taking combined oestrogen/progestagen therapy, as distinct from oestrogen alone, must be studied as progestagens *per se* may increase the risk of death from ischaemic heart disease.

By the age of 75 years, 50% of Caucasian women have radiological evidence of vertebral compression fracture (Greenblatt, 1979) and fractures of the proximal femur are a major cause of mortality and health service expenditure (Gallanaugh *et al.*, 1976) in the postmenopausal age group. The increasing awareness of the serious clinical and financial consequences of osteoporosis has generated demand for effective, prophylactic therapy. Regrettably, a reliable screening test to detect the population most at risk from accelerated bone loss is still not available and no widely applicable and truly sensitive method for measuring bone density has been developed. Oestrogens are known to conserve bone mass and at present are the most effective treatment available. It is likely that they will be increasingly used to prevent against the development of osteoporosis especially as their greatest hazard, the development of endometrial carcinoma, may be prevented.

Hormone treatment will not retard the ageing process although the woman with severe climacteric symptoms will often feel, look, and act older than those of her peers who receive oestrogen. The early development of gonadal failure results in a prolonged period of hypo-oestrogenism which in turn leads to severe atrophic changes in genital tract tissues, the early development of osteoporosis and an increased risk of ischaemic heart disease consequent upon changes in blood lipid concentrations. It is vitally important to treat this group to protect against the development of these adverse effects at a socially and medically unacceptable age.

WHO SHOULD BE TREATED?

Gonadal dysgenesis and premature ovarian failure, whether idiopathic or surgical are absolute indications for hormone treatment although patient numbers are small. Climacteric and postmenopausal disturbances are seen much more commonly but are only relative indications for hormone treatment. Therapy may be prescribed if laboratory or clinical evidence indicates that the symptoms are due to oestrogen deficiency and if the benefits outweigh the risks for that individual.

The "benefit/risk" analysis is the pivot of good clinical practice. As climacteric symptoms are seldom life-threatening the benefits of treatment are largely subjective and these will therefore be assessed more by the patient than by the doctor. The risks of treatment are now better understood than previously and it is possible for every patient to receive accurate information on which to base her decision to accept or reject treatment.

At King's College Hospital and the Chelsea Hospital for Women we try to steer a middle course between the overwhelming enthusiasm of the media for oestrogens and the entrenched opposition of some members of the profession. Our philosophy is liberal and reflects our view of the climacteric as an inevitable event which is "natural" but not necessarily "desirable". This is supported by an increasing ability to miminize the hazards of treatment as our knowledge of the pharmacology and biochemistry of sex steroids advances. Universal treatment, however, is not advocated as not all climacteric women have significant symptoms and the hazards of therapy, although of low incidence, can be serious.

It is clearly important to prescribe oestrogens only for those symptoms which are caused by oestrogen deficiency or are known to respond to oestrogen treatment. The majority can be predicted from our knowledge of the intra-cellular mechanisms of steroid action. All steroid responsive tissues contain specific receptor proteins and these have been detected in the vagina (Wiegerink, 1980), endometrium and myometrium (Gerschenson *et al.*, 1977), fallopian tube (Flickinger, 1974), distal urethra (Wilson, 1981), liver (Duffy and Duffy, 1978) and hypothalamus (McEwen *et al.*, 1978). Therefore, it is to be expected that these tissues would be the sites of oestrogen-deficiency symptoms. The centrally-mediated symptoms associated with the climacteric, such as nocturnal sweating and day time flushing, are most difficult to explain but may result from disordered catechol oestrogen metabolism. In addition, oestrogens modify hepatic metabolism and cause changes in the rate of production of various clotting factors and alter lipid and lipoprotein metabolism.

The two major symptoms of the climacteric, vasomotor instability and urogenital atrophy, responded significantly better to oestrogen than placebo in major, controlled studies (Coope, 1976; Campbell and Whitehead, 1977; Thompson and Oswald, 1977; Whitehead and Campbell, 1978). The response to oestrogen of many of the minor symptoms of which climacteric women complain is more difficult to assess. Objective measurement is difficult and is confounded by the "mental tonic" effect of oestrogen (Utian, 1972) which alters the subjective evaluation. The "domino" effect (Campbell and Whitehead, 1977), whereby oestrogens increase well-being by relieving flushing, makes these minor symptoms seem less troublesome. It is stressed that climacteric women are notoriously placebo responsive (Campbell and Whitehead, 1977).

Despite these difficulties oestrogen treatment has been shown to improve sleep patterns (Taylor, 1923), the urethral syndrome (Silverberg *et al.*, 1977) and coital satisfaction (Townsend *et al.*, 1980). There is no evidence of any beneficial effect on skin, hair, nails, breast atrophy, headache, libido or arthritis. Nor is there any evidence that oestrogen is useful in depressive illness, although certain psychological symptoms such as memory loss, lack of confidence and anxiety respond better to oestrogen than placebo (Campbell and Whitehead, 1977). In summary, vasomotor symptoms and urogenital atrophy will respond to oestrogen treatment. Isolated minor symptoms are probably best treated symptomatically and combinations of minor symptoms may justify treatment in certain individuals.

WHAT ARE THE HAZARDS?

Again, the majority are predictable and are an increase in the risk of endometrial cancer, breast cancer, gall-bladder disease and cardiovascular disease. Much effort has been expended in an attempt to establish and quantify these risks and the validity of the relevant epidemiological studies has been debated *ad nauseam*. Clinically, it is more useful to accept that there may be a potential risk and to minimize this by modifying treatment.

Endometrial Cancer

Several authors have suggested that there is a progression from endometrial hyperplasia through atypical hyperplasia to adenocarcinoma (Taylor, 1923; Novak and Yui, 1936; Gusberg, 1947; Shanklin, 1978). There is a clear association between conditions which result in increased oestrogenic stimulation of the endometrium and both endometrial hyperplasia and carcinoma, e.g., polycystic ovaries (Wood and Boronow, 1976), low progestin sequential oral contraception (Lyon and Frisch, 1976; Silverberg *et al.*, 1977), theca and granulosa cell tumours of the ovary (Mansell and Hertig, 1955) and metropathia haemorrhagica (Brown *et al.*, 1959). By extrapolation, it seems likely that unopposed oestrogen treatment would increase the incidence of hyperplasia and carcinoma and the many epidemiological studies reporting on this association have been elegantly reviewed (Cramer and Knapp, 1979). Although these studies are subject to various methodological faults, it is quite clear that prolonged unopposed oestrogen exposure increases the incidence of stage I, well-differentiated adenocarcinoma of the endometrium.

There is also clinical evidence that unopposed oestrogen treatment is associated with an increased incidence of endometrial hyperplasia (Sturdee, 1978; Whitehead, 1978). This highly undesirable situation can be avoided by the addition of a progestagen each month. This modification, together with regular endometrial sampling, has resulted in the incidence of endometrial carcinoma being reduced to below that observed in the normal population (Gambrell, 1978).

Breast Carcinoma

If prolonged unopposed oestrogenic stimulation results in endometrial hyperstimulation, may similar changes occur in the breast? The normal breast responds to sex hormones at puberty and during pregnancy but this response cannot be used to support a relationship between oestrogen treatment and breast cancer. Other factors such as growth hormone, thyroxine and prolactin, are important regulators of breast growth (McGuire *et al.*, 1977) and the responses of the breast
p.492

to attribute changes in breast tissue solely to the influence of oestrogen. In addition, there is no clear histological model of an oestrogen associated pre-malignant condition analagous to atypical endometrial hyperplasia nor is there any alternative theoretical model for such a development.

The epidemiological data on oestrogen treatment and breast cancer incidence are shown in Table I. None of the 12 studies published to date show an increase in the incidence of carcinoma of the order of magnitude seen in the studies of endometrial cancer and one study actually reported a reduction in risk. The least flawed study, (Hoover *et al.*, 1976) suggested an increase in risk after 15 years oestrogen usage but no dose-dependent relationship was observed. All of these studies are subject to the methodological flaws present in the studies of endometrial cancer risk (Cramer and Knapp, 1979). On the evidence available no clear association has been demonstrated between postmenopausal oestrogen treatment with natural oestrogens and the development of breast cancer, and if such a risk exists then it is likely to be of small magnitude and will possibly be reduced by the precautions outlined below. It remains to be determined whether the small risk demonstrated after prolonged use by Hoover *et al.* (1976) will be present in patients who have received treatment with smaller dosages of natural oestrogens to which a progestagen has been added.

Cardiovascular Risks

Cardiovascular risks in patients receiving hormone therapy have largely been predicted, but not proven, from the known adverse effects of combined oral contraceptives. This extrapolation, however, must be interpreted with caution as oral contraceptive users have a different endocrine background and receive synthetic oestrogens at higher dosages than postmenopausal women taking natural oestrogens. Nonetheless, the oral contraceptive studies have provided useful information which must not be ignored.

The epidemiological studies of oral contraceptive usage, although subject to methodological criticisms (MacRae, 1980) have reported an increase in risk of cardiovascular events such as cerebro-vascular accident, pulmonary embolism and myocardial infarction with increasing age, oestrogen dose and duration of therapy. Further analysis of the data suggests that the arterial complications correlate better with the progestagen dose whereas the oestrogen dosage is related more closely to the incidence of venous thrombosis (Meade, 1980).

The biochemical studies suggest ways in which the clinical sequelae might be mediated. Synthetic oestrogens cause an increase in platelet aggregation and the plasma concentrations of factors I, II, VII, VIII, IX and X (Poller *et al.*, 1971) and lower the level of antithrombin III which in normal concentrations is thought to reduce the risk of thrombosis (Von Kaulla *et al.*, 1971). Progestagens exert no effect on these factors (Poller *et al.*, 1969) but reduce the plasma concentration of HDL cholesterol (Larsson-Cohn *et al.*, 1979) and low levels are associated with an increase in risk of atheromatous disease (Meade, 1980).

The major lesson to be drawn from the above epidemiological and biochemical studies is that the adverse effects of synthetic oestrogens and progestagens appear to be dose-related. It is stressed that the synthetic oestrogens used in oral contraceptives are between 30 and 50 times more potent than the natural oestrogens

Table I. Studies of association between climacteric therapy and breast cancer.

Type of study	Reference
Case control	Boston Collaborative Drug Surveillance Program 1974. *New England Journal of Medicine* **290**, 15.
Case control	Sartwell *et al.*, 1977. *Journal of the National Cancer Institute* **59**, 1589. Wynder *et al.*, 1978. *Cancer* **41**, 2341.
Case control	Henderson *et al.*, 1974. *Journal of the National Cancer Institute* **53**, 609.
Case control	Casagrande *et al.*, 1976. *Journal of the National Cancer Institute* **56**, 839.
Case control	Craig *et al.*, 1974. *Journal of the National Cancer Institute* **53**, 1577. Ravnihar *et al.*, 1979. *European Journal of Cancer* **15**, 395–405.
Case control	Mack *et al.*, 1975. *New England Journal of Medicine* **292**, 1366. Brinton *et al.*, 1979. *Journal of the National Cancer Institute* **62**, 37.
Prospective cohort	Burch *et al.*, 1971. *Annals of Surgery* **174**, 415. Hoover *et al.*, 1976. *New England Journal of Medicine* **295**, 401. Byrd *et al.*, 1977. *Annals of Surgery* **185**, 574. Hammond *et al.*, 1979. *American Journal of Obstetrics and Gynecology* **133**, 537.

used commonly at the climacteric. Although natural oestrogens alter clotting factors in a similar way to oral contraceptives (Poller *et al.*, 1977), the spectrum of activity is less as they do not depress antithrombin III levels (Notelovitz and Greig, 1976) and therefore the thrombogenic potential is probably much reduced. Similarly, in climacteric therapy the daily dosage of progestagen and the duration of administration each month are only one half of that with oral contraceptive usage and any adverse effects are likely to be correspondingly reduced.

This expectation of a reduced cardiovascular risk has been confirmed by the epidemiological studies which have failed to show any increase in risk of arterial and venous thromboembolic disease in climacteric women taking natural oestrogens (Hulka, 1979). The magnitude of any risk, if one exists, must be small and is outweighed by the beneficial effects of oestrogens.

Gall-bladder Disease

One published epidemiological study reported a 2.5 times increase in incidence of gall-bladder disease during hormone treatment (Boston Collaborative Drug

Surveillance Program, 1974). Morbidity was related more to surgical intervention than to the development of gall stones and this side-effect does not constitute a major hazard and requires confirmation.

MINIMIZING THE HAZARDS

From the discussion above it is evident that unopposed oestrogen treatment is associated with a definite risk of endometrial cancer; with a possible risk of breast cancer in susceptible individuals after long-term exposure and with small dose-dependent changes in blood clotting factors and lipid concentrations which are of uncertain clinical significance. Five general precautions can be taken to reduce these risks.

Adequate Pretreatment Evaluation

This should include screening for evidence of existing or past endometrial, cardiovascular and breast disease. Endometrial status is best assessed by histo-logical examination of an adequate sample obtained by suction currettage as an out-patient procedure. In one series, 2% of symptomatic perimenopausal women had endometrial carcinoma and 7% had various forms of hyperplasia prior to treatment (Wenderlein, 1980).

Weight and blood pressure should be measured and cervical cytology evaluated. Desirable additional investigations when risk factors are present include mammo-graphy for breast dysplasia and a lipid profile when there is a strong family history of arterial disease. Gross varicose veins should be treated appropriately. Oestrogens *must never* be prescribed following abnormal vaginal bleeding until this has been fully investigated.

Use the Lowest Possible Dose of Oestrogen

The adverse effects of oestrogens on the endometrium and blood clotting factors are increased with higher dosages (Sturdee, 1978; Whitehead, 1978; Meade, 1980). Although any possible relationship with breast cancer remains controversial it seems prudent to prescribe the minimum effective dosage.

Add a Progestagen to the Treatment

Progestagens oppose the mitogenic activity of oestrogens (Gerschenson *et al.*, 1977). Unopposed oestrogen stimulation is not physiological and the profound beneficial effects on endometrial status that follow the addition of a progestagen have been discussed previously. We believe that prolonged unopposed oestrogenic stimulation of breast tissue is also undesirable and think it wise to prescribe a progestagen even to those patients who have undergone hysterectomy. Whilst there is no evidence that this policy protects against the development of breast cancer, the unpleasant mammary discomfort which sometimes results from oestrogenic hyperstimulation of breast tissue can be relieved in this way.

Maintain Regular Surveillance of Patients on Therapy

Review should be every 9 to 12 months. Direct questioning may elicit symptoms suggestive of early breast, endometrial or cardiovascular disease. Weight, blood pressure and breast status should be checked every 9 months and an endometrial biopsy should be obtained every 18 to 24 months. Histological examination will confirm that the progestagen dose is adequate and exclude hyperplasia and carcinoma. Although it is now possible to prescribe combined oestrogens/progestagen regimens with a very low incidence of hyperplasia (Sturdee, 1978) there is insufficient data at present to justify cessation of the practice of regular curettage. This need for serial biopsies is under review and the currently recommended management is likely to be modified within the next 2 years as safer forms of therapy become more widely available.

THE PHARMACOLOGY OF HORMONE TREATMENT

The first therapies were of unopposed synthetic oestrogens such as stilboestrol and ethinyloestradiol. Although effective in relieving symptoms, an increasing awareness of their potential hazards and a better understanding of the pharmacodynamics of sex steroids has led to the development of more "physiological" regimens of lower potency.

Oestrogens

Oestrogens may be administered orally, by subcutaneous implantation or percutaneously using the skin of either the vagina or abdominal wall. Suppositories and intra-muscular depot preparations are available but the former have low patient compliance and the latter achieve therapeutic plasma levels of only short duration and have to be repeated every 4 to 6 weeks.

The activity of oestrogen is buffered, in part, by the degree of binding to plasma proteins. Oestriol is not strongly bound but circulates largely as the glucuronide and this facilitates rapid renal excretion (Englund, 1979). Oestrone and oestradiol are 30% bound to sex hormone binding globulin (Mercier-Bodard, 1970) and thus have a longer half-life in plasma. An oral dose of oestriol is absorbed and largely excreted within 3 h whereas oestrone and oestradiol remain in plasma for up to 24 h (Englund and Johansson, 1978).

The route of administration partially determines which oestrogen will predominate in plasma. Orally administered oestradiol is converted by 17-oxidase activity in the small bowel and liver to oestrone (Adlercreutz *et al.*, 1976) and consequently oral administration of oestradiol gives rise to a marked increase in plasma oestrone concentrations (Whitehead and Campbell, 1978). However, when oestradiol is administered percutaneously by implantation or vaginally as either a cream or in a ring, plasma oestradiol values are markedly elevated. Table II shows

Table II. Hormone levels after drug administration.

Drug, dose and route	Plasma E_1 pmol/l	Plasma E_2 pmol/l	Progesterone	Comments	Reference
Normal menstrual cycle days 1–10	250	439			Chakravarti et al. (1976)
Conjugated equine oestrogens 1.25 mg daily orally	555	148		Mean peak at 8 h	Englund and Johansson (1978)
Oestradiol valerate 2 mg orally	925	222		Mean peak at 4 h	Englund (1979)
Conjugated equine oestrogens ointment 1.25 mg vaginally daily	1018	777		Mean peak after 3 weeks	Whitehead and Campbell (1978)
Oestradiol 3 mg percutaneously as ointment	900	1000		Mean peak	Whitehead (1980)
Oestradiol 200 μg vaginally daily from intra vaginal ring	370–700	370–740		Stable	Englund (1979)
Oestradiol implant 50 mg	210	306		Mean sustained level	Thom, M. H. Personal Communication
Progesterone 100 mg daily			29.81	Mean peak at 4 h on 7th day of treatment	Whitehead (1980)
Progesterone 100 mg vaginally			42	Mean peak at 8 h after start of dose	Nillius and Johansson (1971)

typical plasma oestrogen concentrations obtained by the different routes of administration. The oral route leads to a predominance of oestrone over oestradiol but with the other routes the increase in oestradiol values is greater and the resultant oestradiol/oestrone ratio more closely approximates the premenopausal, physiological range.

Progestagens

Until recently it was believed that progesterone was not well absorbed but plasma levels within the luteal phase range have been reported with both oral and vaginal administration (Nillius and Johansson, 1971; Whitehead, 1980). The synthetic progestagens, which are alternatives to progesterone, contain either 19 or 21 carbon atoms and all are well absorbed orally and excreted in bile and urine. Comparisons of their plasma concentrations are meaningless but their end-organ effects can be quantified by comparing the intra-cellular changes which they induce on target tissues such as the endometrium. Simultaneous measurements of the increase in activities of various progestagen sensisitive enzymes, such as isocitric dehydrogenase, acid phosphatase and oestradiol 17β-dehydrogenase, and of the reduction of nuclear oestrogen receptor have shown that equivalent and optimal biochemical effects are produced by norethisterone 2.5 mg daily and d-norgestrel 150 μg daily. Comparative data for dydrogesterone, medroxyprogesterone acetate and progesterone are urgently required as they are less androgenic and therefore are less likely to cause effects on HDL cholesterol.

CHOICE OF REGIME

Although the clinician may be confused by the numerous therapies available the choice of regimen will be determined by deciding the type and dosage of oestrogen to be prescribed and the preferred route of administration. If a progestagen is added, the type and duration of administration each month must be considered.

As discussed above, natural oestrogens are preferable to synthetic oestrogens as they appear to be less potent and therefore are less likely to cause cardiovascular side-effects. This is probably true for all patients requiring hormone treatment whether young and suffering from gonadal dysgenesis, premature ovarian failure and castration, or middle-aged and troubled by climacteric disturbances. It could be argued that younger patients may be equally effectively treated with cheaper, combined, oral contraceptives but as the number of such patients is small the financial savings are minimal. The duration of therapy in the younger age group will be longer and therefore the need to minimize the risks of side-effects is greater.

At adequate dosages oestrone, oestradiol and oestriol all effectively relieve the acute symptoms of oestrogen deficiency. It is stressed that because of the rapid clearance from plasma, oestriol must be administered 8 hourly if beneficial effects are to be achieved and failure to do so may explain why oestriol has been reported as being less effective at conserving bone mass. A single daily dosage imparts little oestrogenic stimulus and this may explain the absence of endometrial proliferation observed in one series (Tzingounis, 1980). When given at therapeutic dosages the uterotrophic and endometrial proliferative effects resemble those of oestrone and oestradiol (Fishman and Martucci, 1980) and 2 mg oestriol given 8 hourly has been associated with the development of endometrial hyperplasia (Englund, 1979).

There are no data to indicate whether oestrone or oestradiol is of more therapeutic benefit. Their individual effects are difficult to assess as the interconversion of these two primary oestrogens is considerable (Whitehead, 1980; Greenblatt et al., 1980) and the concentrations of both are elevated when either is given by any route. Target cells exhibit a different affinity for these two oestrogens and the endometrium is capable of selectively incorporating oestradiol despite a plasma excess of oestrone (King et al., 1980).

The different routes of administration appear equally effective in relieving symptoms. It is stressed that vaginally applied oestrogens do not only act locally but are systemically absorbed in amounts sufficient to stimulate distant target tissues such as the endometrium (Whitehead et al., 1978). The major potential disadvantage of the oral route is that the oestrogen is absorbed as a "bolus" and it has been suggested, but is as yet unproven, that it is these high concentrations of oestrogen rather than the steroid per se which are responsible for unwanted changes in clotting factors, lipid moieties and bile constituents. Additionally, the high "first-pass" clearance of oestrogen by the liver results in much of the steroid being metabolized, and therefore rendered inactive, before it has reached the systemic circulation.

At present, there is insufficient evidence to justify the use of "natural" progesterone in preference to one of the synthetic progestagens to suppress endometrial stimulation. Although the use of progesterone is appealing it remains to be established whether the same clinical results can be achieved as those reported for synthetic progestagens (Sturdee, 1978; Whitehead, 1978). Studies of endometrial biochemistry have not only provided useful information on optimal daily dosages of progestagens but have defined some of the mechanisms whereby progestagens modify intracellular machinery (King et al., 1981). The conclusion from these biochemical studies that progestagens will have to be given for at least 12 days each calendar month to totally suppress against excessive endometrial stimulation (Whitehead et al., 1980) is supported by histological data. Prospective studies have clearly shown that 7 days progestin therapy each month is insufficient to completely prevent against the development of endometrial hyperplasia (Whitehead, 1978) but this can be achieved with 13 days administration (Sturdee, 1978). Such a regimen, which is now in use in our clinics, closely approximates the events occurring during the normal ovulatory cycle where the stimulatory effects of endogenous oestradiol are opposed by 12 days of endogenous progesterone, and endometrial carcinoma seldom, if ever, arises.

SPECIAL PROBLEMS

Patients with severe oestrogen-deficiency symptoms pose special problems when there is a history of hypertension, thrombo-embolic disease and breast or endometrial cancer as the accepted principles of management dictate that hormone therapy is contra-indicated. No really effective alternative forms of therapy are available for the relief of urogenital atrophy although norethisterone may help vasomotor instability. The additional risks to which these patients are exposed if oestrogens are prescribed are mainly putative and the majority are unproven.

Effectively controlled hypertension is not common; in our opinion, an absolute contra-indication. Marked increases in blood pressure have been reported with hormone therapy but these are uncommon and the diastolic blood pressure of hypertensive patients can even be reduced by exogenous oestrogens (Campbell and Whitehead, 1977).

Tobacco consumption, a strong family history, diabetes and hypertension are all more significant risk factors than natural oestrogens for myocardial infarction and cerebrovascular accident. Hormone treatment may actually reduce the incidence of thrombo-embolic disease (Reti, 1978).

Although the role of oestrogens in the development of breast cancer remains unresolved it is quite clear that some breast tumours are hormone sensitive. Alterations in the endocrine environment are often associated with remission and for many years oestrogens have been administered, therapeutically, with good results when carcinoma develops postmenopausally. Thus, we believe that hormone treatment is not contra-indicated in this situation. Patient management when breast cancer arises premenopausally is more difficult but hormone responsiveness of the tumour may be predicted from measurement of oestradiol and progesterone receptor content (McEwen *et al.*, 1978). Logically, hormone therapy is not contra-indicated if the breast cancer is receptor negative.

Adenocarcinoma of the endometrium usually presents early and the probability of metastatic disease can be predicted on the basis of the histological grade of the lesion and degree of myometrial invasion. Well-differentiated stage I lesions with little myometrial invasion are unlikely to have metastasized and appropriate surgery, with or without irradiation, is almost invariably curative. Withholding hormone therapy under these circumstances is, in our opinion, unnecessary.

We believe that the presence of risk factors should not alter the principles of clinical management stated previously, namely to inform every patient of all possible advantages and hazards so that a reasoned "benefit/risk" assessment can be made for that individual. In our opinion, hormone treatment may safely be prescribed to patients with severe symptoms and classical contra-indications providing adequate surveillance is undertaken.

REFERENCES

Adlercreutz, H., Martin, F. and Pulkkinem, H. (1976). *Journal of Clinical Endocrinology and Metabolism* **43**, 497.

Boston Collaborative Drug Surveillance Program (1974). *New England Journal of Medicine* **290**, 15.

Brown, J. B., Matthew, G. D. and Kellar, R. (1959). *Journal of Obstetrics and Gynaecology British Empire* **66**, 177.

Campbell, S. and Whitehead, M. I. (1977). *In* "Clinics in Obstetrics and Gynaecology" (R. B. Greenblatt and J. W. W. Studd, Eds), Vol 4, 1, 31–47. Saunders, Philadelphia and London.

Chakravarti, S., Collins, W. P., Forecast, J. D., Newton, J. R., Orian, D. H. and Studd, J. W. W. (1976). *British Medical Journal* **2**, 784.

Coope, J. (1976). *In* "The Management of the Menopause and the Post-menopausal Years", (S. Campbell, Ed.) 159–168. M.T.P. Press, Lancaster.

Cramer, D. W., and Knapp, R. C. (1979). *Obstetrics and Gynecology* **54**, 521.

Duffy, M. J. and Duffy, G. J. (1978). *Journal of Steroid Biochemistry* **9**, 233.

Englund, D. E. (1979). *Acta Universitatis Upsaliensis.* **335**.

Englund, D. E. and Johansson, E. D. B. (1978). *British Journal of Obstetrics and Gynaecology* **85**, 957.

Fishman, J. and Martucci, C. P. (1980). *In* "The Menopause and Postmenopause" (N. Pasetto, R. Paoletti and J. L. Ambrus, Eds), 43–54. M.T.P. Press, Lancaster.

Flickinger, G. L. (1974). *Fertility and Sterility* **25**, 900.

Gallanaugh, S. C., Martin, A. and Millard, P. H. (1976). *British Medical Journal* **ii**, 1496.

Gambrell, R. D. (1978). *Maturitas* **1**, 107.

Gerschenson, L. E., Connor, E. and Murai, A. Jr (1977). *Endocrinology* **100**, 1468.

Greenblatt, R. B. (1979). *Journal of American Geriatric Society* **27**, 481.

Greenblatt, R. B. *et al.* (1980). *Maturitas* **2**, 29.

Gusberg, S. B. (1947). *American Journal of Obstetrics and Gynecology* **54**, 905.

Hoover, R., Gray, L. A., Cole, P. and MacMahon, B. (1976). *New England Journal of Medicine* **295**, 401.

Hulka, B. (1979). Effect of exogenous Estrogen on Postmenopausal Women, The Epidemiologic Evidence. Paper read at the Consensus Conference on Estrogen use and Postmenopausal Women. National Institute on Ageing. September 1979.

King, R. J. B., Dyer, G., Collins, W. P. and Whitehead, M. I. (1980). *Journal of Steroid Biochemistry* **13**, 377.

King, R. J. B., Townsend, P. T. and Whitehead, M. I. (1981). *Journal of Steroid Biochemistry* (in press).

Larsson-Cohn, U., Wallentine, L. and Zador, G. (1979). *Acta Obstetrica Gynecologica Scandinavica* **88**, 57.

Lyon, F. A. and Frisch, M. J. (1976). *Obstetrics and Gynecology* **47**, 639.

MacRae, K. D. (1980). *Workshop on Fertility Control.* Royal Society of Medicine International Congress and Symposium. Series 31, pp. 13–20. Academic Press, London.

Mansell, H. and Hertig, A. T. (1955). *Obstetrics and Gynecology* **6**, 385.

McEwen, B. S., Krey, L. C. and Luine, V. N. (1978). *In* "The Hypothalamus". (S. Reichlin, R. J. Baldessarini and J. B. Martin, Eds), 255–267. Raven Press, New York.

McGuire, W. L., Horwitz, K. B., Pearson, O. H. and Segaloff, A. (1977). *Cancer* **39**, 2934.

Meade, T. W. (1980). *Workshop on Fertility Control.* Royal Society of Medicine International Congress and Symposium Series 31, pp. 39–48. Academic Press, London.

Menard, J. (1973). *Endocrinology* **93**, 747.

Mercier-Bodard, C., Alfsen, A. and Baulieu, E. E. (1970). *Acta Endocrinologica* **147**, 204.

Nillius, S. J. and Johansson, E. D. B. (1971). *American Journal of Obstetrics and Gynecology* **110**, 470.

Notelovitz, M. and Greig, H. (1976). *Journal of Reproduction and Medicine* **16**, 87.

Novak, E. and Yui, E. (1936). *American Journal of Obstetrics and Gynecology* **32**, 674.

O'Herlihy, C., Pepperell, R. J. and Evans, J. H. (1980). *British Medical Journal* **281**, 1447.

Poller, L., Thompson, J., Tabiowo, A. and Priest, C. (1969). *British Medical Journal* 1, 554.

Poller, L., Thompson, J. and Thomas, W. (1971). *British Medical Journal* 4, 648.

Poller, L., Thompson, J. and Coope, J. (1977). *British Medical Journal* 1, 935.

Reti, L. L. (1978). *British Journal Obstetrics and Gynaecology* 85, 11: 857.

Ross, R. K. (1981). Submitted for publication.

Shanklin, D. R. (1978). *Pathology Annual Review* 13, 233.

Silverberg, S. G., Makowski, E. L. and Roche, W. D. (1977). *Cancer* 39, 2, 592.

Smith, P. (1980). *In* "The Menopause and Postmenopause" (N. Pasetto, R. Paoletti and J. L. Ambrus, Eds), 91-106. M.T.P. Press, Lancaster.

Sturdee, D. W. (1978). *British Medical Journal* 1, 1575.

Taylor, H. C. (1923). *American Journal of Obstetrics and Gynecology* 23, 309.

Thompson, J. and Oswald, I. (1977). *British Medical Journal* 2, 1317.

Townsend, P. T., Whitehead, M. I., McQueen, J., Minardi, J. and Campbell, S. (1980). *In* "The Menopause and Postmenopause". (N. Pasetto, R. Paoletti and J. L. Ambrus, Eds), 75-84. M.T.P. Press, Lancaster.

Tzingounis, V. A., Aksu, M. F. and Greenblatt, R. B. (1980). *Acta Endocrinologica* 233, 45.

Utian, W. H. (1972). *South African Medical Journal* 46, 1079.

Vermeulen, A. and Verdonck, L. (1979). *Journal of Steroid Biochemistry* 11, 899.

Von Kaulla, E., Droegemuller, W. and Aoki, N. (1971). *American Journal of Obstetrics and Gynecology* 109, 868.

Weinstein, M. C. (1979). Paper read at the Technical and Consensus Conference on Estrogen use and Postmenopausal Women. September 1979. US National Institute on Ageing.

Wenderlein, J. M. (1980). *In* "The Menopause and Postmenopause" (N. Pasetto, R. Paoletti and J. L. Ambrus, Eds), 63-73. M.T.P. Press, Lancaster.

Whitehead, M. I. (1978). *Maturitas* 1, 87.

Whitehead, M. I. (1980). *In* "Percutaneous Absorption of Steroids" (C. H. Vickers, Ed.), 231-248. Academic Press, New York.

Whitehead, M. I. (1980). *British Medical Journal* 1, 825.

Whitehead, M. I. and Campbell, S. (1978). *In* "Endometrial Cancer" (M. Brush, R. W. T. Taylor and R. J. B. King, Eds), 65-80. Balliere Tindall, London.

Whitehead, M. I., Minardi, J. Kitchin, Y. and Sharples, M. J. (1978). *In* "The Role of Oestrogen/Progestogen Therapy in the Management of the Menopause". (I. Cooke, Ed.), 63-71. M.T.P. Press, Lancaster.

Whitehead, M. I., King, R. J. B. and Campbell, S. (1980). *In* "Proceedings of IX World Congress of Obstetrics and Gynaecology", pp. 61-65. Excerpta Medica, Amsterdam.

Wiegerink, M. A. H. M. (1980). *Maturitas* 2, 59.

Wilson, P. D. (1981). Submitted for Publication.

Wood, G. P. and Boronow, R. C. (1976). *American Journal of Obstetrics and Gynecology* 124 (2), 140-142.

OESTROGEN SUPPLEMENTATION IN CLINICAL PRACTICE

G. B. Serra and A. Bompiani

Istituto di Clinica Ostetrica e Ginecologica, Università Cattolica del S. Cuore, Rome, Italy

INTRODUCTION

Theoretically oestrogen supplementation should aim to prevent or to correct specific and reversible disorders or discomforts related to a pathological oestrogen deficiency. This may occur, between menarcheal and menopausal ages, in women presenting a series of diseases, such as ovarian dysgenesis, premature ovarian failure, either spontaneous or acquired, amenorrhoea with negative MAP test, etc. All these conditions, however, represent a small group of women whose major complaints are more often related to sterility problems rather than to discomforts due to pathological hormone deficiency. In addition to these patients, a larger group of women requires oestrogen therapy to supplement the physiological menopausal decline of ovarian activity. The effort to correct this natural event and the fear of climacteric inconveniences make debatable whether the menopause is a pathological rather than a natural condition.

As a physiological phenomenon until 80 years ago, when the mean length of the life was no longer than 47 years, only a minority of women experienced it. Nowadays, with a life expectancy much longer than ever before, almost 95% of women easily surpass the "critical age". The great increase in population, especially in industrialized countries, has produced inevitable cultural biases. As examples of opposite socio-cultural influences on the consequences of the

Serono Symposium No. 39, "The Menopause: Clinical, Endocrinological and Pathophysiological Aspects", edited by P. Fioretti, L. Martini, G. B. Melis and S. S. C. Yen, 1982. Academic Press, London and New York.

menopause, on the one hand may be considered the mythical idea of "feminine forever", claimed by Wilson in the early sixties to prevent all kinds of frustrations and, on the other hand, the Indian condition where women regard menopause as the beginning of freedom from sexual segregation and as a very rewarding period of life (Flint, 1979). Cultural biases, however, are deeply radicated and slow to change. As a result, in our clinical practice, we have to solve their effects and face the women's needs, whether they are originally of a biological or social nature.

The current literature on the treatment of menopausal disorders suggests several drugs. Many of them, however, appear to have been tested with poor criticism and scarcely indicative clinical trials. Since every drug should be considered dangerous if not appropriate, it should be important, before starting therapy, to know if a specific correlation does exist between symptoms and pathology, in our case oestrogen deficiency, or between symptoms and therapy, in our case oestrogens. In fact, many symptoms appear merely due to the aging process, while others represent an amplification of continuous stresses acting upon a previously vulnerable person, and finally others appear specifically due to the waning of oestrogen levels. Unfortunately, in spite of extensive studies on meno-pause and the wide use of oestrogens, definitive conclusions remain uncertain and contradictory. This makes our choice quite hazardous and empirical, based more on the pressure of request than on the rationale of therapy.

OESTROGEN THERAPY AND POSTMENOPAUSAL PSYCHOLOGICAL SYMPTOMS

Among subjective discomforts, vasomotor effects appear predominant, mainly consisting of hot flushes and sweats. In addition, sleep disorders, loss of vaginal lubrication with dispareunia, mood disorders (particularly depression) and retarded orgasm frequently occur. Objective changes consist of genito-urethral atrophy, with shortening and narrowing of the vagina, different fat distribution with prevalence on the abdomen and thighs, osteoporosis and statistical equaliza-tion between men and women of the risk rate for severe cardiovascular diseases. For the majority of these symptoms oestrogen administration has been claimed to be a sort of panacea. However, since the syndrome itself appears to be hetero-geneous and altered by socio-cultural biases no wonder the results of hormonal therapy are less rewarding than expected. For instance, although many physicians still prescribe oestrogens against anxiety and depression, no real advantages are appreciable with this approach (George *et al.*, 1973; Abe *et al.*, 1976; Detre *et al.*, 1978). The use of antidepressants appears to be more indicated, avoiding sedatives and minor tranquillizers which can mask or aggravate mood disorders leading to an increased suicidal risk. Likewise, the trust placed by some clinicians in oestrogen effectiveness to prevent or correct atrophy of the breasts, or to modify adipose tissue distribution, or to reverse some cosmetic symptoms, is completely unjustified (Utian, 1972). This is because the greater part of these changes are age-related and by no means reversible with the use of oestrogens. Actually it appears that physical activity, standard of life, appropriate diet, climatic conditions, as well as occupational and recreational activities and smoking habits, may modify to a greater extent some of these characteristics, and even certain genetic influences, at least in a more efficacious and safe way.

OESTROGEN THERAPY AND HOT FLUSHES

Oestrogens are very effective in the management of flushing attacks and sweating episodes. Although the origin of these symptoms remains uncertain, and despite some temporary results obtainable with the use of placebo, the administration of oestrogen remains the best remedy to reduce vasomotor discomforts. Both patients and physicians share the idea of such benefits. However there is no evidence yet of a sure pathogenetic relation between these symptoms and oestrogen deficiency. Among women with equivalent hormonal levels only a portion of them will suffer flushing episodes. Among oophorectomized patients, all characterized by an acute and severe oestrogen decrease, only one third will suffer these symptoms (Chakravarti *et al.*, 1977).

OESTROGEN THERAPY, VAGINAL ATROPHY AND OSTEOPOROSIS

On the contrary, atrophy of the genito-urinary tract, with consequent itching or painful coitus, represents a clear consequence of hormonal deficiency. Its decrease under oestrogen treatment is prompt and dose-related.

Osteoporosis represents today a serious health problem with high mortality due to frequent fractures, whose cost in the United States can be estimated at approximately $1 billion annually (Riggs, 1979)..Its occurrence in postmenopausal women has elicited one of the most important and debated indications for oestrogen therapy. In current opinion oestrogens seem to inhibit aspecifically parathyroid activity, preventing bone resorption. Although oestrogen therapy seems to produce a significant improvement, its beneficial effect is accompanied to a lesser extent, by reduction of new bone formation. Therefore, far from replacing the bone already lost, oestrogen administration aims only to be preventive, and needs to be precocious. Once oestrogens are discontinued, accelerated bone loss occurs and the patient's condition becomes almost equal to that which it would have been without supplemental therapy. As a consequence, the hormonal supplementation should not only be precocious, but also of long duration. Although there have been several salutary reports of response to oestrogen therapy, some women continue to substain skeletal fractures and progressive loss of skeletal mass despite long-term hormonal therapy. This in part may be due to the habit of considering menopause as the unique cause of osteoporosis, and oestrogen treatment as the only therapeutic resource. Among other causes of skeletal loss, it would be wise to consider subtle forms of thyreotoxicosis, manifested by unusual elevation of T3, and cases of multiple myeloma, or metastatic carcinoma, or particular forms of bilateral cortical adrenal nodular hyperplasia, without any other signs of Cushing syndrome, cases of primary hypoparathyroidism, or cases of osteomalacia superimposed on the senescent osteopenic process, or some predisposing conditions such as the alcohol habit or diabetes mellitus, which may accelerate the bone loss which attends the aging process (Avioli, 1978). For the therapeutic pattern a diet may be appropriated which insures a calcium to phosphate ratio greater than 1.0, for example with doses of 1.0 to 2.0 g/day of elemental calcium. Moreover, its long-term skeletal effects could be increased by vitamin D in doses of 50 000 U twice a month, for 2 to 4 months. Finally, the importance of appropriate physical exercise must not be forgotten.

THE CHOICE OF OESTROGEN PREPARATION

There is a great deal of controversy concerning the choice of different oestrogen preparations. The first difficulty concerning "natural" and synthetic preparations consists in knowing what doses of each will represent a proper quantity for comparison (Bye, 1978), and what biological parameter may be examined to have an optimal basis for clinical evaluation. Much of the comparison between synthetic and so-called "natural" oestrogens has been based on coagulation factors. The *in vitro* studies of these factors have given a strong preference to natural products. However, whilst laboratory studies of clotting may provide an early warning of the dangers, it is evident that only long-term and epidemiological investigation will produce definitive answers (Aylward, 1978). Despite this limitation, the use of natural oestrogens has steeply increased in the last 5 years, accounting for over 83% of all preparations sold in 1977 (Bye, 1978). The duration, dosage and route of oestrogen therapy depend on the goals the physicians and the patient would like to achieve. If the major concern remains limited to flushing attacks, then the therapy will usually be relatively short-term. Since vasomotor symptoms do not appear to be strongly related to the level of endogenous oestrogens, it may be difficult to indicate a satisfactory theoretical dosage. Some physicians are convinced that treatment has to be balanced against symptoms, and that the optimal dose will be the one which halts flushing attacks. Others, on the other hand, argue that this index may not be a measure of oestrogen activity, since it is poorly related to oestrogen levels, and warn about the danger of switching from a supplementary treatment to a heavy pharmacological one.

For genital atrophy and dispareunia, the hormonal preparations may be applied locally. Although their innocuousness still remains debated, they may have some advantages over the orally-active oestrogens, whose A-alkylation may not only increase their efficacy, but also affect several metabolic systems, including the production of clotting factors (Bye, 1978). In the remaining cases of osteoporosis prevention, or in patients with natural or exogenous premature ovarian failure, the treatment must be long-term. In this regard, the use of large doses to achieve the so-called "oestrogen replacement therapy" appears ambitious and deceptive. High dosages of oestrogens in the clinical trials have produced little, if any, improvement in patients at the risk of, and sometimes, even increased, thromboembolic complications. Moreover, they stimulated a list of side-effects, for example unpleasant tenderness of the breasts, and gastric upsets, as well as a hazardous fluid retention or recurrent bleedings with the possibility of endometrium overstimulation. It appears to be much safer to prescribe the minimal doses sufficient to relieve some of the disorders, remaining in a range between 0.3 and 0.625 mg/day of conjugated equine urinary oestrogens, or 0.01 and 0.02 of ethinyloestradiol. In spite of being too low to be efficacious, even these dosages may prove to be too high to be considered a physiological replacement. Measurements of SHBG significantly show that treatment with 0.625 mg of conjugated oestrogens produces levels of the binding protein higher than those observed either in untreated postmenopausal women, or in normal ovulating patients, suggesting that even with these dosages over-treatment may occur (Pogmore and Jequier, 1979).

Although several benefits are apparent, the percentage of women who would definitely benefit from preventive oestrogen treatment after menopause is very difficult to estimate. The chief controversy regarding long-term use concerns a possible risk of cancer. The study of Burch *et al.*, (1975) performed on hysterectomized women failed to show an increase in the mortality rate. However, in women who have not had the uterus removed, continuous regimens of unopposed oestrogens are associated with the development, within 7 months, of both cystic glandular and atypical hyperplasia (Campbell *et al.*, 1978). This implies the necessity to use oestrogen therapy intermittently rather than continuously in order to allow regression of the endometrium and to avoid endometrial hyperplasia, eventually adding progesterone to produce a deeper shedding of the endometrium. The possibility that long-term use of oestrogens may increase the risk of endometrial cancer seems to receive support by the net augmentation of cancer incidence in the last 10 years. In spite of this, however, the mortality rate for endometrial cancer has not seemed to have increased, suggesting that, besides early detection and higher cure rate, there may be some bias both in retrospective studies as well as in histological reporting, resulting in over-diagnosis of carcinoma. This may well be possible, considering that a true distinction between a severe atypia and an endometrial carcinoma may need repeated curettage specimens before and after progestogen administration. In these conditions only severe atypia will reverse to the secretory form of endometrium (Greenblatt, 1976).

Everyone is in agreement that some kind of regular screening should be required for patients receiving oestrogens, but few of us agree as to the kind of examinations and how often they should be performed. Since almost 1% of patients with cystic glandular hyperplasia will subsequently develop an endometrial carcinoma, and this risk increases to more than 40% in women with severe atypical hyperplasia, it would seem useful to recognize the cases of hyperplasia before starting with oestrogen supplementation. In this regard, bleeding episodes or break-through spottings have no diagnostic value; normal endometrium as well as hyperplasia were both found in patients with scheduled withdrawal bleeding, with break-through spotting, and in the absence of any vaginal bleeding (Whitehead *et al.*, 1978). Therefore, the detection of pathological transformations seems to rely on repeated curettages, at regular intervals. This will take into account that *de novo* development of hyperplasia may be delayed for as long as 24 months, and that after its regression following an oestrogen withdrawal, a reappearance in an even more severe form, may still be possible (Campbell *et al.*, 1978). Some concern should be noted regarding suction-curettage, widely used in outpatient examinations, because the pathological areas may be excluded, producing errors of under-diagnosis. In this regard, it must be considered that traditional curettage also usually removes no more than 50% of endometrial tissue, and therefore may miss a relatively large number of pathological lesions if of focal extension.

CONCLUSIONS

In conclusion we must admit that oestrogen therapy may represent a very costly and palliative relief for menopausal women, whose discomforts, although requiring socio-cultural remedies, when brought into our offices receive only questionable pharmacological support. Clinical practitioners are, and more frequently will be, asked to give oestrogen therapy. However, as long as basic questions remain unsolved and precise guidelines remain undetermined, it must be considered that these drugs may represent a further form of pollution. In these conditions we are asked to evaluate the correct priority of the patient's risks and needs, and try to make the best use of remedies that are, in all cases, inadequate and limited.

REFERENCES

Abe, T., Furuhashi, M., Qhashi, I. and Suzuki, N. (1976). *Tohoku Journal of Experimental Medicine* **119**, 197.

Avioli, L. V. (1978). *American Journal of Medicine* **65**, 881.

Aylward, M. (1978). *Postgraduate Medicine Journal* **54** (Suppl 2), 7.

Burch, J. C., Byrd, B. F. and Vaughm, M. K. (1975). *In* "Estrogens in the Post-menopause" (P. A. van Keep and C. Lauritzen, Eds), Frout. Hormone Res. 3, pp. 208. Karger, Basle.

Bye, P. G. T. (1978). *Postgraduate Medicine Journal* **54** (Suppl 2), 7.

Campbell, S. (1978). *In* "Female and male climacteric" (P. A. van Keep, D. M. Serr and R. G. Greenblatt, Eds.) p. 111. MTP Press, Lancaster.

Campbell, S., Minardi, J., McQueen, J. and Whitehead, M. I. (1978). *Postgraduate Medicine Journal* **54** (Suppl 2), 59.

Chakravarti, S., Collins, W. P., Newton, J. R. and Studd, J. W. W. (1977). *British Journal of Obstetrics and Gynaecology* **84**, 769.

Detre, T., Hatashi, T. T. and Archer, D. F. (1978). *Annales of Internal Medicine* **88**, 373.

Elliot, J. (1979). *Journal of the American Medical Association* **242**, 1951.

Flint, M. P. (1979). *In* "Psychosomatics in Peri-Menopause" (A. A. Hospels and H. Musaph, Eds.) MTP Press Limited, International Medical Publishers.

George, G. C. W., Utian, W. H., Beumont, P. J. U. and Beardwood, C. J. (1973). *South African Medical Journal* **47**, 2387.

Greenblatt, R. B. (1976). *In* "The Menopause" (R. J. Beard, Ed.), p. 247. MTP Press Lancaster.

Pogmore, J. R. and Jequier, A. M. (1979). *Clinical Endocrinology* **86**, 568.

Riggs, B. L. (1979). *Endocrinologica Japonica* S. R. Ho 1, 31.

Utian, W. H. (1972). *South African Medical Journal* **46**, 732.

Whitehead, M. I., Minardi, J., McQueen, J. and Campbell, S. (1978). *Postgraduate Medical Journal* **54**, 69.

OESTROGEN REPLACEMENT THERAPY AND
PSYCHOSOMATIC ALTERATIONS

D. M. Serr and M. Atlas

Division of Obstetrics and Gynecology, the Sheba Medical Centre Tel Hashomer, Sackler School of Medicine, Tel-Aviv University, Israel

INTRODUCTION

No more than 130 years ago, the postmenopausal period was viewed in a fatalistic way, tragically depicted in the statements of Colombat de L'Isere (1850) who describes the "Change of Life" as a kind of gloomy corridor to complete retirement: "Compelled to yield to the power of time, women now cease to exist as for the species, and henceforward live only for themselves. Their features are stamped with the impress of age, and their genital organs are sealed with the signet of sterility . . . It is the dictate of prudence to avoid all such circumstances as might tend to awaken any erotic thoughts in the mind and reanimate a sentiment that ought rather to become extinct . . . in find, everything calculated to cause regrets for charms, that are lost, and enjoyments that are ended forever".

The average age of the menopause in most European communities is about 50. As life expectancy increases, a great majority of women may expect to reach this age. While the so-called "change of life" was experienced in the 17th century by no more than 28% of European women, about 95% reach menopause in the contemporary society of developed countries (Studd *et al.*, 1976), and it is estimated that about 5% of the world population are women of 45 to 54 years of age.

Premenopausal women in the modern era are entitled to look forward to a brighter future, owing much to a more scientific approach which tends to devoid

Serono Symposium No. 39, "The Menopause: Clinical, Endocrinological and Pathophysiological Aspects", edited by P. Fioretti, L. Martini, G. B. Melis and S. S. C. Yen, 1982. Academic Press, London and New York.

the menopause of its fatalistic, somewhat mystical connotation, and favours consideration of the climacteric syndrome as being the expression of a hormone deficiency state to be looked upon just as are hypothyroidism or insulin deficiency in diabetes. Viewed as such, there can be little doubt that ovarian hormone deficiency deserves, in theory at least, replacement therapy. However, this deficiency being a "physiological" one, whether or not to treat it in every case remains partly a philosophical issue. Since occurrence of the climacteric syndrome correlates best with decreasing oestrogens and increasing gonadotropin levels (Rogers, 1956; Adamopoulos *et al.*, 1971; Utian, 1972a; Colston Wentz, 1976; Studd *et al.*, 1976), it is but logical to assume that they may be alleviated by oestrogen replacement therapy. This is probably the case for the climacteric vasomotor symptoms, namely hot flushes, palpitations and perspiration bouts, together with vaginal atrophy and dryness. Indeed, most authors agree upon the beneficial effect of oestrogen replacement therapy on patients exhibiting these specific symptoms (Campbell, 1975; Utian, 1975; Coope, 1976; Studd *et al.*, 1976; Campbell and Whitehead, 1977; Detre *et al.*, 1978).

Attempts to resist the curse of senium are as ancient as mankind and have been the subjects of innumerable popular legends and mythologies. They took a more precise form with the various kinds of organo or glandular therapies which consisted of ovarian or testicular juices, believed for many centuries to possess the power of rejuvenation (Ricci, 1945). But purification of oestrogenic hormones was not achieved until the 3rd and 4th decades of the 20th century (Butenandt, quoted by Utian, 1977).

Today, three groups of oestrogenic agents are therapeutically available (Tzingounis *et al.*, 1978). These are (1) the natural oestrogens (e.g. 17-β-oestradiol or piperazine-oestrone-sulphate); (2) the synthetic oestrogens (e.g. ethinyloestradiol); (3) non-steroidal agents with oestrogenic activity (e.g. diethylstilbestrol). Side-effects and complications of therapy are apparently more frequent with synthetic medications as compared with the natural substances (Lauritzen, 1973; Borglin and Staland, 1975; Utian, 1977; Tzingounis *et al.*, 1978; Davies *et al.*, 1979).

The natural oestrogens are costlier and consist mainly of oestradiol, whereas the main oestrogen derivative in the postmenopausal period is considered to be the weaker oestrogen, oestrone (Dalton, 1977).

DO CLIMACTERIC PSYCHOLOGICAL ALTERATIONS EXIST?

Whether or not oestrogen replacement therapy has a place in the treatment of the psychosomatic alterations of the menopause is still a subject of debate among gynaecologists, internists, psychiatrists and psychologists. The primary question is, in fact, whether psychosomatic alterations characteristic of the menopause exist at all. As was stressed before, only a fraction of menopausal women will experience any kind of disturbance, while the other's entry into this period of life is likely to occur smoothly and uneventfully. Weissman and Klerman (1977) found no evidence that menopausal women are at a higher risk for depression, including those with surgically induced menopause. Also, no correlation could be established by Ballinger (1976) between menopausal status of women defined as "possible psychiatric cases" and anxiety, depression and impaired concentration. Neither could any significant difference between the risk of developing depression during the menopause as compared to other periods of life be demonstrated by Winokur (1973). By the same token, Achte (1970) stressed the lack of evidence that schizophrenia or presenile brain syndrome are in any way linked to the involution of the female reproductive system. Studying individual profiles during the menopause with aid of the MMPI (Minnesota Multiphasic Personality Inventory) Kruskemper (1975) found them to be remarkably constant over 5 years, thus minimizing the impact of the climacteric on the woman's personality.

These observations pertaining to the lack of correlation between psychological alterations and menopause explain why many authors were not able to demonstrate any consistent beneficial effect of oestrogen medication upon menopausal symptoms other than those due to vasomotor instability (Utian, 1972a; Ballinger, 1975a). The results displayed in a double blind study of Thomson (1976) fail to show any difference between oestrogens and placebo in relieving depression, anxiety and hot flushes in perimenopausal women. According to Utian (1975) symptoms such as depression, irritability and insomnia do not represent an indication for oestrogen therapy as they are equally improved by placebo. Since we are dealing with the treatment of symptoms whose specific relation to menopause and to its hormonal deficiency hallmarks is doubtful and with an age group in which the mere idea to be cared for may prove beneficial in itself, it must be kept in mind that most studies will inevitably be complicated by a profound placebo effect, making their interpretation difficult (Thomson, 1976).

Still, the emotional impact of menopause upon at least a certain percentage of women is not to be denied. An age which for males frequently coincides with the summit of their achievements and career is most often linked in the female with such depressing processes as loss of charm, decrease in physical attractiveness and loss of the social role of motherhood as the home is transformed with the departure of grown up children into an "empty nest" (Thomson, 1976; Furuhjelm and Fedor-Freybergh, 1976; Fedor-Freybergh, 1977). Despite the growing understanding of the process of ageing and its rationalization, society as a whole still displays a punitive attitude toward menopause, well reflected by the overgrowing success of cosmetics and plastic surgery meant to combat the dreadful stigmata of ageing. To these stresses a particular female subject will react differently according to her premorbid personality, her education, the social class she belongs to and even such variables as the age at menarche, parity, age at last delivery and marital status (Jeffcoate, 1960; Ballinger, 1975a; Flint, 1976; Humphrey, 1976; Jaszmann, 1976; VanKeep and Kellerhals, 1976). Jeffcoate (1960) regards the climacteric as a "physiological test of personality"—the distressing symptoms being less severe to totally inexistant in emotionally stable women (Greenblatt, 1952; Fedor-Freybergh, 1977; Detre *et al.*, 1978). The concept of "psychosomatic socio-cultural syndrome" was proposed to describe the clinical result of all these variables (Maoz, 1976).

POSTMENOPAUSAL PSYCHOSOMATIC SYMPTOMS: ROLE OF OESTROGEN THERAPY

Psychogenic alterations of the climacterium include varying degrees of irritability, diminished energy, tendency to depression, introversion, nervous exhaustion, frustration and lability of mood (Forman, 1968; Kopera, 1973). The somatization of subjective feelings, mainly of loss of self-esteem, results in psychosomatic reactions (Fedor-Freybergh, 1977). Ballinger (1975b) points out an increase in psychiatric morbidity occuring before the menopause and lasting for about a year after it. Kruskemper (1975), studying a group of climacteric women free of somatic diseases, demonstrated in them a higher rate of hypochondriasis and anxiety, expressed by fears and limitations usually observed in patients with physical disorders. The doctor's attitude towards the vague symptoms of climacteric undoubtedly plays an important role in their interpretation by his patient. It was demonstrated that women between 45 and 55 years of age are underrepresented in outpatient clinics of Internal Medicine, suggesting that symptoms are often attributed to climacteric, and too often dismissed as such, rather than to organic problems, which must first and foremost be cautiously excluded (Kepes, 1976; Serr, 1976; Utian, 1977; van Seumeren, 1978).

In dealing with the question of whether or not there is justification for the use of oestrogen replacement therapy in the psychogenic and psychosomatic alterations of the female climacteric period, one must first try to discern between those symptoms arising directly from the hormonal deficiency and those resulting from the psychological stresses which are to be expected in most women passing through that specific phase of life. The coincidence between the decrease in endogenous oestrogen output and social and environmental changes occurring in the woman's life, distressing by themselves, makes this separation difficult. It is to be kept in mind that we are dealing with drugs carrying the potential of causing definite complications, some of them severe, which contraindicate their use in a substantial group of women (Klopper, 1976; Studd *et al.*, 1976; Utian, 1977; Tzingounis *et al.*, 1978). On the other hand there are claims that oestrogens exert a positive effect on the climacteric psychological alterations *per se* by relieving the anxiety, fatigue and so forth (Hawkinson, 1938; Malleson, 1953; Cameron, 1966; Fligelman *et al.*, 1974). In our work, part of which was previously published (Serr *et al.*, 1968), only four out of 66 women still complained of depression after having been treated for 6 months with combined therapy of mestranol and ethynodiol diacetate and all patients reported a feeling of "freshness and vitality" following treatment. It was stressed that any long-term treatment of menopausal symptoms should take into account the individuality of the patient's social background and ethnic influences.

Durst and Maoz (1978) found oestrogen therapy to be definitely superior to placebo in relieving depression, anxiety and hypochondriasis. Utilizing several psychological tests as parameters, Fedor-Freybergh (1977) demonstrated a change in a positive direction among oestrogen treated women, as well as an improvement in mental performance. Oestrogen was superior to placebo in a double blind study designed by Vanhulle and Demol (1976) in improving attention, alertness and subjective estimation of the state of health. Similar results were achieved in post-oophorectomy oestrogen treated women (Rauramo *et al.*, 1975). Premarin significantly improved 12 psychological and symptomatic scores in 20 menopausal patients studied by Campbell (1975). The superiority of oestrogens vs placebo in producing a feeling of well-being was also pointed out by Utian (1972b) and it proved not to be a placebo effect *per se*. An amelioration of psychosomatic target symptoms and a "mental tonic effect" of oestrogens is evoked by several authors and it was postulated that this effect may be dose-related (Kuperman *et al.*, 1959; Wilson and Wilson, 1963; George *et al.*, 1973; Kerr, 1975).

Physiologically, these encouraging results might be based upon hormonal and more specifically oestrogenic influences on the psyche. Psychosomatic changes are observed in other periods of hormonal alterations as well, such as the premenstrual and menstrual days, pregnancy and post-partum (Kerr, 1975). Performance generally improves at mid-cycle when oestrogen levels are increasing. The fact that only roughly 30–40% of postmenopausal women exhibit psychological modifications has been tentatively attributed to differences in the extent of peripheral conversion of delta-4-androstenedione to oestrone, the main postmenopausal oestrogen derivative (La menopause. Enquête International Health Foundation, 1969). A significant positive correlation has been demonstrated between oestrogen concentration and the concentration of free tryptophan, which in turn affects the rate of serotonin synthesis, a well-known cerebral transmitter (Coppen *et al.*, 1972; Aylward, 1973; Aylward, 1975; Thomson, 1976). Moreover a negative correlation was found between oestrogen levels and monoamine-oxidase (MAO) activity causing degradation of cerebral transmitters. Thus, low MAO activity was detected at the height of oestrogen levels in the preovulatory period of the menstrual cycle, vs high activity in instances of oestrogen deficiency, as in amenorrhoea or the menopause. Oestrogen therapy in these cases brought about a drop in MAO activity (Klaiber *et al.*, 1971). Conversely, exogenous conjugated oestrogens exhibited, just like oral contraceptives, a disturbing effect upon tryptophan metabolism, leading to vitamin B-6 deficiency and to psychic disturbances such as depression, fatigue and irritability. This observation explains why in certain cases oestrogen medication to the postmenopausal women may paradoxically bring about the same negative psychic alterations against which the treatment was applied. Interestingly, the symptoms disappear upon correction of the vitamin deficiency (Haspels *et al.*, 1975).

On the other hand, it might be assumed that at least part of the alleged beneficial effect of oestrogen upon climacteric psychological and psychosomatic variables are but "secondary gains" or "domino effect" of an improvement in general well-being in the purely physical sense and especially in the most disturbing vasomotor symptoms (Campbell and Whitehead, 1977; Campbell, 1976). This relationship is quite plausible in the sense that those women handicapped by a limited tolerance to the hormone dependent physical discomfort are likely to be the most psychosomatically affected.

CONCLUSIONS

Primary or secondary as it might be, there remains little doubt that oestrogens possess, in selected cases and after the possibility of organic disease has been eliminated, a positive effect upon the psychological and psychosomatic changes occuring in a certain proportion of climacteric women unable to cope successfully with the organic symptoms of hormone deficiency. However, with or without oestrogen therapy the biological process of ageing will continue its inexorable progression, and failure of adaptation to it may require addition of psychotherapy.

REFERENCES

Achte, K. (1970). *Acta Obstetricia et Gynecologica Scandinavica (Suppl)* **49**, 3.

Adamopoulos, D. A., Loraine, J. A. and Dove, G. A. (1971). *Journal of Obstetrics and Gynaecology of the British Commonwealth* **78**, 62.

Aylward, M. (1973). *Medical Sciences* **1**, 30.

Aylward, M. (1975). *In* "The Management of the Menopause and Post-Menopausal Years" (S. Campbell, Ed.), 135–147. MTP Press, Lancaster.

Ballinger, C. B. (1975a). *In* "The Management of the Menopause and Post-Menopausal Years" (S. Campbell, Ed.), 117–125. MTP Press, Lancaster.

Ballinger, C. B. (1975b). *British Medical Journal* **3**, 344.

Ballinger, C. B. (1976). *British Medical Journal* **1**, 1183.

Borglin, N. E. and Staland, B. (1975). *Acta Obstericia et Gynecologica Scandinavica (Suppl)* **43**, 1.

Cameron, W. J. (1966). *General Practitioner* **33**, 110.

Campbell, S. (1976). *In* "Management of the Menopause and Post-menopausal Years" (S. Campbell, Ed.), 149–158. MTP Press, Lancaster.

Campbell, S. and Whitehead, M. (1977). *British Medical Journal* i, 104.

Colombat de L'Isere, M. (1850). Diseases of Women. American edition translated by Meigs, C. D. Cited by Ricci, J. V. One Hundred Years of Gynaecology 1800–1900, p. 532. Blakiston Co., Philadelphia, 1945.

Colston Wentz, A. (1976). *Annals of Internal Medicine* **84**, 331.

Coope, J. (1976). *Postgraduate Medical Journal* **52** (Suppl. 6), 27.

Coppen, A., Prange, A. J. Jr and Whybrow, P. C. (1972). *Archives of General Psychiatry* **26**, 424.

Dalton, K. (1977). *Proceedings of the Royal Society of Medicine* **70**, 431.

Davies, T., Fieldhreuse, G. and McNicol, G. P. (1979). *Thrombosis and Haemostasis* **35**, 403.

Detre, T. (1968). *Psychosomatics* **9**, 31.

Detre, T., Hayashi, T. T. and Archer, D. F. (1978). *Annals of Internal Medicine,* **88**, 373.

Durst, N. and Maoz, B. (1978). *In* "Female and Male Climacteric" (P. A. van Keep, D. M. Serr and R. B. Greenblatt, Eds), 15. MTP Press, Lancaster.

Fedor-Freybergh, P. (1977). *Acta Obstetricia et Gynecologica Scandinavica (Suppl)* **64**, 5.

Fligelman, S., Cahana, A. S., Nathan, T. and Gardosh, M. (1974). *Harefuah, Journal of the Israeli Medical Association* **87**, 147.

Flint, M. (1976). *In* "Consensus on Menopause Research" (P. A. van Keep, R. B. Greenblatt and M. Albeaux-Fernet, Eds), 73–83. MTP Press, Lancaster.

Forman, J. B. (1968). *Psychosomatics* **9**, 17.

Furuhjelm, M. and Fedor-Freybergh, P. (1976). *In* "Consensus on Menopause Research" (P. A. van Keep, R. B. Greenblatt and M. Albeaux-Fernet, Eds), 84–93. MTP Press, Lancaster.

George, G. C. W., Utian, W. H., Beumont, P. J. V. and Beardwood, C. J. (1973). *South African Medical Journal* **47**, 2387.

Greenblatt, R. B. (1952). *Geriatrics* **7**, 263.

Haspels, A. A., Goelingh Bennink, H. J. T., van Keep, P. A. and Schreurs, W. H. P. (1975). *In* "Estrogens in the Post-Menopause" Frontiers of Hormone Research (P. A. van Keep and C. Lauritzen, Eds), 3, 199–207. Karger, Basel.

Hawkinson, L. F. (1938). *Journal of the American Medical Association* 111, 390.

Humphrey, M. (1976). *In* "Consensus on Menopause Research" (P. A. van Keep, R. B. Greenblatt and M. Albeaux-Fernet Eds), 7. MTP Press, Lancaster.

Jaszmann, L. (1976). *In* "Consensus on Menopause Research" (P. A. van Keep, R. B. Greenblatt and M. Albeaux-Fernet, Eds), 7. MTP Press, Lancaster.

Jeffcoate, T. N. A. (1960). *British Medical Journal* 1, 340.

Kepes, S. (1976). *In* "Consensus on Menopause Research" (P. A. van Keep, R. B. Greenblatt and M. Albeaux-Fernet Eds), 7. MTP Press, Lancaster.

Kerr, M. Dorothea (1975). *In* "The Management of the Menopause and Post-Menopausal Years" (S. Campbell, Ed.) 127–133. MTP Press. Lancaster.

Klaiber, E. L., Kobayashi, Y., Broverman, D. M. and Hall, F. (1971). *Journal of Clinical Endocrinology and Metabolism* 33, 630.

Klopper, A. (1976). *British Medical Journal* 2, 697.

Kopera, H. (1973). *In* "Ageing and Estrogens" Frontiers of Hormone Research. (P. A. van Keep and C. Lauritzen, Eds), 2, 118–133. Karger, Basel.

Kruskemper, G. (1975). *In* "Estrogens in the Post-Menopause" Frontiers of Hormone Research. (P. A. van Keep and C. Lauritzen, Eds), 3, 105–115. Karger, Basel.

Kuperman, H. S., Wetchler, B. B. and Blatt, M. H. (1959). *Journal of the American Medical Association* 171, 1627.

Lauritzen, C. (1973). *In* "Ageing and Estrogens" Frontiers of Hormone Research. (P. A. van Keep and C. Lauritzen, Eds), 2, 2–21. Karger, Basel.

Malleson, J. (1953). *Lancet* 11, 158.

Maoz, B. (1976). *In* "Consensus on Menopause Research" (P. A. van Keep, R. B. Greenblatt and M. Albeaux-Fernet, Eds), 2. MTP Press, Lancaster.

Rauramo, L., Lagerspetz, P., Engblom, P. and Punnonen, R. (1975). *In* "Estrogens in the Post-Menopause" Frontiers of Hormone Research (P. A. van Keep and C. Lauritzen, Eds), 3, 94–104. Karger, Basel.

Ricci, J. V. (1945). One Hundred Years of Gynaecology 1800–1900. Blakiston, Philadelphia.

Rogers, J. (1956). *New England Journal of Medicine* 254, 697.

Serr, D. M. (1976). *In* "Consensus on Menopause Research" (P. A. van Keep, R. B. Greenblatt and M. Albeaux-Fernet, Eds), 2. MTP Press, Lancaster.

Serr, D. M., Rabau, E. and Mannor, S. (1968). *Clinical Trials Journal* (London) 5, 91.

van Seumeren, E. (1968). *In* "Female and Male Climacteric" (P. A. van Keep, D. M. Serr and R. B. Greenblatt, Eds), 14. MTP Press, Lancaster.

Studd, J. W. W., Chakravarti, S. and Oram, D. (1976). *Postgraduate Medical Journal* 52 (Suppl. 6), 60.

Thomson, J. (1976). *Proceedings of the Royal Society of Medicine* 69, 829.

Tzingounis, V. A., Aksu, M. and Greenblatt, R. B. (1978). *Journal of the American Medical Association* 239, 1638.

Utian, W. H. (1972a). *South African Medical Journal* 46, 732.

Utian, W. H. (1972b). *South African Medical Journal* 46, 1079.

Utian, W. H. (1975). *In* "Estrogens in the Post-Menopause" Frontiers of Hormone Research. (P. A. van Keep and C. Lauritzen, Eds), 3, 74–93. Karger, Basel.

Utian, W. H. (1977). *Obstetrical and Gynecological Survey* 32, 193.

Vanhulle, G. and Demol, R. (1976). *In* "Consensus on Menopause Research" (P. A. van Keep, R. B. Greenblatt and M. Albeaux-Fernet, Eds), 94–99. MTP Press, Lancaster.

Van Keep, P. A. and Kellerhals, J. M. (1976). *Acta Obstetrica et Gynecologica Scandinavica (Suppl)* **51**, 17.

Weissman, M. and Klerman, G. (1977). *Archives of General Psychiatry* **34**, 98.

Wilson, R. A. and Wilson, T. A. (1963). *Journal of the American Geriatric Society* **11**, 347.

Winokur, G. (1973). *American Journal of Psychiatry* **130**, 92.

CALCITONIN DEFICIENCY AND POSTMENOPAUSAL OSTEOPOROSIS: THE RESPONSE TO OESTROGEN THERAPY

P. T. Townsend[1], J. C. Stevenson[2], C. J. Hillyard[2], O. M. Young[1] and M. I. Whitehead[1]

Department of Obstetrics and Gynaecology, King's College Hospital Medical School, University of London, Denmark Hill, London, UK[1]; and Endocrine Unit, Royal Postgraduate Medical School, Hammersmith Hospital, Ducane Road, London, UK[2]

INTRODUCTION

Osteoporosis and the associated skeletal fractures are the major causes of morbidity and mortality in elderly women. Approximately 30% of 75 year old women have fractured a wrist, hip or vertebra (Crilley *et al.*, 1978). The majority of these fractures occur in osteoporotic bones. Following bilateral oophorectomy there is rapid loss of cortical bone (Aitken, 1976). This loss can be retarded by treatment with synthetic or natural oestrogens (Meema *et al.*, 1975; Lindsay *et al.*, 1976). After discontinuing therapy, however, bone loss may resume at an increased rate (Lindsay *et al.*, 1978). A retrospective case control study has demonstrated a reduced risk of osteoporosis and of hip fractures in postmenopausal women who have used exogenous oestrogen (Hutchinson *et al.*, 1979).

Neither the mechanism leading to the development of osteoporosis nor that of the protective action of oestrogens has been elucidated. We have investigated these problems by assessing the plasma levels of calcitonin in postmenopausal women, before, during and after treatment with a natural oestrogen and a synthetic oestrogen.

Serono Symposium No. 39, "The Menopause: Clinical, Endocrinological and Pathophysiological Aspects", edited by P. Fioretti, L. Martini, G. B. Melis and S. S. C. Yen, 1982. Academic Press, London and New York.

Postmenopausal women have lower plasma levels of calcitonin than normal men of similar age (Hillyard *et al.*, 1978). A major action of calcitonin is to protect against skeletal resorption (Stevenson *et al.*, 1979). We therefore felt that the relative deficiency of calcitonin in women could be a factor involved in the pathogenesis of postmenopausal bone loss.

PATIENTS AND METHODS

To date 12 postmenopausal women have been studied. Their ages range from 48 to 60 years. Two patients had undergone hysterectomy with ovarian conservation and the remaining 10 patients had a natural menopause between 6 months and 13 years previously. Postmenopausal status was confirmed by measuring plasma FSH, oestrone and oestradiol. None of the patients had used any exogenous steroids during the year prior to the study.

Seven patients were treated with Oestrogel cream (Laboratoires Besins Iscovesco); 5g of cream containing 3 mg of oestradiol 17β being administered percutaneously each evening for 12 weeks. The remaining five patients took oral ethinyloestradiol 20 μg daily for a similar period.

Blood samples were obtained by venipuncture before, at the end of 12 weeks of treatment and 2 weeks after discontinuing treatment. On each occasion a fasting blood sample was taken at 09.00 h and a second sample at midday. Blood was taken into cold lithium heparin tubes cooled in ice and centrifuged within 30 min of collection. The plasma was stored at $-20°$C.

Calcitonin was measured on the midday sample by an extraction technique and 7 day incubation radioimmunoassay (Stevenson *et al.*, 1979). The sensitivity of this technique is 2 ng/l with intra and inter assay variations of less than 10% and 14% respectively. Fasting calcium and phosphate levels were measured by an auto-analyser technique.

RESULTS

Calcitonin

Figure 1 shows midday plasma calcitonin values for each patient in the two treatment groups. The mean plasma calcitonin levels ($\pm$ SE) prior to treatment was low, 15.3 $\pm$ 2.07 ng/l. After 12 weeks of treatment plasma calcitonin levels had increased in all 12 patients. The mean value ($\pm$ SE) for the seven patients who had used percutaneous oestradiol cream was 33.8 $\pm$ 5.9 ng/l. This rise was statistically significant ($P < 0.01$). A similar increase was observed in the five patients using ethinyloestradiol with a mean calcitonin value ($\pm$ SE) of 32.6 $\pm$ 6.1 ng/l during treatment. This increase was also significant ($P < 0.05$). Two weeks after discontinuing treatment plasma calcitonin levels had returned to the pretreatment levels.

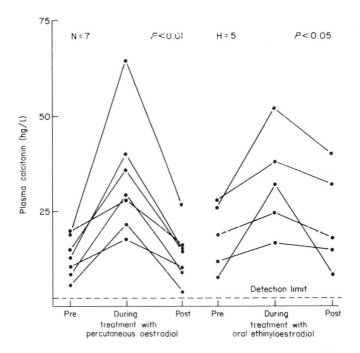

Fig. 1. Changes in plasma calcitonin in 12 patients during oestrogen treatment.

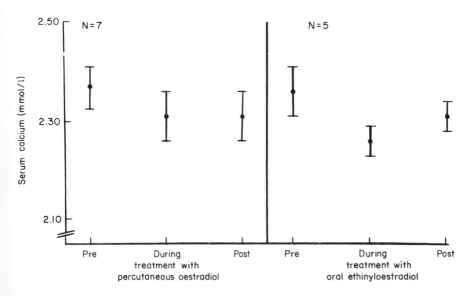

Fig. 2. Mean values (± SE) of serum calcium before, during and after oestrogen treatment.

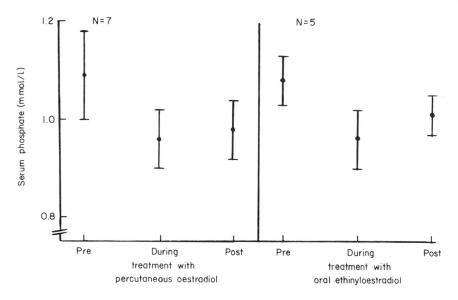

Fig. 3. Mean values (± SE) of serum phosphate before, during and after oestrogen treatment.

Calcium and phosphate

Figures 2 and 3 illustrate the mean serum calcium and phosphate levels before, during and after treatment. There was a small fall in both serum calcium and phosphate during treatment. These changes are within the physiological ranges and similar to those that have been previously reported (Gallagher and Nordin, 1973; Townsend *et al.*, 1980).

DISCUSSION

The major action of calcitonin is to inhibit bone resorption by reducing osteo-clast activity and numbers (MacIntyre *et al.*, 1967; Foster *et al.*, 1969). The fall in oestrogen production that occurs at the menopause may accelerate the decline in calcitonin that occurs with age (Samaan *et al.*, 1975), thus allowing physiological bone resorption to proceed unchecked. Together with a presumed post-menopausal reduction in bone matrix synthesis due to oestrogen deficiency this additional lowering of calcitonin will tip the balance further towards bone loss.

It is known that oestrogens prevent postmenopausal bone loss and reduces the risk of skeletal fractures. Our results demonstrate conclusively that treatment with either a natural oestrogen or a synthetic oestrogen will increase calcitonin levels. It seems likely that at least part of the beneficial effect of oestrogens on bone is mediated via calcitonin and that the combined deficiency of oestrogen and calcitonin may be of major importance in the development of postmenopausal bone loss.

ACKNOWLEDGEMENT

We thank Ayerst International and Laboratoires Besins Iscovesco for their financial support. The secretarial help of Mrs Judith Thow is much appreciated.

REFERENCES

Aitken, J. M. (1976). *In* "The Management of the Menopause and Postmenopausal Years" (S. Campbell, Ed), 225–240. MTP Press, Lancaster.

Crilley, R. G., Horsman, A., Marshall, D. H. and Nordin, B. E. C. (1978). *In* "Frontiers in Hormone Research" (C. Lauritzen and P. A. van Keep Eds), Vol. 5, 53–75. S. Karger, Basel.

Foster, G. V., Doyle, F. H., Bordier, P. and Matryajt, H. (1969). *In* "Les tissues calcifiés, V", Symposium Européen. (G. Milhaud, M. Owen and H. J. J. Blackwood, Eds), 173–177. Société d'Edition d'enseignement supérieur.

Gallagher, J. C. and Nordin, B. E. C. (1973). *In* "Frontiers in Hormone Research", (P. A. van Keep and C. Lauritzen, Eds), Vol. 2, 98–117. S. Karger, Basel.

Hillyard, C. J., Stevenson, J. C. and MacIntyre, I. (1978). *Lancet* 1, 961–962.

Hutchinson, T. A., Polansky, S. M. and Feinstein, A. R. (1979). *Lancet* 2, 705–709.

Lindsay, R., Aitken, J. M., Anderson, J. B., Hart, D. M., MacDonald, E. B. and Clarke, A. C. (1976). *Lancet* 1, 1038–1041.

Lindsay, R., Hart, D. M., Maclean, A., Clark, A. C., Kraszewski, A. and Garwood, J. (1978). *Lancet* 1, 1325–1327.

MacIntyre, I., Parsons, J. A. and Robinson, C. J. (1967) *Journal of Physiology* (London) 191, 393–405.

Meema, S., Bunker, M. L. and Meema, H. E. (1975). *Archives of Internal Medicine* 135, 1436–1440.

Samaan, N. A., Anderson, G. D. and Adam-Mayne, M. E. (1975). *American Journal of Obstetrics and Gynecology* 121, 622–625.

Stevenson, J. C., Hillyard, C. J., MacIntyre, I., Cooper, H. and Whitehead, M. I. (1979). *Lancet* 2, 769–770.

Townsend, P. T., Whitehead, M. I., McQueen, J., Minardi, J. and Campbell, S. (1980). *In* "Menopause and Postmenopause" (N. Pasetto and N. Paoletti, Eds), 75–84. MTP Press, Lancaster.

OESTRIOL AND THE MENOPAUSE: CLINICAL RESULTS FROM A PROSPECTIVE STUDY

H. P. G. Schneider

Department of Obstetrics and Gynaecology, the University of Münster, Münster, West Germany

INTRODUCTION

The careful weighing up of the benefits and hazards of exogenous natural oestrogens in the treatment of menopausal symptoms is a continuum. Good prospective studies on the hazards of oestrogen therapy have rarely been produced. In a double blind randomized cross-over placebo trial Campbell and Whitehead (1977) recently demonstrated conclusive evidence for improvement in wellbeing, both psychological and symptomatic, of patients with severe or moderate menopausal symptoms, whenever conjugated equine oestrogens 1.25 mg daily in three weekly courses with one treatment-free week between each course or a placebo in identical manner were given. Besides an increase in minor side-effects, which is of no significant relation to the overall benefits, an "unacceptably high incidence of endometrial hyperplasia" had been observed. A full secretory dose of progestagens has been suggested as additional protective therapy.

Studies in the literature and reports during this conference have shown that oestriol is beneficial with respect to the risks of human breast and endometrial cancer. The oestriol/oestrone + oestradiol ratio increases in women with higher parity and less breast cancer. On the other hand there is a downward shift of oestriol blood production rates with age and breast cancer.

Bergink (1979) has presented good evidence that only one type of oestrogen receptor binds oestriol without preference due to tissue differences. Proliferation

Serono Symposium No. 39, "The Menopause: Clinical, Endocrinological and Pathophysiological Aspects", edited by P. Fioretti, L. Martini, G. B. Melis and S. S. C. Yen, 1982. Academic Press, London and New York.

of the endometrium is unlikely since the binding time for oestriol in the nucleus is too short to allow full oestrogenic activity.

Oestriol may also act competitively and antagonisticly to oestradiol in that it may inhibit nuclear uptake of oestradiol. Oestriol will however not deplete the endometrial cell of progesterone receptors (Bergink, 1979). In view of this current knowledge the clinical application of oestriol seems increasingly attractive.

A prospective multicentre longitudinal trial had been devised by the late Dr Wenner from Switzerland. Menopausal patients were allocated 2 mg oestriol-succinate b.i.d. per os continuously over a period of 2 years. On admission to this study every patient filled in a questionnaire and every patient's general practitioner or gynaecologist kept detailed records when the patients were recalled at 4-6 week, 3, 6, 9, 12, 18 and 24 month intervals. Out of 801 patients who started the trial, 148 completed the 2 year period. Of these, 42% belonged to the age group of 51 to 55 years, 16% to the group or 56 to 60 years and 28% to the group of 46 to 50 years. Eight-one per cent of these patients were married, only 3% were divorced and 10% were widows. It should also be noted that 43% of these women were housewives, the others professionally active. Sixty per cent of them belonged to the higher income bracket and about 25% were lower or middle income workers.

At each visit the vaginal cytology (oestrogen index) of all patients was measured. The primary aim of this control was to correlate changes in vaginal cytology with changes in symptomatology. It would also enable us to determine whether the patients had taken the tablets or not.

After 2 years of treatment, a eutrophic vagina with a karyopycnotic index varying from 50-70% was found in 89% of the cases, a eutrophic vulva in 91% of cases. Atrophic changes were seen in 6% of each. Thus, we could encounter a very reasonable compliance.

SYMPTOMATIC AND PSYCHOLOGICAL CHANGES

Symptometric and psychometric evaluation in part of the study was carried out by graphic rating scales. For every symptom and emotional factor studied a line of fixed length acts as a scale (Lader and Wing, 1966). By marking the line the patient makes a self-assessment of her present state and this is repeated at given intervals. With respect to the long range of the study no placebo control could be included. Therefore, the psychological changes are only accepted as indicating oestriol effects, when they reach proportions far beyond the range of placebo effects.

With respect to skin appearance, 76% of the patients looked their age at the beginning of the treatment, whereas at the end it was 84% (Table I). However, while 16% believed to appear older, it was not because of the 24 months of treatment. Interestingly, the number of those who felt to appear younger remained unchanged (7% vs 5%). Thyroid function remained unaltered, there was definitely no hypothyroidism or goiter. Varicosis did not develop or disappear. Note that fibroids of the uterus were detected on palpation in only 42% of the patients as compared to the control situation at the beginning of the study. No definite conclusions can be drawn on whether or not oestriol inhibits fibroid growth, but obviously it is not promoted.

Table I. Organic changes during treatment with oestriol succinate.

				Skin appearance (N = 148)				
	Control	4-6 weeks	3 months	6 months	9 months	12 months	18 months	24 months
Older	24	3	1	2	1	1	–	–
According to age	113	131	131	123	124	131	124	125
Younger	11	10	8	8	13	8	5	7
Not identified	–	4	4	15	1C	8	19	16
Goiter	7	5	4	4	4	3	2	1
Varicosis	40	32	28	32	32	32	31	33
Fibroids	12	9	8	8	8	8	5	5

Urinary frequency returned to normal, while dysuria almost disappeared (Fig. 1). Both effects are statistically significant at the 1% level. Vaginal discharge remained unaltered.

Identically dyspareunia and vaginal dryness as well as pruritus improved drastically (Fig. 2).

Hirsutism improved in 77% of those patients who at the beginning of the treatment complained of a deterioration (Fig. 3).

Also a significant improvement in memory and the ability to concentrate was seen in those patients who rated themselves betwen 7 and 10 before treatment (Fig. 4). Similar mental stabilization can be deduced from the very impressive

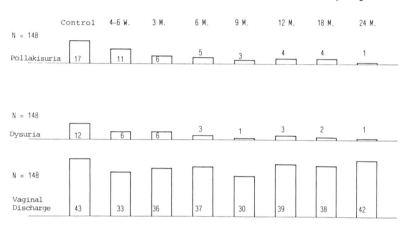

Fig. 1. Symptoms of the urinary and vaginal tract before and during continuous treatment of menopausal women with 4 mg oestriol succinate daily.

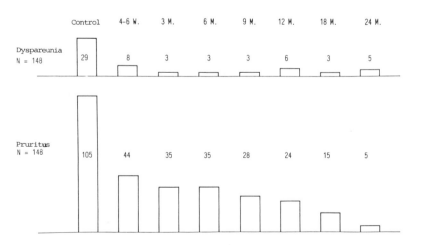

Fig. 2. Incidence of dyspareunia and pruritus before and during continuous oestriol succinate treatment as above.

disappearance of stronger and medium rated degrees of irritability (Fig. 5). The incidence of sweating also was drastically reduced from 60.8% in the strong and medium category to 10.1% at the end of treatment. There was a relative increase in occasional sweating (Fig. 6).

Headaches were already reduced by two-thirds after only 3 months of treatment, whereas the depressive mood (self-rating questionaire) had also disappeared

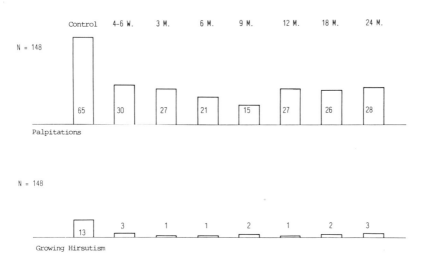

Fig. 3. Palpitations and hirsutism improve by continuous oestriol succinate treatment as above.

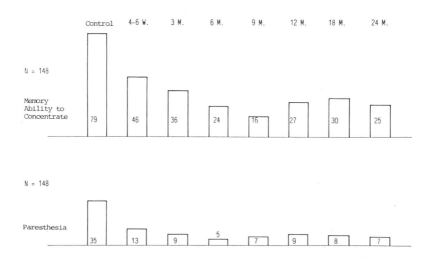

Fig. 4. "Mental tonic" effects and paresthesia before and during continuous oestriol succinate treatment as above.

H. P. G. Schneider

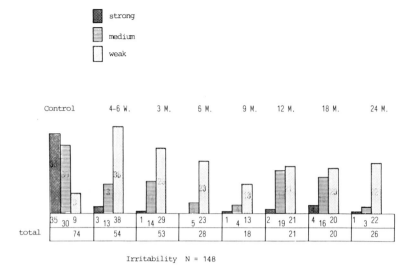

Fig. 5. Effect on various self-rated degrees of irritability of oestriol succinate treatment as above.

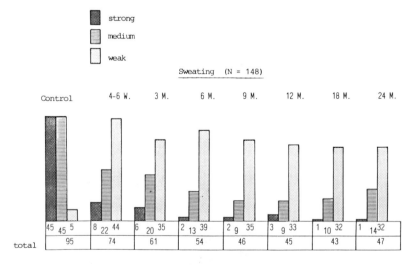

Fig. 6. Various self-rated degrees of sweating before and during continuous oestriol succinate treatment as above.

in two-thirds of these women after three months and still ameliorated for the continuation of the treatment (Fig. 7). Thus, only seven out of 45 patients still rated themselves as being depressive at the end of 2 years' treatment. The improvement in such a large number of symptoms is, as observed by others, to some extent a domino effect, i.e. a reduction in vasomotor symptoms will create a

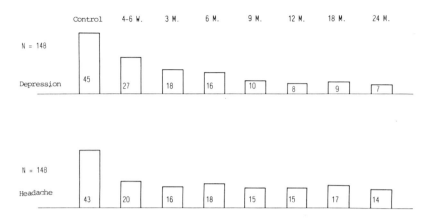

Fig. 7. Depression and headache in relation to continuous oestriol succinate treatment as above.

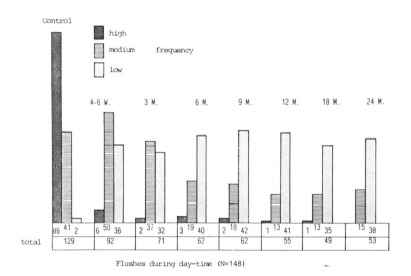

Fig. 8. Daytime flushes before and during continuous oestriol succinate treatment as above.

favourable response in a large number of other associated symptoms. This is demonstrated in the next figures, which characterize the incidence of hot flushes.

As seen in Fig. 8, during day-time high frequency flushes (more than 10, hatched bars) had disappeared after only 3 months of treatment, while the incidence of between five and 10 flushes per day (lined bars), because of the shift, slightly increased after 4 to 6 weeks; but these medium frequent flushes were also reduced to almost one-third at the end of the treatment period. Low frequency flushes (less than five), however, remained fairly constant over the treatment period.

A similar picture is seen in nocturnal flushes (Fig. 9). It appears that some 40% of the patients still experience flushes after 2 years of treatment with 4 mg of oestriol succinate. Therefore, the improvement in memory and remarkable disappearance of irritability as seen from this study suggest that oestriol exerts a "mental tonic" effect independent of the incidence of vasomotor symptoms. This has as yet only been reported for conjugated oestrogens by Hunter *et al.* (1973) and Utian (1972).

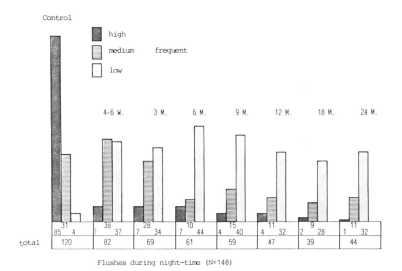

Fig. 9.   Night-time flushes under conditions as Fig. 8.

MEAN CHANGES IN WEIGHT AND BLOOD PRESSURE

The changes in weight and blood pressure at each visit were compared with control values and are illustrated in the following figures. The changes in systolic and diastolic blood pressure are depicted in Fig. 10. Both systolic as well as diastolic blood pressure vary within a range of 5 to 10 mmHg, the pulse rate within 5–10 bpm. In 98 to 99% of the patients diastolic blood pressure stays under the level of 100 mmHg. Systolic blood pressure elevation of over 135 mmHg before treatment went from 53% to 31% by the end of the 2 year trial. Final conclusions shall not be drawn before completion of 5 years. The apparent stabilization or tendency to a reduction in systolic blood pressure, however, should be noted. We do not confirm von Eiff's (1975) claim that oestrogens cause a significant reduction in diastolic blood pressure in postmenopausal women under resting conditions which Campbell and Whitehead (1977) also failed to observe in their doubleblind study with Premarin.

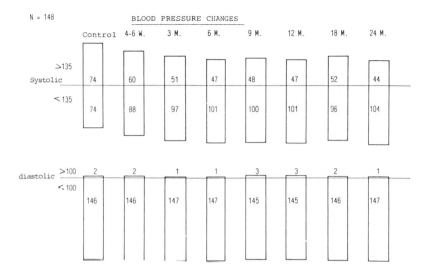

Fig. 10. Blood pressure before and during continuous oestriol succinate treatment as above.

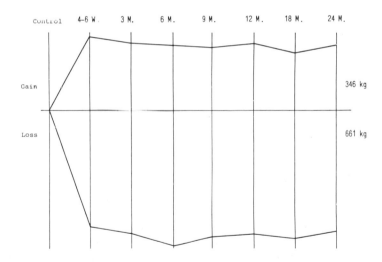

Fig. 11. Weight changes before and during continuous oestriol succinate treatment as above (N = 148).

There were also apparent changes in body weight during the course of the study (Fig. 11). Increments account for a total of 346 kg in all patients, whereas the decrements amount to 661 kg. Thus, of all weight changes observed, about two-thirds (65.6%) represent a weight-loss, whereas only one-third (34.4%) represent a weight-gain, both of which stay fairly constant from 4–6 weeks up to 24 months of treatment.

BREAKTHROUGH BLEEDING

Vaginal bleeding occurred in six patients after 4 to 6 weeks of treatment, whereas after continuation the frequency was extremely low; two patients at 6 months and 9 months; five patients at 12 and 18 months and only one patient after 24 months of treatment. The duration of these breakthough bleedings varied from 1 to 3 days. Thus, the incidence varies from 0.6 to 4%. In these patients, endometrial biopsies had been taken. There was no histological evidence for hyperplastic or neoplastic alterations.

CONCLUSIONS

According to questionnaires or a graphic rating scale system, oestrial succinate caused significant improvements in nine out of 12 severe or less severe symptoms. No elevation is systolic and diastolic blood pressure was seen. The relief of organic symptoms such as dysuria, high urinary frequency, vaginal dryness and headaches did not significantly improve libido. However, improved memory and decreased irritability in view of only a reasonable reduction of the frequency of hot flushes and sweating prove to be a satisfactory "mental tonic effect". Oestriol has been demonstrated to be an oestrogen capable of inducing metabolic responses in oestrogen-receptor containing target tissues, but not always producing identical effects to other oestrogenic substances.

In particular, oestriol appears to be associated with a reduction in potential adverse responses, notably on the endometrium and blood clotting factors. It does suffer from one major drawback, namely the minimal effect on bone. The main place for oestriol therapy after menopause would appear to be the patient who requires exogenous oestrogens, but is considered "high risk" by virtue of the well known absolute or relative contraindications such as obesity, reduced glucose tolerance, hypertension, latent hypothyroidism, nulliparity or other reproductive insufficiency. Thus, oestriol has the potential for reduced risk, but a similar benefit to alternating oestrogen or oestrogen–progestagen combinations, especially with respect to long-term therapy.

ACKNOWLEDGEMENT

I would like to thank W. Schröder, Ph.D., of Nourypharma, Munich, FRG, for running the computerized data collection from the multicentre protocols.

REFERENCES

Bergink, E. W. (1979). Seminar on Current Views on Estriol. Oss, Holland, 28th–30th September, 1979. *Acta Endocrinologia (Kbh.)* (in press).
Campbell, S. and Whitehead, M. (1977). *In* "The Menopause" (R. B. Greenblatt and J. Studd, Eds) Clinics in Obstetrics and Gynecology, 31–47. W. B. Saunders Ltd., London, Philadelphia, Toronto.

Hunter, D. J. S., Akande, E. O., Carr, P. and Stallworthy, J. (1973). *Journal of Obstetrics and Gynaecology of the British Commonwealth* **80**, 827.

Lader, M. H. and Wing, L. (1966). Institute of Psychiatry. Maudsley Monographs. Oxford University Press, Oxford.

Utian, W. H. (1972). *South African Medical Journal* **46**, 1079.

Von Eiff, A. W. (1975). *In* "Frontiers in Hormone Research: Estrogens in the Post-Menopause" (P. A. Van Keep and C. Lauritzen Eds), 177–181. S. Karger, Basel.

CREAM CONTAINING OESTRIOL FOR THE TREATMENT OF MENOPAUSAL VAGINAL ATROPHY

W. H. M. van der Velden[1], R. Trevoux[2] and D. Popović[3]

Department of Gynaecology and Obstetrics, St. Joseph Hospital, Eindhoven, The Netherlands[1], Rue de l'Assomption 31, Paris XVI[e], France[2]; and Department of Gynaecology and Obstetrics, Clinical Centre Dedinje, Belgrade, Yugoslavia[3]

INTRODUCTION

The gradual thinning of the vaginal mucosa in menopausal women is the result of long-standing oestrogen deficiency and in many cases leads to a syndrome consisting of vaginal soreness, dryness, irritation, dyspareunia, itching and susceptibility to infection. Local application of oestrogen-containing preparations has been used with success to treat this syndrome. The most frequently used local preparation contains conjugated equine oestrogens, the principal component being oestrone sulphate. However, the latter has been shown to be readily absorbed from the vagina, leading to high circulating levels of oestrone and oestradiol which in turn produce endometrial proliferation and even glandular cystic hyperplasia (Widholm and Vartiainen, 1974; Englund and Johansson, 1978; Whitehead *et al.*, 1978; Luisi *et al.*, 1980). However, the weak oestrogen oestriol was first shown by Gitsch and Golob as early as 1962 to be an efficient means of treating vaginal atrophy and related complaints, but no attention was paid to this finding until the recent work of Lauritzen (1979). This investigation showed that 1 mg/day of oestriol indeed cures patients suffering from vulvo-vaginal atrophy and related complaints without stimulating the endometrium.

Serono Symposium No. 39, "The Menopause: Clinical, Endocrinological and Pathophysiological Aspects", edited by P. Fioretti, L. Martini, G. B. Melis and S. S. C. Yen, 1982. Academic Press, London and New York.

In the present study the effect of daily intravaginal application of oestriol cream (Ovestin Cream®)* was investigated in a large number of menopausal or ovariectomized patients.

MATERIALS AND METHODS

Sixty patients, 36-70 years old, were divided into two groups. One group (26 patients) received 1 mg/day of oestriol for 3 weeks. The second group (34 patients) received 0.5 mg/day of oestriol for 3 weeks. Eleven of these patients applied a maintenance dose of 0.5 mg of oestriol twice a week during weeks 4-16. A calibrated plastic applicator was used to apply the cream before retiring.

The parameters studied were: clinical and colposcopic findings, vaginal smears (Maturation Index—MI, and Maturation Value—MV), cervical mucus (ferning and spinnbarkeit), and endometrial biopsies.

Vaginal smears were stained according to the Papanicolau method; ferning was scored as 0, 1, 2 or 3; spinnbarkeit was measured immediately in cm; endometrial biopsies were evaluated by routine histological methods.

RESULTS

1 mg/day of oestriol

The effect of 1 mg/day of oestriol on the MI and MV, ferning and spinnbarkeit, is shown in Table I. There was a pronounced effect on the MI/MV and a slight to moderate effect of ferning and spinnbarkeit.

Table I.   Mean values of the Maturation Index (MI), Maturation Value (MV), Ferning (F) and Spinnbarkeit (S) in patients treated with 1 mg/day of oestriol.

| | Pretreatment | | | | | | At 3 weeks | | | | | |
| | MI | | | MV | F | S | MI | | | MV | F | S |
	PC	IC	SC				PC	IC	SC			
x̄	18.2	80.0	1.8	41.8	0	0.45	0	44.1	55.9	77.9	1.42	1.71
N		26		26	12	12		26		26	12	12

PC = parabasal cells; IC = intermediate cells; SC = superficial cells; MV = PC × 0 + IC × 0.5 + SC × 1.

Endometrial biopsies obtained at pretreatment and after 3 weeks of treatment from 15 patients were atrophic in all cases. Clinical and colposcopic examinations showed the therapy to have had a beneficial effect in all 26 patients. Symptoms like dryness, irritation and/or itching were cured and vaginal mucosa had a normal

*Ovestin Cream®, Organon International B. V., Oss, The Netherlands.

appearance. In view of such an excellent effect seen at 1 mg/day, it was decided to investigate a dose of 0.5 mg/day of oestriol. It can be seen from Table II that the effect on the MI/MV was similar to that obtained with the 1 mg dose. Furthermore, the maintenance effect was achieved with a dose of 0.5 mg twice weekly. Similarly, Table III shows that the effect on ferning and spinnbarkeit was slight to moderate.

Table II. Mean values of the Maturation Index (MI) and Maturation Value (MV) in patients treated with 0.5 mg/day of oestriol

	MI			MV	N
	PC	IC	SC		
Pretreatment	17.1	81.2	1.7	42.2	34
Week 3	0	42.9	57.1	78.2	34
Week 5	0	56.0	44.0	72.0	11
Week 8	0	53.8	46.2	73.1	10
Week 12	0	52.9	47.1	73.6	8
Week 16	0	53.2	46.8	73.4	11

Endometrial biopsies obtained at pretreatment and after 3 weeks of treatment from 11 patients were atrophic in all cases. Clinical and colposcopic examinations showed the effects of this dose to be equal to those of 1 mg/day of oestriol. A complete normalization of the appearance of vaginal mucosa was seen in all 34 patients. Regarding clinical effects, a particular improvement in difficulties related to sexual intercourse was reported by the majority of the patients.

Tolerance was good in all 60 patients. However, one patient from each dose group experienced slight transitory breast tenderness. No other side-effects were reported and patients commented favourably on the treatment.

Table III. Mean values of Ferning and Spinnbarkeit in patients treated with 0.5 mg/day of oestriol.

	Ferning	Spinnbarkeit	N
Pretreatment	0	0.9	20
Week 3	1.3	2.6	20
Week 5	0.9	1.7	11
Week 8	0.9	1.6	10
Week 12	0.9	1.6	8
Week 16	0.9	1.7	11

CONCLUSIONS

Oestriol Cream has a significant clinical effect on postmenopausal vaginal atrophy and related complaints at a daily dose of 0.5 mg. A twice weekly maintenance dose of 0.5 mg of oestriol is sufficient to maintain the initial beneficial effect. The therapy does not induce endometrial proliferation.

REFERENCES

Englund, D. E. and Johansson, E. D. B. (1978). *British Journal of Obstetrics and Gynaecology* **85**, 957.

Gitsch, E. and Golob, E. (1962). *Zentralblatt für Gynäkologie* **12**, 454.

Lauritzen, C. (1979). *Therapie der Gegenwart* **118**, 567.

Luisi, M., Franchi, F. and Kicovic, P. M. (1980). *In* "International Symposium on the Menopause: Clinical, Endocrinological and Pathophysiological Aspects", p. 90. Viareggio, Abstract Book.

Whitehead, M. I., Minardi, I., Kitchin, Y. and Sharples, M. J. (1978). *In* "The Role of Estrogen/Progestagen in the Management of the Menopause" (I. D. Cooke, Ed.) pp. 63–75. MTP Press Ltd., Lancaster.

Widholm, O. and Vartiainen, E. (1974). *Annales Chirurgiae et Gynaecologiae Fenniae* **63**, 186.

OESTRIOL AND THE MENOPAUSE: CLINICAL AND ENDOCRINOLOGICAL RESULTS OF VAGINAL ADMINISTRATION

A. R. Genazzani[1], P. Inaudi[1], R. La Rosa[2], V. De Leo[2], M. G. Ricci-Danero[2]
S. Danero[1] and P. M. Kicovic[3]

Cattedra di Patologia Ostetrica e Ginecologica, Università degli studi di Cagliari, Cagliari, Italy[1];
Clinica Ostetrica e Ginecologica, Università degli studi di Siena, Siena Italy[2]; and
Reproductive Medicine Programme, Medical Unit, Organon, Oss, The Netherlands[3]

INTRODUCTION

One of the major complaints in postmenopausal women is that of vaginal atrophy as a consequence of the reduction in endogenous oestrogen production (Jaffe, 1978). Vaginal atrophy is the principal cause of dispareunia occurring in this age group, and which may have negative effects on mood and behaviour due to the consequent impairment of sexual activity. The treatment used up to the present time for this condition has been the oral or intravaginal administration of oestrogens (Lauritzen and Van Keep, 1978).

However, several clinical observations have shown that oestradiol (E_2) or oestrone (E_1) normally used for this purpose not only stimulate the proliferation of the vaginal cells, but also that of the endometrial cells (Whitehead *et al.*, 1978). Oestriol (E_3) seems to be the safer oestrogen on the basis of its weak biological activity (Huggins and Jensen, 1955; Miller, 1969; Myhre, 1978). Recently it has been shown (Schiff *et al.*, 1978) that the route of E_3 administration may interfere in its biological potency and it has been shown that "rapid conjugation of the

Serono Symposium No. 39, "The Menopause: Clinical, Endocrinological and Pathophysiological Aspects", edited by P. Fioretti, L. Martini, G. B. Melis and S. S. C. Yen, 1982. Academic Press, London and New York.

orally administered E_3 renders it a weakly potent oestrogen". On the contrary, "E_3 administered vaginally is conjugated less rapidly than orally administered E_3, thus rendering it more biologically potent" (Schiff *et al.*, 1978).

On the basis of these considerations, we have studied the effect of intravaginal administration of 0.5 mg E_3 daily for 3 weeks on the circulating free and conjugated E_3 and E_2, LH, FSH, prolactin (PRL), cortisol and dehydroepiandrosterone sulphate (DHAS) concentrations and on the vaginal cellularity, comparing two pharmacological forms of E_3: the vaginal cream and the vaginal suppository.

MATERIAL AND METHODS

In the present study, 14 healthy females aged from 49 to 76 years, all of whom had undergone spontaneous menopause (menopausal age ranging from 2 to 26 years), were studied together with four patients (43–48 years) who had undergone surgical castration for uterine fibroids or ovarian cyst (menopausal age ranging from 2 to 10 years). All patients were suffering from vaginal atrophy, and none had received previous oestrogen treatment. The subjects were randomly subdivided into three groups and were treated with 0.5 mg E_3 vaginal cream (Ovestin cream, Organon, Oss, Holland) (six subjects), or 1 mg E_3 vaginal cream (five cases), or 0.5 mg E_3 ovule (Ovestin vaginal suppository, Organon, Oss, Holland) (seven cases) daily for 3 weeks. Basal blood samples and vaginal smears were taken prior to treatment, and were repeated after the second and third week of treatment in the two groups of patients receiving 0.5 mg E_3.

Basal blood samples were also collected in these last two groups of subjects, 0.5, 1, 2, 4 and 8 h after the first medication. LH, FSH, PRL, cortisol, DHAS, free and conjugated E_2 and E_3 were determined in each blood sample. Vaginal smears were stained according to Papanicolau and the results were expressed as percentage of basal–parabasal, intermediate and superficial cells. Absence or presence of vaginal infections was also observed. LH, FSH and PRL were measured using Biodata kits (Rome, Italy), cortisol using CEA-IRE-SORIN kits (Saluggia, Vercelli, Italy), DHAS was measured directly in the plasma by radioimmunoassay (RIA) using the antibody purchased from Dr G. Abraham (Rolling Hills, Ca, USA), tritiated molecules from NEN (Boston, Mass, USA) and purified standard hormones from Merck (Darmstadt, Germany).

To evaluate free and conjugated E_2 and E_3 plasma levels, the samples (1.5 ml) were extracted with diethylether (15 ml) to remove the unconjugated form. After extraction, the residual plasma was submitted to enzymatic hydrolysis (overnight at 37°C) using β-glucuronidase (5000 IU) isolated from Elix-Pomatia and the recovered free E_2 and E_3 were then extracted and assayed by RIA. The highly specific antibodies were from CEA-IRE-SORIN, tritiated hormones from NEN and purified standard hormones from Vister (Milan, Italy). The steroid RIAs were characterized by overnight incubation at 4°C and dextran-coated charcoal separation. Statistical analysis was performed using the paired *t*-test.

RESULTS

Basal Hormone Levels and Cytological Picture

Basal hormone levels, evaluated in the two groups of subjects treated with 0.5 mg E_3 intravaginally, showed no significant differences between the two groups in any of the indices measured (Table I). The range of free E_3 was 3.9–21.7 pg/ml, while conjugated E_3 ranged from 66.0–152.0 pg/ml. Free E_2 ranged from 15.2–63.5 and conjugated E_2 from 145.0–284.0 pg/ml, in the same subjects.

Table I. Basal hormone and cytological data of the subject treated with 0.5 mg oestriol/day.

	Cream	Suppository
Hormones	Mean ± SE	Mean ± SE
E_3 F	8.5 ± 2.7	6.6 ± 0.75
E_3 C	104.8 ± 11.6	108.0 ± 14.0
E_2 F	28.4 ± 5.3	28.5 ± 6.0
E_2 C	249.0 ± 9.3	194.0 ± 15.6
FSH	76.9 ± 13.7	54.7 ± 19.4
LH	109.1 ± 18.9	70.2 ± 23.4
PRL	10.5 ± 0.7	11.5 ± 0.8
DHAS	1.55 ± 0.12	1.62 ± 0.25
Cortisol	110.0 ± 8.4	118.6 ± 5.0
Vaginal cytology	Mean ± SD	Mean ± SD
Basal–parabasal	59.2 ± 23.8	25.7 ± 19.8
Intermediate	39.2 ± 22.8	70.4 ± 19.3
Superficial	1.4 ± 3.7	3.2 ± 3.6

Vaginal cytology showed a high incidence of basal–parabasal and intermediate cells (Table I) with very few superficial cells. Several subjects showed evidence of vaginal infections (Fig. 1).

Effect of Acute Administration of 0.5 mg Intravaginal E_3

The intravaginal administration of 0.5 mg E_3 in the form of either a cream or suppository, was followed 30 min later by a significant increase in free and conjugated E_3 (Fig. 2). The highest concentration of free E_3 was reached after 1 h, and remained more or less constant until the 4th hour, later declining to lower levels.

The conjugated form of plasma E_3 (Fig. 2) showed a similar pattern, and highest values were observed after treatment with vaginal cream. No changes were found in free or conjugated E_2 plasma levels (Fig. 3) in either group of subjects.

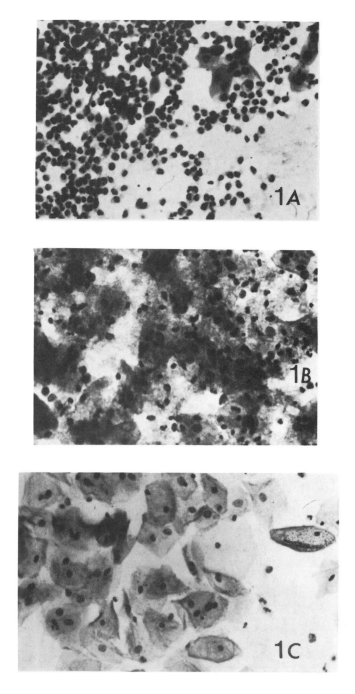

Fig. 1. Vaginal smears in two patients (1, this page; 2, facing page) before treatment (1A, 2A) after 14 (1B, 2B) and 21 days (1C, 2C) of 0.5 mg intravaginal oestriol (E$_3$) treatment.

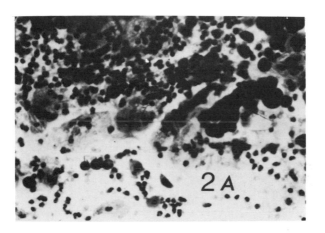

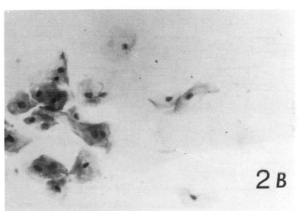

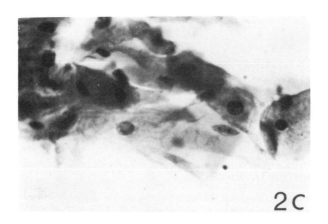

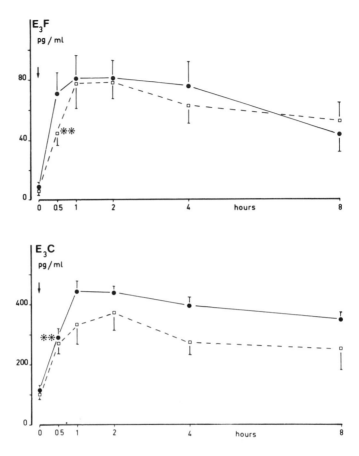

Fig. 2. Mean (± SE) plasma levels of free (E_3F) and conjugated oestriol (E_3C) after 0.5 mg intravaginal E_3 treatment (↓) as cream (solid line) or suppository (dotted line) (** $P < 0.01$).

Mean LH and FSH plasma levels showed a decrease which, in the subjects treated with vaginal cream, ranged between 30 and 78% (LH) and 3.4 and 65.6% (FSH) of the baseline values; in the subjects treated with vaginal suppositories, this decrease ranged between 3.3 and 59% (LH) and between 2.1 and 44% (FSH). Only the LH levels determined 4 h after application of the vaginal cream were found to be significantly lower than the basal values (Fig. 4).

Effect of Long-term Treatment

The long-term intravaginal administration of 0.5 mg E_3 (3 weeks), in the form of either a cream or suppository, was accompanied by a significant increase in plasma E_3 levels (Fig. 5), while no significant changes were observed in free and conjugated E_2 concentrations (Fig. 5).

The LH levels (Fig. 5) declined during treatment, but this decrease was not

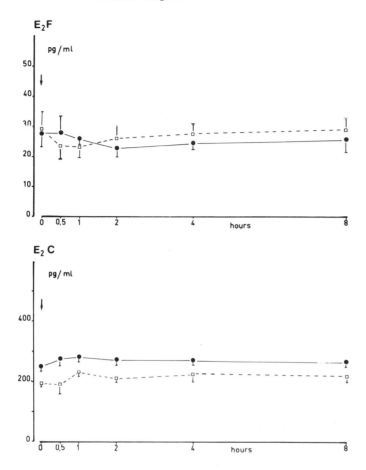

Fig. 3. Mean (± SE) plasma levels of free (E_2F) and conjugated oestradiol (E_2C) after 0.5 mg intravaginal E_3 treatment (↓) as cream (solid line) or suppository (dotted line).

significant in view of the wide range of basal levels in each individual case. A similar trend was also observed in the FSH plasma levels (Fig. 5). No significant variations were observed in basal concentrations of cortisol, DHAS or PRL after 2 to 3 weeks of daily treatment with 0.5 mg E_3 (Fig. 6).

Vaginal Cytological Changes during E_3 Administration

Figure 7 (A and B) reports changes in basal–parabasal (open bars), intermediate (dotted bars) and superficial cells (pointed bars) observed after 2 and 3 weeks of daily treatment with 0.5 mg E_3 as cream or suppository.

The basal–parabasal cells are markedly reduced after 2 weeks and disappear after 21 days of treatment. On the other hand, the superficial cells increase progressively and significantly to reach 34.3 ± 10.9 and 24.3 ± 5.9% after 21 days of E_3 suppository or cream treatment respectively.

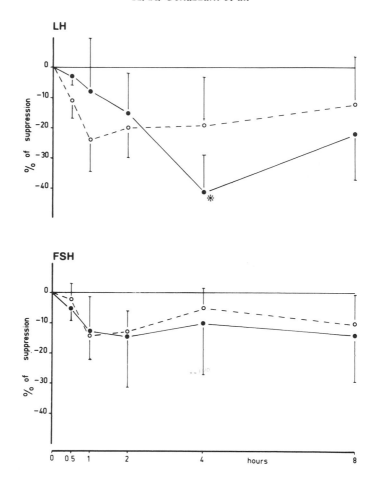

Fig. 4. Mean (± SE) percentage variation of LH and FSH plasma levels after 0.5 mg intra-vaginal E_3 treatment as cream (solid line) or suppository (dotted line). Mean basal values are reported in Table I (* $P < 0.05$).

The daily administration of 1 mg E_3 cream (Fig. 7 C) is accompanied by a more marked stimulation of vaginal cell proliferation, as shown by the presence of 44.0 ± 25% and 78 ± 13% superficial cells after 2 and 3 weeks, respectively.

Clinical Evaluation

All subjects reported a marked improvement in vaginal dryness and irritation after 5 to 10 days of therapy; moreover, dispareunia disappeared in five out of five subjects. Vaginal infections which were present in eight cases, disappeared without any other treatment (Fig. 1).

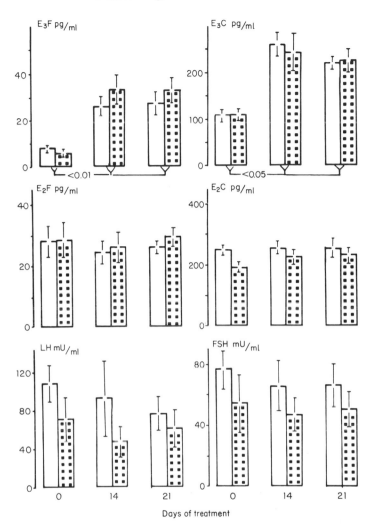

Fig. 5. Mean (± SE) basal plasma levels of free (E_3F) and conjugated oestriol (E_3C), free (E_2F) and conjugated oestradiol (E_2C), LH and FSH before treatment (day 0) and at the 14th and 21st day of 0.5 mg intravaginal E_3 treatment as cream (open bars) or suppository (pointed bars).

DISCUSSION

The present data clearly indicate that E_3 is equally active when administered, by vaginal route, either as a cream or suppository. E_3 is very rapidly absorbed in both forms, and free E_3 levels increase after 30 min from 6.6 ± 0.75 to 44.9 ± 8.7 pg/ml (suppository form) and from 8.5 ± 2.7 to 71.0 ± 14.0 pg/ml (cream form).

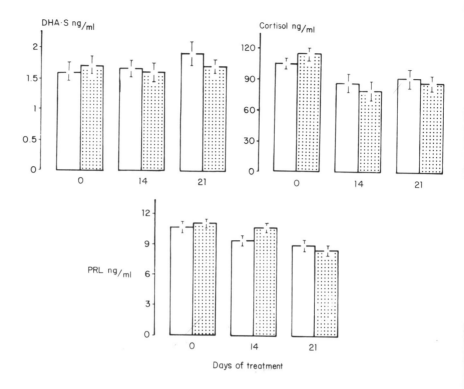

Fig. 6. Mean (± SE) basal plasma levels of dehydroepiandrosterone sulphate (DHAS) cortisol and prolactin (PRL), before treatment (day 0) and at the 14th and 21st day of 0.5 mg intravaginal E_3 treatment as cream (open bars) or suppository (pointed bars).

Moreover, free E_3 levels remain significantly elevated in both cases until 8 h after administration (53.1 ± 11.8 as suppository and 43.9 ± 10.5 as cream). A similar trend was also evident in the case of conjugated E_3, and plasma levels rose in the two groups of patients after 2 h, from 109.6 ± 10.3 to 372.2 ± 5.3 pg/ml (suppository) and from 108.0 ± 13.1 to 436.0 ± 14.6 pg/ml (cream form). The increases found in both free and conjugated E_3 are in agreement with those previously reported by Schiff *et al.* (1978) using a similar dose of E_3 dissolved in 2 ml of saline and administered vaginally. The weak activity of the oestrogen molecule on the central control of gonadotropin secretion is demonstrated by the slight decrease in LH observed when studying either the acute effect or when monitoring long-term treatment, and corresponds to the results of Schiff *et al.* (1978).

Four out of six cases treated with vaginal cream, and five out of seven subjects treated with suppositories, showed an LH decrease after 3 weeks which ranged from 14 to 88%. The biological activity of the medication on vaginal cells was clearly evident after a few days (Fig. 7), and the activation of cell proliferation was also accompanied by a clear improvement in vaginal infections when present (Fig. 1).

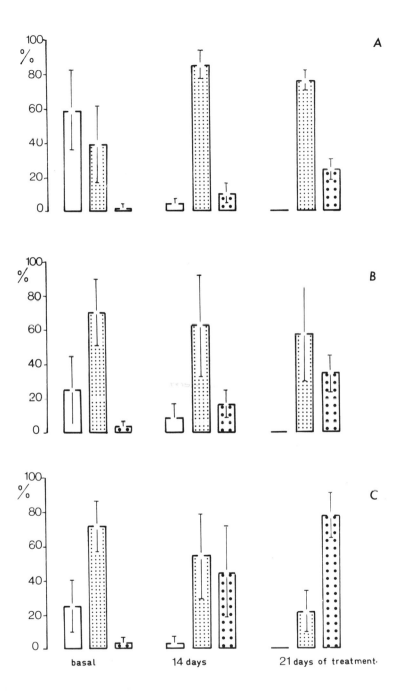

Fig. 7. Mean percentage (± SD) of basal–parabasal (open bars) intermediate (dotted bars) and superficial (pointed bars) cells, in basal condition (day 0) and after 14 and 21 days of 0.5 mg intravaginal E_3 cream (A) or suppository (B) or 1 mg E_3 cream (C) treatment.

These changes in vaginal cellularity are probably the cause of the disappearance of dispareunia and the improvement in sexual activity reported by the sexually active patients. The present data also indicate that steroid secretion by the adrenal glands is not affected by this oestrogen medication. It is also reconfirmed, interestingly, that E_3 administration is not accompanied by any change in conjugated or free E_2 plasma concentrations.

In conclusion, the present study confirms the clinical and biological validity of the intravaginal administration of E_3 at the very low dose of 0.5 mg daily; it also shows evidence that this treatment does not interfere in the secretion of adrenal steroids or PRL, while plasma gonadotropins appear to be slightly reduced by treatment in the majority of cases. These observations lead to the conclusion that when vaginal atrophy is the major complaint in a menopausal subject, the intravaginal administration of small doses of E_3 may be recommended as the safer treatment at the present time.

ACKNOWLEDGEMENTS

This research was partially supported by the CNA project "Biology of Reproduction".

REFERENCES

Huggins, C. and Jensen, E. V. (1955). *Journal of Experimental Medicine* **102**, 335-346.

Jaffe, R. B. (1978). *In* "Reproductive Endocrinology" (S. S. C. Yen and R. B. Jaffe, Eds), pp. 261-270. W. B. Saunders Company, Philadelphia, USA.

Lauritzen, C. and Van Keep, P. A. (1978). "Frontiers of Hormone Research— Estrogen Therapy". S. Karger, Basel.

Miller, B. G. (1969). *Journal of Endocrinology* **43**, 563-570.

Myhre, E. (1978). *In* "Frontiers of hormone research" (C. Lauritzen and P. A. Van Keep, Eds), pp. 126-144. S. Karger, Basel.

Schiff, I., Wentworth, B., Koos, B., Ryan, K. J. and Tulchinsky, D. (1978). *Fertility and Sterility* **30**, 278-282.

Whitehead, M. I., Minardi, J., Kitchin, Y. and Sharples, M. J. (1978). *In* "The role of Estrogen/Progestogen in the management of the menopause" (I. O. Cook, Ed.), pp. 63-70. MTP Press Ltd, Lancaster.

HORMONE REPLACEMENT THERAPY IN POSTMENOPAUSAL WOMEN WITH OESTROGEN, PERIODICALLY SUPPLEMENTED WITH CLOMIPHENE CITRATE

A. Kauppila, O. Jänne, S. Kivinen, E. Kokko, T. Lantto, R. Tuimala
and R. Vihko

*Departments of Obstetrics and Gynecology, Biochemistry and Clinical Chemistry
University of Oulu, Oulu, Finland*

INTRODUCTION

Postmenopausal hormone replacement therapy with oestrogen alone increases the incidence of endometrial hyperplasia (Thom *et al.*, 1979) and the risk of endometrial carcinoma (for review, see Jick *et al.*, 1979). Prevention of these side-effects by cyclic administration of progestin may be successful (Hammond *et al.*, 1979; Thom *et al.*, 1979) but may also fail (Jick *et al.*, 1979; Rosenwaks *et al.*, 1979), and is commonly complicated by uterine bleeding (Lind *et al.*, 1979). Many clinical and experimental studies suggest that non-steroidal anti-oestrogens, e.g. clomiphene citrate (CC), effectively inhibit and reverse the stimulatory action of oestrogen on the endometrium (Jordan *et al.*, 1978). Therefore, this study was designed to explore the clinical, endocrine, metabolic and endometrial effects of postmenopausal hormone replacement therapy with oestrogen periodically supplemented with CC.

Serono Symposium No. 39, "The Menopause: Clinical, Endocrinological and Pathophysiological Aspects", edited by P. Fioretti, L. Martini, G. B. Melis and S. S. C. Yen, 1982. Academic Press, London and New York.

PATIENTS AND METHODS

Twenty-five postmenopausal women participated in this investigation. Three of them had previously undergone an abdominal hysterectomy with bilateral salpingo-oophorectomy.

The study was initiated by clinical examination and cytological screening of vaginal smear and endometrial aspiration sample. The hormonal therapy consisted of daily administration of 1.25 mg of conjugated oestrogen (oestrogen sulphate 84%, oestradiol sulphate 2%, equilin sulphate 14%) for 6 months. This treatment was supplemented three times with daily ingestion of 50 mg of CC for 10 days at 7 week intervals. Fifteen patients used CC alone, whereas 10 patients continued oestrogen administration during the supplementation with CC.

The Kupperman index (1964) was used in the estimation of the severity of the climacteric symptoms before and during the trial. Endometrial histology, and concentrations of cytosol oestrogen and progestin receptors (for methods, see Jänne *et al*., 1979) were determined from samples taken by strict *curettage* at the end of the first oestrogen treatment and then after the first and third CC supplementation periods. On these occasions, as well as before the start of the trial, venous blood samples were taken for determination of serum concentrations of LH, FSH, prolactin, oestradiol, progesterone, testosterone, cholesterol, HDL-cholesterol, triglycerides, free fatty acids, glucose, insulin, albumin, transferrin, ferritin, phospholipids, creatinine, aminotransferases, alkaline phosphatase, γ-glutamyltranspeptidase, sodium, potassium, calcium and iron. Student's *t*-test and paired *t*-test were employed in the statistical analysis of the results.

RESULTS

The Kupperman index showed a significant improvement in the climacteric symptoms during all phases of the study (Fig. 1). The alleviation was good in 22 women and minor in the other three women. There was a slight worsening of the symptoms during CC treatment periods, especially if CC was administered together with oestrogen. Uterine bleeding occurred five times during oestrogen treatment periods, but never during or immediately after CC supplementations. Bodyweight or blood pressure of the subjects did not change during the trial.

All findings in vaginal and endometrial cytological samples prior to the trial were normal. Endometrial stimulation (proliferation or hyperplasia) was evident at the end of the initial oestrogen treatment period in 59% of the samples, and after the first and third CC supplementations in 23% and 27%, respectively (Fig. 2).

Oestrogen receptor concentrations in endometrial cytosol after the first and third CC supplementations were significantly lower than at the end of the initial oestrogen treatment (Fig. 3). The progestin receptor concentration in endometrial cytosol after the first CC treatment was also significantly lower than at the end of the preceding oestrogen period, whereas the concentration of progestin receptor after the third CC supplementation was again increased and close to that after the first oestrogen period (Fig. 3).

The serum concentration of FSH significantly decreased from the pretreatment

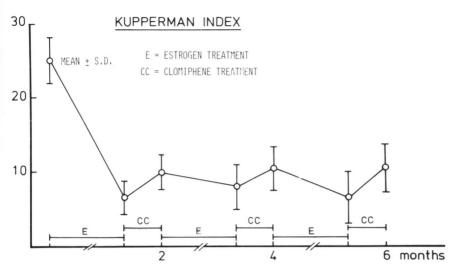

Fig. 1. Mean (± SD) values of Kupperman indices before and during each phase of the trial.

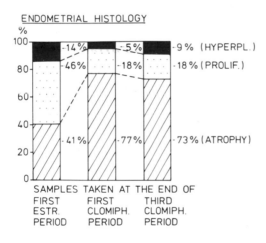

Fig. 2. Findings in histological examination of the endometrial samples.

level during oestrogen and CC treatment periods (Table I). LH and other hormones studied did not change during the investigation. The serum concentration of free fatty acids significantly increased during oestrogen and CC treatments, whereas the serum concentration of triglycerides after the first CC supplementation was lower than the pretreatment level in women receiving CC together with oestrogen (Table I). The other laboratory parameters studied did not change during the treatments with oestrogen alone or CC alone or CC in combination with oestrogen.

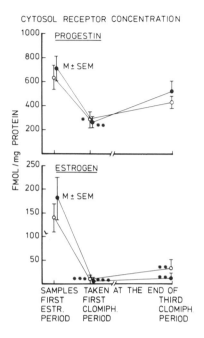

Fig. 3. Mean (± SEM) concentrations of cytosol progestin and oestrogen receptors in endometrial samples. Statistical comparison is made with the values received after the first oestrogen period. ●– –● Clomiphene citrate (clomiph.) alone; ○–○ Clomiph. with estrogen. * = P < 0.05; ** = P < 0.01; *** = P < 0.001.

Table I. Mean (± SD) values of FSH, triglycerides, and free fatty acids (FFA) before and during the hormone replacement therapy with conjugated oestrogen and clomiphene. Other laboratory parameters did not change (data not shown).

		Before treatment	After first oestrogen period	After first clomiphene period	After third clomiphene period
FSH	A(15)[c]	101.1 ± 34.3	62.4 ± 28.3[b]	75.5 ± 34.8[a]	66.9 ± 16.0[b]
IU/l	B(10)	100.1 ± 47.1	77.3 ± 48.4	44.8 ± 38.8[b]	60.2 ± 27.4[a]
Triglycerides	A(15)	1.0 ± 0.3	1.1 ± 0.4	1.1 ± 0.5	1.2 ± 0.5
mmol/l	B(10)	1.5 ± 0.5	1.3 ± 0.6	0.9 ± 0.2[a]	1.1 ± 0.6
FFA	A(15)	0.4 ± 0.2	0.6 ± 0.4[a]	0.6 ± 0.5	0.6 ± 0.2[a]
mmol/l	B(10)	0.3 + 0.1	0.5 ± 0.2[a]	0.5 ± 0.2[b]	0.5 ± 0.2[a]

A = Group of patients without oestrogens during clomiphene administration; B = Group of patients with oestrogens during clomiphene administration; [a] P < 0.05; [b] P < 0.01; comparison is made with the pretreatment values; [c] the number of patients studied, is in parenthesis.

DISCUSSION

In the present new treatment regimen, oestrogen therapy was periodically interrupted or supplemented with a non-steroidal and anti-oestrogen, clomiphene citrate. Previous studies have shown that anti-oestrogens compete with oestrogens for binding to the cytosol oestrogen receptor, and that this antioestrogen-receptor complex is translocated to the nucleus, where it is retained for a prolonged period of time (Clark *et al.*, 1973; Katzenellenbogen and Ferguson, 1975; Ruh and Baudendistel, 1977; Katzenellenbogen *et al.*, 1978). The prolonged nuclear retention of the anti-oestrogen-receptor complex abolishes the reappearance of cytosol oestrogen receptors, and thereby renders the endometrium less responsive to the action of oestrogen.

The relief of the climacteric symptoms was good during the oestrogen treatment period. Reappearance of mild vasomotor symptoms during the supplementation with CC alone was well tolerated by all women. There were no episodes of bleeding during or immediately after the CC treatment periods, which is in marked contrast to the observations showing regular bleedings in about 80% of postmenopausal women on oestrogen therapy periodically supplemented with progestin (Lind *et al.*, 1979).

The findings in histological examination and determinations of cytosol oestrogen and progestin receptor concentrations demonstrated that the stimulatory action of oestrogen on the endometrium was at least partly suppressed by CC. For example, the frequency of hyperplasia (14%) in the endometrial samples after the initial oestrogen treatment period decreased to 9% at the end of the trial, and the frequency of atrophic endometrium increased from 41% to 73% during the same observation period.

The negative feedback effect of oestrogen on the hypothalamic-pituitary axis results in a decrease in the serum concentration of FSH, as is also evident in our study. This change without a simultaneous LH decrease has also been reported previously (Franchimont *et al.*, 1972; L'Hermite *et al.*, 1979). Clomiphene supplementation did not alter these effects of oestrogen on the pituitary gonadotrophins. The serum concentration of prolactin has either increased (Robyn and Vekemans, 1976) or remained unaltered (Lind *et al.*, 1978; L'Hermite *et al.*, 1979) during postmenopausal oestrogen therapy, the latter finding being confirmed in the present study. The changes recorded in the concentrations of free fatty acids and triglycerides were within the normal range of our laboratory. These minor changes in the peripheral concentrations of only a few of the above parameters suggest that this kind of treatment is not associated with any significant metabolic side-effects.

The employed treatment regimen alleviates climacteric symptoms, without pronounced endometrial stimulation. The endometrial histopathological and steroid hormone receptor changes indicate that CC, in the above dose, behaves as a pure anti-oestrogen and thus seems to provide an alternative to progestin for interruption of possible harmful oestrogenic effects. Because nuclear retention of the oestrogen receptor-anti-oestrogen complex may last as long as 19 days (Clark *et al.*, 1973), administration of CC more frequently and for shorter time periods is indicated to be explored in future.

ACKNOWLEDGEMENT

We thank Star Ltd, Tampere, Finland, for the supply of the drugs used in this study.

REFERENCES

Clark, J. A., Anderson, J. N. and Peck, E. J. Jr (1973). *Steroids* 22, 707.
Franchimont, P., Legros, J. J. and Meurice, J. (1972). *Hormone and Metabolic Research* 4, 288.
Hammond, C. B., Jelovsek, F. R., Lee, K. L., Creasman, W. T. and Parker, R. T. (1979). *American Journal of Obstetrics and Gynecology* 133, 537.
Jänne, O., Kauppila, A., Kontula, K., Syrjälä, P. and Vihko, R. (1979). *International Journal of Cancer* 24, 545.
Jick, H., Watkins, R. N., Hunter, J. R., Dinan, B. J., Madsen, S., Rothman, K. J. and Walker, A. M. (1979). *New England Journal of Medicine* 300, 218.
Jordan, V. C., MacDonald, R. R. and Prestwich, G. (1978). *In* "Endometrial Cancer" (M. G. Brush, R. J. B. King and R. W. Taylor, Eds), 323–340, Baillière and Tindall, London.
Katzenellenbogen, B. S. and Ferguson, E. R. (1975). *Endocrinology* 97, 1.
Katzenellenbogen, B. S., Katzenellenbogen, J. A., Ferguson, E. R. and Krauthammer, N. (1978). *Journal of Biology and Chemistry* 253, 697.
Kupperman, H. S., Wetchler, B. B. and Blatt, M. G. H. (1964). *Journal of American Medical Association* 171, 1627.
L'Hermite, M., Badawi, M. M., Michaux-Duchene, A. and Robyn, C. (1979). *Clinical Endocrinology* (Oxford) 11, 173.
Lind, T., Cameron, E. H. D. and Hunter, W. M. (1978). *British Journal of Obstetrics and Gynecology* 85, 138.
Lind, T., Cameron, E. C., Hunter, W. M., Leon, C., Moran, P. F., Oxley, A., Gerrard, J. and Lind, U. C. G. (1979). *British Journal of Obstetrics and Gynaecology* 86, suppl. 3.
Robyn, C. and Vekemans, M. (1976). *Acta Endocrinologica* 83, 9.
Rosenwaks, Z., Wentz, A. C., Jones, G. S., Urban, M. D., Lee, P. A., Migeon, C. J., Parmley, T. H. and Woodruff, J. D. (1979). *Obstetrics and Gynecology* 53, 493.
Ruh, T. S. and Baudendistel, L. J. (1977). *Endocrinology* 100, 420.
Thom, M. H., White, P. J. and Williams, R. M. (1979). *Lancet* II, 455.

MANAGEMENT OF LOWER GENITAL TRACT ATROPHY WITH A VAGINAL CREAM CONTAINING OESTRIOL

C. Babuna[1], M. F. Aksu[2] and R. Erez[3]

Department of Obstetrics and Gynaecology, Istanbul Faculty of Medicine, University of Istanbul, Istanbul, Turkey[1]
Department of Obstetrics and Gynaecology, Cerrahpasa Faculty of Medicine, University of Istanbul, Istanbul, Turkey[2]; and
Department of Psychiatry and Endocrinology, Cerrahpasa Faculty of Medicine, University of Istanbul, Istanbul, Turkey[3]

INTRODUCTION

After menopause, oestrogen deficiency leads to complaints of vaginal dryness, dyspareunia, irritation, itch and inflammation. Local application of oestrogen-containing creams, such as conjugated oestrogens (mostly oestrone sulphate) (Korte, 1973) and diethylstilbestrol (Widholm and Vertianen, 1974), has been successfully used in the management of these disorders. Nevertheless it has been reported that these oestrogens are absorbed from the vaginal mucosa in amounts sufficient to produce endometrial proliferation (Speert, 1948). Moreover, recent works have shown high circulating serum oestrogen concentrations (Schiff *et al.*, 1977; Rigg *et al.*, 1978) and high urinary excretion values (Widholm and Vertianen, 1974), after vaginal administration of the above mentioned oestrogens. On the other hand, more recently it has been demonstrated by Tzingounis *et al.* (1978), that oral oestriol fails to induce endometrial proliferation when 6 to 8 mg/day is administered to postmenopausal women. The alleged relationship between oestrogens and endometrial cancer stimulated further investigations on

Serono Symposium No. 39, "The Menopause: Clinical, Endocrinological and Pathophysiological Aspects", edited by P. Fioretti, L. Martini, G. B. Melis and S. S. C. Yen, 1982. Academic Press, London and New York.

oestriol treatment effects and justified its use in postmenopausal patients. The present preliminary study demonstrates the effectiveness and long-term safety of oestriol vaginal cream on postmenopausal atrophic colpitis.

MATERIALS AND METHODS

This study was performed on 28 postmenopausal or ovariectomized women, aged 33–85 (mean age 56), with vaginal atrophy, dyspareunia, vaginal dryness and other related symptoms. They were all free from any oestrogen treatment for at

Table I. Ferning.

Patient No.	Pretreatment	2 weeks	5 weeks	8 weeks	12 weeks	16 weeks
1	0	1	1	2	1	1
2	0	0	3	3	3	3
3	Hys.	—	—	—	—	—
4	0	2	3	3	2	2
5	0	1	1	1	1	2
6	0	1	1			
7	0	1	1			
8	0	1				
9	0	1	—	1	1	1
10	0	1	—	1	1	
11	0	3	2	2	2	2
12	Hys	—	—	—	—	—
13	0	1	—	2	2	2
14	0	2	2	2	2	2
15	—	—	—	—	—	—
16	0	2	2	3	2	2
17	0	1	1	2	2	2
18	0	2	2	2	2	2
19	0	2	2	—	2	2
20	0	1	1	1	1	
21	0	1	1	2	1	
22	Hys.	—	—	—	—	—
23	0	2	1	2		
24	0	1	2	2		
25	0	1	2	2	2	—
26	0	1	1			
27	0	1	1			
28	0	2	2			
Mean	0	1.29	1.6	1.9	1.68	1.9

Table II. Spinnbarkeit.

Patient No.	Pretreatment	2 weeks	5 weeks	8 weeks	12 weeks	16 weeks
1	0	3	4.5	6	6	5
2	0	0	11	9	9	9
3	–	–	–	–	–	–
4	0	4.5	5.5	6	6	5.5
5	0	2	3.5	5	5	4.5
6	0.5	1	1.5			
7	1	1.5	1.5			
8	0.5	1				
9	0.2	1	–	2	1.5	2
10	0.5	0.8	–	1.5	2	
11	0	5	5	5	6	6.5
12	–	–	–	–	–	–
13	0	6	–	6	6	6
14	0	4	6	6	6	6
15	–	–	–	–	–	–
16	0	5	5	6	6.5	6.5
17	0	4	4	5	6	6
18	0	6	6	5.5	6	6.5
19	0	5	5.5	–	6	6.5
20	0	2	1.5	1.5	2	
21	0	1.5	2	1	1.5	
22	–	–	2	–	–	
23	0	1.5	1.5	1.5		
24	0	1.5	1.5	2		
25	0	6	6	6.5	6.5	–
26	0	0.5	1			
27	0	1	1.5			
28	0.5	2	2			
Mean	0.1	2.7	3.7	4.4	5.1	5.8

least 1 year prior to the present administration of oestriol. Absence of malignancies was ascertained prior to treatment. A complete clinical examination was carried out in all cases.

Oestriol (0.5 mg) vaginal cream was applied daily over a 2 week period. Thereafter a maintenance dose of 0.5 mg oestriol twice a week was applied up to 5, 8, 12 and 16 weeks respectively in 10, 1, 2 and 15 subjects.

The effects of treatment on vaginal epithelium were assessed by means of Maturation Index (MI) and Value (MV) prior to and during treatment. The effects on cervical mucus were assessed by evaluation of ferning (crystallization denoted in terms of 0–3) and spinnbarkeit (measured in cm) in all cases who had not undergone hysterectomy. Endometrial biopsies were performed before and during treatment.

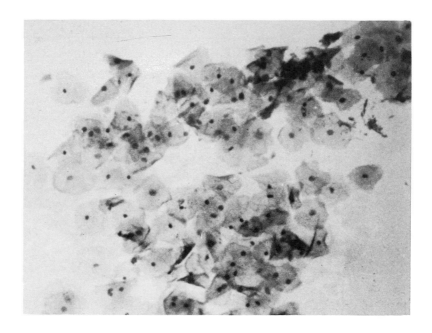

Fig. 1a. Vaginal smear before therapy.

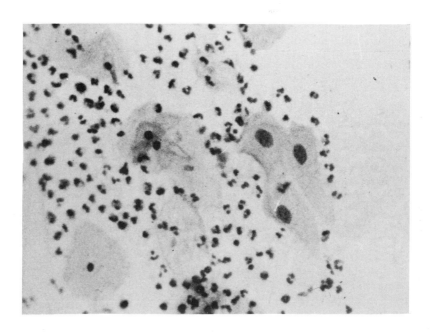

Fig. 1b. Vaginal smear after therapy.

RESULTS

Vaginal smears taken before treatment showed a severely atrophic picture, but after 2 weeks of daily treatment there was a very pronounced increase in superficial cells indicating a marked oestrogenic effect. This initial beneficial effect persisted during maintenance therapy. Mean values for ferning and spinnbarkeit indicated that the treatment had a moderate effect on the former and a marked effect on the latter (Tables I and II).

Colposcopic and clinical examinations showed that the treatment had a beneficial effect in all patients after 2 weeks, the improvement being maintained or increased during maintenance therapy (Fig. 1, a and b). In fact after 2 weeks, the vaginal mucosa was normal in 20 patients, almost normal in one patient and improved in seven patients. Nineteen out of 20 patients suffering from dyspareunia were cured after 2 weeks and the condition was improved in the remaining patient. All patients had a normal vaginal mucosa and were free from complaints after 5, 8, 12 or 16 weeks of maintenance therapy.

Table III. Endometrial biopsy

Patient No.	Pretreatment	2 weeks	5 weeks	8 weeks	12 weeks	16 weeks
1	Atrophic	Atrophic	—	Atrophic	—	Atrophic
2	Atrophic	Atrophic	—	Atrophic	—	Atrophic
4	Atrophic	—	Atrophic	--	Atrophic	Atrophic
5	Atrophic	Atrophic	Atrophic	...	—	Atrophic
6	—	—	—			
7	—	—	—			
8	—	—				
9	—	—	—	—	—	Atrophic
10	Atrophic	Atrophic	—	—	...	
11	Atrophic	—	—	—	—	Atrophic
13	Atrophic	—	—	Atrophic	—	Atrophic
14	Atrophic					Atrophic
16	Atrophic	—	—	Atrophic	—	Atrophic
17	Atrophic	—	—	—	—	Atrophic
18	Atrophic	—	—	Atrophic	—	Atrophic
19	Atrophic	—	Atrophic	—	Atrohpic	Atrophic
20						
21	—	—				
23	—					
24	—	—				
25	Atrophic	—	—	—	Atrophic	
26	Atrophic	—	Atrophic			
27	Atrophic	—	Atrophic			
28	Atrophic	—	Atrophic			

Endometrial biopsies were performed in 16 patients before and 16 weeks after treatment. All specimens showed atrophic endometrium (Table III). No side-effects were noted and tolerance was excellent.

CONCLUSION

Treatment with E_1 and E_2 or synthetic oestrogens may result in endometrial proliferation and abnormal uterine bleeding depending on the dose and mode of administration (Greenblatt *et al.*, 1979). Equine oestrogens and 17-β-oestradiol (stark-oestrogens) can easily be absorbed from vaginal mucosa and they induce endometrial hyperplasia (Schiff *et al.*, 1977).

On the contrary, intravaginally applied 0.5 mg oestriol, daily for 2 weeks, showed positive effects on vaginal atrophy, dyspareunia and vaginitis in post-menopausal women. A maintenance dose of 0.5 mg oestriol twice a week for 8, 12 or 16 weeks was sufficient to maintain or increase the initial effects of daily treatment without inducing endometrial proliferation.

ACKNOWLEDGEMENT

We acknowledge the kind help of Organon International BV., Medical Unit, in providing us with Ovestin Cream and in extending support for the study.

REFERENCES

Greenblatt, R. B., Bryner, J. R., Tzingounis, V. A. and Aksu, M. F. (1979). *In* "Endocrinology of the ovary" (R. Scholler, Ed.), p. 621–637. Editions Sepe, Paris.
Korte, W. (1973). *Fortsch. Med.* **91**, 921.
Rigg, L. A., Hermann, H. and Yen, S. S. C. (1978). *New England Journal of Medicine* **298**, 195.
Schiff, I., Tulchinskey, D. and Ryan, K. I. (1977). *Fertility and Sterility* **28**, 1063.
Speert, H. (1948). *Physiological Review* **28**, 23.
Tzingounis, V. A., Aksu, M. F. and Greenblatt, R. B. (1978). *Journal of the American Medical Association* **293**, 1638.
Widholm, O. and Vertianen, E. (1974). *Annales Chirurgiae et Gynaecologiae Fermiae* **63**, 186.

MEDROXYPROGESTERONE ACETATE IN THE TREATMENT
OF THE POSTMENOPAUSAL SYNDROME

J. Andor, E. Vögelin, P. Schneider and K. Tscherne

Women's Hospital, University of Basle, Switzerland;
1st Women's Hospital, University of Vienna, Austria; and
Women's Hospital, University of Graz, Austria

INTRODUCTION

Recently, the possible connections between oestrogen medication and endo-metrial cancer have been widely discussed everywhere. In short, we can summarize the research results and reports on clinical experience in hand as follows: in physio-logic situations, the proliferative effect of oestrogens is limited by progesterone; if oestrogens are unopposed or given continuously, persistent proliferation of glandular and stromal cells may lead to endometrial hyperplasia from which a malignant process could develop through increased dedifferentiation and selective proliferation of glandular elements; the unopposed continuous oestrogen medica-tion should be regarded as a risk factor for the development of an endometrial carcinoma.

There are relatively few reports on the combined oestrogen-gestagen treatment of postclimacteric complaints. The basic idea of the oestrogen–gestagen combina-tion is to take advantage of the anti-oestrogenic effect of the gestagen with simul-taneous atrophic effect on the endometrium. In other words, to inhibit the shortly discussed hyperproliferative effect of oestrogens. The combined oestrogen-gestagen treatment in cyclic fashion leads to monthly menstruation-like withdrawal bleedings. Our questioning of 100 women has shown that the maintenance of artificial menstruation until old age is neither desired nor welcomed by them. The majority of these women experience these artificial menstruations as unnatural and annoying.

Serono Symposium No. 39, "The Menopause: Clinical, Endocrinological and Pathophysio-logical Aspects", edited by P. Fioretti, L. Martini, G. B. Melis and S. S. C. Yen, 1982. Academic Press, London and New York.

Quite a number of patients with climacteric complaints, especially hot flushes, cannot be treated with oestrogens for different reasons, some of which are outlined below. Some experience contraindications, namely mammary carcinoma, endometrium carcinoma and uterus myomatosus. I have to class the thrombo-embolic diseases with the relative contraindications, either for the oestrogen only medication or for the combined oestrogen–gestagen medication. On the contrary, there is no evidence to date that this risk applies to medroxyprogesterone acetate, either in oral or in injectable form. In some patients, even low-dosage oestrogen produces intolerable side-effects, such as mastodynia, exacerbation of fibrocystic breast disease, breakthrough bleeding and nausea. In other patients exogenous oestrogen simply does not produce complete alleviation of hot flushes.

Clinical experience has shown that in women being treated with Provera for endometrial cancer, the hot flushes from which they suffered at the same time, disappeared completely or improved considerably (Bullock *et al.*, 1975). On the basis of these clinical observations medroxyprogesterone acetate was tried in the treatment of postmenopausal complaints. The objective of this study is to test the efficacy and clinical usefulness of Provera given alone, in the treatment of the postmenopausal syndrome.

METHOD

The patients for this clinical study were selected by the following criteria: patients having had their last spontaneous menstrual bleeding 6 months previously older than 45 years; no hormone medication for at least 6 months; and pronounced postmenopausal complaints, especially hot flushes. Criteria for exclusion were: mammary or endometrial carcinoma: serious liver function disturbances: any hormone medication.

The daily dose was 10 mg medroxyprogesterone acetate (Provera) per os, without interruption. Duration of the study was 4 months for each patient—3 months medication with medroxyprogesterone acetate followed by 1 month therapy break (control month).

Evaluation criteria were: vaginal cytology; hormone determination in the blood: E_2, LH, FSH and prolactin (RIA), liver function tests: SGOT, SGPT, alkaline phosphatosis behaviour of blood pressure; vaginal bleedings; recording of clinical picture, especially hot flushes and recording of side-effects.

Control checks were made before initiating the therapy, after 1 and 3 months of therapy and at the end of the medication-free month.

RESULTS AND CONCLUSIONS

At present we have 35 completed cases which correspond to 105 treatment months. We wish to report the preliminary findings obtained.

The average age of our patients was 57.2 years. Vaginal cytological examinations did not reveal any significant changes in the course of the treatment. The behaviour of the hormone parameters before, during and after gestagen treatment was as follows.

With regard to the hormone parameters, the E_2 and prolactin values did not show any changes. The FSH and LH concentrations decreased during the medication as result of the central inhibitory effect of medroxyprogesterone acetate, whereby the inhibitory effect of the LH was more pronounced (Table I).

Table I. Hormone assays.

	E_2 PG/ML	FSH mIU/ML	LH mIU/ML	Prolactin NG/ML
Before start of therapy	39.9	74.7	60.9	6.4
After 1 month	32.9	61.0	42.6[a]	6.2
After 3 months	37.7	67.9	40.2[a]	8.2
After 4 months control without medication	33.7	70.6	54.7	6.0

[a] $p < 0.001$ (Student's T-test).

The liver function was not impaired by the gestagen medication. Blood pressure remained practically unchanged during and after treatment.

Two of the 35 patients had had a hysterectomy. Of the remaining 33 women, which corresponds to 99 treatment months, one suffered from spotting which spontaneously disappeared. Thus, bleeding frequency under medroxyprogesterone acetate was 2.9%. Compared to this, according to various bibliographic data, the bleeding rate after cyclic oestrogen treatment lies between 10-30%.

Prior to the initiation of gestagen medication, 22 patients (62.8%) complained about severe, 11 patients (31.4%) about moderately severe and two women (5.2%) about light hot flushes.

After 3 months of Provera treatment, none of these women suffered any more from severe hot flushes, six (17%) still had moderately severe and 15 women (43%) only had slight hot flushes. Fourteen patients (40%) were symptom-free.

The following side effects were observed: weight gain (3 cases); dry vagina, pruritus (1 case); tiredness (1 case); gastric disorder (1 case); and headache (1 case).

Our preliminary results suggest that the uninterrupted oral medication of medroxyprogesterone acetate in daily doses of 10 mg results in a reliable alleviation or relief of postmenopausal hot flushes. The tolerance of the preparation is very good. The decisive advantage of this treatment is that unlike oestrogen treatment, this medication does not lead to hyperproliferation of the endometrium.

REFERENCES

Bullock, J. L., Massey, F. M. and Gambrell, R. D. Jr (1975). Obstetrics and Gynecology **46**, 165–168.

EFFECTS OF DIFFERENT NATURAL OESTROGENS ON CLOTTING FACTORS, PLASMA LIPIDS AND ENDOMETRIAL PROLIFERATION IN POSTMENOPAUSAL WOMEN

C. Campagnoli, L. Prelato Tousijn, A. M. Dolfin, L. Ferruzzi,
P. Belforte and G. Morra

Ospedale Ostetrico Ginecologico Sant'Anna, Turin, Italy

INTRODUCTION

Natural oestrogens currently used for the treatment of climacteric complaints do not seem to produce a higher cardiovascular risk in women (Boston Collaborative Drug Surveillance Program, 1974; Pfeffer and Van Den Nort, 1976; Rosenberg *et al.*, 1976). However much attention has been given to this point by epidemiologic reports of a higher risk in women on oral contraceptives, especially when over 40 years of age (Mann, 1978; Masi, 1978; Vessey, 1978). Natural oestrogens, unlike synthetic oestrogens employed in oral contraceptives, do not seem to exert any negative influence on lipemic pattern (Bolton, 1976; Larsson-Cohn, 1976; Utian and Gordan, 1979) and only make small alterations to blood coagulation (Amrbus, 1976; Bonnar *et al.*, 1976; Toy *et al.*, 1978a). There is some disagreement on the real extent and meaning of these latter changes (Poller, 1976; Notelovitz, 1977). There are indications that the action of different oestrogens on blood clotting is dose-related (McKay Hart *et al.*, 1978; Hunter *et al.*, 1979).

Another crucial point concerns the possible adverse effects exerted on endometrium by the various oestrogen preparations. This is a consequence of the growing evidence of a higher risk of adenocarcinoma in postmenopausal women treated for a long time with oestrogens able to induce endometrial proliferation (Cramer and Knapp, 1979). It was suggested that this risk might be lowered or

Serono Symposium No. 39, "The Menopause: Clinical, Endocrinological and Pathophysiological Aspects", edited by P. Fioretti, L. Martini, G. B. Melis and S. S. C. Yen, 1982. Academic Press, London and New York.

avoided by using additional cyclical administration of progestogens (Gambrell, 1976; Campbell and Whitehead, 1979) or oestrogens with a low activity on endometrium (Myhre, 1978; Tzingounis et al., 1978).

In this study we have confronted, in two comparable randomized groups of selected patients, the effects on blood clotting, plasma lipids and endometrial proliferations of two formulations of peroral oestrogens, similarly effective on climacteric complaints in most patients (Lauritzen, 1973).

PATIENTS AND METHODS

All the patients admitted in this study were over 45 years of age, they had had their last spontaneous menstrual period at least 6 months before, and had not been submitted to hormonal therapies for at least 3 months. Likewise patients with a personal or familiar history stating thromboembolic or vascular risk were excluded; women having blood pressure values of over 150/85, smokers and those 20% above average weight for their age and height were also excluded. Nobody had contraindications to oestrogen replacement therapy so they were allocated randomly to one of the two following groups: Group A: conjugate equine oestrogens (CEE), 0.625 mg b m daily for cycles of 3 weeks followed by a week with no treatment, and Group B: oestriol 2 mg b m daily continuously.

Before starting treatment, routine haematological evaluations (normal in all cases) and FSH levels (by RIA, using CEA-IRE-SORIN kits) were determined. Blood coagulation and plasma lipid examinations were carried out before treatment and at the same time intervals for the two groups during treatment: first control in the last days of the third cycle for group A and at the corresponding time (73rd–78th day) of therapy for group B; second control in the last days of the fourth cycle for group A and at the corresponding time (102nd-106th day) for group B.

Endometrial proliferation was indirectly evaluated with the biological progestogen test (Speroff et al., 1978) using medroxyprogesterone acetate (MPA), 10 mg daily for 10 days. The test had been carried out before therapy started (but after basal exams), and was repeated after 124–133 days from the beginning of the therapy (last 10 days of the fifth cycle for group A). The results were classified according to Hull et al. (1979).

Twelve patients of group A and ten patients of group B had the whole set of investigations performed. Five more patients (one in group A and four in group B) could not be tested completely with regard to the haematological examinations; however they received the complete course of treatment as in the protocol, and were therefore informative with respect to the endometrial proliferation (by the MPA test). In both groups one subject was in surgical menopause; two women were aged 48 and 45 and had been respectively submitted to hysterectomy and oophorectomy 38 and 34 months previously. Statistical analysis did not point out any difference between the two groups with regard to age, months from the last menstrual period, value of FSH, and severity of climacteric complaints.

Preliminary MPA test was negative in 10 out of 12 patients group A and in 10 out of 13 patients in group B. Two patients in group A had a postive preliminary MPA test. One patient in group B gave an impaired response and two others a positive one.

Blood Coagulation

Blood coagulation was measured in the following ways: activity of the factor II-VII-X complex, by Boehringer Mannheim kits (n.v.. 70-120%), antithrombin III, by a method of the chromogenic substrates using Boehringer Mannheim kits (n.v.: 15-21 IU/ml); euglobulin lysis time, by the method of the euglobulin fraction precipitation (n.v.. total lysis among 120-300 minutes).

Plasma lipids

Plasma lipids were measured in the following ways: total serum cholesterol, by enzymathic method using Boehringer Mannheim kits (n.v.: 140-270 mg/100 ml); triglycerides, by enzymathic method using Minileiser-Technicon (n.v.. 60-175 mg/100 ml); lipoprotein electrophoresis on Sepraphore III, Gelman Instrument.

Blood was drawn with plastic syringes, between 8 and 9 a.m., after a fasting of at least 12 h.

RESULTS

Blood Coagulation

In basal conditions groups A and B did not differ significantly in any of the considered parameters.

During treatment group A (CEE therapy) displayed a certain trend for an increase of the factor II-VII-X complex but it did not reach a significant level, and the values remained in the normal range for all patients except in two at the second control; there were no changes with oestriol therapy (group B). A shorter euglobulin lysis time was found during therapy with CEE, but again the deviation was not significant; two cases of group B showed an abnormal lengthening of euglobulin lysis time at the first control during the therapy, but normal values at the second control, whereas the patients treated with oestriol did not show any significant variation. Antithrombin III did not show substantial changes in either group, and reached normal values in two women (one for each group) with reduced basal levels.

None of the parameters under study showed any signficant difference between the two groups in the controls during treatment.

Plasma Lipids

In basal conditions groups A and B did not show significant differences with regard to cholesterol, triglycerides and lipoprotein electrophoresis.

Patients treated with CEE showed a heterogeneous behaviour of total cholesterol values: some subjects had a decrease, some an increase over the normal values and most did not show any alterations; this made the overall values during therapy not significantly different from the basal condition. Similarly, in group B (oestriol therapy), some patients displayed a decrease of cholesterol levels and others a certain increase. Altogether the cholesterol values observed during therapy were not significantly different from the basal ones. A similar finding was also obtained for triglycerides which did not show significant changes from pre-therapy values in either group; in both groups some patients showed a clearcut decrease, others a slight increase, and most showed no significant alterations. Only lipoprotein electrophoresis disclosed a significant effect of CEE therapy, i.e. a decrease in the beta fraction and an increase in the alpha fraction, with a decrease in the beta/alpha ratio; all these changes were statistically significant. Similar changes, though less important, were noted in group B; in this case, the difference from basal values was significant only for the beta/alpha ratio in the second control during treatment.

No significant difference between groups A and B was observed during treatment, either for cholesterol and triglycerides, or for lipoprotein electrophoresis.

Endometrial Proliferation

Progestogens given in the second phase of the fifth cycle of CEE produced a withdrawal bleeding in all the patients, both in the two who were positive and in the 10 who were negative in the preliminary MPA test. On the contrary MPA, given from day 124 to 133 of continuous therapy with oestriol, produced a withdrawal bleeding (positive response) only in the three patients who already had a response (one impaired and two positive) to the prior treatment.

DISCUSSION

Many studies have been made on the effects of CEE on blood coagulation, leading to different results: some did not show any alteration (Notelovitz and Greig, 1975, 1976); others found an increase in the factor VII-X complex, but no influence on antithrombin III levels (Bonnar et al., 1976); and still others pointed out a hypercoagulability, due either to a reduction of prothrombin time along with an increase in factors VII and X (Cooper et al., 1975; Poller, 1976) or to a decrease in antithrombin (Von Kaulla et al., 1975; Stangel et al., 1977). Euglobulin lysis time does not seem to be altered (Von Kaulla et al., 1975; Notelovitz and Greig, 1975). All these data are referred to the use of 1.250 mg daily of CEE. We used 0.625 mg daily of CEE, and found no significant alterations of the parameters investigated (activity of factor II-VII-X complex, antithrombin III and euglobulin lysis time). No alterations have been found either using 2 mg daily of oestriol. Some studies reported about the action of oestriol succinate on blood coagulation. This drug showed a moderate increase of factor VII only with doses of 6 mg daily or more (Davies et al., 1976; McKay Hart et al., 1978) and a more important increase of factors VII and X with doses of 12 mg daily (McKay Hart et al., 1978). No changes in clotting factors and in antithrombin III were found during long-term therapy with oestriol succinate, while an increased fibrinolitic activity is proven (Toy et al., 1978b).

The action of oestrogenic therapies also seems to be dose-related on plasma lipids. In a study by Robinson and Lebeau (1965), doses of 1.25–2.50 mg daily of CEE decrease cholesterol but increase triglyceride levels; the same happens with 20–40 µg daily of mestranol (Aitken et al., 1971). Other studies report no change of triglycerides nor cholesterol levels with 0.625–1.250 mg daily of CEE

(Bolton, 1976); likewise no changes were found using 1 mg daily of oestriol (Walter and Jensen, 1977). In agreement with those data, in the present study 0.625 mg daily of CEE and 2 mg daily of oestriol did not significantly affect total cholesterol and triglycerides; nevertheless we found a decrease in the beta/alpha lipoproteins ratio, more important in the group of patients treated with CEE, but also significant in the group treated with oestriol. An improvement of the beta/alpha lipoproteins ratio was found by Nachtigall *et al.*, (1979) after 10 years' therapy with CEE.

Withdrawal bleeding produced by the progestogen treatment is considered a good index of endometrial proliferation (Gambrell, 1976, 1977; Speroff *et al.*, 1978). CEE, even with doses as low as 0.625 mg daily, give an endometrial proliferation in most cases and the addition of progestogens gives a withdrawal bleeding in 90% of cases (Gambrell, 1977). In our study all the previously MPA test negative patients treated with CEE (group A) showed withdrawal bleeding following the assumption of progestogens at the fifth cycle: this shows that the treatment induces a renewal of endometrial proliferation. On the contrary, all the patients of group B previously MPA test negative did not show any withdrawal bleeding even after the assumption of progestogens from the 124th to 133rd day of continuous oestriol therapy. In fact no endometrial proliferation has been noticed even after 6 months of therapy with doses up to 8 mg daily of oestriol (Tzingounis *et al.*, 1978). In three patients in group B, who had 7, 11 and 24 months of menopausal amenorrhoea respectively, progestogen test was positive either before or after oestriol therapy; this might derive from a residual endogenous oestrogenic stimulation, as a positive MPA test is considered a good index of it (Hull *et al.*, 1979).

ACKNOWLEDGEMENTS

The authors express their appreciation to the staff of the AVIS laboratory and the central laboratory of the Sant'Anna Hospital who performed the blood clotting evaluations and FSH and plasma lipids evaluations respectively.

REFERENCES

Aitken, J. M., Lorimer, A. R., McKay Hart, D., Lawrie, T. D. and Smith, D. A. (1971). *Clinical Science* **41**, 597.
Ambrus, F. L. (1976). *In* "Consensus on Menopause Research" (P. A. Van Keep, R. B. Greenblatt and M. Albeaux-Fernet, Eds) 55–58. MTP Press, Lancaster.
Bolton, C. H. (1976). *In* "The Management of the Menopause & Post-Menopausal Years" (S. Campbell, Ed.), 185–194. MTP Press, Lancaster.
Bonnar, J., Haddon, M., Hunter, D. H., Richards, D. H. and Thornton, C. (1976). *Postgraduate Medical Journal* **52**, 30.
Boston Collaborative Drug Surveillance Program (1974). *New England Journal of Medicine* **290**, 15.
Campbell, S. and Whitehead, M. I. (1979). *In* "Female and Male Climacteric" (P. A. Van Keep, D. M. Serr and R. B. Greenblatt, Eds), 111–120. MTP Press, Lancaster.

Cooper, J., Thomson, J. M. and Poller, L. (1975). *British Medical Journal* **4**, 139.
Cramer, D. W. and Knapp, R. C. (1979). *Obstetrics and Gynecology* **54**, 521.
Davies, T., Fieldhouse, G. and McNicol, G. P. (1976). *Thrombosis and Haemostasis* **35**, 403.
Gambrell, R. D. Jr (1976). *In* "Consensus on Menopause Research" P. A. Van Keep, R. B. Greenblatt and M. Albeaux-Fernet, Eds), 152–163. MTP Press, Lancaster.
Gambrell, R. D. Jr (1977). *Clinics in Obstetrics and Gynaecology* **4**, 129.
Hull, M. G. R., Knuth, U. A., Murray, M. A. F. and Jacobs, H. S. (1979). *British Journal of Obstetrics and Gynaecology* **86**, 799.
Hunter, D. S., Anderson, A. B. M. and Haddon, M. (1979). *British Journal of Obstetrics and Gynaecology* **86**, 488.
Larsson-Cohn, U. (1976). *In* "Consensus on Menopause Research" (P. A. Van Keep, R. B. Greenblatt and M. Albeaux-Fernet, Eds), 51–54. MTP Press, Lancaster.
Lauritzen, C. (1973). *In* "Ageing and Estrogens", Frontiers of Hormone Research Vol. 2 (P. A. Van Keep and C. Lauritzen, Eds), 2–19. Karger, Basel.
Mann, J. I. (1978). *In* "Risks Benefits, and Controversies in Fertility Control" (J. J. Sciarra, G. I. Zatuchni and J. J. Speide, Eds), 129–137. Harper & Row, Hagerstown.
Masi, A. T. (1978). *In* "Risks, Benefits, and Controversies in Fertility Control" (J. J. Sciarra, G. I. Zatuchni and J. J. Speide, Eds), 138–155. Harper & Row, Hagerstown.
McKay Hart, D., Lindsay, R. and Purdie, D. (1978). *In* "Estrogen Therapy. The Benefits and Risks", Frontiers of Hormone Research Vol. 5 (C. Lauritzen and P. A. Van Keep, Eds), 174–191. Karger, Basel.
Myhre, E. (1978). *In* "Estrogen Therapy. The Benefits and Risks" Frontiers of Hormone Research Vol. 5 (C. Lauritzen and P. A. Van Keep, Eds), 126–144. Karger, Basel.
Nachtigall, L. A. Nachtigall, R. H., Nachtigall, R. D. and Beckman, M. (1979). *Obstetrics and Gynecology* **54**, 74.
Notelovitz, M. (1977). *Clinics in Obstetrics and Gynaecology* **4**, 107.
Notelovitz, M. and Greig, H. B. W. (1975). *South African Medical Journal* **49**, 101.
Notelovitz, M. and Greig, H. B. W. (1976). *Journal of Reproductive Medicine* **16**, 87.
Pfeffer, R. I. and Van Den Nort, S. (1976). *American Journal of Epidemiology* **103**, 445.
Poller, L. (1976) *In* "The Management of the Menopause & Post-Menopausal Years" (S. Campbell, Ed.), 313–320. MTP Press, Lancaster.
Robinson, R. W. and Lebeau, R. J. (1965). *Journal Atherosclerosis Research* **5**, 120.
Rosenberg, L., Armstrong, B. and Jick, H. (1976). *New England Journal of Medicine* **294**, 1256.
Speroff, L., Glass, R. H. and Kase, N. G. (1978). "Clinical Gynecologic Endocrinology and Infertility", 97–98. Williams & Wilkins, Baltimore.
Stangel, J. J., Innerfield, I., Reyniak, J. V. and Stone, M. L. (1977). *Obstetrics and Gynecology* **49**, 314.
Toy, J. L., Davies, J. A. and McNicol, G. P. (1978a). *British Journal of Obstetrics and Gynaecology* **85**, 359.
Toy, J. L., Davies, J. A. and McNicol, G. P. (1978b). *British Journal of Obstetrics and Gynaecology* **85**, 363.

Tzingounis, V. A., Feridun Aksu, M. and Greenblatt, R. B. (1978). *Journal of the American Medical Association* **239**, 1638.

Utian, W. H. and Gordan, G. S. (1979). *In* "Female and Male Climacteric" (P. A. Van Keep, D. M. Serr and R. B. Greenblatt, Eds.), 89–102. MTP Press, Lancaster.

Vessey, M. P. (1978). *In* "Risks, Benefits, and Controversies in Fertility Control" (J. J. Sciarra, G. I. Zatuchni and J. J. Speide, Eds), 113–121. Harper & Row, Hagerstown.

Von Kaulla, E., Droegmueller, W. and Von Kaulla, K. N. (1975). *American Journal of Obstetrics and Gynecology* **122**, 688.

Walter, S. and Jensen, H. K. (1977). *British Journal of Obstetrics and Gynaecology* **84**, 869.

REDUCTION OF THE FREQUENCY OF CLIMACTERIC FLUSHING AND LH PULSES BY BLOCKADE OF OPIATE RECEPTORS

S. L. Lightman[1], G. McGarrick, A. K. Maguire[1], S. L. Jeffcoate and H. S. Jacobs[1]

St Mary's Hospital Medical School, London, UK[1]; and Chelsea Hospital for Women, London, UK

INTRODUCTION

Hot flushes are considered a characteristic symptom of the menopause, and have been thought to be a direct consequence of oestrogen withdrawal, and subsequent gonadotropin excess. This view, however, is no longer tenable since plasma concentrations of unconjugated oestrogens (oestrone and oestradiol) are similar in those postmenopausal women who do flush and those who do not (Hutton *et al.*, 1978), and climacteric flushing has been reported after hypophysectomy (Mulley *et al.*, 1977). We have therefore looked at a different intrahypothalamic mechanism which we felt might be an important factor in mediating the climacteric flush. We hypothesized that an imbalance in hypothalamic opiate activity might be related to the incidence of climacteric flushing. Circumstantial evidence for the involvement of the endogenous opiate system comes from several studies in totally different areas. It has been shown that a proportion of diabetic subjects, on the drug chlorpropamide, will exhibit a facial flush when they take alcohol (Leslie *et al.*, 1979). This flush can be blocked by the opiate antagonist naloxone, suggesting that it is opiate mediated. The second line of evidence comes from the incidental finding that the administration of a synthetic opiate agonist causes a facial flush, which can again be blocked by naloxone (Stubbs *et al.*, 1978). Finally, it is known that LH reaches high levels during the menopause, and since we have

Serono Symposium No. 39, "The Menopause: Clinical, Endocrinological and Pathophysiological Aspects", edited by P. Fioretti, L. Martini, G. B. Melis and S. S. C. Yen, 1982. Academic Press, London and New York.

shown that LH secretion is at least partially under endogenous opioid control (Jacobs and Lightman, 1979), we have further evidence that opiates may be concerned with the changes of the menopause.

METHODS

Our study was performed on six women who had had severe climacteric flushing (7–12 per 12 h) for between 10 months and 25 years. They were admitted to a metabolic ward on the day prior to the study. The following day a cannula was inserted into an antecubital vein. Blood samples were taken at 15 or 30 min intervals, and at the initiation of each flushing episode, whilst a record was kept of all flushing episodes.

The following day was divided into eight periods of 90 min. Four of these periods were allocated to infusions of naloxone (22.2 μg/min) in 40 ml normal saline, and the other four periods to 40 ml normal saline alone. The order in which these eight separate infusions were given had been previously randomized, and the contents of the numbered syringes were unknown to the patient, the nurses or the doctors overseeing the infusions. Fifteen or 30 min blood samples, plus additional samples at the initiation of each flushing episode, were also taken on this day.

RESULTS

The six subjects had 48 flushing episodes on the control day between 10 a.m. and 10 p.m. and 29 episodes on the treatment day. Moreover, on the treatment day itself there were only eight flushes during the four 90 min naloxone infusion periods as against 24 flushes during the saline infusion period ($2P < 0.01$; Students' t-test for paired data).

The endocrine correlates of flushing also proved to be of interest. Analysis of variance revealed a highly significant increase in LH after the flushing episodes ($P < 0.001$), although there were no significant changes in plasma FSH, prolactin or noradrenaline. Plasma noradrenaline did indeed fall in most subjects at the immediate time that the flush began, but presumably because only a small proportion of blood sampled from the antecubital fossa comes from cutaneous vessels, this failed to reach significance.

During the day of naloxone infusions there was also a marked fall in LH secretory episodes, falling from 44 on the control day to 30 on the infusion day. Interestingly this fall in LH secretory episodes correlated very well with the decrease in the number of flushes on the infusion day ($r = 0.90$, $2P < 0.001$). The number of FSH pulses was not altered by the infusions, neither was there any effect on plasma levels of prolactin or noradrenaline.

CONCLUSIONS

In conclusion we have shown that naloxone significantly reduces the frequency of climacteric flushing, and this reduction is closely paralleled by a decreased frequency of LH secretory episodes. Since we have also shown that climacteric flushes are followed by LH secretory episodes, these two phenomena are obviously closely associated. We believe that opiate receptor activity has an important role in the neurohumoral organisation of climacteric flushing and that opiate receptor blockade may provide a non-hormonal treatment.

REFERENCES

Hutton, J. D., Jacobs, H. S., Murray, M. A. F. and James, V. H. T. (1978). *Lancet*, **1**, 678.

Jacobs, H. S. and Lightman, S. L. (1979). *Journal of Physiology (London)* **300**, 53P.

Leslie, R. D. G., Pyke, D. A. and Stubbs, W. A. (1979). *Lancet* **1**, 341.

Mulley, G., Mitchell, J. R. A. and Tattersall, R. B. (1977). *British Medical Journal* **2**, 1062.

Stubbs, W. A., Jones, A., Edwards, C. R. W., Delitala, G., Jeffcoate, W. J., Ratter, S. J., Besser, G. M., Bloom, S. R. and Alberti, K. G. M. M. (1978). *Lancet* **11**, 1225.

PATTERNS OF HORMONAL THERAPY DURING THE MENOPAUSE: A RETROSPECTIVE SURVEY ON 500 WOMEN IN LOMBARDY

S. Franceschi, C. La Vecchia, A. Tudisco and G. Tognoni

Istituto di Ricerche Farmacologiche "Mario Negri", Via Eritrea, Milan, Italy

INTRODUCTION

Menopausal disturbances, mainly vasomotor symptoms, atrophic changes in the urogenital system, osteoporosis and various psychological disturbances, are reported with varying degrees of frequency in 75–85% of women over 50 years of age (Utian, 1977). The pathogenesis of all these disturbances is still far from being understood; social and cultural factors play a definite role in conditioning a woman's behaviour in seeking relief through medical treatment. As oestrogen deficiency has been proposed as the underlying cause of the problems, an oestrogen-based replacement therapy gained wide acceptance, beginning in the sixties (mainly in the USA where the oestrogen market tripled from 1965 to 1970) (Current Industrial Reports, 1977).

MATERIALS AND METHODS

Detailed medical histories of 500 in-patients (40 to 69 years) were taken by two trained interviewers from May 1979 to February 1980. The sample population was the control group of a larger epidemiological case-control study and

Serono Symposium No. 39, "The Menopause: Clinical, Endocrinological and Pathophysiological Aspects", edited by P. Fioretti, L. Martini, G. B. Melis and S. S. C. Yen, 1982. Academic Press, London and New York.

comprised sequential female admissions with acute disease (diagnosed not more than 1 year before); 35% were surgical patients (174), 36% orthopedic (178) and 29% ENT (148). Patients with surgical menopause were not included.

The reliability of the interviewing techniques used has been tested both for completeness and freedom from important bias and is documented elsewhere (Rosemberg *et al.*, 1979). Whenever a patient could not remember past treatments with precision, colour photographs of pharmaceutical preparations were provided to optimize recall.

Specific attention was given to the number of medical contacts (out-patient and hospital admissions), as these situations could be considered as one factor in increased prescription (Feinstein and Horwitz, 1978).

RESULTS

In our sample 19.4% (97) reported having used oestrogens at some time in the past; 5% (25) for less than 3 months; 7.4% (37) for more than 3 months but less than 1 year; 3.6% (8) for more than 1 but less than 3 years and 3.4% (17) for more than 3 years (mean: 16.2 months; median: 10 months; mode: 2 months — Table I).

Among users 63% were able to specify the type of product used: conjugated oestrogens 23.6%, natural oestrogens 13.3%, synthetic oestrogens 7.8%, oestrogens + androgens 13.7%, oestrogens + progestins 2.9% (Table II).

Among women aged from 50 to 59 years, 27% (57) reported use of oestrogens, 18.7% (21) in the group aged from 60 to 69 years, and 10.8% (19) among women aged 40 to 49 years (Table IIIA). Oestrogen consumption was reported at an age ranging from 40 to 49 in 56.7% of cases (55), at 50–59 in 41.2% (40), and at 60–69 years in 2% (2) (Table IIIB). A history of menopausal symptoms was given by 81.3% of users (flushes and/or sweating), 65% of which were severe (in non-users these values were lower: 63% and 40% respectively); 18.7% of users reported no vasomotor disturbance and had probably taken oestrogens for more controversial indications.

Oestrogen use was commoner among better educated women: 23% (58) in the group with more than 5 years education (that is more than the old obligatory school period in Italy), 15.7% (39) in the group with 5 years' or less education (Table IV).

Table I. Hormonal therapy during natural menopause (500 women in Milan).

	N	%
Non-users	403	80.6
Users < 3 months	25	5
Users > 3 months < 1 year	37	7.4
Users > 1 year < 3 years	18	3.6
Users > 3 years	17	3.4

Mean: 16.2 months; median: 10 months; mode: 2 months.

Rates of replacement therapy differed significantly according to the intensity of contacts the patient had with medical care. A larger percentage of users than non-users reported four or more visits to the physician in the preceding year (62% against 49%, Table V). Similarly, 51.4% of users (50 out of 97) but 32.8% of non-users (132 out of 403) had been in hospital four or more times (pregnancies excluded) (Table VI).

Table II. Type of hormonal therapy.

	N	%
Conjugated oestrogens	24	23.7
Natural oestrogens	13	12.9
Synthetic oestrogens	8	7.9
Oestrogens + androgens	14	13.8
Oestrogens + progestins	3	2.9
Others not specified	31	30.6
Total	101[a]	

[a]Some women took more than one type.

Table IIIA. Hormonal therapy in the different "cohorts" of age.

	N	Users	%
40–49	176	19	10.8
50–59	206	57	27.7
60–69	118	21	18.7

Table IIIB. At at the beginning of hormonal therapy.

	N	%
40–49	55	56.7
50–59	40	41.2
60–69	2	2

Table IV. Hormonal therapy vs education years.

	"Non-users"		"Users"	
	N	%	N	%
0–5 years	209	84.3	39	15.7
> 5 years	194	77	58	23

Table V. Hormonal therapy vs number of medical visits (as an out-patient) during the last year.

Visits per year	"Non-users"		"Users"	
	N	%	N	%
0	51	85	9	15
1–3	155	84.7	28	15.3
4–8	101	74.3	35	25.7
> 9	96	79.4	25	20.6
Total	403		97	

Table VI. Hormonal therapy vs number of previous hospitalizations.

Hospitalizations (N)	"Non-users"		"Users"	
	N	%	N	%
0	37	90.2	4	9.8
1–3	234	84.5	43	15.5
4–8	112	72.7	42	27.3
⩾ 9	20	71.4	8	28.6
Total	403		97	

DISCUSSION

The therapeutic role of oestrogens in controlling the wide range of menopausal disturbances should still be regarded as controversial (mainly in relation to osteoporosis) (Gordan and Eisenberg, 1963; Lindsay *et al.*, 1976; Landau, 1979; Quigley and Hammond, 1979). General agreement appears to have been reached that oestrogen therapy is only justified with a lower dosage schedule over short periods of time and possibly combined with progestins, in the control of vasomotor and vaginal atrophic symptoms (NIH, 1979; Cramer and Knapp, 1979; Thom *et al.*, 1979).

Clinical practice, however, does not reflect these stricter indications, if a recent report could show that in the USA non-contraceptive oestrogens gained widespread popularity (one out of six women from 30 to 69 years of age), as a deceptive attempt to prevent the course of ageing (Rosemberg *et al.*, 1979). In the study quoted, conducted in the Boston area, 35% of users had taken oestrogens for more than 5 years. Most women (70%) took unopposed conjugated oestrogens (Premarin), whose metabolite—Equiline—is now looked at with maximum suspicion because of its extremely long half-life (Whittaker *et al.*, 1980).

This pattern of use is no longer admissible in the light of the undeniable increased risk of endometrial cancer in oestrogen users (RR = 3–15, depending on duration) (Ziel and Finkle, 1975; Horwitz and Feinstein, 1978; Antunes *et al.*, 1979; Weiss *et al.*, 1979), not to mention other suggested associations with breast cancer (Hoover *et al.*, 1976) (RR = 2 with long-term therapy), gall-bladder diseases (RR = 2.5) and perhaps thromboembolic phenomena (BCDSP, 1974).

Young ovariectomized women may constitute a different problem as regards benefit/risk evaluation, as they face severe oestrogen deprivation and usually lack the first organ at risk, the uterus (Lindsay *et al.*, 1976). The situation in Italy is characterized by lower oestrogen consumption and shorter therapeutic schedules. This seems to correspond with the recommendations of the FDA, which has had considerable success in promoting stricter rules for oestrogen use since 1977. The reasons behind the prescription pattern in Italy are unfortunately not linked with a better awareness of the benefit–risk issue for these drugs. On the contrary, it is interesting to recall the position recently taken by the Italian Consiglio Superiore di Sanità which, stressing efficacy, strongly minimized the risks connected with replacement therapy in menopause (Consiglio Superiore di Sanità, 1979).

CONCLUSIONS

From our data, we can draw the following conclusions.

Oestrogen consumption appears to be lower and total exposure shorter in Italy. Only 3.4% of our sample population used them for more than 3 years, since the average duration of therapy is about 2 months in Italy. As the Relative Risk associated with short-term therapy is low (Cramer and Knapp, 1979), the attributable risk must also be low in Italy, even for endometrial cancer.

Oestrogen usage is higher in more educated women and correlates with the number of previous hospital stays, out-patient visits and severity of menopausal symptoms.

For the period covered in our interviews, the most commonly prescribed compounds were conjugated oestrogens.

Despite numerous suggestions in recent literature (Thom *et al.*, 1979), the more prudent and "natural" combination of oestrogens and progestins is still rarely prescribed in Italy. The similarly rare use of progestins alone, suggested as a first attempt to control menopausal symptoms and even osteoporosis, should also be better evaluated (Gambrell *et al.*, 1979; Lindsay *et al.*, 1978).

REFERENCES

Antunes, C. M. F., Stolley, P. D., Rosenshein, N. B., Davies, J. L., Tonascia, J. A., Brown, C., Burnett, L., Rutledge, A., Pokempner, M. and Garcia, R. (1979). *New England Journal of Medicine* **300**, 9–13.

BCDSP—Boston Collaborative Drug Surveillance Program (1974). *New England Journal of Medicine* **290**, 15–19.

Consiglio Superiore di Sanità (1979). *Bollettino e Informazione Farmaceutica* **7**, 5.

Cramer, D. W. and Knapp, R. C. (1979). *Obstetrics and Gynecology* **54**, 521–526.

Current Industrial Reports (1977). Series MA 286 (62)–1 to MA 286 (77)–1. US Department of Commerce Bureau of the Census, Industry Division, Washington, DC.

Feinstein, A. R. and Horwitz, R. I. (1978). *Cancer Research* **38**, 4001–4005.

Gambrell, R. D. Jr, Massey, F. M., Castaneda, T. A., Ugenas, A. J. and Ricci, C. A. (1979). *Journal of American Geriatrics Society* **27**, 389–394.

Gordan, G. S. and Eisenberg, E. (1963). *Proceedings of Royal Society of Medicine* **56**, 1027–1029.

Hoover, R., Gray, L. A., Cole, P. and MacMahon, B. (1976). *New England Journal of Medicine* **295**, 401–405.

Horwitz, R. I. and Feinstein, A. R. (1978). *New England Journal of Medicine* **299**, 1089–1094.

Landau, R. L. (1979). *Journal of American Medical Association* **241**, 47–51.

Lindsay, R., Hart, D. M., Hitken, J. M., MacDonald, E. B., Anderson, J. B. and Clarke, A. C. (1976). *Lancet* **1**, 1038–1040.

Lindsay, R., Hart, D. M., Purdie, D., Ferguson, M. M., Clark, A. S. and Kraszewski, A. (1978). *Clinical Science and Molecular Medicine* **54**, 193–195.

NIH—National Institute of Health (1979). *Annales of Internal Medicine* **91**, 921–922.

Quigley, M. M. and Hammond, C. B. (1979). *New England Journal of Medicine* **301**, 646–648.

Rosemberg, L., Shapiro, S., Kaufman, D. W., Slone, D., Miettinen, O. S. and Stolley, P. D. (1979). *American Journal of Epidemiology* **109**, 676–686.

Thom, M. H., White, P. J., Williams, R. M., Sturdee, D. W., Paterson, M. E., Wade-Evans, T. and Studd, J. W. (1979). *Lancet* **2**, 455–457.

Utian, W. H. (1977). *Obstetric and Gynecology Survey* **32**, 193–204.

Weiss, N. S., Szekely, D. R., English, D. R. and Schweid, A. I. (1979). *Journal of American Medical Association* **242**, 261–264.

Whittaker, P. G., Morgan, M. R. A., Dean, P. D. G., Cameron, E. H. D. and Lind, T. (1980). *Lancet* **1**, 14–16.

Ziel, H. K. and Finkle, W. D. (1975). *New England Journal of Medicine* **293**, 1167–1170.